Preparing for Life and Career

Seventh Edition

Louise A. Liddell

Author of Family and Consumer Sciences Textbooks
Germantown, Tennessee

Yvonne S. Gentzler, Ph.D

College of Education and Human Development
University of Minnesota
Minneapolis, Minnesota

Publisher
The Goodheart-Willcox Company, Inc.
Tinley Park, Illinois
www.g-w.com

Library of Congress Catalog Card Number 2011045455

ISBN 978-1-60525-625-2

2 3 4 5 6 7 8 9 – 13 – 18 17 16 15 14

The Goodheart-Willcox Company, Inc. Brand Disclaimer: Brand names, company names, and illustrations for products
and services included in this text are provided for educational purposes only and do not represent or imply endorsement or
recommendation by the author or the publisher.

The Goodheart-Willcox Company, Inc. Safety Notice: The reader is expressly advised to carefully read, understand, and
apply all safety precautions and warnings described in this book or that might also be indicated in undertaking the activities and
exercises described herein to minimize risk of personal injury or injury to others. Common sense and good judgment should also be
exercised and applied to help avoid all potential hazards. The reader should always refer to the appropriate manufacturer's technical
information, directions, and recommendations; then proceed with care to follow specific equipment operating instructions. The reader
should understand these notices and cautions are not exhaustive.

The publisher makes no warranty or representation whatsoever, either expressed or implied, including but not limited to equipment,
procedures, and applications described or referred to herein, their quality, performance, merchantability, or fitness for a particular
purpose. The publisher assumes no responsibility for any changes, errors, or omissions in this book. The publisher specifically
disclaims any liability whatsoever, including any direct, indirect, incidental, consequential, special, or exemplary damages resulting,
in whole or in part, from the reader's use or reliance upon the information, instructions, procedures, warnings, cautions, applications,
or other matter contained in this book. The publisher assumes no responsibility for the activities of the reader.

The Goodheart-Willcox Company, Inc. Internet Disclaimer: The Internet listings provided in this text link to additional resource
information. Every attempt has been made to ensure these sites offer accurate, informative, safe, and appropriate information.
However, Goodheart-Willcox Publisher has no control over these websites. The publisher makes no representation whatsoever,
either expressed or implied, regarding the content of these websites. Because many websites contain links to other sites (some of
which may be inappropriate), the publisher urges teachers to review all websites before students use them. Note that Internet sites
may be temporarily or permanently inaccessible by the time readers attempt to use them.

Library of Congress Cataloging-in-Publication Data

Liddell, Louise A.
  Preparing for life and career / by Louise A. Liddell, Yvonne S. Gentzler.
     p. cm. -- (Skills for living)
  Rev. ed. of: Building life skills / by Louise A. Liddell, Yvonne S. Gentzler.
  Includes index.
  ISBN 978-1-60525-625-2
  1. Life skills--United States. 2. Home economics--United States.
  I. Gentzler, Yvonne S. II. Liddell, Louise A. Building life skills. III. Title.
HQ2039.U6L53 2013
646.7--dc23

                                                            2011045455

Cover image: © Monkey Business Images/Shutterstock

Introduction

Preparing for Life and Career gives you the tools you need to manage your life while learning about possible future careers. As you grow and change, you are gaining independence. This time can be exciting for you, but it also brings new challenges and responsibilities. Being prepared with the right skills and knowledge can help you get the most satisfaction from the changes you face.

This text can help you develop skills that will be useful throughout your life and in your career. You will learn how to develop and keep successful relationships, as well as how to be a good family member and contribute to your community. Managing your resources—time, energy, money, and technology—to achieve your goals is critical for success in life.

You will learn how to research different careers and apply for jobs—plus how to develop the qualities and skills employers are seeking. The text also focuses on understanding children and parenting issues. Managing your health and nutrition to stay fit and make healthful choices is covered, and you will learn how to select, prepare, and serve a variety of foods.

All aspects of your clothing, from building a wardrobe to caring for your clothes, is presented. You will find ways to improve your home environment, care for your home, and be environmentally responsible in your everyday life. Learning about your transportation options and how to buy a car will help you both now and in the future. This is an exciting time to be a teen and preparing for life and career.

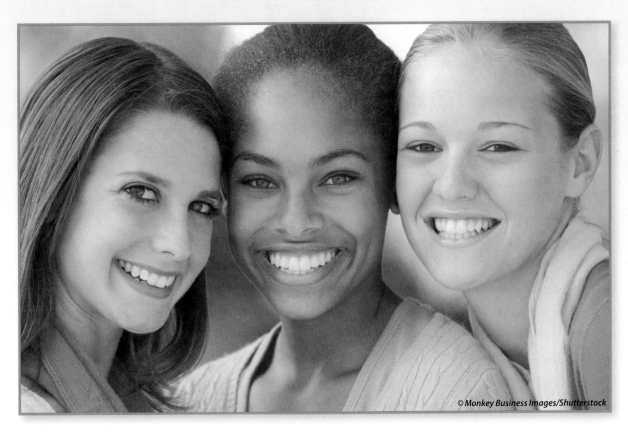

© Monkey Business Images/Shutterstock

About the Authors

Louise Liddell taught high school Family and Consumer Sciences courses for 15 years in the state of Tennessee. As Assistant Superintendent for a youth development center, she continued her work with teens. Louise's leadership roles in professional organizations include service at local, regional, state, and national levels. As president of the Tennessee Association for Career and Technical Education, she received a Life Membership award in ACTE for outstanding leadership. Louise is also the author of *Apparel: Design, Textiles & Construction*, (previously published as *Clothes and Your Appearance*), as well as many magazine and newsletter articles.

Yvonne Gentzler is an Associate Professor in the College of Education and Human Development at the University of Minnesota. She has taught Family and Consumer Sciences courses in secondary and university settings. Her innovative approaches to instruction have captured the attention of audiences nationwide. Yvonne is a popular life skills authority for television, radio, and print media personnel. She has maintained an active record of leadership in professional organizations and has been the recipient of numerous teaching, service, and research awards. During her tenure as a secondary school educator, she led seven groups of students to achieve national recognition in Family and Consumer Sciences related projects.

Reviewers

The authors and Goodheart-Willcox Publisher would like to thank the following professionals who provided valuable input to this edition of *Preparing for Life and Career*.

Doreen Cechnicki

Family and Consumer Sciences Educator
Mont Pleasant Middle School
Schenectady, New York

Susan Fajatin

Family and Consumer Sciences Educator
Hazelwood North Middle School
Florissant, Missouri

Vikki Jackson

Family and Consumer Sciences Teacher
Kathleen Middle School
Lakeland, Florida

Nancy Paulson

Family and Consumer Sciences Teacher
Hueneme High School
Oxnard, California

Organized for Successful Learning

Sections

An easy-to-read format presents the chapter's main themes.

Reading Prep

Quick, easy activities expand reading skills for college and career readiness.

Concept Organizer

Concept organizers challenge students to present chapter information in logical ways.

Companion Website

The website **www.g-wlearning.com** includes activities that extend learning beyond the classroom and downloadable concept organizers.

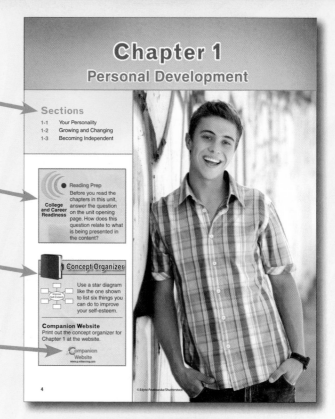

Objectives

Objectives summarize the learning goals for each section.

Key Terms

Presents the new terms you will learn in this section to expand your vocabulary.

Activities Enhance and Extend Learning

Common Core

For college and career readiness, these activities link chapter content to skills students need to master, such as writing, speaking, listening, and math.

Journal Writing

Writing opportunities help you learn about yourself and practice and develop writing skills.

FCCLA

Individual and team activities suggest ways to expand projects for competitive events.

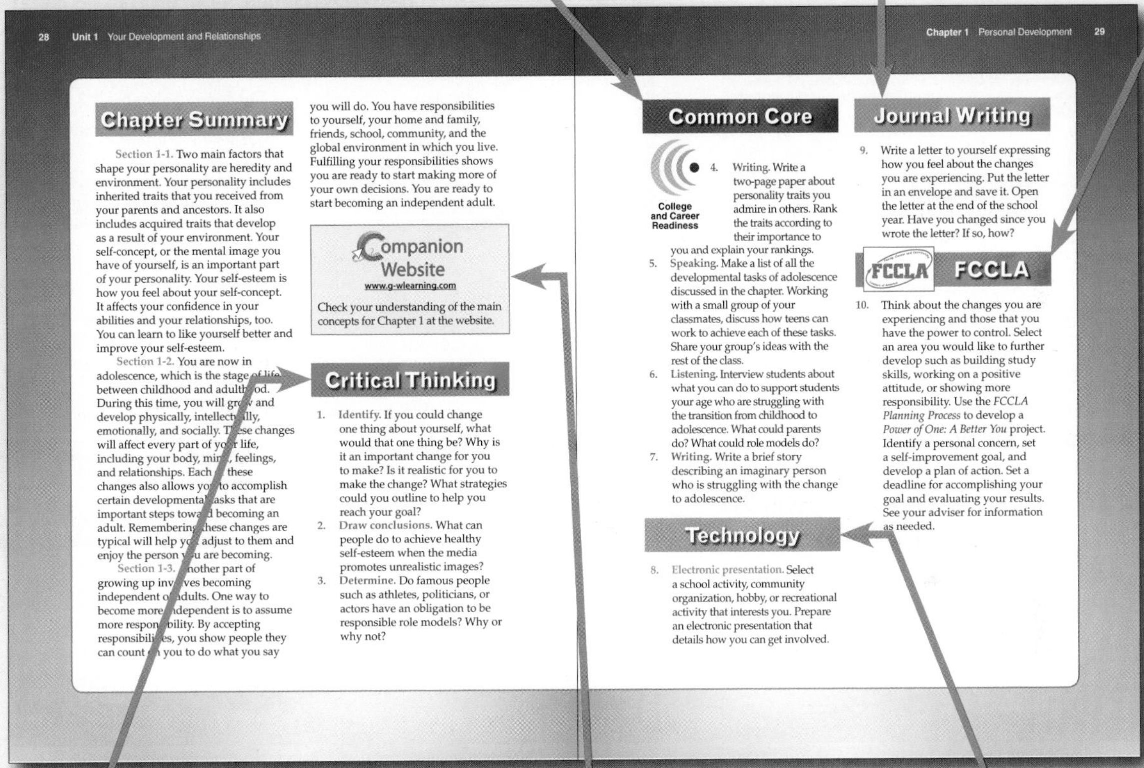

(Textbook page spread shown)

28   Unit 1   Your Development and Relationships

Chapter Summary

Section 1-1. Two main factors that shape your personality are heredity and environment. Your personality includes inherited traits that you received from your parents and ancestors. It also includes acquired traits that develop as a result of your environment. Your self-concept, or the mental image you have of yourself, is an important part of your personality. Your self-esteem is how you feel about your self-concept. It affects your confidence in your abilities and your relationships, too. You can learn to like yourself better and improve your self-esteem.

Section 1-2. You are now in adolescence, which is the stage of life between childhood and adulthood. During this time, you will grow and develop physically, intellectually, emotionally, and socially. These changes will affect every part of your life, including your body, mind, feelings, and relationships. Each of these changes also allows you to accomplish certain developmental tasks that are important steps toward becoming an adult. Remembering these changes are typical will help you adjust to them and enjoy the person you are becoming.

Section 1-3. Another part of growing up involves becoming independent of adults. One way to become more independent is to assume more responsibility. By accepting responsibilities, you show people they can count on you to do what you say

you will do. You have responsibilities to yourself, your home and family, friends, school, community, and the global environment in which you live. Fulfilling your responsibilities shows you are ready to start making more of your own decisions. You are ready to start becoming an independent adult.

Companion Website
www.g-wlearning.com

Check your understanding of the main concepts for Chapter 1 at the website.

Critical Thinking

1. Identify. If you could change one thing about yourself, what would that one thing be? Why is it an important change for you to make? Is it realistic for you to make the change? What strategies could you outline to help you reach your goal?
2. Draw conclusions. What can people do to achieve healthy self-esteem when the media promotes unrealistic images?
3. Determine. Do famous people such as athletes, politicians, or actors have an obligation to be responsible role models? Why or why not?

Chapter 1   Personal Development   29

Common Core

College and Career Readiness

4. Writing. Write a two-page paper about personality traits you admire in others. Rank the traits according to their importance to you and explain your rankings.
5. Speaking. Make a list of all the developmental tasks of adolescence discussed in the chapter. Working with a small group of your classmates, discuss how teens can work to achieve each of these tasks. Share your group's ideas with the rest of the class.
6. Listening. Interview students about what you can do to support students your age who are struggling with the transition from childhood to adolescence. What could parents do? What could role models do?
7. Writing. Write a brief story describing an imaginary person who is struggling with the change to adolescence.

Technology

8. Electronic presentation. Select a school activity, community organization, hobby, or recreational activity that interests you. Prepare an electronic presentation that details how you can get involved.

Journal Writing

9. Write a letter to yourself expressing how you feel about the changes you are experiencing. Put the letter in an envelope and save it. Open the letter at the end of the school year. Have you changed since you wrote the letter? If so, how?

FCCLA

10. Think about the changes you are experiencing and those that you have the power to control. Select an area you would like to further develop such as building study skills, working on a positive attitude, or showing more responsibility. Use the *FCCLA Planning Process* to develop a *Power of One: A Better You* project. Identify a personal concern, set a self-improvement goal, and develop a plan of action. Set a deadline for accomplishing your goal and evaluating your results. See your adviser for information as needed.

Critical Thinking

Questions challenge you to use higher-level critical thinking skills when reviewing chapter concepts.

Companion Website

Link to the text's Companion Website at **www.g-wlearning.com** to check your understanding of the chapter material.

Technology

Apply various technologies to explore chapter topics and complete activities.

Reading Review

1. The combination of traits that makes a person unique is his or her _____.
2. What two factors shape a person's personality?
3. What is the difference between inherited and acquired traits?
4. Distinguish between *self-concept* and *self-esteem*.
5. List six ways to improve your feelings about yourself.

Reading Review

Questions at the end of each section test your reading comprehension.

Lively Features and Charts

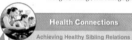

Life Connections

Explore life skills that promote success now and in the future. An activity connects each life skill with a real-world scenario.

Financial Literacy Connections

Develop money management skills.

Health Connections

Focus on how to make healthful decisions.

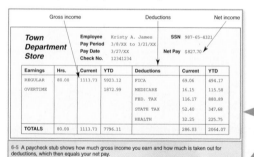

Global Connections

Learn about other countries and cultures as related to the text material.

Tables

Colorful tables bring chapter content to life and make concepts clearer.

Go Green

Green features suggest ways to raise awareness about the environment and how to make sustainable decisions.

Complex Concepts Presented Simply

Math Connections

Calculating Unit Price

Suppose you are shopping for cereal. The store offers the following sizes and prices of your favorite cereal:
- 9-oz. box for $2.50
- 14-oz. box for $2.84
- 18-oz. box for $2.98

Calculate the ounce unit price for each box of cereal. Compare the unit prices and select the box size with the lowest unit price. (Round your answers up to the second decimal place.)

(*Answer:* $2.50 ÷ 9 = $0.28/oz., $2.84 ÷ 14 = $0.21/oz., $2.98 ÷ 18 = $0.17/oz.; The 18 ounce box has the lowest unit price.)

Math Connections

Expands chapter content related to math. Gives specific examples demonstrating step-by-step calculations.

Science Connections

Windows of Opportunity

During early brain development, there are *windows of opportunity*, or limited time frames to develop critical skills. If these windows are missed, it is difficult for the child to develop these abilities at a later time. Following are five major developmental tasks and their approximate windows:
- *Vision.* Birth to six months.
- *Vocabulary/speech.* Birth to three months.
- *Emotional control.* Birth to three months.
- *Math/logic.* Birth to four years.
- *Small and large muscle development.* Birth to eight years.

It is crucial for caretakers to stimulate and encourage all types of development. Having interesting objects, lights, sounds, and people will aid in early brain development and help reach goals within these windows of opportunity.

Science Connections

Links chapter content to the field of science.

Social Studies Connections

Learn About the Past

Grandparents can entertain you and enrich your life with stories of their childhoods. They can tell you many stories about your parents when they were younger. Stories about historical events they may have witnessed can also be interesting. They may have visited or lived in places you have never seen. Ask one of your grandparents or another older adult to name a major historical figure that had an impact on his or her life. Read a book about that person and then have a discussion with your grandparent about the person and events that took place at that time.

Social Studies Connections

Links chapter content to relevant social studies topics.

Reading Connections

Electronic Readers

Electronic books were first being developed in the 1970s, when the first document was transferred into a digital format. This laid the foundation for future texts to become digitalized. It was not until the 1990s, however, that the first electronic reader, or *e-reader*, was introduced to the public. Today, e-readers are becoming more prevalent. E-readers have the ability to hold thousands of books, magazines, and newspapers in one lightweight device, and are environmentally friendly because they do not use paper. While there are positive aspects to e-readers, many people still prefer printed books to e-books. Find and read articles to research the growing trend of e-readers along with the pros and cons of going wireless. How do you feel about e-readers?

Reading Connections

Expands reading skills through additional reading-related activities.

Writing Connections

Writing Clear Messages

Like clear speaking, clear writing makes your messages easier to understand. You will want to be certain people can read your handwriting. You will want to use correct grammar, spelling, and punctuation.

Think through what you want to say before you begin to write. Jot down key points to make in the order you want to make them. An outline is helpful when writing lengthy reports for school. You will find the words come easier when you have an outline to guide you.

Writing Connections

Gives you practice forming ideas in writing and making compelling points.

Safety Connections

Provides tips about how to prevent accidents and ensure your physical, emotional, and financial safety.

Safety Connections

Stop Bullying

If a bully is targeting you or someone you know, report the incident to a parent, teacher, or other trusted adult. You can also make plans to be with a friend in areas you think you might run into the bully. Sometimes just ignoring or standing up to the bully will cause the bullying to stop. Do not fight back, however. This may cause someone to get hurt, and you could also get into trouble.

Community Connections

Positive Peer Pressure

Special groups use positive peer pressure to offer support to their members. These groups help people deal with challenges. *Alateen* is a peer group for teens with family members who abuse alcohol. Support from their peers lets these teens know others are coping with the same challenges. Similar peer groups exist for people who are dependent on drugs or who have eating disorders. Your community may have peer groups that help with other challenges as well.

Community Connections

Fosters concern, appreciation, and involvement in your community.

Learn About Careers

Four Career Chapters

Shows content for four chapters covering all aspects of job searching and successful employment.

Exploring Career Pathways

Includes three related career options—from entry level to experienced—and two activities.

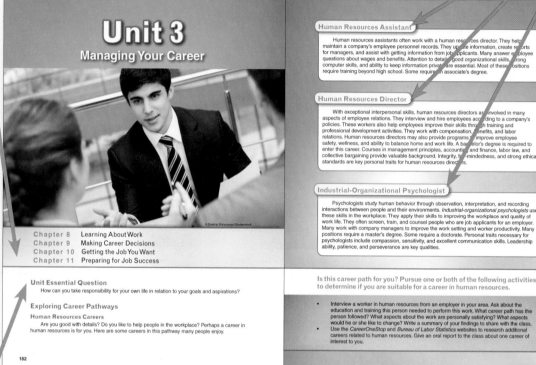

Unit 3
Managing Your Career

Chapter 8   Learning About Work
Chapter 9   Making Career Decisions
Chapter 10   Getting the Job You Want
Chapter 11   Preparing for Job Success

©Dmitriy Shironosov/Shutterstock

Unit Essential Question
How can you take responsibility for your own life in relation to your goals and aspirations?

Exploring Career Pathways
Human Resources Careers
Are you good with details? Do you like to help people in the workplace? Perhaps a career in human resources is for you. Here are some careers in this pathway many people enjoy.

182

Human Resources Assistant

Human resources assistants often work with a human resources director. They help maintain a company's employee personnel records. They update information, create reports for managers, and assist with getting information from job applicants. Many answer employee questions about wages and benefits. Attention to detail, good organizational skills, strong computer skills, and ability to keep information private are essential. Most of these positions require training beyond high school. Some require an associate's degree.

Human Resources Director

With exceptional interpersonal skills, human resources directors are involved in many aspects of employee relations. They interview and hire employees according to a company's policies. These workers also help employees improve their skills through training and professional development activities. They work with compensation, benefits, and labor relations. Human resources directors may also provide programs to improve employee safety, wellness, and ability to balance home and work life. A bachelor's degree is required to enter this career. Courses in management principles, accounting and finance, labor law, and collective bargaining provide valuable background. Integrity, fair-mindedness, and strong ethical standards are key personal traits for human resources directors.

Industrial-Organizational Psychologist

Psychologists study human behavior through observation, interpretation, and recording interactions between people and their environments. *Industrial-organizational psychologists* use these skills in the workplace. They apply their skills to improving the workplace and quality of work life. They often screen, train, and counsel people who are job applicants for an employer. Many work with company managers to improve the work setting and worker productivity. Many positions require a master's degree. Some require a doctorate. Personal traits necessary for psychologists include compassion, sensitivity, and excellent communication skills. Leadership ability, patience, and perseverance are key qualities.

Is this career path for you? Pursue one or both of the following activities to determine if you are suitable for a career in human resources.

- Interview a worker in human resources from an employer in your area. Ask about the education and training this person needed to perform this work. What career path has the person followed? What aspects about the work are personally satisfying? What aspects would he or she like to change? Write a summary of your findings to share with the class.
- Use the *CareerOneStop* and *Bureau of Labor Statistics* websites to research additional careers related to human resources. Give an oral report to the class about one career of interest to you.

183

Essential Career Question

Inspires insight into a career direction that matches your talents and abilities.

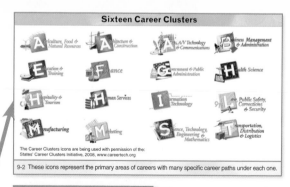

Sixteen Career Clusters

The Career Clusters icons are being used with permission of the: States' Career Clusters Initiative, 2008, www.careertech.org

9-2 These icons represent the primary areas of careers with many specific career paths under each one.

Career Clusters

Presents the 16 Career Clusters and how they relate to Family and Consumer Sciences careers.

Online Career Resources

Lists valuable online sources and their websites for more in-depth career exploration.

Online Career Resources	
Source	**Internet Address**
USAJOBS, the official job site of the U.S. Federal Government	www.usajobs.gov
Occupational Outlook Handbook, U.S. Department of Labor (Bureau of Labor Statistics)	www.stats.bls.gov/oco
Occupational Outlook Quarterly, U.S. Department of Labor (Bureau of Labor Statistics)	www.bls.gov/opub/ooq
U.S. Department of Labor (Employment and Training Administration)	www.doleta.gov
The Occupational Information Network (O*NET™)	www.onetonline.org
CareerOneStop	www.careeronestop.org
Mapping Your Future	www.mappingyourfuture.org

9-4 Take advantage of the many resources available online for your career research.

Emphasize Health and Nutrition

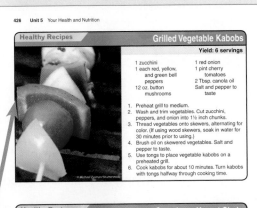

Healthy Recipes

Grilled Vegetable Kabobs

Yield: 6 servings

1 zucchini
1 each red, yellow, and green bell peppers
12 oz. button mushrooms
1 red onion
1 pint cherry tomatoes
2 Tbsp. canola oil
Salt and pepper to taste

1. Preheat grill to medium.
2. Wash and trim vegetables. Cut zucchini, peppers, and onion into 1½ inch chunks.
3. Thread vegetables onto skewers, alternating for color. (If using wood skewers, soak in water for 30 minutes prior to using.)
4. Brush oil on skewered vegetables. Salt and pepper to taste.
5. Use tongs to place vegetable kabobs on a preheated grill.
6. Cook kabobs for about 10 minutes. Turn kabobs with tongs halfway through cooking time.

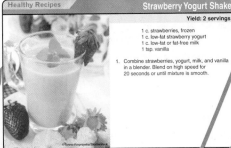

Healthy Recipes

Strawberry Yogurt Shake

Yield: 2 servings

1 c. strawberries, frozen
1 c. low-fat strawberry yogurt
1 c. low-fat or fat-free milk
1 tsp. vanilla

1. Combine strawberries, yogurt, milk, and vanilla in a blender. Blend on high speed for 20 seconds or until mixture is smooth.

Healthy Recipes

Grilled Peach Salad

Yield: 6 servings

1½ Tbsp. vegetable oil
4 firm, ripe peaches
1 oz. Parmesan cheese, large shred
3 Tbsp. pine nuts, toasted
4 oz. baby lettuce
¼ c. balsamic vinaigrette

1. Preheat a grill to medium heat.
2. Halve and pit unpeeled peaches. Cut each half into 3 wedges and lightly brush with oil.
3. Place pine nuts on a sheet pan in a 300°F oven for 10 minutes until lightly browned. Shake pan after about 5 minutes to ensure even browning.
4. Place wedges on grill. Cook for about 2 minutes on each side.
5. Arrange 4 wedges on a bed of lettuce. Sprinkle with cheese and pine nuts. Drizzle with vinaigrette.

Healthy Recipes

Marinated Cherry Tomatoes

Yield: 6 servings

½ tsp. salt
¼ c. lemon juice
¾ c. oil
1 clove garlic, crushed
½ tsp. basil
½ tsp. thyme
1 Tbsp. parsley, chopped
2 pints cherry tomatoes

1. Mix all ingredients except tomatoes in a bowl.
2. Wash cherry tomatoes and remove stems.
3. Add tomatoes to dressing and chill 2 hours or overnight.

Healthful Recipes

Presents twelve easy-to-follow, healthful recipes across the major food groups in Chapter 17.

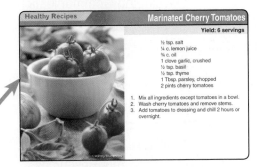

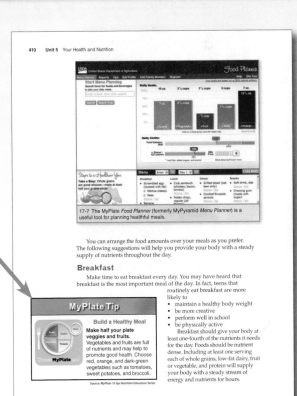

17-7 The MyPlate *Food Planner* (formerly MyPyramid *Menu Planner*) is a useful tool for planning healthful meals.

You can arrange the food amounts over your meals as you prefer. The following suggestions will help you provide your body with a steady supply of nutrients throughout the day.

Breakfast

Make time to eat breakfast every day. You may have heard that breakfast is the most important meal of the day. In fact, teens that routinely eat breakfast are more likely to
- maintain a healthy body weight
- be more creative
- perform well in school
- be physically active

Breakfast should give your body at least one-fourth of the nutrients it needs for the day. Foods should be nutrient dense. Including at least one serving each of whole grains, low-fat dairy, fruit or vegetable, and protein will supply your body with a steady stream of energy and nutrients for hours.

MyPlate Tip

Build a Healthy Meal

Make half your plate veggies and fruits. Vegetables and fruits are full of nutrients and may help to promote good health. Choose red, orange, and dark-green vegetables such as tomatoes, sweet potatoes, and broccoli.

Source: MyPlate 10 tips Nutrition Education Series

MyPlate Information

Provides helpful tips throughout the foods chapters from **ChooseMyPlate.com**. The advice points out healthful options for choosing and preparing nutritional meals.

Contents in Brief

Contents

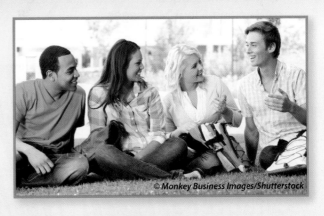

Unit 2
Managing Your Life

Chapter 5
Getting Ready to Manage . . . 100

Chapter 6
Managing Your Resources . . . 126

Chapter 7
Being a Responsible Consumer . . 158

© Monkey Business Images/Shutterstock

Unit 3
Managing Your Career

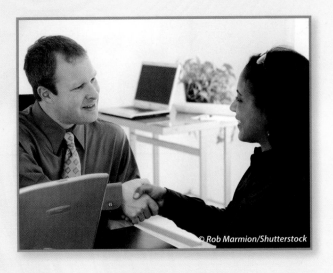

© Rob Marmion/Shutterstock

Unit 4
Understanding Children and Parenting

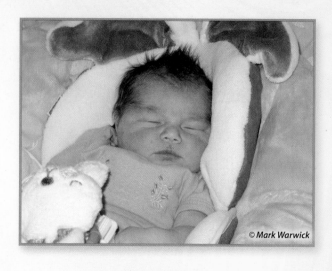
© Mark Warwick

Unit 5
Your Health and Nutrition

Unit 6
Preparing Meals and Dining Out

Chapter 19
Getting Ready to Cook 474

© Bochkarev Photography/Shutterstock

© Paul Matthew Photography/Shutterstock

Unit 8
Housing and Transportation

Chapter 26
Your Personal Living Space . . 624

Chapter 27
Transportation Options 654

Features

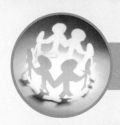

Life Connections

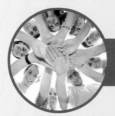

Community Connections

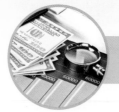

Financial Literacy Connections

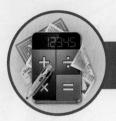

Math Connections

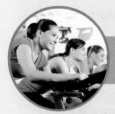

Health Connections

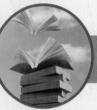

Reading Connections

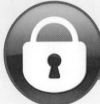

Safety Connections

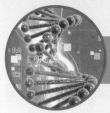

Science Connections

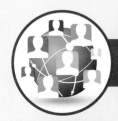

Social Studies Connections

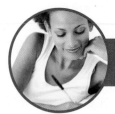

Writing Connections

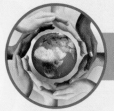

Global Connections

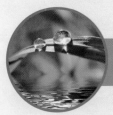

Go Green

Healthy Recipes

MyPlate Tip

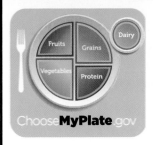

Unit 1
Your Development and Relationships

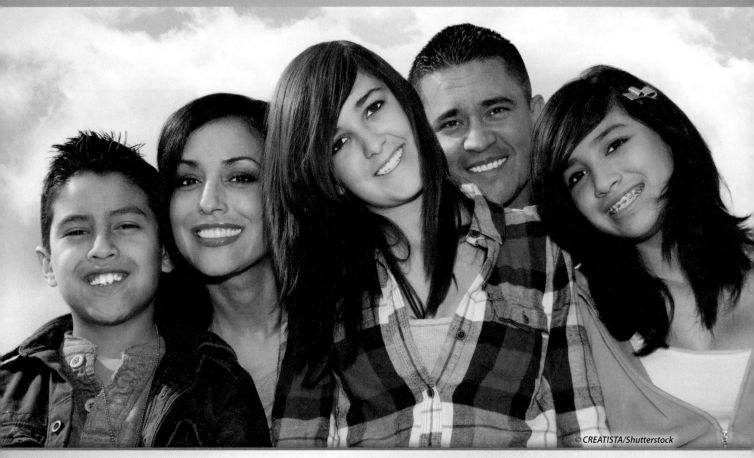

© CREATISTA/Shutterstock

Chapter 1   Personal Development
Chapter 2   Your Family
Chapter 3   Your Friends
Chapter 4   Developing Communication Skills

Unit Essential Question

How can understanding yourself in relation to your surroundings and others help you to become the person you want to be?

Exploring Career Pathways

Human Services Careers

How well do you communicate with and show compassion to others? Are you a good helper? If you enjoy working with people, perhaps a human services career is for you. Here is a possible career path you may find rewarding.

Personal and Home Care Aide

Personal and home care aides serve people with disabilities, older adults, or those with chronic illnesses. Some work includes light housekeeping, laundry, shopping for food, and preparing meals. Other work activities may include helping with daily living activities such as hygiene and grooming tasks. The work can be physically demanding and exposure to illnesses is possible. Following proper sanitary procedures is necessary. Aides generally have a high school diploma. Those who work for agencies that serve Medicare and Medicaid clients must complete a 75-hour training program and a competency evaluation. Some supervised training is also a requirement. Additional certification requirements can vary by state.

Social and Human Service Assistant

Social and human service assistants work under the direction of social workers, health care workers, or other professionals who provide services to people. They may assess client needs, investigate client eligibility for benefits such as food assistance programs, or administrate food banks or emergency fuel-assistance programs. Special certificates or an associate's degree is a requirement in these careers. Course work often includes learning how to observe patients or clients, record information, conduct patient/client interviews, and implement treatment plans. Passion to help others, excellent communication skills, problem-solving skills, and the ability to handle crises are essential.

Social Worker

Social workers may choose to specialize in working with children, families, and schools. Others choose to help people who are dealing with abuse, chronic or terminal illnesses, aging parents, grief, or other life changing events. A bachelor's degree in social work is a minimum requirement. Most positions require a master's degree. Emotional maturity and sensitivity to the needs of others are important. All states require some type of certification, licensing, or registration for social workers. Many require 2 years (or 3,000 hours) of supervised clinical experience before granting licensure of clinical social workers.

Is this career path for you? Pursue one or both of the following activities to determine if you are suitable for a career in human services.

- Plan an ongoing service learning project. Consider serving at local Boys and Girls Clubs, a food pantry, a daycare, or residential facility for older adults. Keep a journal for your project, noting what you learn about helping others.
- Many human service workers serve *nonprofit organizations*. These organizations raise their own funds to support the work they do to help others. Choose a local nonprofit organization and find out how this group raises funds for their work. Arrange to volunteer at a fund-raising event. Create a photo essay about the event to share with the class.

Chapter 1
Personal Development

Sections

Reading Prep

College and Career Readiness

Before you read the chapters in this unit, answer the question on the unit opening page. How does this question relate to what is being presented in the content?

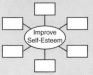

Concept Organizer

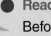 Use a star diagram like the one shown to list six things you can do to improve your self-esteem.

Improve Self-Esteem

Companion Website

Print out the concept organizer for Chapter 1 at the website.

Companion Website
www.g-wlearning.com

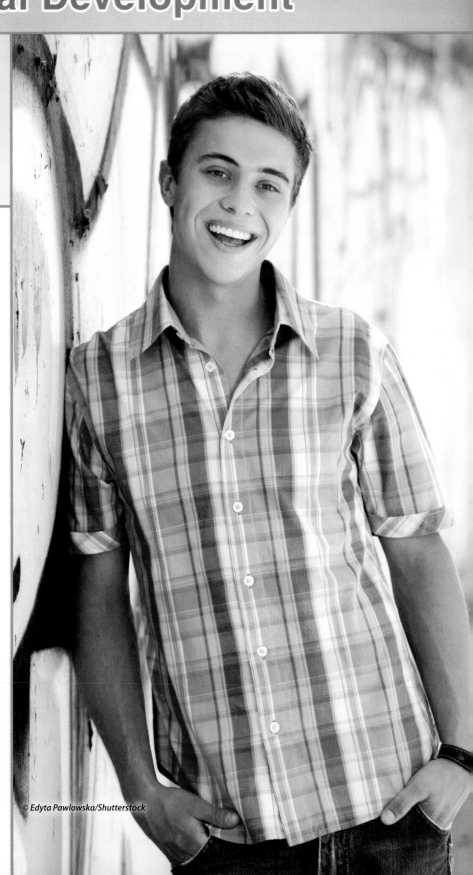

© Edyta Pawlowska/Shutterstock

4

Section 1-1

Your Personality

Objectives

After studying this section, you will be able to
- **explain** how heredity and environment affect personality development.
- **formulate** ways to enhance your personality.
- **compare and contrast** self-concept and self-esteem.
- **identify** suggestions for improving self-esteem.

Key Terms		
personality	environment	self-confidence
traits	acquired traits	attitudes
heredity	self-concept	optimists
inherited traits	self-esteem	pessimists

You are a very unique person—one of a kind. There is no other person in the world exactly like you with the same characteristics. Look around you to see how different people look even though they may have similar features. Even their voices and mannerisms are different.

How Personality Develops

One factor that makes you unique is your personality. Your **personality** is the combination of traits that makes you the person you are. It includes your habits and feelings. Your personality also includes how you think and interact with others.

You have many personality traits. **Traits** are qualities that make you different from everyone else. Certain personality traits are desirable, while others are less desirable. Some of your friends may like your honesty, while others may complain about your laziness. Figure **1-1** lists some typical personality traits.

Personality Traits		
Agreeable	Easygoing	Lazy
Aloof	Excitable	Loyal
Bashful	Faithful	Mature
Careful	Flighty	Moody
Cheerful	Friendly	Nervous
Confident	Generous	Responsible
Cooperative	Grumpy	Silly
Critical	Happy	Sincere
Delightful	Kind	Understanding

1-1 Which of these personality traits would your friends use to describe you?

Personality Differences Among Siblings

Brothers and sisters in the same family often have completely different personalities. One *sibling* (brother or sister) may be easygoing and joyful. Another might be quite serious and shy around other people. How can two siblings be so different?

Remember that everyone begins life with a specific set of inherited traits. No other person, not even a sibling, has the exact same set. These traits can influence behavior. Individuals react differently to similar experiences, and personalities develop from all of a person's experiences. The result can be very distinct personalities among family members.

You are born with certain personality traits. Other traits develop as you grow. Two main factors shape your personality: heredity and environment.

Heredity

Heredity refers to the passing of traits from one generation of family to the next. Parents pass these traits to their children through genes. *Genes* determine the characteristics that will appear as you grow and develop. The traits you receive from your parents and ancestors are **inherited traits**. The color of your eyes, hair, and skin are inherited traits. Your height, body build, and facial features are also inherited. Physical and mental capabilities are inherited traits, too.

From the moment babies are born, they begin to show inherited personality traits. For instance, some babies may only be content to fall asleep when their parents are holding them. They begin crying as soon as they are in their cribs. Some people may describe these babies as having *fussy* personalities. Other babies are more adaptable and may be able to fall asleep easily in unfamiliar settings. People may describe these babies as having *easygoing* personalities.

Environment

Your **environment** includes everything and everyone around you. Your family, home, friends, school, classmates, teachers, coaches, and community are all part of your environment.

Traits that develop as a result of your environment are **acquired traits**. Your acquired traits are not inherited qualities. These traits may include your likes and dislikes, goals, and interests. Your attitudes and abilities are also acquired traits. Your speech and mannerisms are other examples.

Like inherited traits, acquired traits can be seen from a very early age. As babies interact with family members, their acquired traits begin to develop, **1-2**. Later, they will

© Gayvoronskaya_yana/Shutterstock

1-2 These sisters may share similar experiences, yet each has a unique personality.

have contact with the world outside their homes. Neighbors, friends, and teachers will help shape their personalities.

Your inherited and acquired traits have an effect on each other. For instance, your mother may be an accomplished musician. You may have inherited a talent for music. You will need to take lessons, however, to acquire the ability to play an instrument.

Home and Family

Your family, no matter who is included in your family, is the most important environmental force shaping your personality. You have probably spent more time with the members of your family than with anyone else. During the early childhood years, almost all a child's contacts are with family members. The amount of love, care, and concern a child receives in the home influences personality formation.

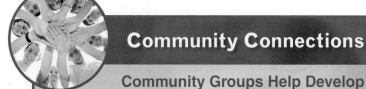

Community Connections

Community Groups Help Develop Positive Traits

The people in your community can affect your acquired traits. For instance, you may join a scout troop in your community. Going on camping trips with the troop might affect your feelings about nature. Your scout leader might help you to develop leadership traits. Other members of your troop might encourage you to enjoy hiking. Sports teams, youth groups, and local clubs are other community groups that might affect your acquired traits in a positive way.

Sometimes family members change with the death of a parent, separation, or divorce. New family members also have an influence on you, as well as you on them.

The size of your family also influences your personality. An only child will often develop different personality traits from children who have brothers and sisters. Your birth order within your family affects your personality, too. *Birth order* indicates whether you are the first, middle, or youngest child in your family. An oldest child may have a leadership personality. This is due to the responsibilities the oldest child may need to assume. Middle and youngest children tend to develop distinct personality traits for similar reasons.

Personality traits acquired from family members are often learned by imitation. If a parent is always calm during a crisis, the children might pick up this trait. On the other hand, if a parent becomes angry easily, the children may develop this form of behavior.

School and Friends

Eventually, children begin to spend more time away from home. As this continues, the family becomes a less powerful force in shaping personality. Other environmental factors, such as television, the Internet, and other media, become more important. School and friends become more of an influence. The size of a school and the kinds of courses offered can affect feelings and opinions about learning, **1-3**.

Your relationships with your friends and classmates affect your acquired traits. Their likes and dislikes may become your likes and dislikes. The activities you enjoy with them may become lifelong interests for you.

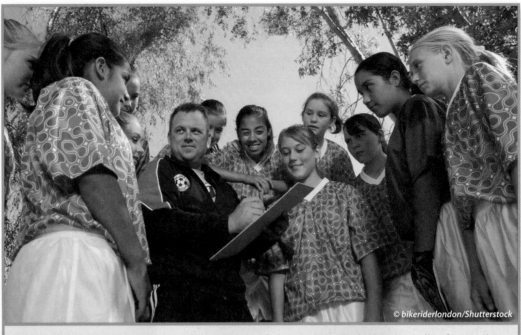

© bikeriderlondon/Shutterstock

1-3 Teachers and coaches often play an important role in personality formation.

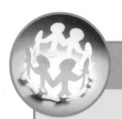

Life Connections

How to Make a Change

When thinking about changing your personality, select only one area for improvement at a time. Do not try to change everything about yourself at once. Then write a specific plan of what you will do to change this quality. As part of your plan, set a realistic goal for yourself. Also, plan a reward for yourself when you reach your goal. This will give you an incentive to try even harder to make a change. The final step is to put your plan in action.

Change does not happen easily. Do not be surprised if you fall into your old habits sometimes. Do not let this discourage you. With time, you will be able to make a positive change if it is really important to you.

Writing Activity

Look again at the list of personality traits in Figure 1-1. Are there some positive changes you would like to make to your personality? Are you as friendly as you could be? Do you complain too often? Do you make fun of someone because he or she is different? Write a list of your traits and identify the one you would most like to improve or change. Then write a plan of what you can do to change this trait.

Changing Your Personality

With so many influences on your personality, you can see why you are such a complex person. The effects environmental factors have on your personality will continue throughout your life. The influence will never be as strong, however, as it was during your early childhood years. Your personality has taken form. Any changes that occur from now on will likely require effort on your part. You can change personality traits, but these patterns are hard to break.

Young people who feel good about themselves generally want to be the best they can be. They know they are not perfect and never will be. They recognize their shortcomings and try to enhance them.

There may be some less desirable personality traits that you would like to improve or change. Changing a quality that has been a part of your personality for a long time may not be easy. It will take time and effort. You can do it, however, if you really want to change. You are in control of your behavior and actions.

Your Self-Concept

Have you ever asked yourself "How do other people see me?" The mental image you have of yourself is called your **self-concept**. Your self-concept is an important part of your personality.

Your self-concept is formed from your contacts with other people. You get an idea of what others think of you from what they tell you and the ways they treat you. Suppose classmates often ask you to help them with their math homework. This might give you the idea they think you do well in math. An experience like this can affect your self-concept because you might become more confident and begin to believe in your ability.

Your mental picture of yourself impacts your decisions and actions, **1-4**. If a boy believes he is shy, he may not try to make friends. If he believes he is outgoing, however, he may find it easier to make friends.

Having a Healthy Self-Esteem

Do you like the person you see in the mental picture of yourself? Is there anything about yourself that you wish you could change? Maybe you like the way you are. How you feel about yourself is called your **self-esteem**. It is how you view your worth as a person.

People who have a healthy self-esteem feel good about themselves. They accept qualities about themselves they cannot change. They are confident they can change what needs to be changed. People who have a healthy self-esteem like who they are. They have a positive outlook on life. These people are fun to be with because they do not let challenges get them down. They do not worry about what other people say. They know how to use suggestions for improvement and overlook the negative. People who have a healthy self-esteem can help others feel good about themselves, too.

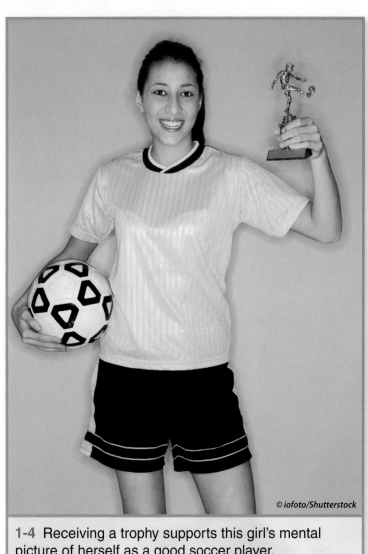

© iofoto/Shutterstock

1-4 Receiving a trophy supports this girl's mental picture of herself as a good soccer player.

People who have a low self-esteem do not feel good about themselves and their abilities. These people worry about their shortcomings and failures. They dwell on their past mistakes. They are often afraid to try anything new. People who have a low self-esteem are often putting themselves down. When they receive a compliment, they usually give reasons for not deserving the remark. They feel and act as though they are worthless. Sadly, most of these feelings have no basis or truth to them.

Families who provide love, appreciation, and encouragement can help children develop a healthy self-esteem, **1-5**. Suppose a young child is trying to learn to tie his shoes by himself. A family member encourages him to try again and again. When he finally learns to tie his shoes, his family praises and compliments him. This makes him feel good about himself. Experiences like these can cause a healthy self-esteem to develop.

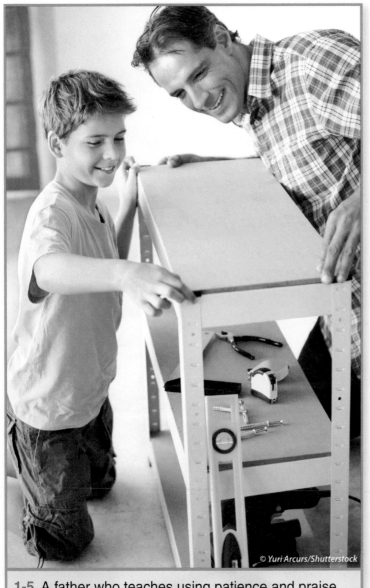

© Yuri Arcurs/Shutterstock

1-5 A father who teaches using patience and praise can help his son develop a healthy self-esteem.

Improving Your Self-Esteem

Even people who have a healthy self-esteem sometimes doubt themselves. This is normal. During these times, they can think about their accomplishments. They realize that doubts and the events that caused them are just a temporary stop. Tomorrow will be a new day and a new beginning. People who have a healthy self-esteem continue to look for solutions to challenges. They make the changes needed to lessen doubts and get back on track.

In the years ahead, you will continue to learn and grow, **1-6**. Your self-confidence may improve as well. **Self-confidence** is the assurance you have in yourself and your abilities. Self-confidence gives you courage to deal with people and events in positive ways. New experiences can be frightening to anyone. As you develop self-confidence, you can face these new experiences with less fear.

If you do not feel good about yourself, you can work to improve your self-esteem. The following ways can help you improve your feelings about yourself.

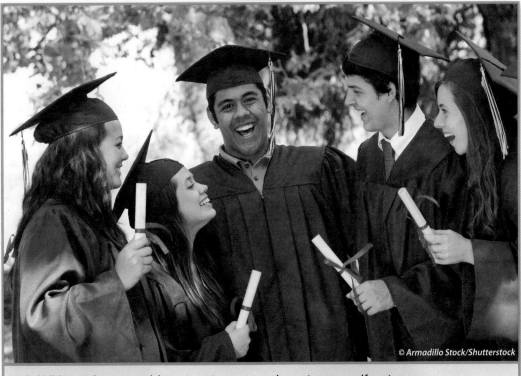

© Armadillo Stock/Shutterstock

1-6 With each new achievement, you can boost your self-esteem.

Look at Your Positive Qualities

One way to develop a healthy self-esteem is to look at all your positive qualities. Of course, everyone has weaknesses. You cannot expect yourself to be perfect. Try not to focus on your weaknesses. Instead, try to improve them.

Take a careful look at yourself as if you are looking into a mirror. What positive qualities do you see? Maybe you are a cheerful person, a responsible student, or a loyal friend. Make a list of your positive qualities. Think about all your past successes and add these to your list, too. You may be surprised at how long your list is. Pull out the list the next time your self-esteem needs a boost. Remind yourself frequently that you have value and worth. No matter what you are facing, tomorrow is a new day. It provides an opportunity for you to see the situation from a different perspective.

Try Not to Compare Yourself with Others

Try not to compare yourself with others, especially personalities portrayed on television and in the media. Learn to accept yourself as you are. If you try to compare yourself with others, you may only compare their strengths to your weaknesses. This is not a fair comparison and will not help to improve your self-esteem.

At the same time, try not to find fault with other people in order to make yourself feel better. People who criticize others only make themselves appear small in comparison. Maybe you have known someone who had a lead in a school play. You may have heard others in the play criticize that person's performance. They may have made remarks such as, "She can't act at all. I could have done a much better job." These statements are not helpful or a true indication of the person's acting abilities. They just make the people who said them appear jealous.

Remember, only one person in the world can be the best snowboarder or the best rapper. These titles are short-lived. There will always be people who can do something better than you. There will also be people who are better looking, smarter, funnier, or more graceful than you are. Just because you may not be as funny as someone else, does not mean you are not funny at all. Try to do the best you can do, and avoid comparing yourself with others, **1-7**.

Learn to Give and Accept Compliments

Giving people compliments builds their self-esteem. Look for strengths in other people. It is easy to see positive qualities in your close friends. If you try, you can find something nice to say about everyone. Compliment people about their strengths. You might even try complimenting someone you do not know very well. You may be pleased at the reaction.

Sometimes accepting compliments is harder than giving them. People often brush off compliments with a negative comment. For instance, Keisha's classmate complimented her on a report she gave in class. Keisha replied, "You're kidding. It's the worst report I've ever given." Keisha may not have realized how her reply put down her classmate's opinion.

You should not sell yourself short on what you have done. You may want to make mental notes on how you can improve the next time. Try to accept that you might have done a good job this time as well. Thank people when they give you compliments and allow their remarks to give your self-esteem a lift.

Develop New Interests

You can improve your self-esteem by getting involved in groups and activities you might enjoy. Pursuing new interests can give you the chance to discover talents you did not know you had. Displaying these talents can help you feel confident about yourself.

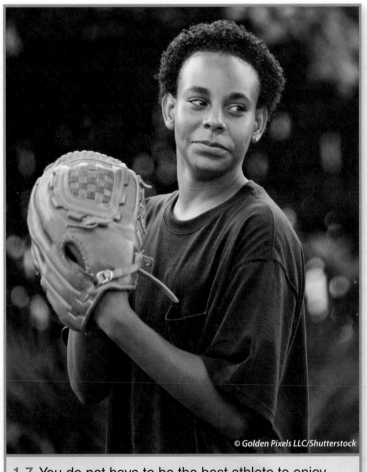

© Golden Pixels LLC/Shutterstock

1-7 You do not have to be the best athlete to enjoy playing a sport.

You can develop interests in a wide variety of areas, **1-8**. Each of these areas includes activities that will give you chances to grow and learn new skills. You can meet people and learn about their interests, too.

As you mature, you will have many opportunities to develop new interests. Keep an open mind and take advantage of these opportunities. Many hobbies you start at a young age will continue throughout your life. The more interests you develop, the more chances you have to improve your self-esteem.

Try Something New

School Activities	Athletics	Hobbies and Recreation
Special Interest Courses	• Baseball/softball	• Bicycling
• Art	• Basketball	• Boating
• Computer programming	• Cross country	• Camping
• Drama	• Football	• Computers
• Music	• Gymnastics	• Cooking
• Photography	• Hockey	• Crafts
• Trade and industrial	• Lacrosse	• Collecting
	• Soccer	• Dancing
Clubs and Organizations	• Swimming	• Fishing
• Activity planning committees	• Tennis	• Gardening
• Band	• Track and field	• Hiking
• Cheerleading	• Volleyball	• Ice skating
• Chess club		• Inline skating
• Choir	**Other Clubs and Organizations**	• Knitting
• Computer club	• Book club	• Model building
• Drama club	• Community volunteer work	• Needleworking
• Foreign language club	• Park district youth programs	• Quilting
• Glee club	• *Athletics*	• Reading
• Mathematics club	• *Exercise programs*	• Robotics
• Robotics	• *Field trips*	• Sewing
• School newsletter/website	• *Hobby instruction*	• Skateboarding
• Science Olympiad	• Family, Career and Community Leaders of America (FCCLA)	• Skiing
• Speech and debate team	• Hospital organizations	• Snowboarding
• Yearbook	• *First aid and child training programs*	• Surfing
	• *Volunteer services*	• Woodworking
Student Government	• Religious organizations	
• Class officer	• SkillsUSA	
• Student council	• YMCA/YWCA	
• *Officer*		
• *Representative*		

1-8 Some of these school activities, organizations, and hobbies might be of interest to you.

Develop a Positive Attitude

Have you ever said "I like her attitude" or "He has a positive attitude"? Everyone has attitudes. What are they though? **Attitudes** are feelings and opinions about someone or something. They determine how you react to situations. Attitudes affect your decisions and actions. They also affect your self-esteem.

You were not born with your attitudes. Just like the other acquired traits that make up your personality, your attitudes are learned. You learn from the people around you and from the experiences you have every day.

People who have positive attitudes are **optimists**. Optimistic teens feel good about life and look on the bright side of situations. They have a *can-do* approach to challenges. They are certain they can find solutions. They feel good about themselves and have a healthy self-esteem.

People who have negative attitudes are **pessimists**. They find something wrong with everything. They often put themselves down, and others as well. You cannot please them. Pessimists would cancel a picnic if there was the slightest chance of rain. Optimists, on the other hand, would go on the picnic and enjoy the excitement of running for shelter if it rained.

Learn to Smile and Laugh

Learning to smile is one of the most effective ways to change a negative attitude into a positive one. A smile reflects healthy self-esteem, **1-9**. A genuine smile comes from the heart by way of the face. It is not just on the face alone. There is a story about a small boy who asked his father if he was feeling good. The father said he was feeling great. The boy replied, "Why don't you tell your face about it?"

A laugh is just a step beyond a smile. It is important to enjoy life. You are able to laugh with, not at, your friends. You are also able to laugh at yourself. This is a sign of healthy self-esteem and a well-rounded personality.

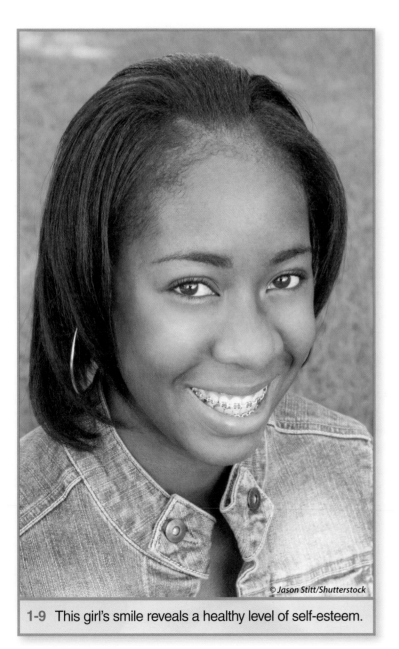

© Jason Stitt/Shutterstock

1-9   This girl's smile reveals a healthy level of self-esteem.

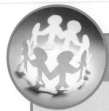

Life Connections

Success and a Positive Attitude

A positive attitude helps improve your self-esteem. When you look for the good aspects in situations, it is also easier to find the good in yourself. People enjoy being around you when you have a positive attitude. You will also find it easier to face the tough times when they come along.

One of the best ways to develop a positive attitude is expressing your thoughts in a positive manner. Say "I have to plan carefully today because I have so much to do," instead of "I'll never be able to get everything done today." If your field hockey team is the underdog, say "If we play hard, remember what we worked on in practice, and get a few good breaks, we can win." Only pessimists say "There's no way we can win tonight."

Reading and Writing Activity

Studies consistently show that people with positive attitudes are more successful both personally and professionally than those with negative attitudes. There are many books available about exactly how positive thinking contributes to a person's success in life. Ask your librarian for a recommendation or conduct an Internet search for one that appeals to you. Read it and write a short report about how you can develop a more positive attitude.

Reading Review

1. The combination of traits that makes a person unique is his or her _____.
2. What two factors shape a person's personality?
3. What is the difference between inherited and acquired traits?
4. Distinguish between *self-concept* and *self-esteem*.
5. List six ways to improve your feelings about yourself.

Section 1-2

Growing and Changing

Objectives

After studying this section, you will be able to
- **describe** physical, intellectual, emotional, and social changes that occur during adolescence.
- **give examples** of ways to handle negative emotions.
- **relate** how the physical, intellectual, emotional, and social changes that take place during adolescence help you achieve certain developmental tasks.

Key Terms

adolescence	emotional changes	hormones
developmental tasks	social changes	emotions
physical changes	growth spurts	role
intellectual changes	puberty	

The teen years are often a challenging and exciting time of life. Your body will be changing in many ways. You will begin to think in new ways. You will begin to have feelings that may be new to you. Your relationships with others will change.

You will also be making choices now that can impact your future. Knowing what to expect can make it easier to adjust to new feelings and changes. Understanding that these changes are normal can help you accept and enjoy what you are feeling and look forward to what's in store for you.

Social Studies Connections

Changes During Adolescence

The changes that take place during adolescence will affect the ways you act and think. Your actions directly relate to your decisions, which can affect your future. The more you know about these changes, the easier it will be to understand them in yourself. Through these changes, you will also realize you are special and unique. There is no one else like you, with your exact feelings and ideas. At the same time, you will know that what you are feeling and experiencing is a normal part of the growth process.

Growth and Development

People pass through three major stages of life. You are entering the stage of life called **adolescence**, which is the stage between childhood and adulthood. Within each stage, **developmental tasks**, or certain skills and behavior patterns, should be achieved, **1-10**. For instance, preparing for your future is a developmental task of adolescence.

Developmental Tasks of Teens
Learn to accept changes in your body
Select and prepare for a career
Achieve emotional independence
Learn to get along with peers
Acquire a set of standards that guide your behavior
Learn what behavior will be expected in adult roles
Accept responsibility
Become more independent at home, school, and in the community
1-10 These developmental tasks are usually achieved during adolescence.

People achieve some developmental tasks as the body physically matures. Achievement of these tasks usually occurs in a certain order. For instance, children will learn to sit, crawl, walk, and run in that order. People achieve other tasks as they learn proper standards of behavior. Learning how to get along with friends is an example.

During adolescence, you can expect to experience four major types of changes as you grow and develop. These include physical, intellectual, emotional, and social changes. **Physical changes** occur as your body grows and matures. **Intellectual changes** take place as you learn more about the world around you. **Emotional changes** affect how you feel about situations and how you express those feelings. **Social changes** occur as you meet more people and learn how to get along with them. Each type of change will help you achieve certain developmental tasks.

Physical Changes

Adolescence usually lasts from about ages 11 to 17. During this time, physical changes involve not only the growth of larger muscles, but also an improved ability to use those muscles. Your skill in sports and other activities often improves. Your eye-hand coordination improves as the small muscles in your fingers and hands develop.

Growth spurts, or rapid periods of growth, often occur. One month your clothes will fit.

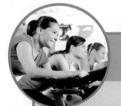

Health Connections

Growing out of Adolescence

The many physical changes that take place during adolescence may make you feel different from others and insecure at times. You may feel you will never get through this period in your life. These feelings are typical. Many people you know may feel the same way from time to time. How you choose to handle these changes is as important as what you are feeling and seeing. Remember that physical changes are a natural part of growing up. Learn to enjoy your new physical strength and grace. Learn to like the person you are and the one you are becoming.

The next month, they may be too tight or too short. You could easily grow several inches in one year.

Many physical changes affect the shape of your body during puberty. **Puberty** is the time when the body begins to mature sexually. You begin to have an adult figure or physique. **Hormones**, or chemicals produced in the body, influence the way you grow and develop. For instance, hormones cause young men's necks to get thicker and their shoulders to broaden. Males also get facial hair and soon have to shave. Their voices become deeper, too. Hormones cause young women's hips to widen and their breasts to enlarge. They begin having menstrual cycles. Their figures become shapelier. Changes that occur inside the body eventually enable a person to become a parent.

Girls usually mature about two years earlier than boys do. The average age when girls stop growing is about age 15. Boys reach this stage at about age 17. Some people continue to grow until 20 years of age.

Everyone grows and develops at an individual rate. Some teens become mature at an earlier age than others. There is no time schedule for these changes. You cannot speed up or slow down the process. What you choose to eat and drink, however, can affect your health, weight, and appearance.

Because your body is changing so rapidly, taking good care of yourself is important. The way you care for your body will affect your physical development. Eat healthful foods and get enough sleep to function your best. Be physically active to improve your strength and coordination. Avoid substances such as tobacco, alcohol, and illegal drugs that can have harmful effects on your physical development.

Intellectual Changes

During adolescence, your intelligence increases. The rate of growth, however, decreases. By the age of eight, 80 percent of adult intellect is already developed.

The ability to reason and solve problems generally develops between the ages of 13 and 15. During this time, you are able to think beyond concrete facts. Thinking through problems becomes easier. You think about options and consequences when solving problems. You are more likely to listen to both sides of an argument. You often gather facts before making decisions. With these new abilities, you can express your thoughts more clearly to others. You are able to see others' viewpoints as well. These skills can help you to better communicate with your friends and the adults in your life, **1-11**.

Another developmental task of adolescence is to select and prepare for a career or profession. Your emerging reasoning skills help you achieve this task. You will be making choices about what activities and potential careers interest you. Using your mental abilities will help you study and enjoy school subjects that prepare you to be a responsible adult.

Emotional Changes

It is easy to see the changes that are happening to you physically. You also know that you are learning every day. You may wonder if all these new and confusing feelings you are having are normal. The answer is "Yes!"

Emotions are feelings about people and events in your life. During adolescence, your emotions may become more intense. Something that never used to bother you before may suddenly cause worry, sadness, or confusion. Perhaps you did not spend much time thinking about your appearance. Now you may change your clothes three times before you decide what to wear. Talking in front of the class may have seemed easy when you were younger. Perhaps you worry more now about what your classmates think and say about you.

You may also notice your feelings change quickly. You begin to understand what people mean when they say someone is *moody*. You may feel happy and carefree one day and sad the next. One day you might enjoy being with people. The next day you may wish they would all go away and leave you alone. Your best friend may hurt your feelings one day and make you angry. You then worry about how to become best friends again, **1-12**.

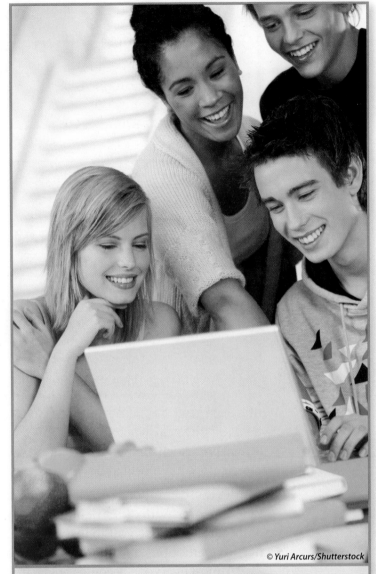

© Yuri Arcurs/Shutterstock

1-11 Communicating your thoughts becomes easier as your intellectual skills improve.

At times, your friends may get on your nerves. You might be angry with a sibling or parent for no apparent reason. You may feel certain that you know exactly what you want. At other times, you may feel like doing something completely different. These constantly changing feelings are normal. There is nothing wrong with you. As you develop, you learn how to handle your emotions. You also learn how to express your feelings and emotions appropriately.

There are both negative and positive emotions. *Negative emotions*, such as anger, jealousy, envy, and fear, can often be hard to handle. *Positive emotions*, such as love, affection, and joy, make life fun and exciting.

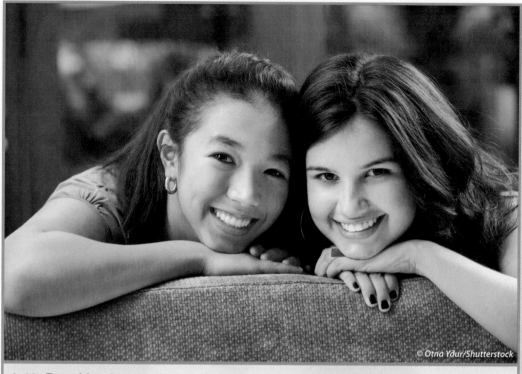

© Otna Ydur/Shutterstock

1-12 Best friends understand each other's moods and can forgive each other.

Negative Emotions

Negative emotions are often hard to understand and control. If you do not handle these emotions properly, you may find yourself in a difficult situation. Relationships with other people may be affected. Uncontrolled jealousy or anger may cause you to lose friends. A well-adjusted person recognizes negative emotions and works to understand and control them.

Almost everyone becomes angry from time to time. Sometimes when people lose their tempers, they say things they do not really mean. They may even hurt the feelings of people they love. They may take their anger out on other people who are not even involved. Venting negative emotions on just anyone is not appropriate.

Getting feelings out in the open can be a good way to deal with anger or frustration. Everyone needs to express feelings. When feeling angry, it is important to remain calm. Waiting awhile before talking with the person involved is sometimes a good tactic. You may often realize the issue is not so important after all. Sometimes you might find out you were wrong or decide to forget about it. An apology, especially for displaying a negative emotion, might clear the air and make everyone feel better.

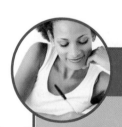

Writing Connections

Express Your Feelings

Writing a letter to express your feelings is another way to deal with anger or confusion. This does not mean you have to send the letter. You may find tearing it into pieces will make you feel better. On the other hand, you may want to save the letters you write when you are upset or confused. If you reread them at a later point, you may realize how much you have matured.

When you feel angry, talking with someone you trust may help, **1-13**. Talk with a friend who is not involved. Do not ask your friend, however, to take sides or tell you what to do. All you may need is for someone to listen while you share your feelings.

Another way to manage your anger is by doing some type of physical activity. Walking, running, swimming, or biking may improve your mood.

Anger is only one negative emotion. You also need to find appropriate ways to deal with other negative emotions, such as envy and fear. You may feel hurt if a close friend spends time with someone else. If you really care about your friend, it will be okay to share him or her with others. Talk with your friend about how you feel. This may be all you need to ease your feelings of jealousy. Sharing your feelings is often a good place to start.

Positive Emotions

Positive emotions are the ones that make everyone feel good. Many of the positive emotions you feel are the result of your relationships with others. You have fun being with your friends. You enjoy doing activities with your family. Happiness and laughter are often the result.

Many of your relationships are based on love. You feel love for your family and close friends. You may feel you are *in love* with someone special. This love may become a strong emotion for you to deal with in your teen years. Learning to express your feelings of love in an acceptable way can be an exciting challenge.

Social Changes

During adolescence, social changes often have to do with how you relate to others. You interact with many people every day. Some are family members and friends. Others are classmates, teachers, and neighbors. Some you know very well. You may only exchange a few words with others. Learning to communicate and get along with others is an important developmental task of adolescence.

Another part of social development is learning how to act in each of your roles. A **role** is a pattern of expected behavior. You already fill many roles. You are a son or a daughter, and possibly a brother or a sister, **1-14**. You are also a student, a friend, and maybe an employee. In each of these roles, people expect you to behave in

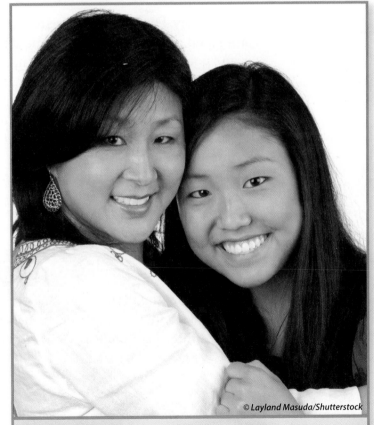

© Layland Masuda/Shutterstock

1-13 Friends of any age provide the support you need for handling emotions.

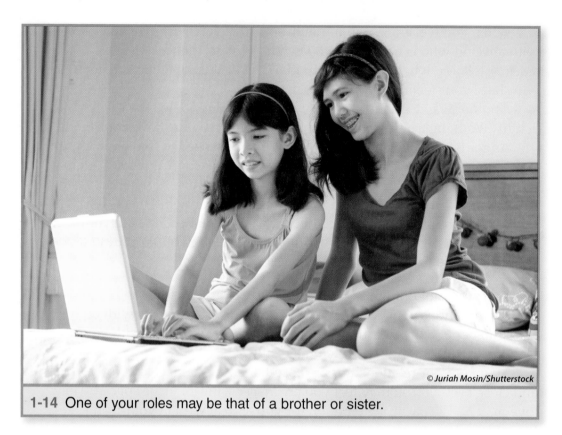

© Juriah Mosin/Shutterstock

1-14 One of your roles may be that of a brother or sister.

a certain way. For instance, as a student, your teachers expect you to attend classes and complete their assignments.

As you get older, you will assume some new roles. You may become a health care provider, a skilled laborer, or an architect. You may also become a spouse (husband or wife) and a parent. At the same time, you will give up some of your present roles. For instance, at some point you will no longer have the role of student. Learning how to act in your new roles can lead to success in your adult life.

The social changes that await you are many. Remember to relax and be yourself. Enjoy each day and look forward to the future.

Reading Review

1. What are the three major stages people pass through in life?
2. What are the four types of changes you experience during adolescence?
3. List three positive ways to deal with negative emotions.
4. Give an example of a developmental task you may achieve during each type of change.

Section 1-3

Becoming Independent

Objectives

After studying this section, you will be able to
- **explain** how to achieve independence.
- **identify** ways to show responsibility at home and at school.
- **demonstrate** how to be a responsible citizen in your local and global communities.

Key Terms		
independence	citizen	authority figures
responsibilities	citizenship	

How many times have you said "I can't wait until I'm old enough to do that"? Maybe you are excited to get a driver's license or have a part-time job. Maybe you are looking forward to going to college. Perhaps you just want to be more independent.

Becoming independent involves forming your own identity. It means preparing for a career. It also means becoming responsible for your decisions and developing socially acceptable behavior, **1-15**. Being responsible means you can be trusted to carry through an assignment, commitment, or job.

Now that you are entering adulthood, it is natural to want to become independent. This feeling is part of growing up and becoming mature. A person does not wake up one morning and decide "This is the day I will be independent." Independence is achieved one step at a time.

Achieving Independence

One of the tasks of adolescence is to start becoming independent of adults. People who have achieved **independence** are those who are responsible for their own actions.

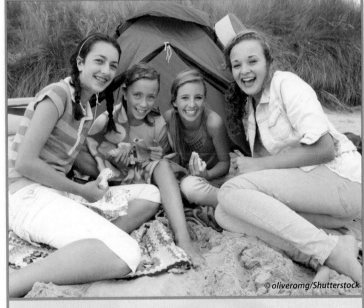

© oliveromg/Shutterstock

1-15 During adolescence, friends share experiences that help them learn socially acceptable behavior.

They provide for their own needs and wants. Independent people are in control of their lives.

Perhaps you would like to show your parents and other adults that you are ready to become more independent. One way to do this is to assume more responsibility. **Responsibilities** are the duties or jobs you must carry through. You have responsibilities to yourself, your family, friends, school, community, and the global environment in which you live.

Accepting Responsibility

The more responsible you are, the more you show you are ready for greater independence. This means others can count on you to do what you say you will do. When you tell your parents you are going to a concert, you go to the concert. If you and your friends decide to go somewhere else, you call your parents and tell them of the change. This type of behavior shows you are responsible.

One way to achieve greater independence might be getting an after school or summer job, **1-16**. When you arrive on time and work hard, you show maturity as well as responsibility.

Another way to show responsibility is to manage money you have been given or earned. If you can manage and use your money without having to ask for more, you are being responsible with money. Managing money wisely is often associated with independence.

Becoming independent gives you more freedom. You and your friends may be looking forward to making your own decisions. As you become more responsible, greater independence will follow.

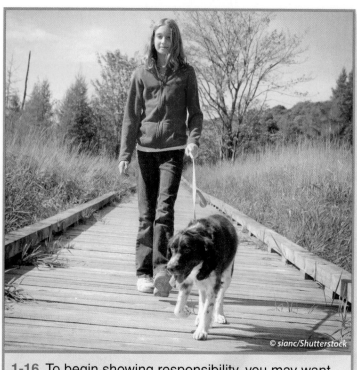

1-16 To begin showing responsibility, you may want to consider a job babysitting, mowing lawns, or walking dogs in your neighborhood.

Being Responsible for Yourself

Part of growing up is accepting responsibility for yourself and your actions. This means making decisions about your actions. It also means accepting the results of your choices. You begin to decide for yourself what is right and wrong. Although many people and events may influence your decisions, you alone are responsible for who you are and the person you will become.

Every day you become responsible for more decisions and tasks. Many of these have to do with your well-being. When you were younger, your family was totally responsible for you. They made the decisions that would influence the person you would become. Now, however, you are entering an age when you will be making more of the decisions that affect you. Will you choose healthy foods? Will you choose to go to bed early enough to feel ready for the day? Will you make informed choices about the use of the Internet or illegal use of tobacco, alcohol, and drugs?

You are responsible for the skills you develop. One of your parents may buy you a guitar and pay for lessons, but you must practice to learn the skill. The responsibility for learning to play the guitar is up to you.

You are responsible for the choices you make. When making decisions, you must consider how they will affect yourself and others. For instance, suppose you promised your youth group that you would help them collect donations for a local community shelter on Saturday. Instead of helping them, however, you chose to go to a movie with some friends. To be responsible, it is important to follow through with what you say you are going to do. Otherwise, people may feel as though they cannot count on you.

Responsibilities at Home

As a member of a family, you have certain responsibilities. Your parents may expect you to help with some of the housework. They also expect you to follow family rules. You may be responsible for getting home by a certain time in the evening. If you are going to be late, you might be expected to call so others will not worry about your safety.

Some of your responsibilities at home may include cleaning your room and taking care of your clothes. You may care for a younger brother or sister after school. If there is a new baby in the family, you may have even more responsibilities. You may also need to prepare some of the family's meals, **1-17**. As you handle these tasks, you show you are ready to take on other responsibilities. Each added responsibility you accept shows you are maturing.

The amount of responsibility you are given is determined by how well you handle those you already have. If your parents and other adults see that you show good judgment, you will probably be able to make more decisions. For instance, your parents may notice you always complete your homework and maintain good grades. Knowing this, they may allow you to schedule your own study time. On the other hand,

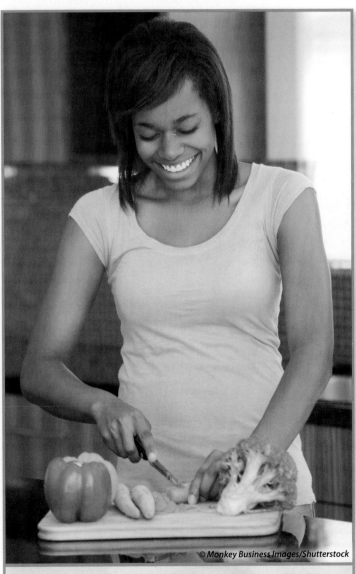

© Monkey Business Images/Shutterstock

1-17 As you get older, you may be responsible for preparing meals for the family.

when your grades are poor and you rarely do homework, your parents may feel you are not responsible enough to set your own study schedule. Instead, they may feel that they must require you to study a certain amount each evening.

Responsibilities at School

You have many responsibilities at school. Your most important responsibility is to learn. You are expected to attend school on a regular basis and arrive on time each day. Teachers expect you to complete work and take part in class projects, **1-18**. Teachers also expect you to bring needed supplies to class. Many rules are necessary for a school to run smoothly. It is also your responsibility to follow these rules.

Your responsibilities at school help prepare you for future ones. Failing to fulfill some of your school responsibilities may not seem to matter much. Failing to meet the future responsibilities they are preparing you for, however, may have greater effects. For instance, doing homework teaches you to complete tasks on time. You may see no harm in turning in some of your homework assignments after they are due. In the future, however, turning in projects late at work could cause you to lose your job.

Responsibilities in the Community

A **citizen** is a member of a community. For instance, you are a citizen of a city, state, and country. As a student, you are a member of a school community. You are also a member of the community in which you live. **Citizenship** is your status as a citizen with rights and responsibilities.

Your responsibilities to your community are much like responsibilities in other areas of your life. You can display good citizenship and fulfill many of your community responsibilities simply by obeying laws. In other cases, you must make a special effort to carry out responsibilities to the community.

One of your responsibilities as a citizen is to respect authority figures. **Authority figures** are people who help guide the behaviors of others in the community. They create and enforce rules designed to help and protect you and all other citizens in the community. Your principal, teachers, and any other faculty are authority figures in your school. You can show respect for authority by following the rules.

Police officers and government leaders are authority figures in larger communities such as your city or country. Their duty is to create and enforce rules that protect the rights

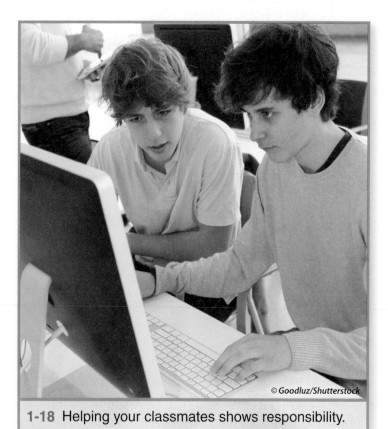

© Goodluz/Shutterstock

1-18 Helping your classmates shows responsibility.

of all community members. For instance, police officers enforce laws. You should respect police officers as representatives of the law.

Respecting other people is another community responsibility. The rights of others are protected by law. For instance, it is against the law for one person to physically harm another. Respect for another's property is also a responsibility. This includes anything from bicycles to homes. If you respect someone's property, you do not damage it or take it without permission.

Respect for community property, such as parks and libraries, is also a responsibility. You have the right to use and enjoy public property. You share public property with everyone in the community, however. You can show good citizenship by using community property carefully. Leave parks and buildings the same way you would want others to leave them for you—free from damage and litter.

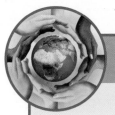

Global Connections

Community Responsibilities

In addition to being a citizen of your local community, you are also a citizen of a global community. The most important responsibility you have to your community is to protect the Earth. Pollution from fuels harms the air you breathe. Waste dumped into waterways contaminates the water. How you protect and care for the planet now will have an impact on the quality of life for future generations.

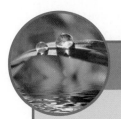

Go Green

Protect the Environment

There are many ways you can do your part to help protect the environment. You could organize a group to help pick up trash in a park or on roadsides. You might use public transportation, ride your bike, or walk instead of riding in a car. You can be more mindful of how much energy and water you use. Learning to be a responsible citizen can help you make a difference in your local and global communities.

Volunteering

One way to demonstrate good citizenship is to volunteer in your community. When you volunteer, you donate money, materials, or time to help other members of your community.

There are many ways you can volunteer in your community. By contributing to a food or clothing drive, you are helping people in need of these items. If you volunteer to organize a drive, you volunteer your time as well as materials.

Hospitals, community centers, and retirement homes offer opportunities for volunteering. You could spend time visiting people in these facilities. Your contributions can include reading to someone or entertaining a group of sick children. Helping clean or prepare meals is another way to volunteer your time.

Reading Review

1. What does becoming independent involve?
2. What is one way to show your parents and others that you are ready to become more independent?
3. What are some of your responsibilities at home? at school? in the community?
4. What does *citizenship* mean? Give an example of a way to show good citizenship.

Chapter Summary

Section 1-1. Two main factors that shape your personality are heredity and environment. Your personality includes inherited traits that you received from your parents and ancestors. It also includes acquired traits that develop as a result of your environment. Your self-concept, or the mental image you have of yourself, is an important part of your personality. Your self-esteem is how you feel about your self-concept. It affects your confidence in your abilities and your relationships, too. You can learn to like yourself better and improve your self-esteem.

Section 1-2. You are now in adolescence, which is the stage of life between childhood and adulthood. During this time, you will grow and develop physically, intellectually, emotionally, and socially. These changes will affect every part of your life, including your body, mind, feelings, and relationships. Each of these changes also allows you to accomplish certain developmental tasks that are important steps toward becoming an adult. Remembering these changes are typical will help you adjust to them and enjoy the person you are becoming.

Section 1-3. Another part of growing up involves becoming independent of adults. One way to become more independent is to assume more responsibility. By accepting responsibilities, you show people they can count on you to do what you say you will do. You have responsibilities to yourself, your home and family, friends, school, community, and the global environment in which you live. Fulfilling your responsibilities shows you are ready to start making more of your own decisions. You are ready to start becoming an independent adult.

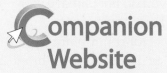

Companion Website
www.g-wlearning.com

Check your understanding of the main concepts for Chapter 1 at the website.

Critical Thinking

1. **Identify.** If you could change one thing about yourself, what would that one thing be? Why is it an important change for you to make? Is it realistic for you to make the change? What strategies could you outline to help you reach your goal?

2. **Draw conclusions.** What can people do to achieve healthy self-esteem when the media promotes unrealistic images?

3. **Determine.** Do famous people such as athletes, politicians, or actors have an obligation to be responsible role models? Why or why not?

Common Core

College and Career Readiness

4. **Writing.** Write a two-page paper about personality traits you admire in others. Rank the traits according to their importance to you and explain your rankings.

5. **Speaking.** Make a list of all the developmental tasks of adolescence discussed in the chapter. Working with a small group of your classmates, discuss how teens can work to achieve each of these tasks. Share your group's ideas with the rest of the class.

6. **Listening.** Interview students about what you can do to support students your age who are struggling with the transition from childhood to adolescence. What could parents do? What could role models do?

7. **Writing.** Write a brief story describing an imaginary person who is struggling with the change to adolescence.

Technology

8. **Electronic presentation.** Select a school activity, community organization, hobby, or recreational activity that interests you. Prepare an electronic presentation that details how you can get involved.

Journal Writing

9. Write a letter to yourself expressing how you feel about the changes you are experiencing. Put the letter in an envelope and save it. Open the letter at the end of the school year. Have you changed since you wrote the letter? If so, how?

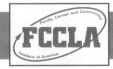 FCCLA

10. Think about the changes you are experiencing and those that you have the power to control. Select an area you would like to further develop such as building study skills, working on a positive attitude, or showing more responsibility. Use the *FCCLA Planning Process* to develop a *Power of One: A Better You* project. Identify a personal concern, set a self-improvement goal, and develop a plan of action. Set a deadline for accomplishing your goal and evaluating your results. See your adviser for information as needed.

Chapter 2
Your Family

College and Career Readiness

Reading Prep

Before you read the chapter, review the objectives for each section. Then look at all the major headings and compare them to the objectives. What did you learn? How can checking this information help you prepare to read new material?

Concept Organizer

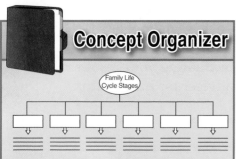

Family Life Cycle Stages

Use a diagram like the one shown to list the six stages of the family life cycle. Then write a short, defining sentence for each stage.

Companion Website

Print out the concept organizer for Chapter 2 at the website.

Companion Website
www.g-wlearning.com

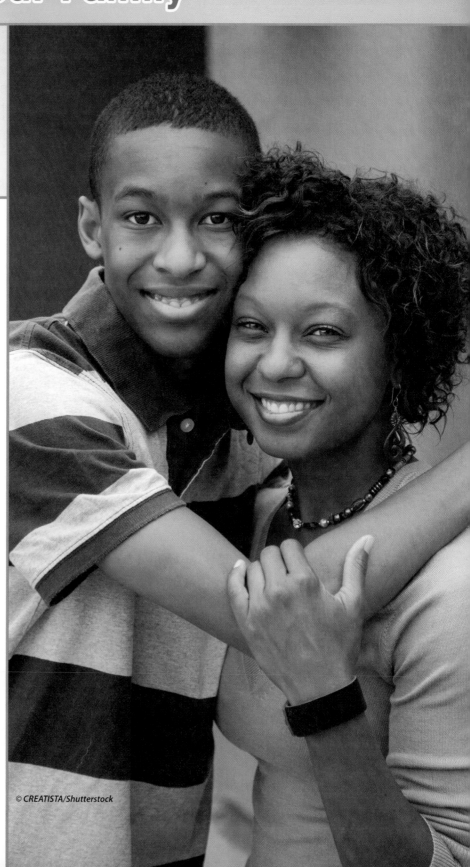

© CREATISTA/Shutterstock

30

Section 2-1

Understanding Your Family

Objectives

After studying this section, you will be able to
- **explain** functions served by the family.
- **describe** the different family types.
- **identify** roles and responsibilities filled by family members.
- **differentiate** between functional and dysfunctional families.

Key Terms		
family	single-parent family	foster family
socialization	stepfamily	childless family
culture	extended family	functional family
nuclear family	adoptive family	dysfunctional family

Families play an important role in the lives of many people. Most families provide for physical needs such as food, clothing, and shelter. They also provide emotional support. Families have a way of sticking together. Family members often come to each other's rescue. Even children show this type of support for family members when they tell their playmates, "My mom is the best cook in the world!" or "My dad is funnier than your dad."

Your family is probably the greatest influence in shaping your personality. You learn much of what you know from your family members. They influence your personality, values, and behaviors. Sometimes you think like other members of your family; sometimes you do not. Many of your goals come from them. You can understand yourself better if you learn more about families. Understanding family dynamics will help you as you select your partner and start your own family.

Functions of the Family

What is a family? A **family** is a group of two or more people related to each other. Some examples of family include people who are related by blood (birth), marriage, or adoption, **2-1**. A baby who is born to a couple is related by blood. The man your sister marries will be related to you by marriage. A child who is legally adopted by an adult is related by adoption.

Every country in the world contains family units of some form. What makes up a family unit, however, can vary. For instance, in some countries, and among certain religious groups, a man may have more than one wife. In other situations, several families may live together as a group. All families, no matter what their makeup, perform similar functions.

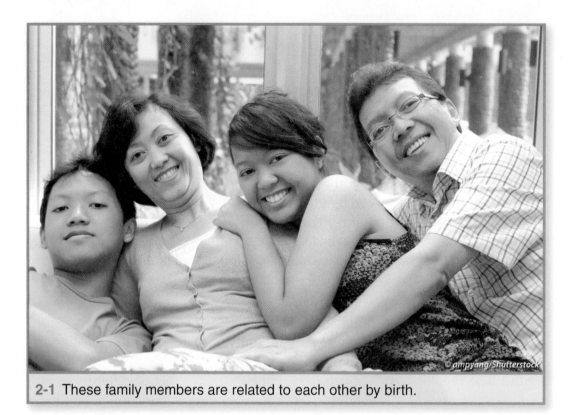

2-1 These family members are related to each other by birth.

Physical Needs

One function of the family is to provide for the physical needs of family members. These needs include food, clothing, and shelter. In years past, serving this function meant growing your own food, canning or preserving it, and preparing it for the family. It also meant making clothes and building your own home. Today, factories produce most food, clothing, and housing materials. Serving this function now means having a job to provide a source of income. Families purchase the food, clothing, and shelter needed for survival.

Emotional Support

Another function the family provides is for the emotional well-being of its members. All people need to feel loved and accepted, even when they make mistakes. They need to feel they belong somewhere. Family members provide the security of someone to turn to—even a shoulder to cry on at times. They recognize each other when they do something well. Families often best provide the emotional support needed for its members.

Socialization

The family also fulfills a socialization function. Socialization means that families teach their children about the culture of the society in which they live. Culture refers to the beliefs and customs of a particular racial, religious, or social group.

Socialization also includes teaching children acceptable forms of behavior. From an early age, children begin to learn how to function effectively in their culture. Parents teach children the appropriate way to act in personal and public situations. Parents also encourage correct manners and deter unacceptable behavior.

Types of Families

Families come in many sizes and combinations. As society changes, different family types often form. Today, there are many different family types in the United States. No one family type is better than another as long as the family performs its necessary functions.

The Nuclear Family

A **nuclear family** consists of a married couple and their biological children. Parents in nuclear families share child care and household responsibilities. They may also both earn incomes. Relatives may not be readily available for guidance and support. They may even live in other parts of the country. This can draw the nuclear family closer together and cause the members to depend more on each other.

The Single-Parent Family

A **single-parent family** includes one parent and one or more children. The parent may be either the father or the mother. The parent could be divorced, widowed, separated, or never married. An adult who has never married may want to be a parent. He or she may then adopt one or more children to form a single-parent family.

In single-parent families, the single parent must play both roles of father and mother, **2-2**. This parent must often provide both emotional and financial support for the family. The parent usually works full time. A working parent must arrange for child care for young children. He or she will need to find time to spend with children, maintain the house,

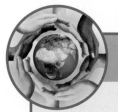

Global Connections

Your Cultural Heritage

Cultural heritage consists of learned behaviors, beliefs, and languages that are passed from one generation to another. The cultural heritage of your family is reflected in the traditions you observe, the foods you eat, and the holidays you celebrate. You will find families of different cultures in communities nationwide.

Ethnic groups help preserve the cultural heritage of a family. *Ethnic groups* are groups of people who share common cultural and/or racial characteristics such as language, traditions, religion, and national origin. Making friends with people from different cultures can help you learn more about other people and the world. Be open to meeting people with different backgrounds. In addition to learning from them, they can learn from you.

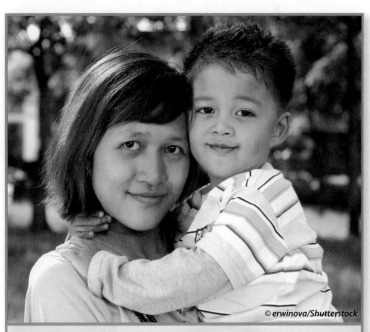

© erwinova/Shutterstock

2-2 The single mother may have to provide for all the needs of her child.

and meet career demands. These many responsibilities can present challenges for the single parent.

Often, a single-parent family forms because of a death or divorce. Either situation creates a great deal of emotional stress for the family members. Children may need help in coping with the loss of the parent. Older children may have to take on extra responsibilities. All members will need to pull together and support one another as they adjust to the changes. The family members can provide love, security, and encouragement for one another.

The Stepfamily

A **stepfamily**, or *blended family*, forms when a single parent marries. In a stepfamily, at least one of the parents is a stepparent to the children. A *stepparent* is a person who marries a child's mother or father. He or she is not related to the child by blood. Stepmothers or stepfathers may legally adopt the children of their spouse.

The blending of two families can present new challenges for the family members. Children have to learn to share their home with another adult, and possibly other children. There will be more people using the same facilities. Adjustments in daily routines may occur. There may be more demands on the family income.

When a stepfamily forms, it is a new beginning for the married couple. Their love for each other can draw all members of the family closer together. The strengths of each member of the family can benefit the family as a whole.

The Extended Family

An **extended family** has relatives other than parents (or stepparents) and children living together in one home. An extended family could include grandparents, aunts, uncles, or cousins.

In an extended family, there are more family members to provide guidance and support for one another, **2-3**. They can take care of small children if the parents work. They can help with household chores and meals. They can be there to listen and advise when others may not be available.

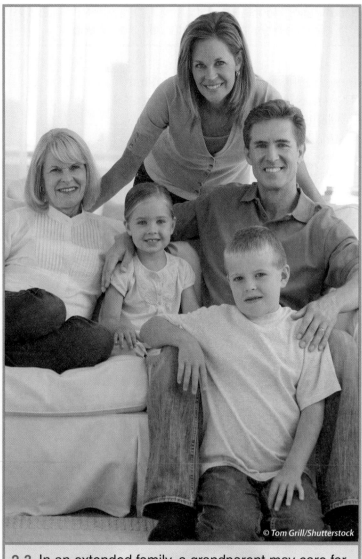

© Tom Grill/Shutterstock

2-3 In an extended family, a grandparent may care for the grandchildren while the parents work.

The Adoptive Family

An **adoptive family** occurs when an adult brings a child from another family into his or her own family through legal means. The child is then a permanent part of the family with similar rights and responsibilities as other family members.

Sometimes couples choose to adopt because they are physically unable to have children. Other couples may wish to add more children to their family. A single person may want to provide a home for a child. In most cases, adoptive families create a loving, stable home life for the child.

The Foster Family

A **foster family** forms when a family temporarily takes care of children because their parents are unable to do so. Foster parents assume the responsibilities of providing care for the children until they can go home to live with their parents. In some cases, the children will stay with the foster parents until they are adopted. Foster families perform the same functions as any family.

The Childless Family

A **childless family** consists of a married couple without children, **2-4**. There are various reasons couples may choose not to have children. Some couples are unable to have children. Other couples may decide to never have children. They may want to apply their time and energy to their careers or other passions. These couples may enjoy spending time with children of friends and relatives. They may not want, however, the full-time responsibility of raising children.

Family Roles and Responsibilities

As a member of a family, you have certain roles. You may be a daughter, son, niece, nephew, aunt, or uncle. These roles describe your relationship to other family members. You also have family roles that are defined by the tasks you perform. Cook, launderer, and shopper are just a few of these roles you might fill. In each role, you assume different responsibilities. Family members expect you to perform certain actions.

In many families, members often exchange roles and responsibilities. For instance, family members may rotate tasks such as cleaning the

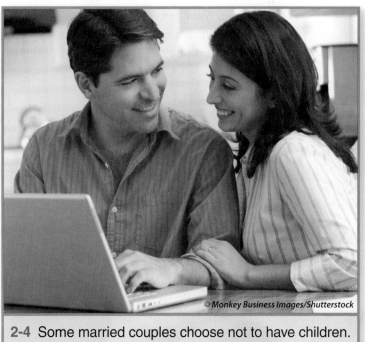

© Monkey Business Images/Shutterstock

2-4 Some married couples choose not to have children.

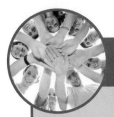

Community Connections

Family and Community

Strong families help make sound communities. Children raised in a loving family are more likely to become caring adults. Their contributions to society will include honesty and compassion. Children who learn peaceful conflict resolution can use those techniques to help solve community problems. If family members respect and support one another, they are likely to respect and support people outside the family as well.

Your community is a lot like a big family. Many people in your community may come from different family situations, backgrounds, and cultures. How you get along with others can help make you and your family happier, and your community a better place to live.

kitchen after dinner. Doing the laundry may be the responsibility of one family member for a limited time, such as a week. Then another member takes the role of launderer.

Your roles will often change as there are changes in your family. If a member of your family leaves, you may need to accept new responsibilities and roles. Your roles may also change as you get older. As a young child, you may have filled the role of pet feeder or table setter. As you got older, however, a younger sibling may have taken over that role. You may have then assumed the role of launderer or cook. You learn your family roles from the members of your family.

Functional and Dysfunctional Families

In a **functional family**, each member contributes to the family unit by fulfilling his or her roles and responsibilities. Each family member is committed to the well-being of the others. The family becomes a **dysfunctional family** when a member does not do his or her part to fulfill responsibilities. For instance, when a parent leaves unexpectedly or a child refuses to do his or her share, the family system becomes out of balance.

Every family faces problems. Strong, functional families are able to solve problems together. They do this through communication and respect for each other. Members of a functional family also trust one another. They spend time together. They make each other feel good and help each other develop self-esteem. Observing family traditions will help link one generation of a family to the next.

Reading Review

1. How does socialization fulfill a function in families?
2. Name seven types of families.
3. What type of family occurs when an adult brings a child from another family into his or her own family through legal means?
4. Distinguish between a functional family and a dysfunctional family.

Section 2-2

Family Relationships

Objectives

After studying this section, you will be able to
- **relate** techniques to help improve relationships with parents.
- **give examples** of ways to achieve good sibling relations.
- **explain** how to keep relationships with grandparents strong.

Key Terms		
relationship	sibling rivalry	cooperation

The first bond most people develop is with their parents. Then their relationships often include siblings and other relatives. Relationships with family members are likely to continue throughout life.

Relationships with Parents

A **relationship** is a special bond or link between people. In relationships, you learn how to get along with others. You also learn more about yourself.

Sometimes relationships with parents become strained during the teen years. Have you ever complained that your parents do not understand you? Have you ever asked "Why don't you trust me?" or "Why can't I go there?" Many conversations between parents and teens include these statements. What happens during the teen years to cause a smooth parent-child relationship to change?

One family member that is changing a lot right now is you. Sometimes your parents do not see these changes right away. Perhaps they do not want to see them. Maybe they are reluctant to see you growing up. Therefore, they may continue to treat you as a child.

This can be a difficult time for both you and your parents. Relations can become strained. You want more independence. They are afraid to give you more freedom. You feel you can be trusted. They are afraid you might make a mistake. You want to be able to go more places and do more things on your own. They are afraid for your safety and well-being. It seems like there is a continual struggle.

It is normal for teens to want to get on with the business of living. It is normal for parents to want what is best for their children. It is also normal for these two desires to cause conflict on occasion. All family members need to work at maintaining harmony within the family. With love, patience, and respect, families can achieve this goal.

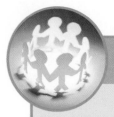

Life Connections

Improving Relations with Parents

The following suggestions may help you improve your relationship with your parents:

- **Share your concerns.** Keep the lines of communication open. Talk with your parents. Let them know how you feel. Then ask them to share their feelings. Try to understand their point of view. Also, explain the reasons for your viewpoint.
- **Show you care.** Adults sometimes think teens only care about themselves. Let your parents know you care about them, as well as others.
- **Show you are responsible.** You have read in this book how you can show that you are responsible at home and at school. Put some of these ideas into practice. Respect your parents' privacy. Remember to do assigned tasks without them needing to ask you. Carry out all your responsibilities. Prove that you are ready for more.
- **Show you can be trusted.** In order to receive more freedom, you must prove that you can handle it. If you say you will be home at a certain time, be home at that time. If you cannot, call and explain your delay. When your parents know they can trust you, they will be more likely to give you greater freedom.

Writing Activity

Think about your relationship with your parents. Are there times you have trouble getting along? What can you do to help relieve the strain? Write a journal entry describing ways you can help improve your relationship with your parents.

Sibling Relationships

Sibling relationships can create either harmony or discord within a family. Special bonds exist among many brothers and sisters. There can be a closeness not found in any other relationship. Brothers and sisters can be best friends. They can enjoy being with one another, **2-5**. They can share thoughts, feelings, and belongings.

On the other hand, sibling relationships can sometimes involve bitterness, jealousy, and fighting. **Sibling rivalry** is competition between brothers and sisters. Siblings try to compete with each other in some ways. When very young, they may compete for their parents' attention. As they get older, they may compete for special privileges. They might try to outperform one another in school or sports, too.

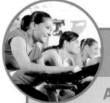

Health Connections

Achieving Healthy Sibling Relations

Siblings often share problems and worries. In order to help siblings with their problems, try to tune into how they are feeling. Hear exactly what they are saying. Try to understand why they are worried. Imagine how you would feel in the same situations. Avoid making judgments by saying "You should have…." Listen instead. Then ask how you can help. Do not give advice to a sibling unless he or she asks for it. When you do give advice, give it in a way that shows you care.

You can achieve good sibling relations by several means. First, listen to what your brothers and sisters are saying. Try to understand their moods and feelings. Also, share your thoughts and concerns with them. Keeping communication lines open is as important in sibling relationships as in others.

Respect the property and possessions of your siblings. Ask before borrowing their belongings. Knock before entering their rooms. If you share a room, show respect by keeping your clothes, books, and other items picked up. Be sure to do your share of the cleaning chores, too.

Cooperation among family members to achieve family goals can help sibling relationships. **Cooperation** means everyone works together and does their share. For instance, your sister may be performing in the school play. The play is going to run three nights. You volunteer to do her chores at home those three nights so she can be in the play. She will return the favor when you have some evening events to attend. Cooperation makes life easier and more enjoyable for all family members. When you cooperate, you are letting others know you care about them.

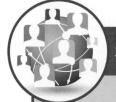

© Galina Barskaya/Shutterstock

2-5 These sisters are very close and enjoy spending time together.

Relationships with Grandparents

Grandparents are special people. They may live far away from you, or they may live in your own home. You may see them a few times a year or every day. Some grandparents work full-time, others are retired. Some may be healthy and others may be very frail. Some play tennis, ski, or swim. Others have hobbies such as woodworking and gardening.

Many teens have very special relationships with their grandparents. Time spent with your grandparents can be very enjoyable. Getting to know your grandparents may give you a better understanding of your parents. You may find it easier to talk about your feelings or problems with your grandparents.

Social Studies Connections

Learn About the Past

Grandparents can entertain you and enrich your life with stories of their childhoods. They can tell you many stories about your parents when they were younger. Stories about historical events they may have witnessed can also be interesting. They may have visited or lived in places you have never seen. Ask one of your grandparents or another older adult to name a major historical figure that had an impact on his or her life. Read a book about that person and then have a discussion with your grandparent about the person and events that took place at that time.

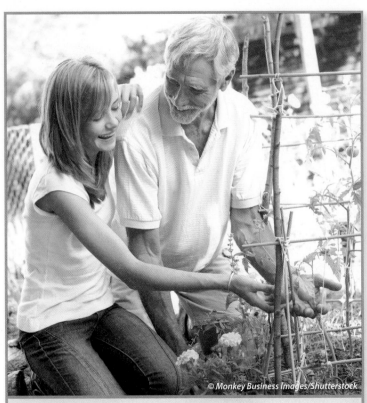

2-6 Grandparents may offer advice based on their many life experiences.

Grandparents are sometimes not as busy as your parents. If they have more time on their hands, they may be able to help you with your activities. They may enjoy taking you shopping or attending a special event with you. They may enjoy hearing about your opinions, interests, and hobbies. A sympathetic grandparent may be able to offer advice or help you solve your problems, **2-6**.

Sometimes, as grandparents get very old, they may not be able to continue their usual activities. You and your family may need to care for them. They may need your help in getting around. You could help them with their shopping or e-mails.

Grandparents who are unable to live alone may move into your home. This situation will require all family members to make adjustments. You will need to help your grandparents feel welcome. You can respect your grandparents' privacy and give them a place for their belongings. Grandparents will need to feel they are not a burden. They need to be as independent as possible.

Grandparents may suffer from poor health. Some grandparents have trouble remembering things. Others may stay mentally alert, but have physical disabilities. Their disabilities may be mild, moderate, or severe. These may cause a grandparent to walk with difficulty or need to use a wheelchair. Your grandparent may need to have special services by trained people. Your visits and attention will be very important at this time.

Your relationship with your grandparents will remain strong as you share your time with them. Your caring concern will help keep them alert and happy for many years.

Reading Review

1. What is a relationship?
2. List four ways that might help you improve your relationship with your parents.
3. Competition between brothers and sisters is called _____. *(2 words)*
4. How can you achieve good sibling relations?
5. Describe how you can have a positive relationship with your grandparents.

Families Face Change

Objectives

After studying this section, you will be able to
- **identify** the stages of the family life cycle.
- **give examples** of changes that may occur within each stage of the family life cycle.
- **describe** crises that can cause families to change.
- **assess** techniques that family members can use to help them cope with or adjust to change.

Key Terms

family life cycle	grief	telephone hotlines
empty nest	substance abuse	support groups
crisis	domestic violence	
chronic	shelters	

Families change through the years. They very seldom stay the same, especially if a couple has children. There are other changes, however, that not all families will face. A *life change* is any event that causes significant change in the way you manage your life. Many factors have an impact on life changes. Situations such as birth, death, accidents, divorce, or job loss can significantly change your life. Because the choices you make have consequences, they also have the potential to change your life. These changes may require special coping skills.

The Family Life Cycle

Many families go through similar changes that are a normal part of life. These changes occur in six basic stages that make up the **family life cycle**.

The first stage in the family life cycle is the *beginning stage*. It generally begins when a couple decides to marry. They establish a home and learn to get along with each other. They have time to pursue interests. Both husband and wife may have jobs outside the home.

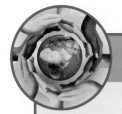

Global Connections

A Ceremony in India

As part of the wedding ceremony in India, the bride's mother and father wash the couple's feet with water and milk in order to purify them for the journey of their new life together. During the ceremony, the couple holds grains of rice and oats and green leaves in their hands to signify good health, wealth, and happiness.

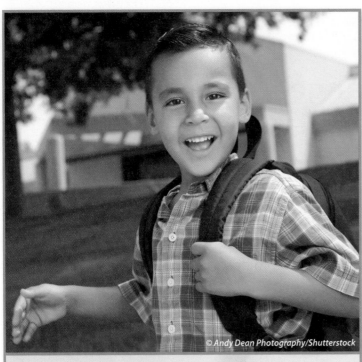

© Andy Dean Photography/Shutterstock

2-7 During the parenting stage, clothing, school events, and new social activities take more of the family's time and money.

A major change in the family occurs when a couple decides to have a child. This is the beginning of the *childbearing stage*. This stage will involve many adjustments as the couple assumes their new roles as parents. There will be increased demands on time, energy, finances, and freedom. These demands will affect the couple's home, work, and social life. This stage continues until all children are born or adopted.

When the first child begins school, the family enters the *parenting stage*. This stage brings new changes for the family, **2-7**. The child's school activities and sports events may alter the family's schedule. As this stage continues, children enter the teen years. Other changes occur during this stage because of teens' social activities. Teens begin to spend more time away from home. They become more involved with their friends. As teens seek more independence, they and their families are affected.

During the *launching stage*, the first child leaves home. Children may leave for college or join the military. They may work full time and want to find their own place to live or move in with friends. They may get married and start families of their own. As children leave, parents will have more space at home. They will have the time and freedom they enjoyed during the first years of marriage. Today, however, it is not uncommon for adult children to return home and live with their parents longer.

During the *mid-years stage*, the couple is faced with an **empty nest** when the last child leaves home. They may feel a void in their lives. The active parenting role is behind them. They may have more time to explore some of their personal interests. Both husband and wife may continue their careers until they retire. Their income may be the highest during this stage. They may travel and become involved in other activities.

After retirement, a couple enters the *aging stage*. This stage lasts until both spouses die. If the couple is financially secure and in good health, they may have many happy years together. They can enjoy pursuing lifelong interests. This can be a very satisfying and rewarding time of life.

As health begins to fail, however, more help from family members and friends may be necessary. Older people may need special services such as transportation, meals, and recreational services provided for them. When one spouse dies, the other may need help adjusting to the loss.

Throughout the family life cycle, stages may overlap. For instance, after the oldest child has started school, the mother may have another baby, adopt, or raise foster children. Thus, the family would be in both the childbearing stage and the parenting stage at the same time.

Family Challenges

All families must face challenges, **2-8**. Some challenges may be small, such as arguing with your parents about what time you should come home from a friend's house. Other challenges are much bigger. A **crisis** is a difficult situation that becomes very serious. Unemployment, relocation, financial setbacks, divorce, and the loss of a family member or friend are just several examples of crises families may face.

Families handle crises in different ways. Some families have a difficult time learning how to adjust and cope to changes that may occur as a result of a crisis. Other families, however, are more prepared to handle the challenges that come their way. They can adapt to change much more easily.

A crisis can occur in your life at any time. Knowing the kinds of crises that might occur and the changes that can result may help you prepare for such events. Knowing what resources you can call on to help you deal with crises will also be helpful.

Unemployment

When a person becomes unemployed, he or she no longer receives an income, which affects the family's finances, **2-9**. If the person has difficulty

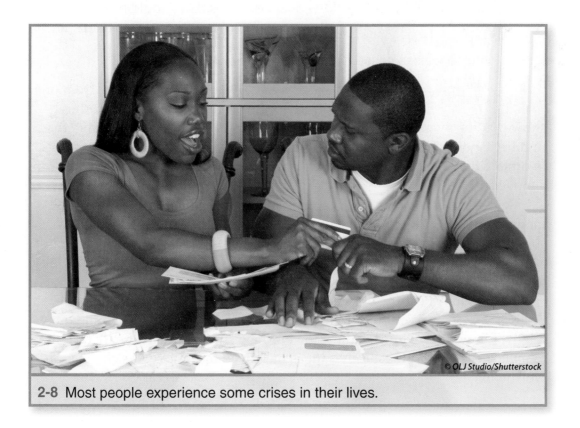

© OLJ Studio/Shutterstock

2-8 Most people experience some crises in their lives.

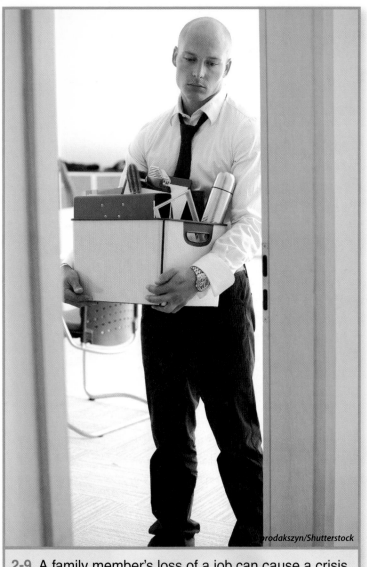

prodakszyn/Shutterstock

2-9 A family member's loss of a job can cause a crisis for many families.

finding another job, any money the family has saved will probably go toward paying bills.

In addition to financial concerns, attitudes of family members may also be affected. When a person loses a job, feelings of low self-esteem may develop. The person may be discouraged and become depressed. Some unemployed people may then turn to alcohol or other drugs. Some might even consider suicide.

When a family faces an unemployment crisis, they should talk with one another about changes they will need to make. The family can make a budget together. Teens or other family members might be able to help by getting part-time jobs. Younger children might be able to help more with chores around the house. All family members should encourage each other and be supportive. Teens might be able to add to the family income by doing odd jobs. They could babysit, shovel snow, or mow lawns to help.

Relocation

Many families move from one home to another, **2-10**. Studies show that the average family moves several times. Some families move to find better jobs. Sometimes employees are transferred to company locations in other cities. Death, divorce, or separation within a family can also result in a move.

Regardless of the reason for moving, it causes changes in the family. A move to another city or state means the family will have to get used to new surroundings. They will have to shop in new stores and make new friends. The children will have to attend new schools. Wage earners will have to adjust to new jobs.

A move may be difficult at first because so many adjustments are necessary. You miss your old friends. You may have moved away from your relatives. It will take time to adjust to your new surroundings. It may take time to make new friends. If a family's life is improved by a move, the changes are worthwhile.

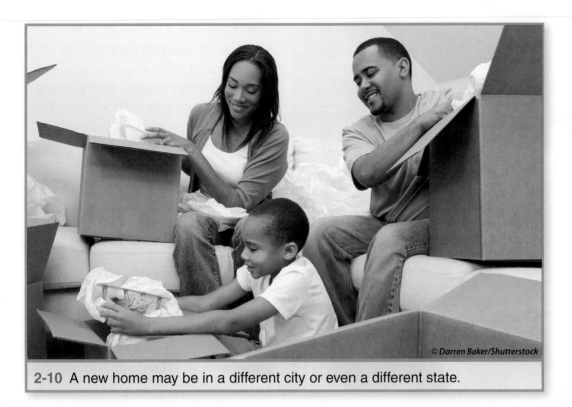

© Darren Baker/Shutterstock

2-10 A new home may be in a different city or even a different state.

Financial Crises

Many families face financial difficulties from time to time. The loss of a job can create money challenges. Sometimes bills begin to pile up and there is not enough money to pay them. A serious illness or death can lead to a financial crisis. Sometimes a job change requires the family to move to a new place. Some financial situations are more widespread than others. Economic crises have always plagued society.

When a family faces a financial crisis, all members should be informed. Everyone in the family can find ways to help deal with the situation. If the family will not have as much income, they can discuss ways to make the money go farther. A family may have to postpone a vacation. Plans for music lessons or new clothes may have to be changed. Sometimes future goals, such as college or a new car, have

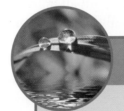

Go Green

Saving Money

Family members need to keep a positive attitude during a financial crisis. Each person can do his or her part to help cut expenses. This may be a good time to institute money-saving practices that are also environmentally friendly or *green*. Instead of buying new clothes, repair or alter items. Adjust thermostats to reduce utility bills. Turn off computers and lights when not in use to lower electric bills. Reduce the use of electrical appliances. Carpooling can help with auto expenses.

Teens could walk or ride their bikes whenever possible so their parents do not have to use the car. They could use their cooking skills instead of buying prepared foods. A financial crisis may bring families closer together. By solving a problem together, the family may develop a new closeness and even help the environment.

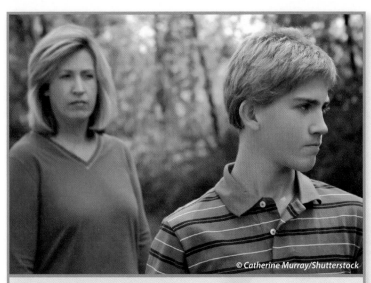

© Catherine Murray/Shutterstock

2-11 Changes in the family structure require family members to make many adjustments.

to be altered. There will be less fear and tension if everyone works together to solve the crisis.

A budget or spending plan can help. If income is limited, a plan can indicate which expenses are most critical. Food and shelter are necessities. Families can reduce recreation expenses, however, until the crisis is over.

Family Structures Change

Several events can occur to cause a family structure to change, 2-11. A nuclear family could become an extended family if a grandparent moves in with them. The couple in a nuclear family could get a divorce, causing a single-parent family to form. A single parent could remarry, forming a stepfamily or blended family.

Family members need to stick together during this time of change. They need to show love, concern, respect, and consideration for one another. With time and patience, everyone can begin to feel comfortable with the new structure.

Divorce

Unlike many fairy tales, not all married couples live happily ever after. When a couple decides to divorce, all family members are affected. This crisis can last for months or even years. It can be a very difficult time for everyone.

A divorce does not usually occur suddenly. Children are often aware of tension building between their parents. Sometimes children feel they are the cause of their parent's divorce. This is seldom the case. Changing interests, values, goals, or financial challenges may cause a couple to grow apart. Sometimes domestic violence may be the cause. Alcohol or drug abuse can also lead to a divorce.

When a couple decides to end their marriage, it can be hard on everyone. Children may feel a mixture of fear, anger, depression, and guilt. Small children may wonder what will happen to them. Older children may become angry with their parents. Teens may feel pulled between the two adults.

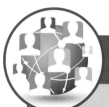

Social Studies Connections

Child Custody

Decisions concerning child custody and support are made during the divorce process. The courts decide who gains custody of the children. The parent who does not have custody of the children may be required to pay child support. In some cases, the mother retains custody. The children would live with her and she would provide for their care. In other cases, the father gets custody. Another arrangement is joint custody.

They may feel pressure to fill the role of the absent parent. Sometimes children try to reunite their parents.

Many changes occur during a divorce. One or both parents may decide to move out of the family home. Possessions and property are usually divided. A move may mean making new friends. Children may have to attend different schools. The mother may become a full-time wage earner for the first time. Child care services may be needed for preschoolers. Older children may have to accept more responsibilities in caring for the home and siblings. There may be less allowance to spend and fewer comforts to enjoy. An older teen may decide to find a part-time job to help ease the strain on the family budget.

For some couples, divorce may seem to be the only way to end tension and arguments. In this sense, the changes caused by a divorce can help a family. Family members can work together to adjust to the new situation. They can use this as an opportunity to become closer. Getting professional advice and help is another healthy way to handle the stress of divorce. Do not be afraid to ask for, or seek, help.

Remarriage

If the single parent remarries, the family unit changes again, **2-12**. Stepfamilies result in new forms of family life for everyone. Often, both

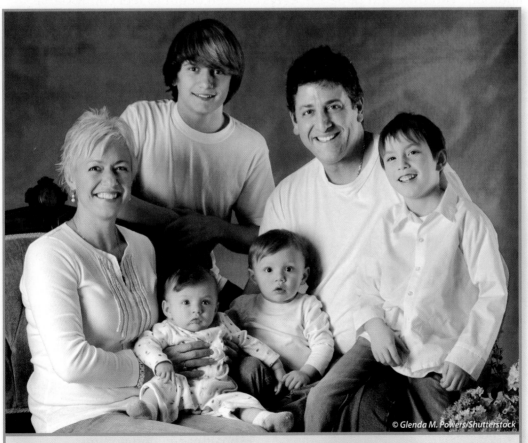

© Glenda M. Powers/Shutterstock

2-12 The addition of a stepparent and stepchildren may require the family to readjust.

families have children. Stepparents and stepchildren begin a new relationship. Children also continue to spend time with their other parent.

If both divorced parents remarry, children may have four parents. This will be in addition to siblings, stepsisters, stepbrothers, and eight grandparents. Adjusting to all these new people can be challenging. The children may also have to accept more responsibilities at home. The amount of income the family has may change.

Guidelines for behavior may be different in each family. Stepparents may find it difficult to discipline stepchildren. The stepchildren may feel they do not have to listen to their stepparents. Stepchildren may feel they are being treated differently from children, whether they are or not.

When families are combined, financial demands may increase. The additional money needed for the new family may cause cutbacks to occur. There may be less money available for items you want, such as new clothes. This will be an adjustment for all members of the family. Families who work together with respect and love for one another can adjust to these many changes. Having a positive attitude can make the adjustments easier.

Family Members Change

Many of the changes families face occur because people change. No one stays the same forever. Some changes cannot be avoided. Serious illnesses and accidents sometimes occur. The death of a family member is also an unexpected change.

These crises mean adjustments for family members. Other family members may need to assume the roles and responsibilities of a family member who is sick, has special needs, or is deceased. A sickness may mean a temporary change. A life altering sickness, disability, or death may cause a permanent change.

Families must work together to cope with these difficult changes. Family members may have to take turns caring for the ill, **2-13**. They will need to comfort one another when there is a life altering sickness or death.

© ampyang/Shutterstock

2-13 When a grandparent is hospitalized, all family members may need to make adjustments.

Health Crises

Family members must deal with illnesses and accidents at times. You may get a cold, the flu, or have an upset stomach. You might break your arm falling off your bike. These challenges are temporary. You are often feeling healthy again in no time.

Some sicknesses, however, can become **chronic**, which means they continue for a long time. They can also be life threatening. Disabilities caused by accidents or illnesses may become permanent.

Family members will need to make adjustments to cope with the health crisis. Parents may have to change their work schedules so they can be home to provide care. Children may need to do more chores or spend more time watching younger siblings. Financial difficulties may arise due to high costs of medical bills. Family members may need to cut expenses.

A life-threatening illness or permanent disability may cause family members to feel worried, helpless, sad, frustrated, or depressed. It is important for family members to offer love and comfort to one another during this difficult time.

Family members may also receive support outside the family. Relatives, friends, or neighbors may provide meals or run errands. People who are going through similar experiences can offer advice and encouragement. Doctors or other organizations can provide information that might help the family to better understand the illness or disability. Families can then work together to provide the type of care needed.

Death

Very few people of any age are comfortable talking about death. Just like birth, death is a part of the life cycle. Death can happen to anyone at any time or any age.

It is natural to feel **grief**, or emotions such as sadness, loss, anger, and guilt, when someone you know or love dies, **2-14**. These feelings are hard to overcome.

There are ways you can help ease the pain you feel about someone's death. You can accept the comfort of friends and the sympathy of the people around you. Special support services available through schools, religious organizations, or counseling services may be a source of comfort. Everyone deals with death differently. Your friends and family may want to comfort you in times like these. Others will not know what to do or say. Either way, it is okay to express your feelings when someone you know or love dies, **2-15**. Talking about the deceased loved one will help you deal with the loss. Talk about the sadness you feel. Cry if you feel like it. This is a normal reaction. Discuss the positive traits of the person. Recall happy times and events you shared together. Soon you will begin to accept that the person has passed. Then the healing process can begin.

Stages of Grief

- **Denial**—refusing to believe the person is leaving you
- **Anger**—directed at the person for leaving you or at others for not understanding your feelings of loss
- **Bargaining**—trying to negotiate with the person who is leaving; for instance, promising to do whatever the other person wants to save the relationship
- **Depression**—feeling sad and lonely and not wanting to be around others
- **Acceptance**—understanding that relationships change and that change is part of the life cycle

2-14 Most people go through a pattern of the stages of grief when a death or other loss occurs.

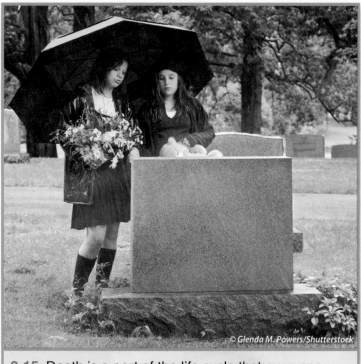

2-15 Death is a part of the life cycle that everyone must face sometime.

Suicide

Losing someone you love is very painful. When that person takes his or her own life, it is even more tragic. People who knew the victim wonder if they might have been able to prevent the suicide. Some even worry they might have caused the tragedy.

Among young people, suicide is a leading cause of death. Experts give a number of reasons for teen suicide. Some young people feel they cannot cope with the pressures to succeed. Some become very depressed when a close relationship ends. Sometimes it is due to problems at home, school, or with peers. The young person feels a great deal of uncontrolled stress and is looking for a way out.

A suicide attempt is usually a cry for help. Most teens do not want to die. They want help. They need someone to listen to them. If young people you know talk of suicide, do not ignore their remarks. Let them know you care. Encourage the person to seek help from a trusted adult. Do not keep the remarks a secret even if the person wants you to. Instead, share your concerns with the parents or another adult who is close to the person. Sometimes the family may not be aware of a problem or the person may be afraid to ask for help. Many communities have suicide hotline numbers people can call for confidential counseling.

Substance Abuse

Substance abuse involves misusing drugs, alcohol, or some other chemical to a potentially harmful level. Like other changes to family members, a drug or drinking problem of one member affects all family members. Extra time and patience will be needed from each family member to help the person overcome his or her problem. Money may be needed for professional treatment and special care.

When a family member develops a drug or drinking problem, help is needed. Family members should not ignore a serious problem or try to cover it up. These behavior patterns are hard to change. It is very difficult for the person to change without help.

Family Violence

As families change, and pressures and demands increase, a family member could sometimes become violent. Domestic violence is physical or emotional abuse of a family member. The victim may be a child, a sibling, or a parent. The violent outburst may involve hitting, kicking, biting, or threatening or causing bodily harm in another way. Because the family is usually a source of love and comfort, violence in the home is damaging to all family members.

People who abuse others are usually angry, frustrated, unhappy, and insecure. They are often afraid and confused. They feel they have lost control of their lives so they strike out at others. Children who have suffered family abuse have the potential to become abusive as adults. They learned a pattern of behavior that involved physical or verbal abuse. Children in abusive situations, however, can also become stronger and find ways to get the help they need.

Coping with Change

Not all changes in a family are sad, confusing, or stressful. Many can be happy and challenging. Some cause minor changes and others major changes. The following techniques can help family members cope with or adjust to change.

- **Accept the change.** Ignoring it will not make it go away. To accept it will be less stressful than if you try to pretend it is not happening. Talk over adjustments you will need to make with your family. Share ideas that will make the change as smooth as possible.

- **Prepare for the change.** Perhaps there is something you can do to get ready. This will make the actual change easier. Suppose you are moving to a new city or state. Find out as much as you can about the new location. Search for someone who once

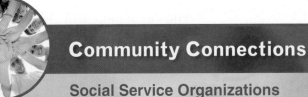

Community Connections

Social Service Organizations

Many local organizations can provide help in cases of family violence. You can find numbers for help organizations online or in the telephone book under "Social Service Organizations" or "Crisis Intervention." Also, look under the county name and the Department of Human Services, Social Services, or Public Welfare. The local police department may have a juvenile officer trained to assist families. Many religious organizations can provide counseling. Do not be afraid to ask for help, support, or guidance for you or your family. People should not have to live in fear.

Life Connections

Coping with Crises

Teens react to family crises events in different ways. Some run away from their problems—they leave home. They believe they can leave their problems behind. These teens soon find a new set of problems on the street. They often become victims of crime. Their money is soon gone or stolen. They cannot afford food and safe shelter. With little education, they cannot get good jobs. By trying to leave their problems behind, personal crises occur from the stress of trying to survive.

Another less-stressful option for dealing with crises is to seek help and support from relatives, friends, or neighbors. A school guidance counselor or another trusted adult might be able to help, as well. People who care about you may be able to provide emotional support during a challenging time.

Writing Activity

Sometimes writing about your feelings helps to ease the stress involved with trying to solve difficulties. Spend some time writing in your journal about any challenges you or your friends face today. Brainstorm all possible solutions, whether or not you think them feasible. New ideas may come out of this exercise that could help everyone dealing with crises.

lived there. Ask about schools, shopping, and recreational facilities. Use the Internet to read about the new area. Be enthusiastic about meeting new friends and having new experiences.

- **Support the change.** Keep a positive attitude about the changes your family will face. Many changes are not by choice. They just happen. A car accident or a job loss may have been unavoidable. Pitch in and help as best you can. Be supportive. Try not to criticize, condemn, or complain. Remember that change is constant. How you handle the change is what is important.

Sources of Help

Sometimes families need help from other sources to cope with a crisis, **2-16**. Shelters provide food, clothing, and housing to families who do not have anywhere else to go. Some shelters offer protection for people who are victims of domestic violence or abuse.

Community Resources	
Resource	**Services**
Al-Anon	A support group for the family and friends of people who abuse alcohol.
Alateen	This support group is specifically for teens who are trying to cope with another person's alcohol abuse.
Alcoholics Anonymous	A support group for people who are trying to quit drinking.
American Red Cross	This organization provides food, shelter, and other necessary items to victims of natural disasters. Also provides community services that help families in need.
Big Brothers Big Sisters	An organization that partners adult volunteers with children from single-parent families. The adult meets weekly with the child to serve as a mentor and offer emotional support and guidance.
Family Counseling Center	This agency provides individual and family counseling services to help with grief recovery, marital and parenting issues, depression, or career counseling.
The National Domestic Violence Hotline	A hotline that offers crisis intervention and referrals for local services to victims of domestic violence. It operates at all times every day of the year with interpreter services for many languages.
Temporary Assistance for Needy Families (TANF)	A government agency that provides assistance and work opportunities to needy families. People must apply for government-sponsored TANF programs at designated agencies within their communities.

2-16 There are many community resources available to help families in times of crisis.

Telephone hotlines are an immediate source of support for people coping with a crisis. Most hotlines are toll-free numbers a person can call at any time of the day or night. Telephone hotline operators are often trained to deal with a specific crisis such as drug and alcohol abuse or domestic violence. They can also refer people to local community resources that might be available.

Support groups consist of a group of people who meet regularly to discuss common challenges and to help one another cope. Support groups are often available for people who abuse drugs and alcohol. Some groups are specifically for the family members of these people. Support groups may also offer help for families coping with life-threatening illnesses, disabilities, or grief over the loss of a loved one.

Reading Review

1. What is a life change?
2. Name the stages of the family life cycle.
3. List the five stages of grief.
4. List five examples of crises families may face.
5. List three techniques that can be used to help family members cope with change.

Chapter Summary

Section 2-1. Families provide for physical needs. They also meet the emotional needs of family members. They provide for the socialization of children. The members who form a family determine the family type—nuclear, single parent, stepfamily, extended, adoptive, foster, and childless. Family members each have certain roles and responsibilities. These roles and responsibilities may change as families and family members change. When family members fulfill their roles and responsibilities, they are a functional family. The family becomes dysfunctional when a member does not do his or her share.

Section 2-2. A relationship is a special bond or link between people. The first relationships most people have are with family members. Relationships with parents, siblings, and grandparents can teach people how to get along with others. Family relationships can also teach people about themselves.

Section 2-3. Many families begin when a couple marries. Couples may have children. The children grow, enter school, and eventually leave home. This natural chain of events is part of the family life cycle. A number of challenges can occur at any stage in the family life cycle. Families can move. A family member can die. Parents can divorce and remarry. Family members can have problems that lead to substance abuse or domestic violence. Family members must work together to face these changes and manage the stress created by the changes.

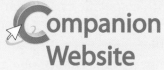

Companion Website
www.g-wlearning.com

Check your understanding of the main concepts for Chapter 2 at the website.

Critical Thinking

1. **Draw conclusions.** Do you think a single person should be allowed to adopt a child?
2. **Evaluate.** Think about the relationships you have between you and members of your family. Evaluate these relationships and describe how you could improve them.
3. **Determine.** If you could be one other person in your family for a day, who would you choose to be and why?

Common Core

College and Career Readiness

4. **Reading.** Read a book about a family. Describe the family. Analyze in what ways the family in the story is like your family and in what ways it is different from your family.
5. **Listening.** Watch three television programs about families. Identify the types of families shown in each show. Compare your findings with those of your classmates.

6. **Speaking.** Role-play various family crises. After acting out each family crisis, discuss how the situations were handled.

7. **Writing.** Write a story about a family that is facing one of the challenges discussed in this chapter. Include how each family member might react to the challenge. How well did the family cope with the crisis?

Technology

8. *Video history.* Interview your grandparents on video about their parents and family members. Discuss how they feel the family has changed over the years. If possible, share the video at a special time such as an anniversary, holiday, or birthday.

Journal Writing

9. Create a calendar with photographs and dates of important events in your family's life history. Write your impressions about the significance of the photographs to your family history.

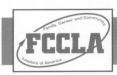

FCCLA

10. Work with your peers to create a *Families First* project—a national peer education program to help you gain a better understanding of how family members can work together to strengthen the family bond. Project topics may include understanding and celebrating diverse families, strengthening family relationships, overcoming obstacles, managing multiple responsibilities, or learning to nurture children. Use the *FCCLA Planning Process* as your guide in planning your project. See your adviser for information as needed.

11. Investigate the relationship between stress and violent behaviors. Create a *STOP the Violence* (Students Taking On Prevention) project that teaches your peers how to appropriately manage the stresses in everyday life. See your adviser for information as needed.

Chapter 3
Your Friends

Sections

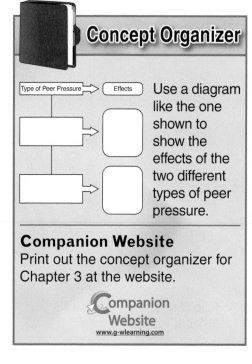

Reading Prep

College and Career Readiness

Before you read the chapter, write all the main headings within each section, leaving space under each heading. As you read the chapter, write three main points that you learned from reading each section.

Concept Organizer

Type of Peer Pressure → Effects

Use a diagram like the one shown to show the effects of the two different types of peer pressure.

Companion Website

Print out the concept organizer for Chapter 3 at the website.

Companion Website
www.g-wlearning.com

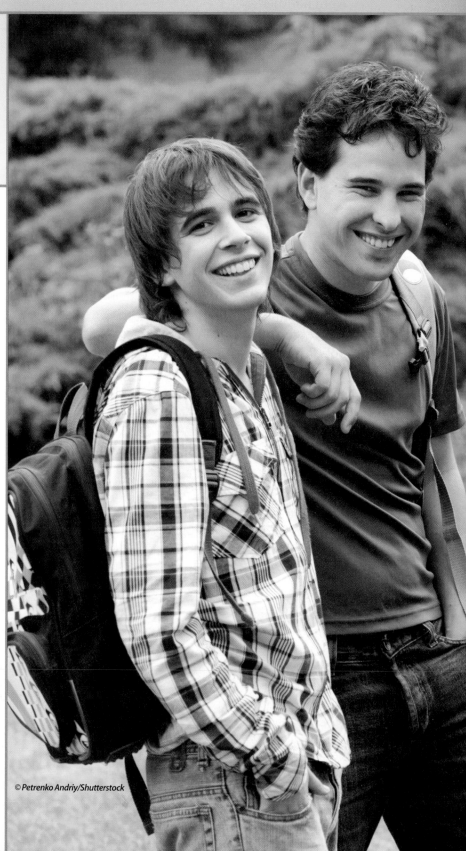

© Petrenko Andriy/Shutterstock

Developing Friendships

Objectives

After studying this section, you will be able to
- **compare and contrast** acquaintances and best friends.
- **give examples** of common qualities of friendship.
- **demonstrate** various ways to make new friends.
- **describe** how to strengthen friendships.
- **identify** reasons friendships may end.

Key Terms	
acquaintances	loyalty

You just found out you made the team. Your sister told you she and her boyfriend became engaged last night. There was a cute new student in your science class today. What is the first thing you do when you have exciting news? You tell your best friend, of course!

When something special happens to you, or you have some important news, it is hard to keep it to yourself. You may tell your parents, but sometimes they are not nearly as excited as you. A friend may be more enthusiastic. He or she can often relate to your news the same way you do.

What Is a Friend?

You have different kinds of friends. Each friend has different qualities that are special to you. You share certain traits with your friends that allow you to enjoy each other's friendships.

Types of Friends

Everyone has friends. Some friends are **acquaintances**, or people you have met, but do not know well. With time, acquaintances may become friends.

A number of your friends may be casual friends. These friends may be of either sex. Most of your

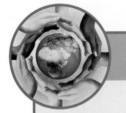

Global Connections

Diversity in Friendships

The United States is a worldwide destination for many people. Most communities have many residents with diverse backgrounds who bring their ethnic cultures and practices with them. Take advantage of opportunities to have diverse friendships inside and outside your school. Make friends with both older and younger people in your community. After all, every person has the same need for good friends. Your friends with different backgrounds from your own give you the gifts of unique experiences, expanded worldviews, and even new foods.

casual friends may be your age, but some may be younger or older. Casual friends share similar interests and enjoy many of the same activities. You may have a group of casual friends with whom you spend a lot of time.

You are likely to have a number of acquaintances and casual friends. You probably have only a few very close friends, however. Best friends develop the closest friendships. You share your deepest thoughts and secrets with these friends.

Qualities of Friendship

All your friends are likely to have certain qualities in common. One such quality is loyalty, which means you show strong support for your friend. Loyal friends stick with each other during good times and bad times.

Friends often show loyalty even though they make mistakes. Maybe one of your friends shared personal information about another one of your friends. You may not approve of the action, but you can still remain loyal. You may try to help your friend see that what he or she did was hurtful, even though it is not your responsibility. If you help your friend understand the consequences of his or her behavior, maybe it will not happen again.

Friends care about each other. They share a special feeling. You feel comfortable being around your friends. You can relax knowing they accept you as you are. You do not have to worry about how you look or act. Friends like you for who you are, not what you can do for them. If you do act crazy sometimes, friends can tell you to straighten up without hurting your feelings. You know they make these remarks because they care about you.

Friends are reliable. Being reliable means doing what you say you will do. If you tell your friends you will meet them after school, you will not forget or change your mind at the last minute. You realize that your friends count on you to do what you promise to do.

Friends can be trusted. If you confide in a friend, you know you can trust your friend to keep your secret. Maybe you need someone to talk with and share your innermost thoughts, **3-1**. You know your friend will not tell anyone else what you say. Your friend will not laugh at your ideas or make fun of you.

Making Friends

Being friendly can help you get to know new students at school. You might feel at home more quickly after a move if you make new friends. Making friends may also help you feel comfortable at social events.

Knowing how to make friends is a skill you can use throughout your life.

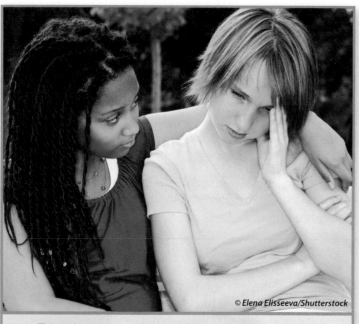
© Elena Elisseeva/Shutterstock

3-1 Friends are people who are there for you when you need them.

There will always be situations where you will be meeting people for the first time. No matter how many friends you have, you can always have more. The following suggestions may help you take advantage of opportunities to make new friends.

Finding Friends

You can find friends wherever you go. People are all around you every day. Think about the people you are with most often. Any of these acquaintances might become close friends. Perhaps you have a classmate that you have not shared a class with before. Maybe a coworker seems to be much like yourself. Perhaps you would like to get to know someone better from your neighborhood.

It may take some work on your part to form a closer friendship with these acquaintances. Good friendships do not form quickly. They take time to develop. You must take the time to learn about the people you meet. Find out if they have interests and ideas in common with you. Getting to know your acquaintances better may seem like a lot of trouble. Forming a close friendship that could last a lifetime, however, is worth the effort.

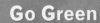

Go Green

Environmentally Friendly Friends

If one of your values is to protect the environment, you may find like-minded friends through volunteering. For instance, your community or school might sponsor recycling projects, food and clothing donation drives, community gardens, or habitat protection projects. Volunteer with the organization or project that appeals to you most. If you cannot find one, start one of your own and advertise for volunteers at your school and through free local media.

The Nature Conservancy coordinates many volunteer projects around the country to protect and preserve nature and extend conservation efforts. Find your state on their website at www.nature.org/volunteer to locate group opportunities near you.

Becoming Involved

Becoming involved is one of the easiest ways to make new friends. You might join a new club or volunteer in your community. You might also get involved in an activity that interests you. Other people in the group are likely to have similar interests, **3-2**.

When you share a common interest, becoming friends is easier. You have something to talk about that will strengthen the friendship. If you enjoy writing, you might want to join the school newspaper staff. You can meet other students who share your interest in writing. You may find you have other interests in common with them as well. They may like the same music you do or share your interest in hiking.

Introduce Yourself

When you were a baby and learned to walk, taking the first step was the hardest. The rest was easy. The same is true about meeting people. For many people, especially those who are shy, meeting new people can be difficult. Such people may have to push themselves a little. With practice, meeting new people will become easier.

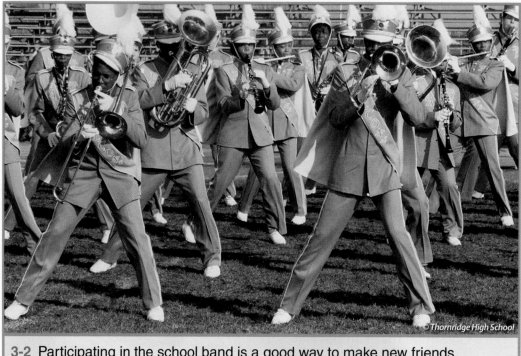

3-2 Participating in the school band is a good way to make new friends.

You can begin by just being friendly to people you meet. Maybe there is a new student in school, or maybe you are the new student. Start with a smile. A sincere smile shows you are friendly and interested in meeting people. It can also show a willingness to start a conversation.

Introduce yourself. Let people know you are interested in them. Ask questions that require more than a yes or no answer. You might ask about their interests or hobbies. You could ask what activities they enjoy or where they live.

You might try inviting a new acquaintance to work with you on a homework assignment. Attending a school function together would be another way to get to know each other. This could be the beginning of a new friendship.

Be Positive

When you are positive, you see the best side of people and situations. You are happy, enthusiastic, and friendly to everyone, **3-3**. A positive person is fun to be around and knows how to make others happy, too.

Having a positive attitude goes hand in hand with having healthy self-esteem. Healthy self-esteem means you feel good about yourself. You feel you have something to offer other people. If you feel good about yourself, your friends will feel the same way about you. They will like you and be glad you are their friend. They will even feel better about themselves when they are with you.

Building Strong Friendships

To be a friend to others, you must offer them the same loyalty, caring, and trust they offer you. After you form friendships, you need to nurture them in order for them to grow and remain strong.

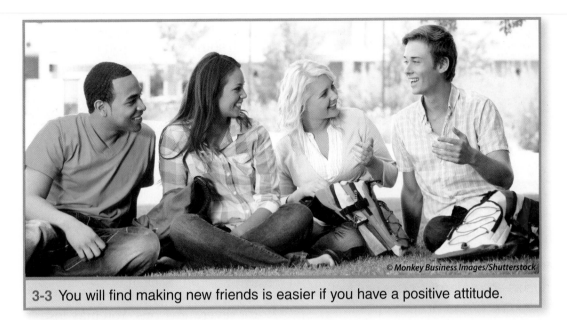

© Monkey Business Images/Shutterstock

3-3 You will find making new friends is easier if you have a positive attitude.

Having someone to talk with is an important part of being a friend. If personal challenges arise, friends help each other solve those challenges. You should be able to share your thoughts and feelings with your friends. You must also be willing to listen when they share their thoughts and feelings with you.

Communication will help you get along with your friends. If you have a temper, you should learn to control it. You must be careful not to make hurtful comments. When a disagreement occurs, communication can help you handle the situation more effectively.

Being a friend means that you must be willing to accept your friends regardless of their opinions. You may not always agree with them. For instance, you may feel a teacher's rules are fair. Your friend may feel the rules are terribly unfair. You and your friend both have reasons for your point of view, yet you respect each other's opinions. You do not allow this difference to change your friendship.

You must allow your friends to have other friends without being possessive or jealous, **3-4**. *Jealousy* is a fear that someone will take your place as a friend. If you let this fear overwhelm you, it could end up hurting your friendship.

You must give your friends freedom to do other activities. Your best friend may not always want to do what you want to do. Sometimes he

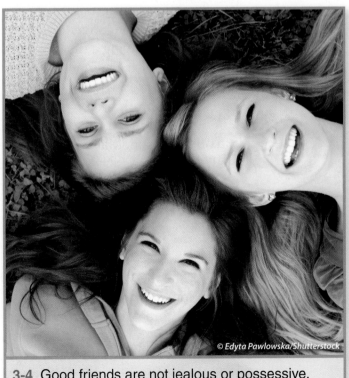

© Edyta Pawlowska/Shutterstock

3-4 Good friends are not jealous or possessive.

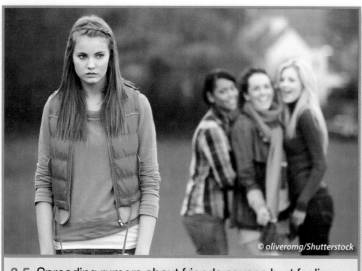

© oliveromg/Shutterstock

3-5 Spreading rumors about friends causes hurt feelings.

or she may want to do something with someone else. You must be willing to accept this without getting upset.

Ending a Friendship

Friendships do not often last forever. Many adults have a few friends they have known since childhood. Most adult friendships, however, form during adulthood.

Some of your friendships may last a long time, but many will eventually end. This can happen for several reasons. You may lose a friend because he or she moves away. When this happens, you need to remember the good things about that friendship. Build new friendships on those same qualities.

Sometimes, as friends grow and change, they find they have less in common with one another. Their interests change. They become involved in different activities and find they have less time to spend together. As they see less and less of each other, their friendship gradually ends.

Sometimes only one person's interests will change. That person may want to spend time with other friends or do other activities. This may make his or her friend jealous. The person whose interests are changing may want to end the friendship. He or she may feel the other is not giving him or her enough space.

Sometimes personalities change. The personal qualities that drew the friends together no longer exist. These friendships may end suddenly, sometimes following a disagreement. A friendship can end quickly if a friend breaks a promise. Failing to keep secrets or spreading rumors about a friend might also cause a friendship to end, **3-5**. Losing a friend in this manner can be bitter and painful.

Before ending a close friendship for these reasons, it is best to talk with the other person. Maybe there was a misunderstanding. Perhaps an apology is all that is necessary. A close friendship should not end on the basis of one bad experience.

Reading Review

1. Someone you have met, but do not know well, is a(n) _____.
2. Name three types of friends.
3. List three qualities people usually seek in their friends.
4. After you form friendships, what do you need to do in order for them to grow and remain strong?
5. Before ending a close friendship, what should you do?

Peers and Peer Pressure

Objectives

After studying this section, you will be able to
- **give examples** of ways conformity can be positive and ways it can be negative.
- **differentiate** between negative and positive peer pressure.
- **demonstrate** ways to handle negative peer pressure.
- **explain** how peer pressure can be positive.

Key Terms

peers	peer pressure	bullying
clique	conformity	empathy

Your friends play a big part in your life right now. Your family is still special to you. Your friends, however, are becoming more important. You may want to spend more time with your friends than with your family. You may think your best friend is more likely to understand your feelings and concerns.

Many teens feel this way. As you face new experiences, it helps to know other teens are having the same experiences. The world does not seem so scary when close friends share your challenges.

Peers

Your **peers** are people who are about the same age as you, **3-6**. Your peers affect your life in many ways. The activities your peers enjoy are often the activities you prefer. The clothes you select are usually the styles worn by members of your peer group. You like to go to the places that are popular with your peers.

Cliques

A group of peers may form a clique. A **clique** is a group that excludes other people. Members of a clique may have their own ways of thinking, dressing, and behaving.

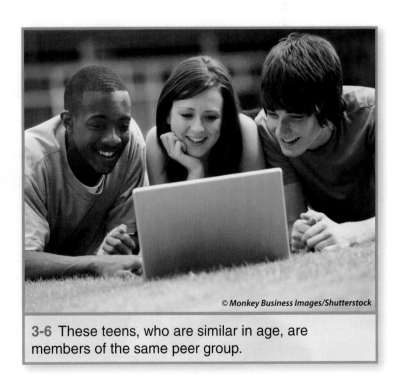

© Monkey Business Images/Shutterstock

3-6 These teens, who are similar in age, are members of the same peer group.

Cliques can be limiting. They may limit friendships, experiences, or even thoughts. Members may begin to think the same way. They may criticize those with differing viewpoints. Members may feel they have to dress a certain way and talk a certain way. They may make fun of people who are not in their clique.

Young people outside a clique may feel left out and wonder why they cannot be a part of the group. They may think there is something wrong with them. Some may imitate the actions of the clique so the group will accept them.

Being left out of a clique you want to belong to can hurt. The clique may be a popular group in school. Perhaps you will find that you have more in common with another group. You will probably enjoy being with teens who have interests and attitudes more like your own. You will feel more comfortable being yourself than trying to be like the members of a clique.

Peer Pressure

Peer pressure is the influence your peers have on you. This influence can affect the way you think and the way you act. Sometimes group members will use peer pressure to get you to conform to the group. Conformity means you look and behave like the other members of your group. Sometimes conformity is positive. For instance, you use good table manners in public to conform to accepted social practices. Conformity is negative when you allow the group to think for you. An example of this would be doing something you do not want to do just to go along with the group.

Peer pressure affects people of all ages. It affects some people more than others. Peer pressure can especially influence teens, **3-7**. They want to make the right impression on their peers so they will fit in with the group.

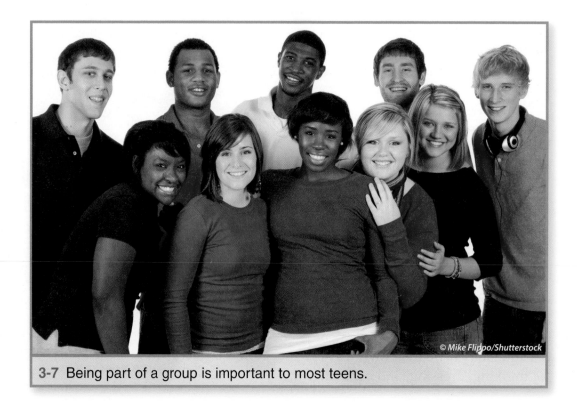

© Mike Flippo/Shutterstock

3-7 Being part of a group is important to most teens.

Negative Peer Pressure

Peer pressure can be either negative or positive. The pressure is negative if it causes you to behave in a way that brings harm to yourself or others. Negative peer pressure can also cause you to feel uncomfortable about yourself. You may like a certain teacher that your friends dislike. You may criticize that teacher because your peers expect you to. This could make you feel uncomfortable. You are saying something you do not believe just to please your friends. When you do this, you are being dishonest with yourself.

Suppose some of your friends use drugs. They want you to join them in using the drugs. Their insistence causes a lot of pressure on you. You know drugs are illegal as well as harmful to the body. Deciding not to take drugs shows others that you have the strength to resist this negative peer pressure.

Bullies

Bullying occurs when a person hurts or threatens another person. Bullying may include pushing, hitting, teasing, as well as verbal insults. More subtle bullying can involve deliberate ignoring or excluding others from a group. Bullying also occurs with the use of technology such as the Internet or cell phones.

Bullying affects many teens. It can happen to anyone at any time. Bullies will often target people who they think are different for some reason, such as the way they look or act. Bullies may also target people who they feel are weaker than they are.

People who bully others are often doing so to gain attention. They may think picking on someone else makes them feel more important or powerful. Sometimes bullies have been victims themselves and are repeating the cycle of violence. Most bullies do not care about the feelings of others and have difficulty showing empathy. **Empathy** means you are able to understand another person's emotions. You can see something from his or her point of view.

Bullying does not stop at a certain age. Sometimes, your parents or other trusted adults can share examples of bullying that they experience in the workplace or in social circles. Talking with them can provide an opportunity to see how adults handle this type of behavior.

Gangs

Gang violence is a growing concern for many people. A *gang* is a group of people who join together for a variety of reasons.

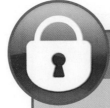

Safety Connections

Stop Bullying

If a bully is targeting you or someone you know, report the incident to a parent, teacher, or other trusted adult. You can also make plans to be with a friend in areas you think you might run into the bully. Sometimes just ignoring or standing up to the bully will cause the bullying to stop. Do not fight back, however. This may cause someone to get hurt, and you could also get into trouble.

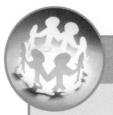

Life Connections

Learn to Say *No*

There are several ways to make saying *no* easier. First, say *no* like you mean it. If you are hesitant or uncertain, people will think they can get you to change your mind. Look the person straight in the eye and firmly say *no*. Do not lose your temper though. Getting angry might make people feel you are challenging them.

When you say *no*, you do not need to give any reasons or excuses. This may lead to an argument. For instance, you might say that you cannot go somewhere because you do not have a ride. If someone offers to drive you, however, then you no longer have an excuse. The person may continue to pressure you. Instead of giving an excuse, suggest another activity. Then the other person has to decide what to do.

It will also help if you can leave a situation as soon as you say *no*. Do not stick around to face a possible argument. No one can pressure you when you are not there.

Speaking Activity

Practice saying *no* using the tips just described. You and your friends can take turns using the various methods. Finding the right words will be easier when and if it becomes necessary.

Members may not have a supportive family or anyone who cares about them except for other members of the gang. These teens are often trying to find the family structure they do not have at home. Some gangs may try to pressure teens into joining. If teens refuse, they may become victims of the gang. Many innocent people are caught in violence between rival gangs. Hotlines and community officials can be helpful if you are unable to discuss this situation with your parent or guardian.

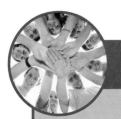

Community Connections

Positive Peer Pressure

Special groups use positive peer pressure to offer support to their members. These groups help people deal with challenges. *Alateen* is a peer group for teens with family members who abuse alcohol. Support from their peers lets these teens know others are coping with the same challenges. Similar peer groups exist for people who are dependent on drugs or who have eating disorders. Your community may have peer groups that help with other challenges as well.

Handling Negative Peer Pressure

Have you ever let a friend talk you into doing something you did not want to do? Peer pressure can put you at risk if it causes you to make poor decisions.

Instead of conforming, you may sometimes need to say *no*. Saying *no* to negative peer pressure is not going to be easy. If you are shy or uncertain of yourself, it can be especially hard.

Remember, it is your life and you have the ability to decide what is best for you. The decisions that affect you are for you to make. Do not let others talk you into doing something you are not comfortable doing.

The best defense against negative peer pressure is to know what you believe. Think through how you feel about certain issues. Know the position you will take before you encounter difficult situations. Then, standing firm for what you believe is right for you will be easier.

Positive Peer Pressure

Peer pressure is positive when it affects your behavior in a beneficial way. As a member of a group, you try to improve yourself in order to meet the standards set by the group. Suppose most of the students in your group get good grades. Their influence may cause you to study hard to get good grades, too. Positive pressure from your peers might also be just the boost you need to run for a class office.

Reading Review

1. True or false. People who are significantly older than you are your peers.
2. What does conformity mean?
3. What does bullying involve?
4. Give an example of how to handle negative peer pressure.
5. Give an example of positive peer pressure.

Dating

Objectives

After studying this section, you will be able to

- **describe** the stages of dating and the types of activities and emotions that may be involved at each stage.
- **differentiate** between love and infatuation.
- **identify** risks associated with sexual relations and state positive ways to show affection that are not physical.
- **give examples** of reasons a relationship may end.

Key Terms		
dating	sexually transmitted	AIDS
love	infections (STIs)	HIV
infatuation	sterility	abstinence

When you were younger, you enjoyed outings and activities with friends of your own sex. Now that you are older, you may be more interested in members of the opposite sex. You may want to begin dating.

Stages of Dating

Dating is participating in an activity with a friend of the opposite sex. It gives people a chance to go places with others. Dating can also teach people how to get along with members of the opposite sex.

A person you date is someone you are attracted to and enjoy being around. You may often be attracted to people very much like yourself. They are more likely to be close to your own age. They might have a family background similar to yours. The people you date may even have personality traits similar to yours. For instance, if you are energetic and outgoing, you may be attracted to someone with a similar personality type.

Social Studies Connections

Dating Practices

There is no specific age to begin dating. It really depends on the young person and his or her family. Some young teens may be eager to begin dating. Others do not develop an interest in dating until they are in their late teens. Some parents may feel it is appropriate for young teens to date. Parents in other families do not allow teens to date until they are older and more mature. Dating practices also vary depending on the community in which you live. It will be up to you and your family to decide the age that is best for you.

Group Dating

Many young teens start dating in groups. Several young people may go together to a ball game or to a concert. This is called *group dating*. Group activities can often take place on the spur of the moment. This is a good way to begin dating. Being yourself and finding topics to talk about is easier when you are in a group. You are less likely to feel awkward or self-conscious. You can relax and become more comfortable with members of the opposite sex.

Casual Dating

When teens begin to feel more confident relating to members of the opposite sex, they often begin to break off into pairs. This leads to the next stage of dating. *Casual dating* involves one couple, not a group of people. During this stage, a person may date several people on a regular basis. This is called *random dating*.

Casual and random dating helps you learn to get along with a variety of people. You learn what personality traits you like in people. You develop your social skills and become more comfortable when meeting new people, **3-8**. You will probably not want to share deep personal feelings with casual dates. This type of sharing is not likely to occur until you enter the next dating stage.

Steady Dating

After you have been dating a while, you may find one person you enjoy being with more than anyone else. You will find yourself having fewer dates with other people. You will begin having more dates with this one particular person. A special feeling may start to grow between the two of you. If you decide to date only each other, you will have entered the steady dating stage. You may say you are "going out with" this person, or you are "going together."

A couple should begin steady dating because they enjoy each other's company, but sometimes there are other reasons. Some teens want to be sure of having a date when they want one. Some couples go together because of peer pressure. All their friends have steady dating partners, so they feel they should, too.

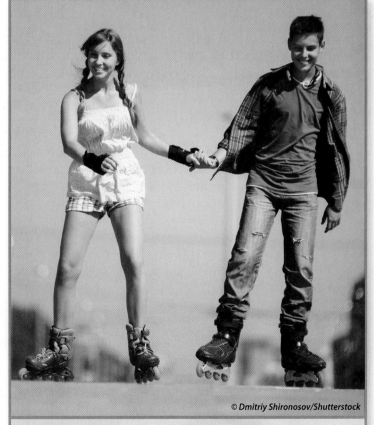

© Dmitriy Shironosov/Shutterstock

3-8 Casual dating gives teens a chance to be with another person and have fun together.

First Dates

You may be nervous about your first real date. If you have already begun to date, you may still be anxious when you date someone new. You may wonder, Will I be dressed right? Will I seem nervous? Will I be able to find enough to talk about with him or her? Will I say the wrong things? Will my date think I am boring? What if I trip or spill food on my clothes?

These are all concerns that most young teens have when they begin to date. Both guys and girls will have many of the same thoughts.

As you continue to date, you will become more relaxed. Your self-confidence will increase. You will be able to worry less about yourself and learn more about the people you date. In the meantime, the suggestions given in **3-9** will help make dates go more smoothly.

Is It Love?

In dating relationships, young people begin to have some strong, new feelings. Some of these feelings have to do with *love*. Although teens have experienced love within the family, this is a new kind of love. What is love? How do you know if you are really in love?

Love is easy to define, but it is sometimes difficult to recognize. **Love** is a strong feeling of affection between two people. It grows stronger with time.

Suggestions to Keep Your First Date from Being Your Worst Date

1. Be yourself. Your date was attracted to you—not someone else.
2. Choose a type of entertainment you both will enjoy, such as a movie or school event. Having something to watch will help calm your nerves during the first part of the date. Then, you will have something to talk about after the event.
3. Before you go out, think about topics that your date may enjoy discussing. You might talk about movies, TV programs, school events, or news items. Let your date do as much talking as you do.
4. Take time to really learn about your date. Ask about his or her thoughts and opinions using questions that require more than a yes or no answer.
5. If you have a mishap, such as tripping or spilling food, try to laugh it off and not dwell on it.
6. If your date has a mishap, try to make him or her feel at ease. In either case, try to forget the incident as quickly as possible.
7. Do not cancel a date unless you absolutely have to. Be honest with your excuse.
8. Be ready at the agreed upon time or call if you must be late.
9. Be in a good frame of mind. Do not tell your date all your problems and troubles.
10. After the date, keep the details of your date to yourself. A date is a personal experience.

3-9 These suggestions can make dating a pleasant experience for you and your date.

Love is unselfish. It is based on the total person, not just the outward appearance. Love is based on trust and openness. It is not jealous or possessive.

The special feeling that exists between two people who are in love is unlike any other they will know. People in love are concerned more for each other than for themselves, **3-10**.

Infatuation

Many young teens feel they are in love from time to time. What they may really be feeling, however, is infatuation. **Infatuation** is an intense feeling of attraction that begins and ends quickly. Many teens are infatuated with TV stars or famous musicians. The attraction is usually based on physical appearance or popularity.

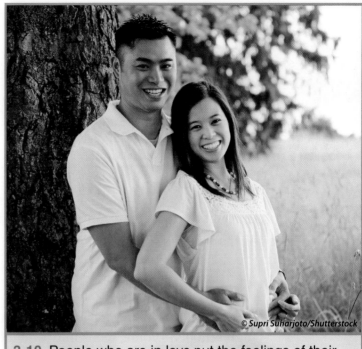

© Supri Suharjoto/Shutterstock

3-10 People who are in love put the feelings of their partners before their own.

An infatuation is sometimes called a *crush*. You may have had a crush on a classmate or friend who was unaware of your feelings. Infatuation is unlike love because love is a shared feeling.

Infatuation can affect the way you normally think about people. When you are infatuated with someone, you may spend a lot of time thinking about him or her. You find it hard to keep your mind on what you are doing. Your infatuation also allows you to see only the person's positive traits. You may overlook his or her flaws.

Infatuation is not unusual among young teens. It is a natural way of exploring new feelings for the opposite sex.

Physical Expressions of Affection

It is natural for teens to have sexual feelings. They want to show and receive affection. They should avoid having sexual relations, however. Sexual activity involves risks. It is important to know what those risks are.

Teen Pregnancy

Pregnancy can occur any time a person has sexual intercourse. Even if a type of contraceptive (birth control) is used, there is always a chance it may fail. A female can get pregnant the very first time she has sex. She can never assume that it is the "wrong time of the month" to get pregnant. Having a baby may be something to look forward to as an adult, but it has the potential to disrupt a teen's life. Teens may have to delay or abandon life goals if they must assume responsibility for a baby. Teen parents must also

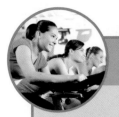

Health Connections

Risks of Teen Pregnancy

Though a teenage girl can become pregnant, pregnancy and birth can be difficult for young teens. Because a young girl may not be fully grown, her body must support her own growth plus the development of the baby. This causes a strain on the mother's body. It is also a risk to the unborn child. Babies of younger mothers are more often born with low birthweights or birth defects. Teen mothers also have more *miscarriages* and *stillbirths*, meaning their babies have died before birth.

rely heavily on their own parents for help. This can cause a strain on the family resources.

Teens accept more and more responsibility as they get older. Caring for a child, however, is a tremendous responsibility. A teen may not yet be able to manage his or her own life independently. Taking responsibility for a child is often more than a teen can handle.

Because raising children is so costly, it is doubtful that a teen is financially ready to become a parent. Most teens who work have part-time jobs. If he or she becomes a parent, it may be necessary to drop out of school to work full time. Without a high school diploma, teens may only be able to work at low-paying jobs. Their chances of further education may also become limited.

Teen parents must often rely heavily on their own parents for help. Teens may borrow money from their parents. They may ask their parents to care for the child while they are at work or school. Many times teen parents continue living with their parents.

Some teen parents choose marriage, which may be difficult to maintain given all the changes they are experiencing. Teens may not yet understand how to create a lasting marriage. They may discover they were not truly in love when they married. People change as they grow, and the couple may decide they are not the right partners for each other. Waiting until a person is an adult to have a baby is the best way to guarantee the health and well-being of the parents and baby.

Sexually Transmitted Infections

Sexually transmitted infections (STIs) are illnesses that spread through sexual contact. STIs are also known as *sexually transmitted diseases (STDs)*. Sexually transmitted infections can jeopardize a person's health. Some STIs cause infections that damage reproductive organs. This may result in **sterility**, the inability to conceive a child. Sometimes, people can be infected with an STI and not even realize it because they do not have any visible infection. This can be dangerous to others if the person has sexual relations.

AIDS (acquired immune deficiency syndrome) is a disease caused by a virus called **HIV** (human immunodeficiency virus). HIV can be spread through sexual contact. Someone can also get HIV by sharing a hypodermic needle with an infected person. AIDS affects the body's immune system. People who have AIDS cannot fight off diseases as healthy people can. These diseases then lead to death.

In addition to AIDS and HIV, there are many kinds of sexually transmitted infections. Figure **3-11** lists some of the most common STIs.

Sexually Transmitted Infections

Infection	Symptoms	Health Effects	Treatment
AIDS/HIV	Early HIV symptoms may include swollen glands, fever, headaches, fatigue, muscle aches; AIDS symptoms include weakened immune system, weight loss, shortness of breath, rashes, sores, decreased mental abilities	Weakened immune system causes inability to fight diseases, which can lead to death	Combinations of medicines called *cocktails* can allow people to live longer, but there is no cure
Chlamydia	Symptoms are often not apparent, but may include abdominal pain, low-grade fever, pain or burning while urinating, bleeding between menstrual periods	If left untreated, may harm reproductive organs and cause sterility	Prescription antibiotics
Genital herpes	Symptoms are often not apparent, but may include blisters, itching, flu-like feelings, open sores	During vaginal delivery, contact with open sores may cause the baby to have a life-threatening infection	Prescription medications, but sores may come back because there is no cure
Genital warts	Cauliflower-shaped warts on surface of genital area that are often painless, but may itch	Often not dangerous, but may cause sores or bleeding, which can increase risk of HIV	Surgical removal or prescription medications, but warts may come back because there is no cure
Gonorrhea	Symptoms are often not apparent, but may include abdominal pain, fever, painful urination, menstrual irregularities, vomiting	If left untreated, may harm reproductive organs and cause sterility	Prescription antibiotics
Hepatitis B	Symptoms are often not apparent, but may include tiredness, loss of appetite, fever, hives, joint pain, abdominal pain, jaundice	May cause severe liver disease or liver cancer; can lead to death	Prevention vaccine, but there is no cure
Human papillomavirus (HPV)	Symptoms are often not apparent, but some types of HPV may cause genital warts; high risk types can cause cell abnormalities	High risk types of HPV can cause cervical cancer and other genital and throat cancers	Prevention vaccine for males and females ages 9–26; surgical removal of abnormal cells
Pelvic inflammatory disease (PID)	Symptoms are often not apparent at first, but as PID worsens it may cause lower abdomen and back pain, flu-like feelings, unusually long or painful menstruation	If left untreated, may harm reproductive organs and cause sterility	Prescription antibiotics
Pubic lice (crabs)	Symptoms are often not apparent, but may include genital itching, fever, lack of energy, irritability	Often not dangerous, but can cause skin damage and infection	Over-the-counter or prescription medications
Syphilis	First stage symptoms may include a small, firm sore (called a *chancre*); second stage symptoms may include body rashes, fever, hair loss, weight loss, swollen glands, muscle pains	If left untreated, may cause serious damage to the nervous system, heart, brain, and other organs; may result in death	Early stages treated with prescription antibiotics

3-11 In most cases, there is no cure for these common sexually transmitted infections.

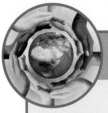

Global Connections

Public Contact

Public contact is not always the same from culture to culture. For instance, many Japanese people strongly disapprove of public expression of affections by males and females through kissing or any form of body contact. In India, public displays of affection are considered taboo and could possibly lead to a punishable offense by law.

Sexual Responsibility

Because of the risks associated with sexual relations, most young teens choose abstinence. **Abstinence** means choosing not to have sex. It is the best way to avoid an unplanned pregnancy and exposure to STIs. It is also the only method of birth control that is 100 percent effective.

There are positive ways to show affection that are not physical. Being thoughtful of your partner is a way to show him or her that you care. Listen when your date expresses feelings. Be supportive when challenges arise. Spending time together is itself a sign of affection.

Being together does not mean you have to be alone together. Sometimes abstinence is harder when you are alone together. Avoid going to each other's home when no adults are present. Instead, join clubs or groups that reflect interests you have in common. Think of activities in which you and your date can become involved. When you go on a date, make a definite plan for what you will do. Decide ahead of time to go to the movies or a teen club. That way, you will not end up in a situation where you feel pressured.

Decide how you feel about having sex. Let your date know how you feel. Practice saying *no*, and be prepared to stand up for what you believe. Be respectful of your partner's decision.

Breaking Up

Many close relationships eventually come to an end. There are various reasons a couple might end a relationship. Personal goals and interests might have changed for one or both members of the relationship. Being together just may not be fun anymore. They may not be as interested in each other as they once were. Communication between them

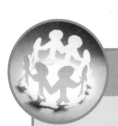

Life Connections

Ending Abusive Relationships

Dating violence happens in some teen relationships if they are not aware of the abusive signs and do not protect themselves. Besides physical violence, it can include emotional abuse. Emotional abuse can involve insulting or humiliating a partner. It can also include jealous and controlling behavior. Ending an abusive relationship is the first step toward stopping a cycle of violence. If you believe a boyfriend or girlfriend is abusing you in any way, talk to a parent, counselor, or friend. Understanding the symptoms and characteristics of abuse is the best way to get out of a potentially painful relationship.

Reading Activity

Sometimes it is helpful to read about how other young people removed themselves from abusive relationships. You many learn how to identify abusive traits in others and strategies for asserting yourself positively. Check the Internet for books that can inform you about these issues.

may not be easy or pleasant any longer. Conflicts may have become a habit. There may be another person one of them would like to date.

When a relationship reaches the point where it is not growing in a positive way, it may be over. Talking honestly can make breaking up less stressful. Being considerate and respectful of each other's feelings is important. Making unkind remarks and causing each other to feel guilty is harmful to each person. Dating partners should tell each other the things they liked and appreciated about each other. It is best if they can remain friends even though they are no longer going together.

After being with only one person, you may feel lost following a break up. You may not feel like dating again for a while. Rather than feeling lonely and depressed, use this time to focus on yourself. Review your goals and develop a plan to reach them. Learn something new, such as a new skill or craft. Visit new places of interest. Spend more time with your friends and family members.

In time, the pain of a break up will be behind you. You will be ready for new friendships to grow and develop. A new relationship can begin at any time.

Reading Review

1. What is dating?
2. List three stages of dating.
3. Describe the difference between love and infatuation.
4. What are two risks involved with sexual activity?
5. List two examples why a relationship might end.

Chapter Summary

Section 3-1. Friends play a big part in your life during the teen years. You feel different levels of closeness toward your acquaintances, casual friends, and best friends. Being able to make friends will help you feel comfortable in a number of situations. Friendships may end for a number of reasons. In such cases, talking about the issue is usually a good idea. Friends may be able to clear up misunderstandings and save the friendship.

Section 3-2. Your friends are your peers. Sometimes friends use peer pressure to influence you and get you to conform. Peer pressure can be negative if it causes you to do things that are harmful to yourself or others. Peer pressure is positive when it causes you to improve yourself in some way. You must learn how to resist negative peer pressure and use positive peer pressure to your advantage.

Section 3-3. During the teen years, some friendships between members of the opposite sex turn into dating relationships. Many teens feel nervous about their first dates. As they mature, most teens gain confidence in relating to members of the opposite sex. Feelings change from infatuation to love as relationships develop with one special person. Being sexually responsible will help keep you safe. Many dating relationships end in breakups. Communication can make a breakup less painful and prepare teens to build new dating relationships.

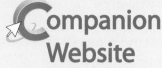

Companion Website
www.g-wlearning.com

Check your understanding of the main concepts for Chapter 3 at the website.

Critical Thinking

1. **Analyze.** What should be done to lessen the impact peer pressure has on teens? Give examples of how peer pressure has affected you or your friends.
2. **Determine.** When would it be a good idea to end a friendship? How can you end a friendship that is harmful to you?
3. **Assess.** If you could go out on a date with anyone in the world, who would it be and why? What qualities would make this person a suitable dating partner?

Common Core

College and Career Readiness

4.   **Writing.** Write an article about a group at your school that uses positive peer pressure, such as Students Against Smoking or Athletes' Study Group. Submit your article to the school newspaper for possible publication.

5. **Speaking.** Role-play each of the following situations:
   A. a teen being influenced by negative peer pressure
   B. a teen saying no to negative peer pressure
   C. a teen being influenced by positive peer pressure

6. **Listening.** Interview three adults. Ask them to list five qualities they think describe a true friend. Compare your findings with those of your classmates.

7. **Reading.** Share articles from popular teen magazines about dating with the class. Do you agree with the ideas/opinions expressed in the articles? Explain.

Technology

8. **Video presentation.** Role-play various friendship and dating situations. Video the role-plays and use them as a basis of a class discussion.

Journal Writing

9. Make a list of your friends. Next to each name, write the qualities that make this person your friend. Write about ways you can enhance each of your friendships.

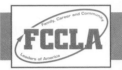

FCCLA

10. Create a *STOP the Violence* project that educates your peers on the differences between healthy and unhealthy relationships and/or love and infatuation. Invite guest speakers from organizations that work with victims of domestic violence to promote positive decision making and healthy relationships. Use the *FCCLA Planning Process* to fully develop your project. Take your project one step further and apply for national recognition for your *STOP the Violence* project. See your adviser for information about the application process.

Chapter 4
Developing Communication Skills

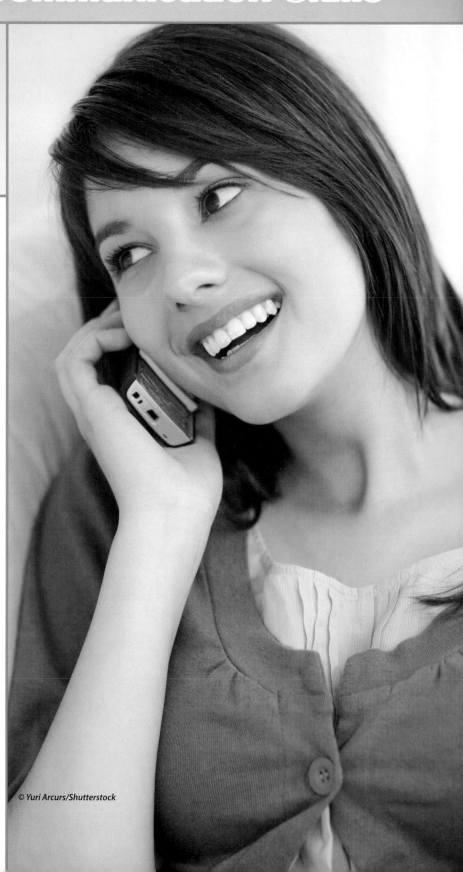

Sections

4-1 Communicating with Others

4-2 Avoiding Barriers to Good Communication

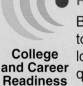

Reading Prep

College and Career Readiness

Before you begin to read the chapter, look at the review questions at the end of the chapter. Keep the questions in mind as you read to help you determine which information is most important.

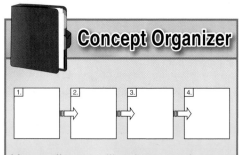

Concept Organizer

1.	2.	3.	4.

Use a diagram like the one shown to identify the four steps of conflict resolution.

Companion Website

Print out the concept organizer for Chapter 4 at the website.

Companion Website
www.g-wlearning.com

Section 4-1

Communicating with Others

Objectives

After studying this section, you will be able to
- **define** verbal and nonverbal communication.
- **compare and contrast** the various forms of verbal and nonverbal communication.
- **demonstrate** active listening techniques.
- **describe** how to give feedback effectively.

Key Terms

communication	body language	active listening
verbal communication	personal space	feedback
nonverbal communication	manners	

Learning to communicate well is a skill you will use throughout your life. You need this skill in your personal life to express your feelings to friends and family members. You need to be able to communicate well in school, too. Your future job success may also depend on your ability to communicate.

Types of Communication

Communication is the process of sending and receiving information. You communicate with the people around you every day. In fact, you probably spend a large percentage of your day communicating in some way.

There are two main types of communication. The first type is verbal communication. **Verbal communication** involves the use of words to send information. It is probably what came to your mind first when you thought about communication. Speaking and writing are both forms of verbal communication.

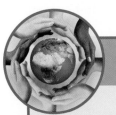

Global Connections

Communication Differences

People from some Asian cultures seldom feel free to say *no* to a request. They believe it is rude to say *no* and creates ill feelings. They will often go to extremes to avoid doing so. Preferring harmony, they generally use indirect communication methods to achieve that goal.

Eye contact is another area in which there are marked culture differences.
- Western cultures value direct eye contact and train children to "look people in the eye."
- Arabic cultures make prolonged eye contact. They believe it shows interest and helps them determine a person's honesty. A person who does not reciprocate is viewed as untrustworthy.
- Japanese, African, and many Latin American cultures avoid eye contact to show respect.

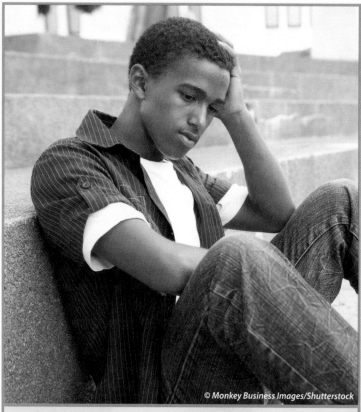

© Monkey Business Images/Shutterstock

4-1 Everything about you gives off some kind of nonverbal messages.

Nonverbal communication includes any means of sending a message that does not use words. Your appearance says something about you. Your facial expressions, gestures, and posture say a lot, **4-1**. The way you react to other people also tells something about who you are and how you feel. All these factors make an impression on other people without you saying a single word.

Verbal Communication

Words used in speaking and writing usually convey precise meanings. Have you ever thought what it would be like if you had no language? How much more difficult would it be to express your wants and ideas?

People are not born with the ability to speak, but they can learn to communicate very quickly. For instance, babies use certain sounds to express their needs and wants to family members. In time, children learn to use real words to communicate with others. As people grow older, they often take speaking for granted. They may even speak without thinking sometimes.

The language you speak is likely to be the language most often spoken in your home. English is the primary language in all parts of the United States. People may pronounce some words differently, however, in different parts of the country. For instance, a person in Maine may say some words differently from someone who lives in Louisiana.

The way you speak to people often depends on the situation. When you are with your friends, you may use slang. *Slang* consists of words used by a certain group of people. The meanings of the words used by the group are different from the usual meanings. It is best to avoid the use of slang when speaking with

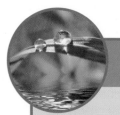

Go Green

Green Technology

Most people have a computer or access to one for school or work. Have you ever considered computers to be green technology? Much of what you learn in school comes from written words in books and papers. You write assignments in school. You write answers to test questions. You prepare written papers and reports. You keep journals. Think about all the trees needed to make paper for books and your written activities. The ability to transfer these tasks to a computer makes it quite an environmentally friendly invention. Some schools now provide both the textbooks and homework assignments online. Perhaps the future of education will be on the computer.

people outside the group. The use of such words can lead to a lack of communication with people who do not know the slang meanings. Therefore, it may be wise to avoid the use of slang when speaking with anyone outside your group.

Sometimes the emphasis you place on a word can change the meaning of what you are saying. Read each of the sentences in Figure **4-2**, emphasizing the italicized word. Notice how each question conveys a different meaning. Be certain the tone of your voice conveys the message you are trying to send.

You can use what you know about spoken communication to send clear messages to others. Use language and pronunciations they understand. Use words with meanings that are familiar to everyone. Use your voice to emphasize your message.

The way you use your voice can also help you send clear messages. Speak in a clear voice without mumbling. You should not speak too loudly, or too softly. Try not to speak too slowly. You may lose the attention of your listener. On the other hand, if you speak too fast, your listener may not be able to follow what you are saying.

If people often ask you to repeat what you say, you may want to try to improve the way you speak. You might ask a friend or family member to suggest how you could speak more clearly. You might also record a conversation with a friend. Then listen to the recording to identify speech patterns you may want to change.

Writing

A second form of verbal communication is writing. You still use words to communicate, but you write them instead of speaking them. You use your writing skills in school many times each day. You also communicate personal information by writing. You may send text messages or even write a letter to a friend or relative you do not see very often. You may send cards and notes to friends on special occasions or when they are ill. You may also write to pass along information to family members who are not at home.

Communication

Emphasis can change the meaning of a message. Read each of these sentences aloud, emphasizing the italicized word. Notice how the message varies.

What do you want me to do?

What *do* you want me to do?

What do *you* want me to do?

What do you *want* me to do?

What do you want *me* to do?

What do you want me to *do*?

4-2 The emphasis placed on each word in a sentence can change the message.

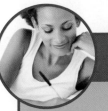

Writing Connections

Writing Clear Messages

Like clear speaking, clear writing makes your messages easier to understand. You will want to be certain people can read your handwriting. You will want to use correct grammar, spelling, and punctuation.

Think through what you want to say before you begin to write. Jot down key points to make in the order you want to make them. An outline is helpful when writing lengthy reports for school. You will find the words come easier when you have an outline to guide you.

Many jobs require writing skills. You may have to write orders or reports. You may have to develop business letters. Therefore, your skill at writing may be very important to your success on the job.

Nonverbal Communication

Sometimes people communicate without even speaking. You often know when friends are worried or unhappy without them saying anything. You may know by the way a person sits or stands, or by facial expressions. Likewise, if a friend has had a good experience, you may see it in the way he or she walks or smiles.

Sometimes the nonverbal messages you send about yourself are not typical of you. Perhaps you are walking slower, your shoulders are sloping, or you are slumping in your seat. Maybe your eyes do not have their usual sparkle, or you are frowning. Your family members and friends may question the change in you. Their comments may surprise you if you are not aware you are sending uncharacteristic messages.

Taking a closer look at nonverbal forms of communication will help you become aware of the messages you send. You will be able to decide if you are sending true messages about yourself.

Appearance

When you meet new people, you should want their first impression of you to be good and one that says, "You'll like knowing me." If the first impression you give turns people off, you may never get to know them. They will not get a chance to know the person you really are. If this happens at a job interview, you may not get the job. You will not be able to prove you can handle the job and be a good employee.

People often base their first impressions of you on the way you look. Before you get a chance to say a word, your appearance sends an instant message, **4-3**. The people you meet may often notice tattoos, piercings, and your hairstyle. They notice if you are well groomed. The people you meet can make these

© Phase4Photography/Shutterstock

4-3 Every aspect of your appearance communicates a message about you.

observations quickly, and may not even be aware of the judgment they are making. For this reason, you need to think about your appearance and the message you want it to send to others.

Body Language

Another form of nonverbal communication is body language. **Body language** is the sending of messages through body movements. These movements include gestures, facial expressions, and posture. A wave of the hand is an example of body language. This gesture communicates recognition and friendship.

Body language can communicate both positive and negative messages. For instance, suppose your mother meets you after school. She has her hands on her waist. She has a frown on her face. It would probably not take you long to figure out that she is upset. On the other hand, she may smile and nod her head to communicate approval of something you say or do.

An important form of body language is eye contact. When talking with people, try to look them in the eye, **4-4**. This shows interest in what they have to say. It lets them know that what they are saying is important to you. If you often look away, someone could interpret your action to mean you do not care about what he or she is saying.

Your posture is another part of body language. It can tell others how you feel about yourself. Having good posture sends a nonverbal message that you are self-confident and care about yourself. Your posture also tells people how you feel about situations. Leaning forward in a chair indicates interest in what someone is saying. On the other hand, slouching back in a chair with your arms crossed communicates a lack of interest.

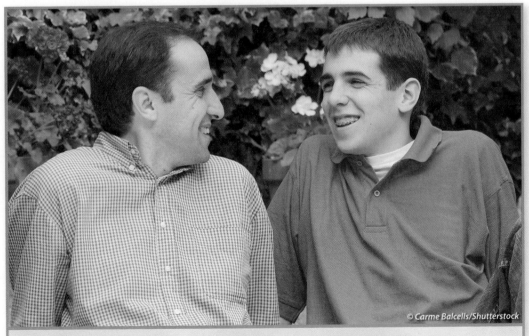

© Carme Balcells/Shutterstock

4-4 Maintaining eye contact lets others know that you care about what they have to say.

Sometimes the messages people convey are not the messages they mean to send. A new student who does not talk to others may convey that she is aloof and stuck-up. Perhaps she is really just shy. A classmate who sits with his head on his desk may send a message that he is bored. Instead, he may be sick.

Be aware of the body signals people send. Be careful, however, not to make judgments only on the basis of body language. You may need to use verbal communication to really find out how someone feels.

Personal Space

Each person has a personal space. Your **personal space** is the area around you. When someone enters this space, you react in different ways. This reaction is a form of nonverbal communication.

The way you react to someone entering your personal space depends on how well you know the person. If you are crowded into an elevator with many strangers, you may feel uneasy. Often, no one may even speak. On the other hand, suppose you and several friends are in an elevator together. In this case, you would probably talk freely and enjoy the closeness. See **4-5**.

The situation you are in may also affect how comfortable you feel when you are in close contact with others. For instance, if you are at home and a family member enters your personal space, you may welcome the closeness. You may even touch, hug, or kiss. If you were in a public place, however, this type of close contact might embarrass you.

You can convey nonverbal messages by entering a person's personal space. A light touch on the hand or arm or even a hug lets someone know you care. A formal handshake shows a stranger that he or she is welcome.

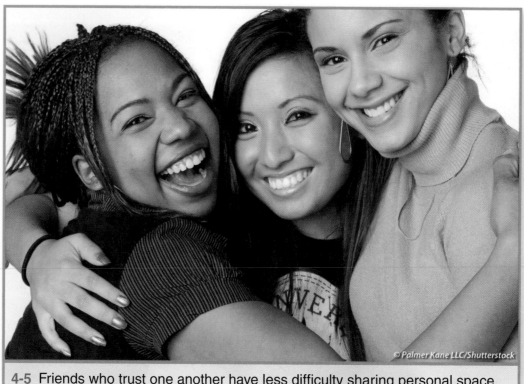

© Palmer Kane LLC/Shutterstock

4-5 Friends who trust one another have less difficulty sharing personal space.

Manners

Manners are rules for proper conduct. Your manners are a form of nonverbal communication. You send a message about yourself in the way you behave around others.

When you use good manners, you act in a way that makes people feel comfortable. Your manners reflect your attitude toward others. Using good manners sends a message that you care about others' feelings. This clears the way for good communication.

Good manners are appropriate at every age. You do not have to wait until you are an adult to start practicing good manners. In fact, the sooner you learn to practice good manners, the sooner you will start sending clearer messages. Being knowledgeable of manners that are unique to different cultures will show respect for others.

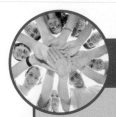

Community Connections

Display Good Manners

It is easy to have good manners if you try to think of others first. If someone new joins your group of friends or moves into your neighborhood, introduce yourself. Make him or her feel welcome. Help someone who needs a favor. Hold the door open for the person behind you. Show respect for the possessions and property of others. Remember to say *please* and *thank you*. These are only a few of the many ways you can show courtesy for others.

Being an Active Listener

Communication is a two-way process. Sometimes you are the sender and sometimes you are the receiver. To receive messages clearly, it helps to be an active listener. **Active listening** is a communication technique in which the listener shows a clear understanding of what a person is saying. You can do this in several ways.

Restate what the speaker says. To be certain you understand the message, repeat what you think the speaker is saying. You may begin by saying, "I understood you to say…" or "Do you mean…." Letting the speaker know you receive the message correctly is called **feedback**.

Let the speaker know you are listening by sending signals. This is another form of feedback. Nod your head when you agree with the speaker or shake your head if you disagree. Lean toward the speaker and maintain eye contact.

If the message you receive is not clear, ask questions. Do not be afraid to ask questions when you do not understand. Ask the speaker to explain more fully or to clear up certain points.

If you are learning a new job, it is especially important to ask questions because you need to perform the job as instructed. It is normal to ask questions when you are being trained. You can then avoid making mistakes later.

Listen before answering. You may think of questions or comments while the speaker is talking. Allow the speaker to complete his or her remarks before you respond. If you are not listening closely, you might ask a question the speaker has just answered. That can be embarrassing.

Do not interrupt. Allow the speaker to finish what he or she has to say. Your turn will come. It is impolite to begin talking before the speaker finishes, **4-6**. It shows you are not really listening.

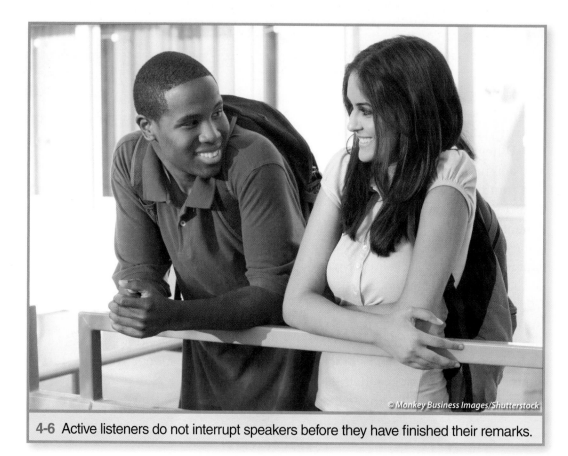

© Monkey Business Images/Shutterstock

4-6 Active listeners do not interrupt speakers before they have finished their remarks.

Keep your mind on what the speaker is saying. Try not to let your thoughts wander. It is sometimes hard to do this, especially if you are worried or excited about some upcoming event. If the speaker is a teacher or employer, however, it is a good idea to pay attention.

Reading Review

1. The process of sending and receiving information is called _____.
2. Differentiate between verbal and nonverbal communication.
3. List four ways to send clearer messages when speaking.
4. Give three guidelines for writing clear messages.
5. What is active listening?

Section 4-2

Avoiding Barriers to Good Communication

Objectives

After studying this section, you will be able to
- **describe** how to avoid communication barriers.
- **distinguish** between you-messages and I-messages.
- **explain** how using communication skills can help resolve conflicts.

Key Terms

mixed messages	critic	conflicts
assertive communication	destructive criticism	mediator
nonassertive communication	constructive criticism	compromise
	stereotype	
aggressive communication	prejudices	
criticize	racism	

Communicating clearly with others is not always easy. A number of barriers can get in the way of the communication process. Understanding these hurdles can help you avoid them. Learning to improve your communication skills can also help you avoid these barriers.

Using good communication skills can help you get along with others. Success at a job is more likely to occur if you get along well with your coworkers. You can strengthen your relationships with family members and friends by using good communication skills. Being able to communicate well with people is a key to a satisfying life.

Mixed Messages

It is easy to get messages mixed up when there are so many ways to send and receive them. Sometimes people do not say what they mean. People are sending **mixed messages** when their actions send one message and their words say something else. When this happens, it is difficult to know how a person really feels.

Global Connections

Meanings of Hand Gestures

Hand gestures do not have universal meaning. For people from some parts of the world, such as the Middle East, Nigeria, and Australia, the thumbs-up gesture is considered obscene. Pointing with the index finger is sometimes considered rude to people from outside the United States, especially people from Asian countries. The American "bye-bye" gesture means "come here" to people from Southeast Asia.

Suppose a friend of yours is facing a challenge. You may sense something is wrong, but when you ask him, he says everything is fine. Your friend is sending a mixed message. When he says nothing is wrong, what he really means is that he does not want to talk about it. Maybe he is afraid you will laugh at him. If he communicated that, you could reassure him you would take the issue seriously. By sending a mixed message, however, your friend may not get needed help.

Another kind of mixed message occurs when a person says one thing, but does another. You have probably heard the expression "Actions speak louder than words." This means that what a person does sends a more accurate message than what he or she says.

Sending Clear Messages

You send hundreds of messages to dozens of people every day. Good communication occurs when you send these messages clearly. The people receiving the messages understand what you are communicating and interpret the messages correctly. The listeners clearly understand the facts, feelings, and ideas.

Life Connections

Develop Your Conversation Skills

Some people worry about what to talk about in a conversation. The best topics to discuss are ones you and your friends have in common. This could include favorite TV shows, favorite singers, new video games, or news events. You might talk about an upcoming school event or something that happened at school. A concern, fear, or homework assignment might be a topic to discuss. The list is endless. Avoid getting too personal unless you are close friends. If there is a lull in the conversation, or if someone seems embarrassed, change the subject.

When in groups, encourage everyone to speak. Learn to ask the kinds of questions that draw quiet people into the conversation. Ask for the opinion of a member of the group who has not spoken. Avoid questions people can answer with a simple *yes* or *no*. Instead, ask questions that require an explanation.

Speech Activity

If you are nervous about speaking in front of people, then practicing can help you gain confidence. Work with a small group and have everyone pick topics they would like to discuss. Let each person lead a discussion about his or her chosen topic. When finished, other members of the group can offer suggestions for improvement.

You can use a number of techniques to help you send clear messages.

First, think before you speak. Think about how you feel and what you want to say. You must form your thoughts in your mind before you can express them to others. If you have trouble forming your thoughts, spend more time analyzing them. Spend some time reading and researching your facts. Then you will be ready to share your ideas.

After you have formed your ideas clearly in your mind, you are ready to speak. Be sure you provide all the needed facts. Make your points in a clear and concise manner. Include *who*, *what*, *when*, *where*, and *why* information. Keep your comments brief and to the point.

Presenting your ideas clearly is often referred to as assertive communication. **Assertive communication** means expressing thoughts, feelings, and beliefs in open, honest, and respectful ways, **4-7**. A nonassertive person may have a hard time expressing thoughts and feelings.

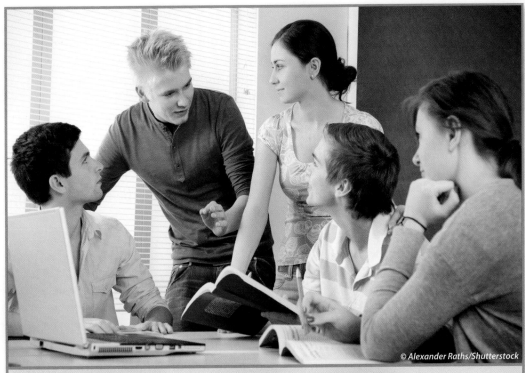

© Alexander Raths/Shutterstock

4-7 An assertive communicator can convey their message clearly while respecting the feelings and beliefs of others.

Passive or **nonassertive communication** describes speaking that is unclear or easily misunderstood. This manner of speaking fails to clearly convey the speaker's beliefs. A nonassertive speaker may use wordy sentences, apologize often, or put oneself down.

Sometimes people express themselves in negative or aggressive ways. **Aggressive communication** means expressing yourself in a forceful way that may step on the rights of others. People who speak in an aggressive manner may often be loud, sarcastic, or use threats.

Be considerate of others' feelings. Choose your words carefully to avoid hurting others. If you are tactful in what you say, you are less likely to offend people. You may need to practice making tactful remarks. This communication skill will help you relate to others.

Listen and pay attention to your tone of voice. People are more likely to respond well to a pleasant tone of voice. For instance, if you pleasantly ask a favor of your parents, they are more likely to agree to your request. If you use a tone that sounds demanding or whining, you may receive an abrupt "No."

Maintain eye contact. Look directly at your listeners. They will be more likely to pay attention to what you have to say. You will also seem more self-confident. If you look at the floor or stare past your listeners, you may lose their attention. They may also feel you are not being completely honest. They may wonder if you are afraid to look them in the eye because you are hiding something.

You-Messages and I-Messages

Try to avoid using you-messages when communicating. *You-messages* are often statements that are more negative and can end up causing a confrontation. An example of a you-message might be, "You made me upset when you told me I could not go to the concert."

Instead, you can use I-messages to send clear messages to others. *I-messages* are statements that can help you take responsibility for how you feel. An example of an I-message might be, "I am feeling sad because I am unable go to the concert." This I-message lets others know you are clearly upset without accusing or belittling anyone. I-messages can be less threatening to others and might encourage further communication.

Criticism

"It seems like someone is always finding something wrong with me. I'm always being picked on!" Almost everyone feels this way at some time or other. You may feel this way when someone criticizes you. To **criticize** means to make judgmental remarks without having sufficient knowledge.

A **critic** is a person who criticizes people, items, or events. A movie critic is paid to watch a movie and comment about its positive and negative points. A food critic comments on the food served in restaurants.

Some people become critics without being paid. They seem to have opinions about any and every subject. Maybe such people have criticized you inappropriately. How did that make you feel?

Some criticisms hurt more than others. If someone you care about criticizes you negatively, it may cause more pain than criticism from a casual friend. For instance, an older brother or sister may laugh at your haircut. This may make you feel worse than when someone you do not know makes a joke about your hair. You may not expect your relatives to be so critical of you. Other's criticism of you should not destroy your self-confidence.

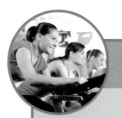

Types of Criticism

Criticism often uses negative comments to poke fun at a person. It makes you feel badly. This type of criticism is **destructive criticism**. Destructive criticism is not helpful.

Destructive criticism can hurt friendships and damage a person's self-esteem. A friend may use destructive criticism to make a hurtful remark about the way you look. The remark may affect the way you feel about your friend. You may resent your friend for saying something so mean. You may feel that he or she is not worthy of your friendship. Your friend's remark may also affect the way you feel about yourself. You may wonder if your friend was right. You may begin to think there *is* something strange about the way you look.

Destructive criticism may be a result of jealousy or resentment. People may be jealous if you have something they do not. Suppose you got a new jacket. When you wore it, your friend said she did not think it looked right on you. Maybe her criticism was because she was jealous. Perhaps she really liked the jacket and just wished she had one herself.

Some people use destructive criticism to make themselves look better. For instance, a friend who tells you your music solo is off-key may feel this makes his solo better.

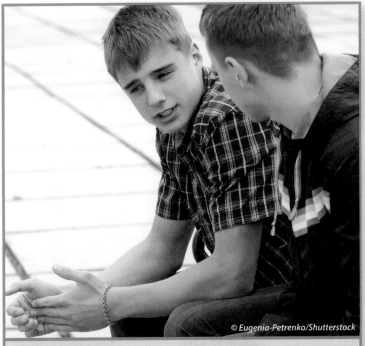

© Eugenia-Petrenko/Shutterstock

4-8 Constructive criticism from a friend can help you become a better person.

If you ask for an opinion, you may receive constructive criticism, **4-8**. **Constructive criticism** helps describe where or how a person could improve. You might ask a friend about the report you gave in class. He might say, "It was okay, but I noticed that you said *you know* a million times." Your friend gave you constructive criticism to help you do better next time. In another instance, you may ask a friend how she likes your new sweatshirt. She may tell you she thinks you would look better in another color. She has given you constructive criticism to help you look your best.

Handling Criticism

Both constructive and destructive criticism can hurt your feelings. Learning to handle criticism can help you manage your feelings and benefit from the criticism.

First, ask yourself who is doing the criticizing. A person who cares about you may give you constructive criticism to help you become a better person. An older friend, brother, or sister who warns you against the dangers of smoking may be trying to save you from an unhealthy addiction.

Decide if you asked for the criticism. If you ask a person's opinion, you may receive a positive comment, or you may receive criticism. If you ask for an opinion, be willing to accept it.

Be cautious of people who are too willing to criticize others. They may be criticizing because they are jealous or do not have a very high self-worth. They criticize others because it makes their weaknesses less obvious. Many times these people do not even realize they are doing this.

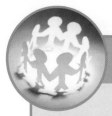

Life Connections

Giving Criticism

Ask yourself if you give criticism in a way you would like to receive it. Sometimes learning to give criticism well is harder than learning to accept it. You should try to give *constructive* criticism without hurting a person's feelings. This requires sensitivity and carefully chosen words.

Rather than just telling someone what is wrong, suggest how the person could improve or change. For instance, if you tell Jackson you do not like his shirt, Jackson has not learned anything that can help him. If you tell Jackson that he looks better in blue than red, however, then you have offered constructive criticism. Remember that he has the right to accept or reject your criticism.

Speaking Activity

Practice giving constructive criticism with a friend. Take turns defining a situation and then giving and receiving critical feedback. After giving criticism, ask your friend if there is a better way to phrase the critical feedback to promote learning. Then trade places so you are the person who hears the critical feedback and comments on its effectiveness. After doing this exercise several times, you both will know how it feels to give and receive constructive (versus destructive) criticism.

Listen carefully to criticism. Ask yourself what is being criticized. Do not feel you are not liked because you have been criticized. A teacher who criticizes your report is not criticizing you, only the report. A friend who criticizes your loud laughter does not dislike you personally—only your way of laughing.

If criticism can make you a better person, learn to accept your critics' remarks. Then try to change, or avoid making the same mistake. If you feel the criticism is unfair, then you may not need to take any action. If another person makes the same remark, though, maybe you should look at yourself again.

Differences

Communicating with someone who is very much like you can be easy. You share many of the same beliefs and opinions. Often, this is because you have had similar experiences. You may even have grown up in the same area.

Many people you meet, however, will have values, beliefs, and opinions different from yours. This may make it difficult for you to understand why they think and feel as they do. These differences can create barriers to good communication if you are not aware of them.

Stereotypes

One type of communication barrier that can arise from differences among people is stereotypes. A **stereotype** is a fixed belief that all members of a group are the same. People may base stereotypes on a group's sex, age, race, work, locality, culture, religion, or looks, **4-9**.

Stereotypes do not allow for individual differences. If people belong to certain groups, then some people believe they will behave in certain ways. For instance, some people believe stereotypes such as "girls like to cook" and "boys like sports."

As you can see, neither statement can be true for all people within these groups. Every person is different. Not all girls like to cook, nor do all boys like sports.

Stereotype attitudes can be hard to change. Stereotypes develop over a long period of time. They are sometimes learned from family members and sometimes from people outside the home. The media can also reinforce stereotypes.

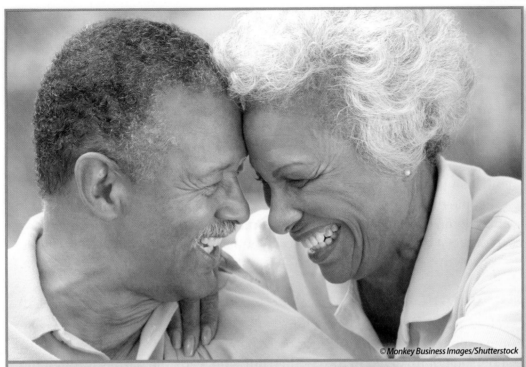

© Monkey Business Images/Shutterstock

4-9 Stereotypes about members of a group, such as older people, block communication.

Stereotypes are caused by a lack of understanding. They continue as long as people fail to see individual differences as valuable. Instead of forming opinions of people as members of a group, look at each person as an individual. Do not let stereotypes get in the way of open communication.

Prejudices

Another type of communication barrier that forms as a result of differences is prejudices. **Prejudices** are opinions people form without complete knowledge. They are not based on facts. Like stereotypes, prejudices often exist about certain groups of people.

Racism is an extreme type of prejudice. It is the belief that one culture or race is superior to another. People who are racists are called *bigots*. Bigots refuse to accept any group but their own. Racism can stir up violence and can hurt many people.

Social Studies Connections

Culture and Prejudices

Cultures in various regions of the world have differing norms and standards. Prejudices, which are often negative, usually come from a lack of knowledge about culture, people, or things that are different. Strong prejudices may cause people to avoid certain people or groups and prevent good communication from happening.

From religion to food to body language, cultures vary. For example, it may be considered rude to avoid eye contact in one culture, but considered inappropriate to hold eye contact in another. To break prejudices, create an information exchange. Learn by asking questions and discussing similarities and differences. You may discover that there is more in common than previously thought.

Learning about beliefs and customs that are new to you can help you understand the people who follow them. Know these differences exist and welcome them. Do not let them block the lines of communication.

Conflicts

Conflicts are disagreements or problems in a relationship. In spite of your best attempts at clear communication, conflicts are bound to happen. Family members and close friends will likely have conflicts because they are together so much of the time.

People think differently. They have different personalities, needs, and wants. Because of these differences, people will sometimes disagree with each other. When conflicts occur, how you handle them is most important to your growth.

Resolving Conflicts

Use a method of resolving conflicts that will result in positive feelings. Some people may have a mediator help them solve the problem. A **mediator** is a person not involved in the conflict, but who leads the parties through the steps of conflict resolution. The mediator uses negotiation to get both sides to come to an agreement.

Sometimes, the outcome of a conflict may disappoint the people involved. Even so, they find a way to solve their problem that is fair to all. In a **compromise**, both sides give up some of what they want in order to settle the conflict. For instance, you and a brother may be responsible for preparing the evening meal three nights a week. Neither of you, however, likes to set the table. You could compromise by deciding that you will set the table one night and he sets it the next. You might also decide to set it together.

Compromise is a very effective way to resolve conflicts. There are often several ways to reach a compromise. Finding the most agreeable one requires good communication skills.

To keep hurt feelings to a minimum, avoid angry yelling and physical violence. Choose methods for resolving conflicts that allow you to maintain positive self-concepts, **4-10**.

Find the right time to resolve conflicts. Discussing a problem when other people are around is not a good idea. Suppose you see your sister and her friends walking home from school. You notice she is wearing your sweater and this upsets you. If

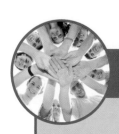

Community Connections

Communicate Clearly to Prevent Conflicts

Being able to communicate well will help you get along with people at home, at school, at work, and in your community. Poor communication is often the reason people get into disagreements. During an argument, one person may say, "You don't understand!" Both people may not have communicated their thoughts and feelings clearly. Even though your family members and friends love and care about you, they are not able to read your mind. You need to convey your thoughts and feelings clearly to prevent conflicts from occurring.

Steps to Resolving Conflicts

- **Voice your concerns.** The other person needs to know what is bothering you. Keeping silent does not resolve a conflict. Angry glares and slammed doors only cause ill will. After a problem is recognized, all concerned can discuss the issue calmly.
- **Decide what the problem is.** When discussing the problem, the facts become clear. Everyone can see where the disagreements lie. Stick to the problem at hand. State only the facts that relate to the current problem. Do not bring up past misdeeds.
- **Listen to the other side.** You need to listen to what the others involved in the conflict have to say. When resolving conflicts, it is important to try to view things from someone else's point of view. Respecting another point of view will go a long way toward resolving the conflict. After everyone has a chance to speak, you can begin finding a solution.
- **Suggest all possible solutions.** Evaluate the suggestions and choose the best one. Everyone must agree on how to make the solution work. All parties can then act on the solution.

4-10 These steps may help you resolve conflicts in positive ways.

you confront her in front of her friends, she may be embarrassed and become defensive. It would be better to wait until you get home to discuss the matter with her.

Avoid bringing up a conflict when people are busy with other activities. If your parents are getting dressed to go out, it is not a good time to discuss your curfew. You probably will not have much success. Wait until they have time to listen and can discuss the issue with you.

Deal with issues—not personalities. Name-calling is destructive. It causes hurt feelings and resentment. It does not resolve the conflict. In fact, it may make matters worse.

Do not allow a conflict to go on without being resolved. Constant arguing without solutions can hurt relationships. Identify the particular problem. Then find a solution that everyone can agree to before the issue is pushed aside.

Reading Review

1. Explain the difference between assertive communication, nonassertive communication, and aggressive communication.
2. Compare you-messages and I-messages.
3. How can learning how to handle criticism help you?
4. Explain the difference between stereotypes and prejudices.
5. List four steps for resolving conflicts.

Chapter Summary

Section 4-1. All forms of communication are either verbal or nonverbal. Verbal communication involves the use of words. Speaking and writing are verbal forms of communication. Nonverbal communication involves sending messages without the use of words. Your appearance, body language, use of personal space, and manners are examples of nonverbal communication. Communication is a two-way process. Sometimes you are the sender and sometimes you are the receiver. To receive messages clearly, it helps to be an active listener.

Section 4-2. A number of barriers can get in the way of the communication process. Sometimes people send mixed messages or allow others' differences to interfere with the lines of communication. You can use a number of methods to help you send clearer messages. Many conflicts arise as a result of poor communication. Improving your communication skills can help you resolve conflicts. Through communication, you can learn to handle conflict in a positive way. You can reach a compromise that is agreeable to all involved in the conflict.

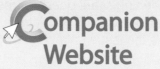

Companion Website
www.g-wlearning.com

Check your understanding of the main concepts for Chapter 4 at the website.

Critical Thinking

1. **Draw conclusions.** Give examples of how communication can have a positive or negative effect on people's lives. Discuss the advantages and disadvantages of communication.

2. **Identify.** If you could receive a message from one person in history, whom would it be from and what would it say?

3. **Recognize points of view.** Read some editorials in the newspaper. What message is the writer trying to convey? Do you agree or disagree with the writer?

4. **Analyzing behavior.** Sometimes it is more important to think about how you say something than what you actually say. The timing of a comment or the tone of your voice can have a lot to do with what a person might actually hear. Can you think of a time when someone might have completely misunderstood you because of how you said something? How did this make you feel? How do you think the other person felt?

Common Core

College and Career Readiness

5. **Writing.** Try to communicate a message to a classmate using only verbal communication. Then try to communicate a message using only nonverbal communication. Switch roles, having your partner send a verbal and a nonverbal message for you to receive. After completing this exercise, write a one-page report about your experience. Describe how easy or difficult it was to send and receive messages using only one type of communication.

6. **Speaking.** Role-play a situation in which a person sends mixed messages. Then discuss with the class how this situation created a barrier to communication. Discuss ways to improve communication in this situation.

7. **Writing.** Describe a problem that concerns the student body of your school. Using clear communication, write a letter to the school paper or website addressing the issue. Apply the steps of conflict resolution to the problem to offer a possible solution.

8. **Speaking.** Select a partner for a role-play. Plan a demonstration of how not to give and receive criticism. Then show how you should give and receive criticism. Present your role-play before the class.

Technology

9. **Website development.** Create a website that explains the steps people can take to resolve conflicts in positive ways. List the steps of conflict resolution and suggestions about how to implement them.

Journal Writing

10. Find a poem or song that you like. Write about what you believe the author was trying to communicate. How does the poem or song make you feel?

FCCLA

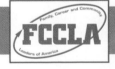

11. Analyze areas where you and your peers need strong communication skills in one of the following areas: community, employment, family, peer groups, or school groups. Create a case study that illustrates the issue and an oral presentation that addresses how specific communication skills can improve your relationships in one of the chosen areas. Submit your project in the *STAR Event, Interpersonal Communications* competition. See your adviser for more information about competitions.

Unit 2
Managing Your Life

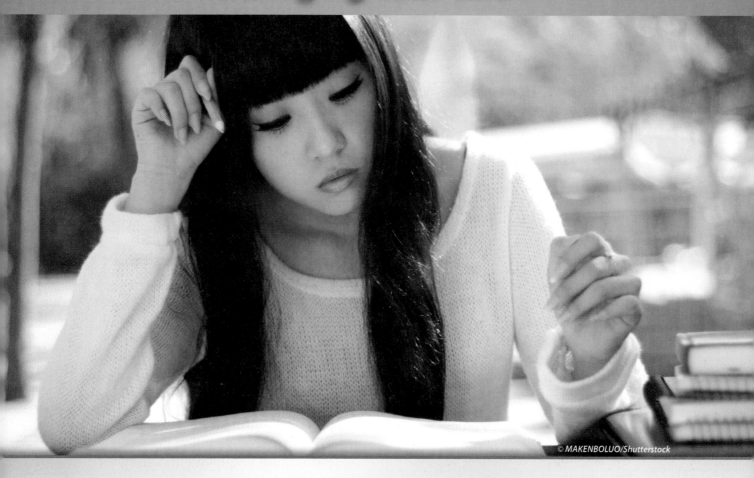

© MAKENBOLUO/Shutterstock

Unit Essential Question

What role can a life plan have in managing your daily life and planning for the future?

Exploring Career Pathways

Finance-Related Careers

Are you good at math? Do you like to analyze and solve complex problems involving numbers? Perhaps a career related to finance is for you. Here are some careers in this pathway many people enjoy.

Teller

Working quickly and accurately are essential skills for tellers. They conduct routine transactions such as cashing checks and making deposits, withdrawals, or loan payments for customers of a financial institution. A high school diploma and a background check are the main requirements for this career. Financial institutions provide on-the-job training for tellers. Tellers may work a variety of weekday and weekend hours due to customer demand.

Bookkeeping, Accounting, or Auditing Clerk

Detail-oriented, organized, trustworthy, a strong aptitude for numbers, and good communication skills—all describe the traits of bookkeeping, accounting, and auditing clerks. Responsible for maintaining accounting records, these clerks calculate expenditures and deal with accounts receivable and payable and profit and loss. Strong computer skills are necessary for calculating and recording data. Although some positions require a high school diploma, many require at least an associate's degree in accounting or business. Achieving the Certified Bookkeepers (CB) designation requires two years of bookkeeping experience, passing a rigorous four-part exam, and adherence to a strict code of ethics. Bookkeepers need regular continuing education.

Financial Analyst

Assessing the performance of various investments are key responsibilities of financial analysts. They also study a company's financial statements and other financial data to project the company's future earnings. There are two types of financial analysts. *Buy side analysts* work with companies that have a lot of money to invest. In contrast, *sell side analysts* help banks and other financial institutions sell investments such as stocks and bonds. Financial analysts must have strong math, analytical, and communication skills. Maturity and self-confidence are key traits. A bachelor's degree is a minimum for this career. Many employers, however, require a master's degree in finance or a Master's in Business Administration (MBA). The Financial Regulatory Authority (FINRA) licenses financial analysts. Licensing may vary depending on the type of work.

Is this career path for you? Pursue one or both of the following activities to determine if you are suitable for a career in finance.

- Use reliable Internet resources, such as the *Bureau of Labor Statistics*, to conduct an in-depth study of one or more finance-related careers. What does this job profile look like now? How might it change in the next five to ten years? What personal traits do you have that make you suitable for this career?
- Talk with your school guidance counselor about post-secondary schools that offer finance-related degrees. Investigate the courses these schools offer. How are the courses similar and different among the schools? Write a summary of your findings.

Chapter 5
Getting Ready to Manage

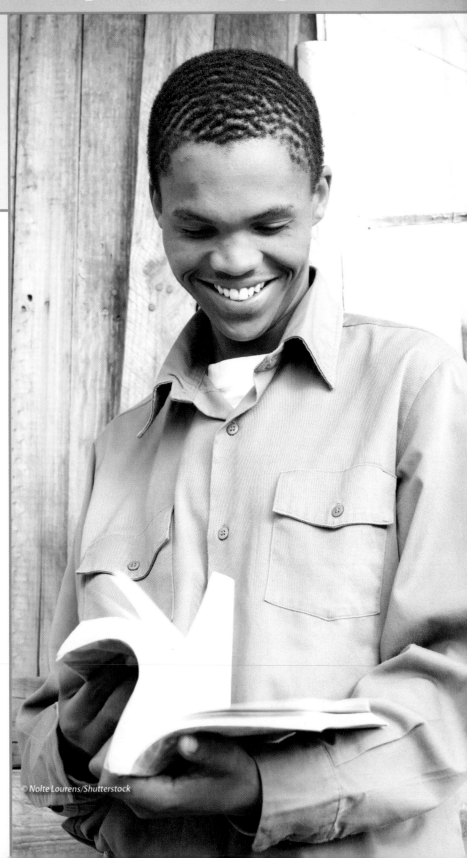

© Nolte Lourens/Shutterstock

Sections

● Reading Prep

College and Career Readiness

Before you read the chapter, read all of the table and photo captions. What do you know about the material covered in this chapter just from reading the captions?

Concept Organizer

Planning Process

Use a diagram like the one shown to list the five steps of the FCCLA planning process in order.

Companion Website

Print out the concept organizer for Chapter 5 at the website.

Companion Website
www.g-wlearning.com

Section 5-1

Needs versus Wants

Objectives

After studying this section, you will be able to
- **differentiate** between wants and needs.
- **give examples** of physical and psychological needs.
- **describe** how a person can achieve self-actualization.

Key Terms		
needs	physical needs	self-actualization
wants	psychological needs	

Your needs and wants affect your behavior every day. They affect what you do with your time and money. They even influence how you get along with others. The way you meet your needs is unique, just as you are unique.

Maslow's Hierarchy of Human Needs

People often confuse the words *needs* and *wants*. Your needs and wants, however, are entirely different. **Needs** are basic items you must have to live. Food is an example of a basic human need. The need to feel love and acceptance is another. **Wants** are items you would like to have, but do not need. You might want a new video game system, a new cell phone, or a pet, but these items are usually not needs.

Abraham Maslow, a noted psychologist, created a theory of human needs. He believed that a person's development is a result of meeting individual needs, **5-1**.

Maslow separates the basic human needs into four groups. The first group consists of the *physical needs* people must meet. The next three groups include basic *psychological needs*. The last level in the hierarchy is for higher-level needs, which Maslow refers to as *self-actualization needs*.

Physical Needs

Physical needs are your most basic needs. You must meet these needs in order to stay alive. Physical needs include food, water, clothing, shelter, and sleep. According to Maslow, you must first meet your physical needs before you can work on any of your other needs and wants.

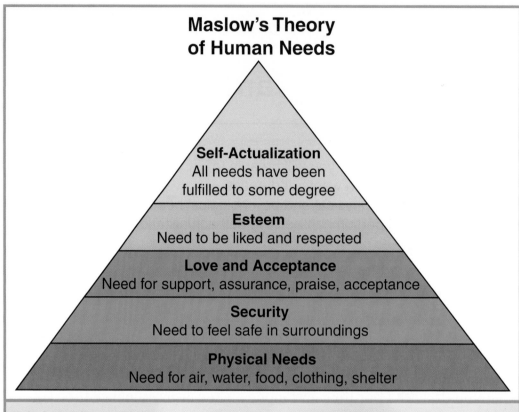

Maslow's Theory of Human Needs

Self-Actualization
All needs have been
fulfilled to some degree

Esteem
Need to be liked and respected

Love and Acceptance
Need for support, assurance, praise, acceptance

Security
Need to feel safe in surroundings

Physical Needs
Need for air, water, food, clothing, shelter

5-1 According to Maslow, everyone works to fulfill basic human needs as well as higher-level needs.

All people need *food* to survive. What you want to eat, however, may differ greatly from what you need to eat, **5-2**. You may want a bag of corn chips, ice cream bar, and soda for lunch. A sandwich, salad, piece of fruit, and glass of low-fat milk would be a more healthful choice, however. These items would satisfy your hunger just as well, too. Eating a variety of nutritious foods will satisfy your body's need for food.

Water is also essential to life. Your body needs plenty of water to function properly. You get water from eating many foods as well as by drinking it in beverages.

Everyone needs some type of *clothing*. The amount and types of clothing you need, however, depend somewhat on where you live. If you live in southern California, your clothing needs will differ from those of someone who lives in Michigan. When you live in a warmer climate, you will probably want to choose fabrics and styles to keep you cool.

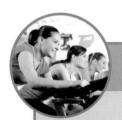

Health Connections

Getting Plenty of Sleep

Lack of sleep at night may cause you to be irritable the next day. You probably know how much sleep you need each night, but have you ever stayed up late to chat with your friends on the computer or watch a television show? If you did, you may not have realized it, but your next day in school was not as productive as it could be. You may have had trouble concentrating on your work. When you tried to listen to your coach, you could only think of how tired you were. Interfering with your body's time clock causes consequences for you physically. (You did not meet your physical need for sleep.) You need plenty of sleep to continue your active life.

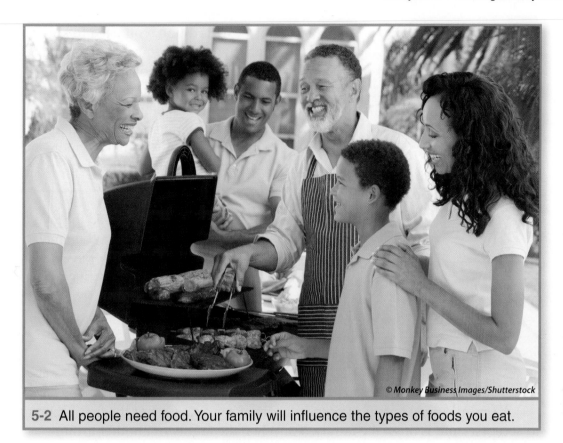
© Monkey Business Images/Shutterstock

5-2 All people need food. Your family will influence the types of foods you eat.

A person in Minnesota, however, will also need fabrics and styles that provide warmth in a cooler climate.

You need *shelter* to protect your body from the environment. In the past, people used caves, covered wagons, and tents as places to live. All these met the basic need for shelter. Today, your family can select from many types of shelter. You might live in a house, apartment, condominium, town house, or mobile home. The type of home you live in is not important as long as it meets your basic need for shelter.

Sleep is another physical need common to all people. The amount of sleep people need varies. You may need less sleep than your younger brother or sister, but more sleep than your parents.

Psychological Needs

Psychological needs are the needs related to your mind and feelings. People need to meet these needs in order to live a satisfying life. According to Maslow, your psychological needs include the need to feel safe and secure and the need to feel love and acceptance. Another psychological need is for esteem, or the need to have self-respect and the respect of others.

Safety and Security

People need to feel safe and free from fear. You need to feel safe from anything that could harm you as you go about your daily activities. This feeling will help you relax and put you at ease. Feeling safe will help you grow and develop into a mature, healthy person.

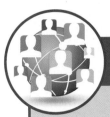

Social Studies Connections

Feeling Accepted

Many young children do not understand acceptance. When they misbehave or fight with other children, their parents may become annoyed. Young children often feel rejected when people are annoyed with them. Children do not understand that a person is only rejecting the action. The child is still accepted.

Even people your own age may feel rejected when they should not. When you bring home a good report card, you feel acceptance and approval. If your grades are not so good, you might feel rejected. Try not to feel this way. Your family is only expressing how they feel about your grades, which reflect your actions. They still accept you.

In addition, you need to know that your important possessions are safe and where you can reach them. Your home should be a safe place to keep your belongings. You can lock your home or have an alarm system, which will make it more difficult for intruders to break in.

Love and Acceptance

People of all ages need the love of others. Without love, a child may not develop normally. People who lack love in their lives may have poor relationships with others. They may not feel worthwhile or accepted by others. On the other hand, people who experience love often have a better sense of security. They may also have a more positive outlook on life.

All people need to feel accepted as part of a group. One of the first groups to accept a child is often the family, **5-3**. When the family or another group accepts you, they take you just as you are.

Your friends are another important group of people who accept you. Friends accept you as you are without trying to change you. Relationships like this with people your own age are important. You may have more or fewer friends than other people you know. That is fine. No one can tell you how many friends you should have. The acceptance of your friends, however, fulfills an important psychological need.

People also need acceptance in social situations. You know how to get along with others. Good manners are important in social situations. You must be polite and respect others for them to treat you well in return. Acceptance in social situations by both your peers and adults can make you feel more comfortable and secure.

© Liunian/Shutterstock

5-3 Family members need to feel accepted and loved by each other. Spending time together gives everyone a good feeling.

Esteem

Esteem needs relate to your feelings of respect. You need to have respect for yourself and the respect of others. People need to feel they are worthwhile and that others think so, too. If you always try to do your best, you probably feel worthwhile and have self-respect.

When you have self-respect, other people might also think of you with higher regard. Having pride in what you do lets other people recognize your accomplishments. They begin to have respect and esteem for you.

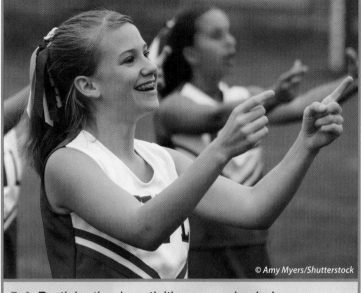

© Amy Myers/Shutterstock

5-4 Participating in activities you enjoy helps you develop a healthy sense of self.

The need to have self-respect and the respect of others is a basic need, **5-4**. This need is satisfied when you behave in a way that you and the people around you accept.

Everybody has the same important psychological needs. Like you, they act in a way that will satisfy their psychological needs. When you meet your psychological needs, you often become more secure and happy with your life.

Self-Actualization Needs

According to Maslow, you must be able to partially fulfill all your basic needs before trying to meet higher-level needs. By the time you reach this level, you have developed an understanding and appreciation for yourself and for others. You are concerned about society as a whole.

Self-actualization is to fully realize your own potential. Achieving self-actualization is a lifelong process. This means you are always trying to improve yourself and be the best person you can be.

Developing new skills and talents, engaging in new hobbies, and becoming more educated about the world around you can help you meet some of your needs for personal growth and self-fulfillment.

Your Wants

While your needs must be met for your growth and development, wants are what you desire. You may think that having your wants met will give you more satisfaction. Everyone has the same basic needs, but each person has different wants.

Each day exposes you to many factors that can make you want something. Sometimes you want to have something because a friend has it. Advertisements can also make you want to buy products. You may want items you see in attractive store displays at the mall, **5-5**. These factors can cause you to become confused about what your needs and wants really are.

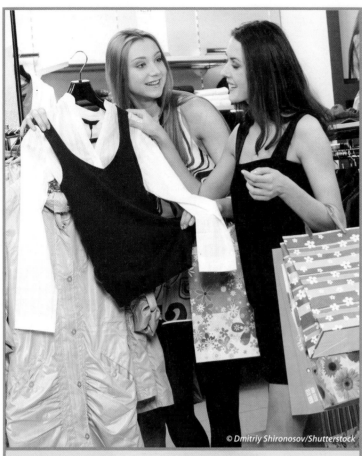

© Dmitriy Shironosov/Shutterstock

5-5 When shopping, it is very easy to confuse needs and wants.

Sometimes wants become so strong you convince yourself they are needs. Suppose you have a cell phone that works, but a new one has just been introduced in the market. You may think you need the new model in the store that has expanded features. Remember that a newer cell phone is not something you must have to live or communicate effectively. It is something that makes your life more satisfying. A cell phone is a want.

Clothing is one item that can be both a need and a want. Of course, you need clothing to cover your body and keep you comfortable. A sweater or sweatshirt satisfies this need in chilly weather. You may decide, however, that you want several sweaters in various colors. You also need shoes to cover your feet, but you may want several styles to go with different outfits.

Throughout life, you will have many wants that do not relate to buying something. You might want to go to the beach next weekend. Maybe you want to go to the basketball game with your friends on Wednesday night. You also want to do well in school.

Most people have many more wants than they could ever satisfy. You must ask yourself which of your wants are most important. Then you can try to satisfy those.

Reading Review

1. True or false. Your needs and wants affect your behavior every day.
2. How can you tell the difference between your needs and wants?
3. According to Maslow, what are the four groups of basic human needs?
4. What is self-actualization?
5. How can you meet some of your needs for personal growth and self-fulfillment?

Your Values and Goals

Objectives

After studying this section, you will be able to
- **identify** the values that are most important to you.
- **discuss** how people's behavior shows their character and ethics to others.
- **distinguish** between short- and long-term goals.
- **explain** how your values and goals affect your standards.

Key Terms

values	goals	priority
character	short-term goals	standards
ethics	long-term goals	

Values help you determine what is right or wrong, important or unimportant. They are the guidelines for how you live your life. Your values affect everything you think, do, or say. They influence the goals and standards you set for yourself. What you decide to do the rest of your life will be a result of your values.

Values

Values are the beliefs, feelings, and experiences you consider important. Do you know where you get your values? Unlike your clothes and your food, you cannot buy values. You learn them. You learned your first values at home. Perhaps your relatives have always celebrated holidays together. If so, you probably value family togetherness. Love, honesty, health, money, religion, or education may be other values you have learned, **5-6**.

Many of the values you learned as a child will stay with you throughout life. When you were a young child, your parents

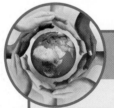

Global Connections

Culture and Values

Different cultures often have different values, which may cause people to plan their lives differently. For instance, in some cultures, education is a primary value. Some other cultures view family as the primary value—even though education is important. No culture's values are right or wrong, they simply may be different. You will not always agree with another person's values. Learning to respect other people's values is important, however. This means that you can have your values and they can have theirs.

Think about your own values. Some of your values are likely to be more important than others. Does your family's cultural heritage affect your values? Ultimately, you are the one who decides and ranks your values.

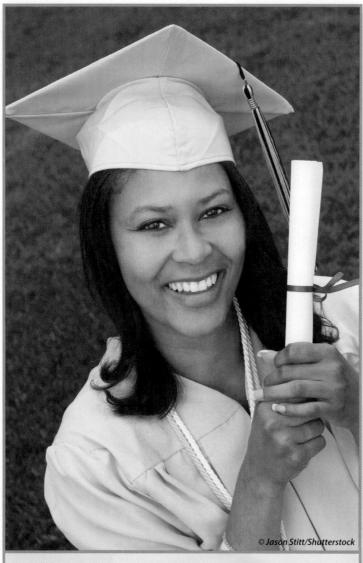

© Jason Stitt/Shutterstock

5-6 Education is a value that many individuals and families share.

may have taught you to put your toys away when you finished playing. Neatness was a value for them. They passed this value on to you. Because of your parents, you prefer to keep your room neat.

As you got older, you also learned values from your school activities and your peer group. If honesty is very important to your best friend, it might also be very important to you. Then you would never consider cheating on a test. Good grades, friendships, and popularity may also be important to you.

Although you and your friends share some of the same values, you also have some that are different. Your friends may prefer to go to the pool, while you would rather spend time with a relative who is visiting. Neither you nor your friends are wrong. You just have different values, **5-7**.

Your community or society helps you form some of your values. A group that collects food for people in need expresses caring for others. If you donate to this cause, you are showing that caring for others is one of your values, too.

What Do You Value?		
Adventure	Health	Pleasure
Appearance	Honesty	Popularity
Comfort	Humor	Power
Education	Independence	Recognition
Family	Intelligence	Religion
Friends	Love	Security
Happiness	Money	Trust

5-7 A variety of values are shown here. Which values would you add to this list?

What you read online or in the newspaper, see on television, or hear on the radio also influences some of your values. Hearing about many unemployed people in your community or state might affect your values. You may feel that making good grades could increase your chances of getting a good job when you finish school. This knowledge of unemployment could make studying a higher value for you.

Your experiences also affect your values. Some personal experiences strengthen your values. If you were burned by a hot pan as a young child, safety probably became important to you. From then on, you probably used a pot holder to avoid being burned. Safety is one of your strong values.

Experiences within a family often change your values. For instance, money is very important to some families. When both parents in a family have high-paying jobs, they may be able to afford to spend money on possessions and activities. If one parent decides to quit his or her job, the family's values might change. They may not be able to spend as much money as they once did. Without extra money to spend, the family might begin to spend time together. Family togetherness could become more important than spending money. You may have had experiences like this that changed your own values.

Character

Character is a description of a person's good qualities, which often include moral strength, honesty, and fairness. Your character helps you decide right from wrong, and then choose what is right. It helps you make choices that support your values. The strong beliefs about what is morally right and wrong that guide your behavior are called **ethics**. The way you behave shows your character and ethics to others.

Like values, character development often begins at home. Parents teach their young children which behaviors are acceptable and which are not. Children then follow these guidelines to receive the approval and praise of their parents. As children grow older, friends and society become more of an influence in deciding what is acceptable and unacceptable.

Throughout life, you will continue to meet many new people who may influence you and help you to build character. You will also face many new situations. How you respond to each of these situations will reveal your character to others.

Goals

Goals are what you endeavor to do or achieve. They provide direction in your life. Your goals are based on your values. If you value a healthful lifestyle, your goals may be to eat well, be physically active, and get plenty of sleep. If you value adventure, one of your goals may be to sail around the world someday.

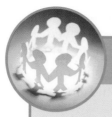

Life Connections

Setting Goals

Before you begin to set goals, you will want to know yourself. What do you want out of life? What type of person are you? What activities and subjects do you enjoy most? What are your values? The way you answer these questions will affect the goals you set.

How will you reach your goals? After you have decided on your goals, you must make plans for reaching them. Begin working on your goals right away. If you do not start working on them, you will have a more difficult time reaching them.

Whenever you reach a goal, try to set a new one. You will need to have goals throughout life. They give your life direction and purpose.

Writing Activity

How would you answer the questions posed in this feature? Write your responses to the questions in your journal. Try setting a realistic goal and think of the changes you need to make to meet that goal. Make a plan and try sticking to it. Be patient, it might not be easy, but sticking to your plan can help you meet that goal.

Types of Goals

There are two types of goals. **Short-term goals** are what you hope to achieve in the near future. They might take hours, days, or weeks. **Long-term goals** are major accomplishments you are trying to achieve. They may take many months, a year, or many years to reach. The goal to have a party for a friend is a short-term goal. The goal to run your family's business is a long-term goal.

Your long-term goal might be to become a journalist, 5-8. You could achieve this goal in several years. In the meantime, you can deliver newspapers in town. This will meet your short-term goal of earning money. You might meet some people from the newspaper company. You might even be able to work for the newspaper during the summer while you attend college. Your short-term goals and experiences will help you reach your long-term goal.

Many of your short-term goals do not relate to your long-term goals. For instance, your goal to buy a new outfit for the Valentine's Day dance will not bring you any closer to your long-term goal of becoming a fashion designer. Your goal to save enough money to buy a new tennis racket will not help you reach your goal of taking a trip to Europe.

You will probably find that specific short-term goals are better than goals that are broad. A goal to lose 10 pounds by the end of the school year is better than just a goal to lose 10 pounds. You will work harder when you have set a deadline for yourself.

Your long-term goals, however, are a little different. As you learn and grow through your life experiences, you may find that some of your goals change. This is perfectly normal. Because of this, you might want to select a broad area of interest as your long-term goal. Then you will not be limiting your options. For instance, do you think you would like a career in athletics? You may want to look at several areas. There are many careers in athletics besides being a professional athlete. Coaches, managers, trainers, sportscasters, and sportswriters are all involved with sports. You may need some experience in several fields before you make a final decision in choosing a specific goal.

Priorities

A **priority** is what is most important to you. Setting priorities based on values can help you decide how to reach your goals. Making a list will help you accomplish the necessary tasks first. When these are finished, you might have extra time to do other activities. Setting your priorities will help you make the best decision.

Whenever you have too many goals, just stop and decide what is most important. Learning to rank your goals in the order of importance can add order to your life. You can gain a sense of where you are going and what you plan to do.

Set Challenging Goals

Have you ever heard of a *sure thing*, or something you know will happen? Some people set their goals on sure things. They want to be safe. They know they can reach these goals. Maybe you always get straight *A's* in biology. Then one day, your teacher asks you to set a goal you want to reach. You set a goal of passing biology. This is a sure thing.

Some people set all their goals like your goal to pass math. Although these goals are easy to reach, they are never very exciting or challenging. People who set easy goals may give up too

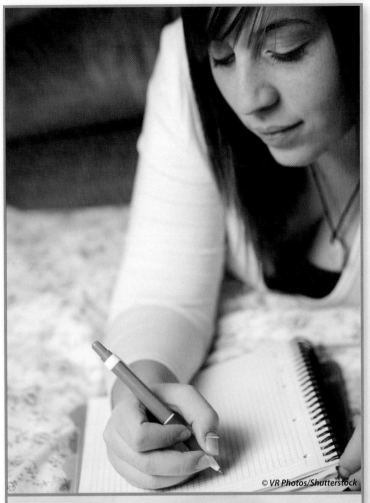

© VR Photos/Shutterstock

5-8 Now is the best time to think about your goals for the future. You may want to put these goals in writing.

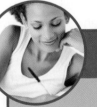

Writing Connections

Creating a Priority List

Have you ever had so many goals that you simply could not begin to work on any of them? You might have short-term goals to learn the lines for your role in a school play, practice your instrument, or clean your computer desktop. You could not meet all these goals at once. You would have to decide which goal needs immediate attention.

One way to determine which task to do first is to create a chronological list, or a list of goals written in order of the date it is due. Once you have the list, it can provide you with a sense of direction. You can also rearrange priorities. As you accomplish goals, you gain the satisfaction of watching your list grow smaller.

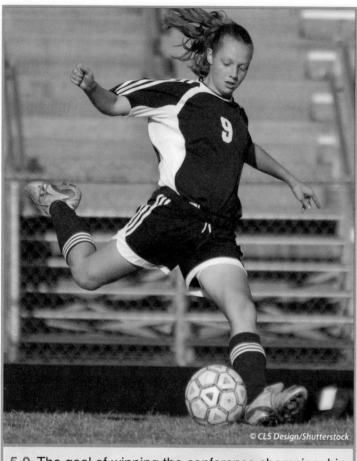

5-9 The goal of winning the conference championship in soccer is a challenging one.

© CLS Design/Shutterstock

soon when they face a difficult goal. Most people enjoy a little challenge. In fact, some people accomplish more when their goals are really challenging.

Think about your own goals. Are they sure things, or will you have to work at them? If you challenge yourself with exciting goals, you might have an easier time achieving goals that are more difficult in the future, 5-9.

Standards

Once you have begun to reach your goals, your standards become important. **Standards** are the way you measure what you have done. You learn your standards from your family, your friends, and other people around you.

Standards are a part of your daily life as a student. Schools have educational standards. You must earn a certain number of credits or units to graduate. Your teachers have standards for evaluating your work in class. They probably expect you to participate in class, complete assignments, and score well on tests.

You also set standards for yourself related to what you do in school. After a test, one of your friends may ask how well you did. You might say that you got a good grade. To some students, a good grade may be anything above passing. To others, a good grade is a *C*. To you, a good grade might mean an *A*.

People may set their standards at different levels. Sometimes these differences cause conflicts. This could happen if your parents asked you to clean your room. They might have a different standard of cleanliness than you do. Your standard of cleanliness might mean that everything is off the floor. Your parents' standard of cleanliness may also include sweeping the floor, dusting the furniture, and changing the sheets.

Reading Review

1. What are values?
2. List three sources of values.
3. What is character?
4. Distinguish between short-term goals and long-term goals.
5. To measure whether you have reached your goals, you use _____.

Your Resources

Objectives

After studying this section, you will be able to
- **identify** your human and nonhuman resources.
- **describe** the ways you can use your resources.
- **determine** how you can develop your resources.

Key Terms

resource	human resources	nonhuman resources

There are many sources available to help you reach your goals. Some of these sources come from within you. They are part of you and are yours alone. Other sources are objects you may own, or items from your environment. When you begin to understand all the ways you can use these sources, you will be better able to manage them.

Types of Resources

Anything that can help you reach a goal is a **resource**. For instance, your endurance and ability to run quickly are resources that can help you reach the goal of winning a race. You may have never thought about all the resources available to you. These resources can be either human or nonhuman.

Human Resources

Resources that come from within yourself or from your relationships with other people are **human resources**. They are also called *personal resources*. Your skills and talents are human resources. Other human resources include knowledge, creativity, time, and energy.

Life Connections

Recognizing Your Resources

Maybe math is a stronger subject for your friend than it is for you. Perhaps you could ask your friend to help you study together throughout the term. Your friend is a resource for knowledge about math. Your teachers are also important resources. They share their knowledge and skills with you each day. Talking with them may help you solve problems.

Your family members may also be valuable resources. They love you, care for you, and help you when needed. They are there for you when you have challenges to solve and when you need to talk with someone. They may help you fix your bike or pick you up after band practice.

Writing Activity

Write a list of every external resource in your life. If you spend some time really thinking about all the people and assets you have in the many different areas of your life, you likely have many more than you first thought.

Friends, family, and other people are also valuable human resources, **5-10**. They can help you achieve goals and manage your life. These people can combine their own resources with yours to reach a goal.

Time is a human resource that is limited to 24 hours each day. Everyone has an equal number of hours in a day. You must decide the best way to use those hours. Young people have the freedom to spend many of these hours as they wish. How do you use your free time? Do you develop new skills? Do you spend all your time watching television? Having fun is important, but you also need to spend time learning and growing.

Your energy is an important human resource. The amount of energy you have varies throughout the day. Your age, what you eat, how long you sleep, and what you do each day affects your energy level. You probably have more energy at a certain time of the day. Some people do their best work in the morning while others do their best at night.

Nonhuman Resources

Nonhuman resources include money, community resources, and possessions. Although everyone has some of these resources, different people have different amounts. Making wise use of your nonhuman resources can help you reach your goals.

People use money to buy goods and services. You may need money to buy your friend a birthday gift or to go bowling. This money may come from your allowance, a paper route, or a babysitting job. Teens usually have a small amount of money and limited ways of making money.

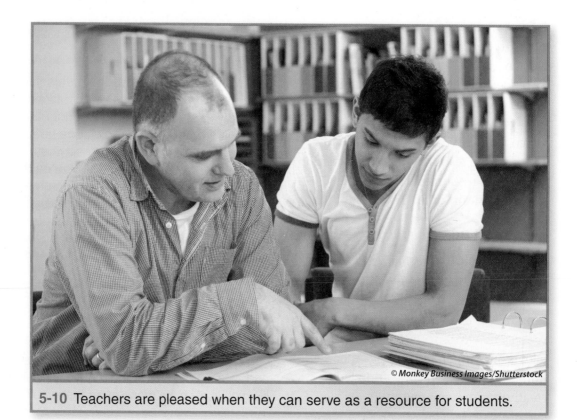

© Monkey Business Images/Shutterstock

5-10 Teachers are pleased when they can serve as a resource for students.

As you get older, you will have the chance to make more money. You will spend your money in different ways. You may begin to save money for special goals, such as your education or a car. Money is an important resource to people of all ages.

Community resources are all around you. Many people share them. Schools, libraries, stores, theaters, parks, zoos, and museums are all community resources, **5-11**. Your school is a resource for knowledge. You can use the library to borrow books instead of buying them. Using your community resources can be both fun and educational.

Your *possessions* are another nonhuman resource. Possessions include anything you own. Clothing is just one example of a typical possession. Many possessions belong to more than one person. For instance, you may share a TV or computer with other family members.

Using Your Resources

You will be able to manage your resources better when you understand all the ways you can use them. You may choose to use a resource alone or to combine it with another resource. You can often combine human and nonhuman resources to get better results. Combining the computer with your skill to write well can help you finish a book report quickly. You can share your resources with others or exchange them. You can substitute one resource for another. You may use some resources to produce other resources.

You may use the same resource for different purposes at different times. One day you might use your free time at school to complete your homework. Another day you might use that time to talk with friends.

Sharing Resources

You share many of your resources, especially with your family, **5-12**. Family members take turns using cooking supplies and appliances. Everyone in the family shares other resources all the time, such as living space and furniture. You also share your skills and attitudes with each other every day.

A good example of shared human resources is a band. Each person shares musical talent with the group. Everyone enjoys this sharing.

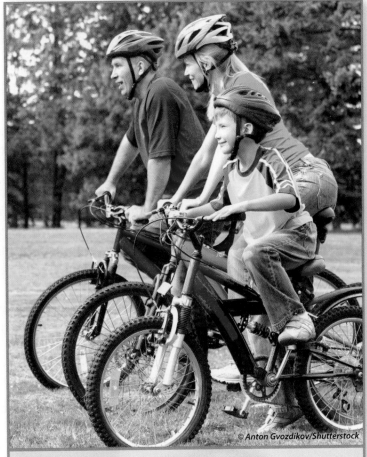

© Anton Gvozdikov/Shutterstock

5-11 A city park is a community resource shared by members of that community.

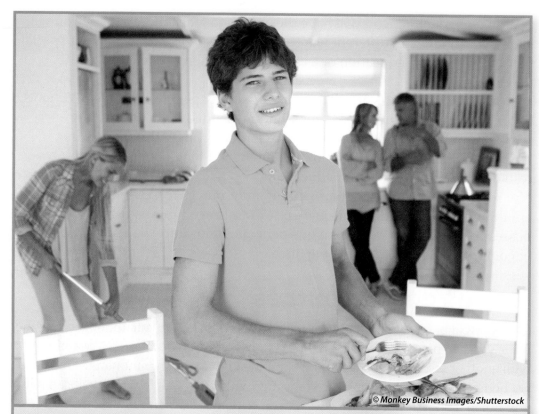

© Monkey Business Images/Shutterstock

5-12 Family members share many resources when cooking or cleaning a kitchen together.

When band members share resources, the band's sound improves and everyone feels satisfied.

People also share community resources. Many people use the banks, stores, zoos, and libraries in your community.

Exchanging Resources

Money is one resource people often exchange. When you buy frozen yogurt, you are exchanging your money (one resource) for food (another resource). Consumers exchange their money for goods and services every day. If you have a car washing and detailing job, you are exchanging your time and skills for money.

People can also exchange human resources. You might agree to teach a friend to ice skate if she teaches you to play tennis. You would be exchanging your skills as resources.

Substituting One Resource for Another

If you have very little of one resource, you may be able to use another resource in its place. If you do not have the money to buy a pair of sweatpants, you might be able to use your sewing skills to make a pair. If you do not have a natural talent for something, you can substitute time and energy so you can learn, 5-13.

Using Resources to Produce Other Resources

You can use some of your resources to produce others. For instance, you may have the ability to play the piano. Having this musical resource might make it easier for you to learn to play other musical instruments, too. Your musical resource could help you get into a band. By playing at parties, your musical resource could produce the resource of money.

Maybe you have good personal qualities as a resource. You are friendly, trustworthy, and eager to help others. Resources like these could produce a new resource—friends.

Developing Resources

You can develop your resources to help you reach more goals. For instance, you can develop your knowledge by taking more classes, reading books, or even talking with other people. You can develop your skills and talents by practicing skills you already have. You can also develop new interests.

People choose to develop their resources differently. Your needs and wants can influence how you decide to develop your resources. Think about what you can do to develop the resources you already have. You might even discover other special talents as you work on developing your resources.

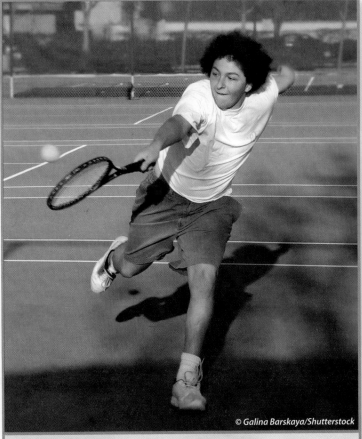

© Galina Barskaya/Shutterstock

5-13 Being willing to learn and practice hard can help you develop skills.

Reading Review

1. What is a resource?
2. Distinguish between human resources and nonhuman resources.
3. Give three examples of how you use your resources.
4. Give three examples of how you can develop your resources.

Management and Decision Making

Objectives

After studying this section, you will be able to

- **describe** the steps of the management process.
- **give examples** of decisions you can make using the decision-making process.
- **demonstrate** how to use the FCCLA planning process to solve a problem or reach a goal.
- **discuss** the importance of accepting the consequences of your decisions.

Key Terms		
management	decision	trade-off
management process	decision-making	FCCLA planning
implement	process	process
evaluate	alternatives	consequences

When you manage, you work to get something done in the best possible way. Making decisions is an important part of management. Good managers understand decision-making and planning processes. They know themselves well enough to make the decisions that are right for them.

The Management Process

Management is using your resources to reach a goal. Reaching goals can be difficult sometimes. You might set a goal for yourself, but you may not be sure about how to achieve it. The **management process** is a method used to achieve a goal using available resources. The steps in the management process include setting a goal, making a plan, implementing the plan, and evaluating it.

Setting a Goal

The first step in the management process is to identify and set the goal. You are more likely to set a realistic goal when you carefully consider your needs, values, and resources, **5-14**. To be successful, be sure to consider your priorities and try to focus on one goal at a time.

For instance, Deon is having difficulty in his science class and was disappointed when he received a *C* on his last test. He needs to maintain good grades to get into college. Deon has another big science test in a month. Therefore, he has set a goal to earn an *A* on the test.

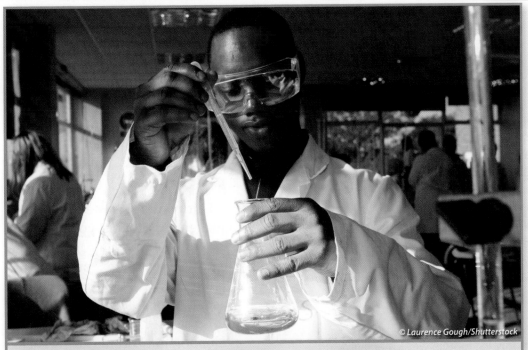

5-14 If one of your values is education, you will try to work hard and get good grades in your classes.

Making a Plan

The second step in the management process is to plan how to achieve the goal. First, you need to determine what you must do to reach the goal. Consider what you need to do and what resources you will be able to use. When you decide which actions to take, you can then organize the plan.

Deon determined that he could use both human and nonhuman resources to reach his goal. These resources included his science teacher, focused time, the local library, and his computer.

Deon developed a plan to talk with his science teacher about finding a tutor who could help him study. He rearranged his schedule to do some activities in the morning. This would give him more time each afternoon to work on his homework. He set up a plan to study at the local library so he would have fewer distractions than at home. Deon recorded the plan on his computer and set up a schedule to check his progress.

Implementing the Plan

After you make a plan, you are then ready to **implement**, or carry out, your plan. Be sure to regularly check your progress. If you realize something is not working, you can always adjust your plan or you can determine a new goal.

Deon put his plan into action. He got several names of possible tutors from his science teacher. He talked with each of them and then chose the one he felt could help him the most. Deon arranged to meet his tutor at the library one day a week after school. He used his computer to set up all his appointments on a calendar.

Life Connections

Multitasking

Students often have very busy schedules. Sometimes, priorities will conflict with one another, which can be overwhelming. A valuable skill to have in tackling a long priority list is the ability to *multitask*, or working on more than one task at a time. For instance, if you need to prepare dinner, read a chapter for class, and go to practice, you can read during practice breaks and while waiting for dinner to bake. You might also eat while you read. Although you could not have done all three things at the same time, multitasking allows you to work on two or more things at once, which can save you time.

Writing Activity

Create a priority list for this week's activities, practices, and assignments. After ranking which projects to work on first, review your list to see if any of these activities can be combined. Using the management process, write a plan of action, implement your strategy, and evaluate the effectiveness of your strategies.

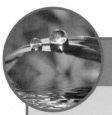

Go Green

Green Decisions

Managing your resources is an important part of making decisions. Many decisions concerning your resources affect your daily life. They relate to your food, clothing, and relationships with family and friends. Your values about the environment affect how you decide. For instance, when going to the mall with friends, you may decide to take public transportation instead of driving. You may decide to eat at a café that serves locally grown organic food instead of a fast-food restaurant serving food in nonrecyclable packaging. Some decisions may be greener than others; it is good to know the difference.

After a week, Deon checked his progress. Even though he studied more on his own, he was still having difficulty understanding the material. Deon realized that he needed to adjust his plan. Therefore, he changed his plan so he could meet with his tutor two days a week.

Evaluating the Plan

During the final step of the management process, you evaluate your plan. **Evaluate** means to judge the value of the plan. You do not need to wait until your plan is finished to evaluate it, however. As you can see by Deon's example, evaluation may occur during each step of the management process.

When you are setting a goal, you must evaluate it to decide if it is realistic. When you make your plan and implement it, you evaluate your resources and check your progress to determine if it is working. After you finish your plan, you should evaluate it again to decide if you would want to do anything differently next time.

Making Decisions

You have already learned about your needs, wants, values, goals, and standards. You also know how to use the management process and your resources to help you reach your goals. Now you are ready to move on to another part of management—learning to make decisions.

A **decision** is a choice. It is making up your mind about what you will do or say. Your values, goals, standards, needs, and wants all affect your decisions. If you value honesty, you will decide to always tell the truth. If buying a pet is one of your goals, you may decide to become a lifeguard to earn the money you need. If your grades do not meet your standards, you may decide to spend more time studying. If your body needs food, you will have to decide what foods to eat. If you want a new gaming system, you will decide how to earn money to afford it.

The Decision-Making Process

The **decision-making process** is a step-by-step approach to help you make a decision, reach a goal, or solve a problem, **5-15**. Whether your decisions are simple or complex, you can use the decision-making process to help you make decisions.

You can also use the decision-making process for problem solving. Suppose your aunt from out of state is coming to visit for the weekend, but you have already made plans to go camping with your friend. To use the problem-solving process, first consider your **alternatives**, or options.

You may need to make a trade-off. A **trade-off** is an exchange of one thing in return for another. You can go camping, but you will miss your aunt's visit and not get to see your aunt again for a long time. If you stay home, you will get to see your aunt. It may not be as much fun as camping, however, and you may disappoint your friend by changing your plans.

You must choose the best alternative for you. If you choose to visit with your aunt, evaluate whether it was a good decision. Are you glad you stayed, or are you sorry you missed the camping trip? Either way, you made a decision and learned from the process.

The FCCLA Planning Process

Family, Career and Community Leaders of America (FCCLA) is a career and technical student organization for family and consumer sciences

---

The Decision-Making Process

1. **State the decision to be made.** Some decisions involve just making a choice. Others also involve solving a problem. Be sure you understand what needs to be done. The best way to do this is to state your decision or problem as a goal. That is a positive approach to making decisions.

2. **List all possible alternatives.** Your alternatives are the possible ways you might reach your goal. For most decisions, you will have more than one option. Always try to list at least two alternatives. Other people may be able to help you think of ideas.

3. **Evaluate your alternatives.** Take a good look at each alternative. Think through the options and see what would happen if you chose each one. Think of the pros and cons of each alternative.

4. **Choose the best alternative.** After you have thought through all the alternatives, you are ready to choose one or more. Sometimes you will only be able to use one. Other times you may be able to try a few at the same time.

5. **Act on your decision.** Now you are ready to take action. This can be the most difficult step in the decision-making process. You will need to do whatever is necessary to follow through on your decision.

6. **Evaluate your decision.** To evaluate your decision means to decide whether you have made a good decision. You will decide whether that decision helped you to reach your goal.

5-15 Using this process will help you make decisions that lead you toward your goal or solve your problem.

students through grade 12. The **FCCLA planning process** is a set of five steps members use to help make decisions, reach goals, and solve problems. The steps include identifying concerns, setting your goal, forming a plan, acting on the plan, and then following up, **5-16**.

1. **Identify concerns.** Brainstorming ideas helps you determine what problem you need to solve or goal you want to achieve. When you have a list of several ideas, it is time to start evaluating your options. You can then narrow your list until you identify a concern you want to address.

2. **Set your goal.** After you identify a specific concern, you are ready to set your goal. Be sure to consider all your available resources. It is important to be specific and set a realistic goal, or one you can achieve.

3. **Form a plan.** Now you are ready to develop a plan. As you are thinking about the plan, answer *who, what, where, when,* and *how* questions. Is there anyone who can help you? What possible challenges might you face? Are there community resources you can use? When do you need to complete tasks? How will you measure your progress along the way? Answering questions such as these can help bring your plan together.

4. **Act.** After you determine everything you need to do, you are ready to carry out your plan. As you review your progress along the way, be sure to change any aspects of your plan that are not working. You can also seek advice from parents, teachers, or other trusted adults when needed.

5. **Follow up.** Follow up includes reviewing and evaluating your plan when you are done. Think about ways you might want to do something differently next time. Share your achievements with others. Also, recognize others by thanking them for any help they provided to you along the way.

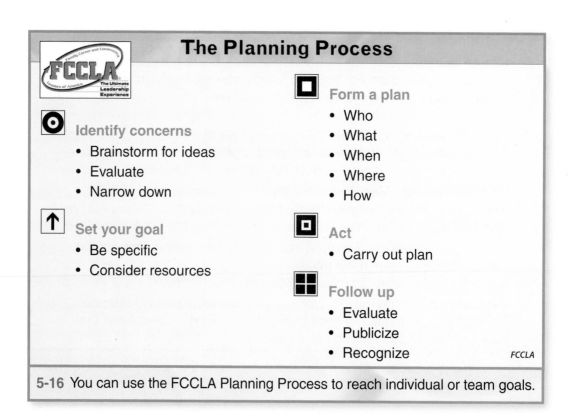

The Planning Process

Identify concerns
- Brainstorm for ideas
- Evaluate
- Narrow down

Set your goal
- Be specific
- Consider resources

Form a plan
- Who
- What
- When
- Where
- How

Act
- Carry out plan

Follow up
- Evaluate
- Publicize
- Recognize

FCCLA

5-16 You can use the FCCLA Planning Process to reach individual or team goals.

Accepting Responsibility for Your Decisions

Being a responsible person involves accepting the **consequences**, or the results, of your decisions. Carefully following the decision-making and planning processes can help you to be better prepared to take responsibility for the consequences of those decisions, **5-17**.

Sometimes your evaluation may tell you that you have made an unwise decision. This decision may have negative consequences. For instance, you may decide not to do your share in a group project. A negative consequence of this decision might be the loss of respect of your group members.

Whether your decisions are wise or unwise, you must be willing to accept the consequences. When the consequences are positive, you can enjoy the credit you deserve. When the consequences are negative, you can learn from them to help you make better decisions in the future. A positive thing about life decisions is that you get to make new decisions daily.

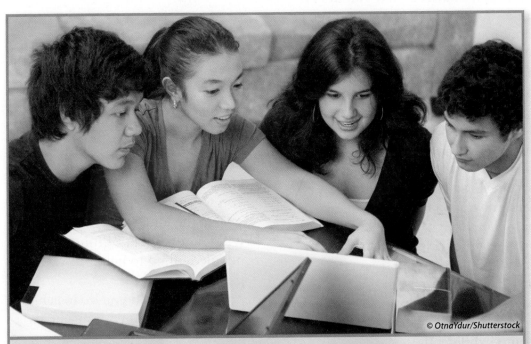

© OtnaYdur/Shutterstock

5-17 Deciding to study and complete assignments brings the positive consequences of learning and doing well on tests.

Reading Review

1. List the four steps in the management process.
2. List the six steps in the decision-making process.
3. What factors affect the decisions you make?
4. What is a trade-off?
5. List the five steps of the FCCLA planning process.

Chapter Summary

Section 5-1. You have many needs and wants. You act in a way that will help you satisfy your needs and wants. Maslow's theory of human needs separates the basic needs into *physical needs* and *psychological needs*. The last level in the hierarchy is for higher-level needs, or *self-actualization needs*. Everyone has the same basic needs, but each person has different wants.

Section 5-2. Your values, goals, and standards also affect what you do. Your values determine the goals you set throughout life. Goals give direction to life. You work to reach your goals that are important to you. The way you set standards depends on the importance of your goals. Setting priorities helps you determine which goals are most important.

Section 5-3. Anything that can help you reach a goal is a resource. Human resources come from within yourself or from your relationships with other people. Nonhuman resources include money, community resources, and possessions. Understanding the many ways you can use your resources will help you to better manage them. People choose to develop their resources differently.

Section 5-4. The decisions you make depend on the way you manage your resources. Using the decision-making and planning processes can help you make the decisions that are best for you. Good managers take responsibility for their decisions. They accept the results of each decision they make.

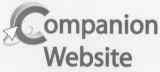

Companion Website
www.g-wlearning.com

Check your understanding of the main concepts for Chapter 5 at the website.

Critical Thinking

1. **Identify.** Think of something you would like to see changed in your school or community. Set this as a long-term goal. List the steps involved in reaching this goal. Find out what short-term goals you would need to accomplish to realize the long-term goal. How will you organize a group of people willing to help put your plan into action?
2. **Assess.** What can you do to achieve your wants when your resources are limited?
3. **Recognize.** What can you do to accept responsibility for an unwise decision?

Common Core

College and Career Readiness

4. **Speaking.** Discuss needs and wants with your classmates and then make a list of needs and wants for each of the following groups of people:
   A. infants
   B. young school-age children
   C. teens
   D. young adults
   E. older adults

5. **Writing.** Select a long-term goal. Write about the values that might cause you to set the goal. Plan how you will reach the goal. What short-term goals will bring you closer to the long-term goal? What standards will you use to measure your achievement of the goal?

6. **Reading.** Visit the library. Read a book about management techniques. How do the management techniques described in the book compare to those described in this text?

7. **Listening.** Interview a store manager. Ask him or her to describe management techniques that he or she finds effective and those he or she finds ineffective. Ask him or her to give examples of how using management techniques can affect successful operation of the store.

Technology

8. **Computer applications.** Computers are an important resource. Invite someone familiar with practical applications of computers to speak to the class. Discuss how you can use computers to manage your other resources and your life.

Journal Writing

9. Think about the future. Write about a big decision that you will face in the next few years. Think of several alternatives and list the pros and cons of each. Choose the best alternative. Explain why you made that choice. If you could have complete success in only one area of your life, what area would you want it to be?

FCCLA

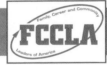

10. Create a portfolio for the *Life-Event Planning STAR Event* that demonstrates your ability to manage resources and develop a plan. This could be anything that will bring changes/challenges and pose specific financial responsibilities such as planning a special trip, planning a birthday celebration, or going to a concert. Select an event and identify the roles of wants versus needs related to the event. Use the *FCCLA Planning Process* to create a plan for achieving your project goals. See your adviser for information as needed.

Chapter 6
Managing Your Resources

Sections

Reading Prep

College and Career Readiness

Before you read this chapter, read the *Reading Review* questions at the end of each section. This will prepare you for the content you will be reading. The review questions at the end of the sections help you evaluate your understanding of the material.

Concept Organizer

Pluses	Minuses	Implications

Use a *PMI* chart like the one shown to list the *Pluses*, *Minuses*, and *Implications* of using credit cards.

Companion Website

Print out the concept organizer for Chapter 6 at the website.

Companion Website
www.g-wlearning.com

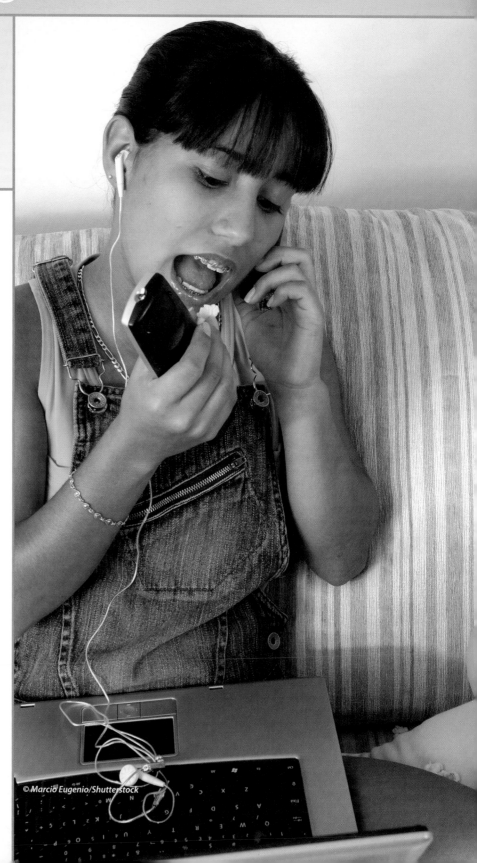
© Marcio Eugenio/Shutterstock

Managing Time and Energy

Objectives

After studying this section, you will be able to
- **identify** ways to manage your time wisely.
- **plan** an effective study schedule.
- **describe** factors that affect your energy level.
- **determine** ways to best manage your energy to reach your goals.

Key Terms	
schedule	procrastination

Your time and energy are two of your most valuable resources. Learning to manage these resources will help you manage every other part of your life. When you make the best use of time and energy, your other resources seem to grow. Learning to manage these resources now will help you throughout life.

Managing Time

Time is unlike any other resource because everyone has the same amount. There are 24 hours in each day for you to use as you wish. Time is a precious resource, yet many people waste it. Other people seem to have plenty of time. They are able to manage their time so they can do everything they need and want to do.

Planning Your Time Use

Have you ever run out of time before you could finish an important project? This can be a frustrating experience. It is hard to know what to do when you run out of time.

Planning is the way to avoid this problem. When you follow a plan for using your time, you know how much you can expect to accomplish, **6-1**.

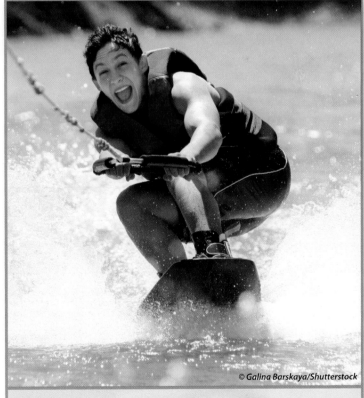
© Galina Barskaya/Shutterstock

6-1 You can make plans to do the activities you want to do as well as those you must do.

The most efficient way to plan the use of your time is to develop and use a schedule. A **schedule** is a written plan for reaching your goals within a certain time. To create effective schedules, write them for short periods, perhaps daily or weekly.

A Daily Schedule

Preparing a schedule is quite simple. Set aside a time each day to make a to-do list for the next day. Just before going to bed is a good time for most people. Making the list at this time helps you mentally prepare for the next day.

When making your list, first block out time for exercise, studying, meals, and other activities you need to do each day. Be sure to have time set aside for all the activities you know you must do, such as chores at home. You can then plan the rest of your schedule around these required activities.

Plan to do important activities first. For instance, you might be required to empty the dishwasher and do your homework before you can check your e-mail. On your daily schedule, place a star or some other mark by these activities so you know they are a priority. Any items on your list that are priorities are the most important and should be taken care of first.

You have no control over how you spend some of your time. You attend school for a large portion of the day, and you sleep for much of the night. Your schedule will have to account for these activities. You cannot plan to clean your bedroom when you will be at choir practice. Keep track of all the jobs and activities you must do, **6-2**. Then estimate how much time each item on your list will take. Put each activity into a time slot. The next day, try to follow your schedule.

Some activities will take more time than you expect, and some will take less. Adjust your schedule accordingly. Try to allow yourself some free time each day. You may need to use it to complete an important activity. The more you use a schedule, the more accurately you will allow time for activities.

Avoid Wasting Time

Using a schedule will make you aware of how you spend your time. If you are not careful, cell phones or computers can cause you to waste time. Be aware if this is happening.

My Schedule	
Wednesday, October 12	
7:30–8:15	Get up, eat breakfast, and get ready for school.
8:15–8:30	Go to school.
8:30–3:30	Attend classes.
3:45–5:00	Volleyball practice.
5:00–5:15	Go home.
5:15–6:15	Do homework.
6:15–7:00	Eat dinner and help clean kitchen.
7:00–8:00	Free time.
8:00–9:00	Study for math test.
9:00–10:00	Watch television.
10:00–7:30	Sleep.

6-2 When you have developed a schedule, you can make better use of your time.

If constant texting with friends is keeping you from getting important chores or homework done, then you may need to limit your own texting. Then you can take responsibility for your time. If spending too much time on the Internet is keeping you from meeting your deadlines, you may want to limit the time you spend on the computer. Keep using a schedule and you will find ways to reach your goals and still have time for other activities.

Many people procrastinate. Procrastination means putting off difficult or unpleasant tasks until later. Sometimes people never complete these tasks, or they hurry and do the job poorly.

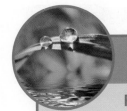

Go Green

Reduce Clutter and Save Time

Sometimes it is easy to become overwhelmed with all the *things* in your life. It is easier to just let your clothes, papers, magazines, books, or stuff in general pile up. Eventually, though, they must be either discarded or stored. Organizing the things in your life takes time. One way to save time, reduce clutter, and help the environment is to decide what to save, reuse, or recycle. Consider giving some of your things away rather than throwing them out. Keep a bin for recyclables like paper, plastic bottles, cans, and magazines in your room. You can immediately discard recyclables in the bin instead of letting them clutter your room. The same principle can apply to your old, outgrown, or damaged clothing.

You can make a task you dislike more pleasant by dividing it into smaller segments. If your job is to vacuum the entire house, you could work on one room or half the house first. Then take a short break and do something you enjoy. After a break, you will probably feel more like vacuuming another room or finishing the job.

As you use a schedule and learn to manage your time, you will more than likely make mistakes. Everyone does. You can become a better time manager when you admit your mistakes and correct them. Managing your time at this point in your life will set the stage for your time management as an adult.

Improving Your Study Habits

Being a student is one of your biggest responsibilities. Managing your study time wisely and improving your study habits will help you meet this responsibility. Everything you have learned about time management so far also applies to your schoolwork. Improving your study habits can help you be more successful in classes you take now and in the future.

A Place to Study

The first step to improving your study habits is to find a special place to study. It could be the corner of a room, a desk in your room, or the table in the dining room. The place you choose should be quiet and without televisions, cell phones, or other distractions. In this place, you can store all the tools you need to study in a bin if you do not have a designated space. You will need a place for paper, pencils, pens, and a computer. A shelf for your books and notebooks will make your study area neater, **6-3**.

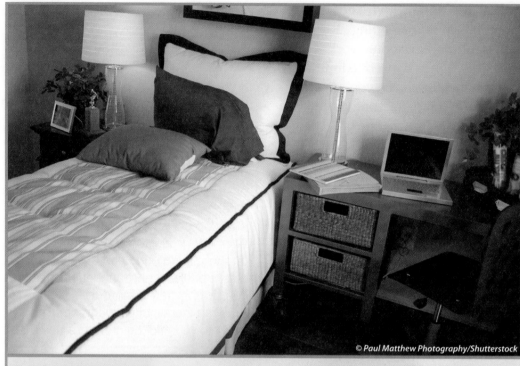

6-3 A small section of your bedroom can be used to create a comfortable study area.

When you study, you do a lot of reading. Therefore, you need plenty of light. A comfortable chair might help you study more effectively. You are more likely to work and study better in pleasant, clean surroundings.

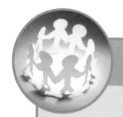

Life Connections

Study Skills

Most people find it is best to study the hardest or longest assignment first. Your mind is often clearer and you are more alert at the beginning of your study period. It may be difficult to start these assignments, however. Just remember that after you finish your longest or hardest job, the smaller assignments often go more quickly.

When studying, be sure to take breaks, especially between subjects. This can clear your mind and relax your body. You must be careful not to take too many breaks though. If you take a break every five minutes, you will not get much studying done.

Research Activity

Developing good study skills are important for success in school and in life. Use the Internet to research tips about how to study and improve your study skills. Share your findings with the class.

Your Study Schedule

You need to schedule study time just as you schedule other activities in your life. Begin by writing a step-by-step plan of what you want to do. This can help you to better organize your time.

Before you prepare a study schedule, be sure you understand your assignments clearly. Then you will be better able to decide how much time to allow for each subject. You might also do better work when you clearly understand what your teachers expect you to do.

Long projects or reports may take several days or weeks to complete. Do not try to handle a huge task in one night. When a big test is coming up, plan to study for an hour or so each night. Then you will not feel so rushed. Most people do better when they have plenty of time to prepare. Do not try to research a big report for school in one day. Break the job into smaller chunks. Do research for an hour each day in study hall or after school. On another day, pull all your information together into a report. Breaking a big job into smaller tasks makes the job seem easier. The quality of your work is often better when you do a job this way, too.

Managing Your Energy

Your personal energy is the resource that allows you to complete a task. Your body must have enough energy for all its systems to function. In addition, you need energy to continue your daily activities. Physical activities such as running, walking, or even sitting take energy, **6-4**. You also need energy to think, read, and sleep. Because the teen years are a period of rapid growth, you need extra energy for your development.

You probably have more energy than some people you know and less energy than others. Each person has his or her own energy level. Whether you have more or less energy than your friends is not important. What is important, however, is that you do your best to manage your energy and use it to reach your goals.

Food and Energy

What you eat affects your energy level. Eating nutritious foods at regular times each day gives you the energy to do what you want to do. Eating right also helps you to manage your health. The amount of food you need varies according to your energy needs. Physically active people need more energy than people who are not as active. It takes more energy to play softball, play tennis, jog, and swim than to read, write, watch television, or hang out with friends. Making healthful choices is especially important during the teen years when you are growing quickly. Making these wise food choices gives your body the energy it needs to develop properly.

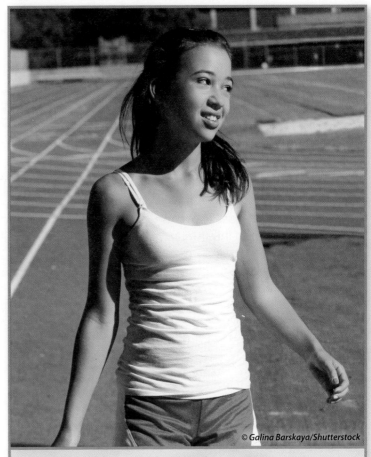
© Galina Barskaya/Shutterstock

6-4 Without enough energy, your body cannot keep growing.

Sleep and Energy

Everyone must get enough sleep to have the energy they need. Many teens need eight to ten hours of sleep each night. There is no way to say

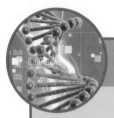

Science Connections

Melatonin

Some people have the ability to maintain high levels of energy with minimal amount of sleep, while others have trouble functioning without eight to ten hours of sleep. Why is that? These people have different levels of *melatonin*, a hormone that helps regulate the sleep cycle. Known as the *sleep hormone*, high levels of melatonin cause you to feel sleepy. At night, the pineal gland releases melatonin into your bloodstream, helping to put you to sleep. During daytime hours, melatonin is low, because bright lights interrupt melatonin levels. Therefore, if you are not tired when going to sleep, shutting off the lights can induce the feeling of tiredness. This might help you maintain a regular sleep schedule.

exactly how much sleep you need, however. Everyone is a little different. You may require more hours of sleep to stay alert and energetic. On the other hand, you may be able to function fine on fewer hours of sleep. To manage your energy, try to get enough sleep every night. Also, make a point of sleeping during the same hours each night to get your body on a regular schedule.

Physical Activity and Energy

Physical activity does not take away your energy. In fact, people who are regularly active often have more energy. Regular physical activity makes your body able to handle a larger workload. Swimming, cycling, and aerobics are just a few examples of healthful physical activities. The more you are physically active, the less quickly you tire. This increases your energy level.

Reading Review

1. A(n) _____ is a written plan for reaching your goals in a given period of time.
2. List three ways you can manage your time.
3. What is procrastination?
4. How can you manage your study time wisely and improve your study habits?
5. List three factors that affect your energy level.

Managing Money

Objectives

After studying this section, you will be able to
- **identify** sources of income.
- **differentiate** between fixed and flexible expenses.
- **create and follow** a budget to manage your money.
- **describe** various options for saving and investing money.
- **demonstrate** how to write a check, endorse a check, make a deposit, and balance a checkbook.
- **list** common online banking features and services.

Key Terms

income	flexible expenses	individual retirement
deductions	interest	account (IRA)
gross income	money market account	endorse
net income	U.S. savings bonds	ATM card
budget	certificate of deposit	debit card
expenses	(CD)	bank statement
fixed expenses		

Money is more important to some people than to others, but everyone in today's world needs money. You cannot get by without it. Money is a resource often exchanged for other resources. You must use money to purchase goods and services. Many activities you enjoy also require money. Your cell phone or access to the Internet costs money. You use money to meet many of your needs and wants. Therefore, learning to manage your money is important. To reach many of your goals, you need to spend your money wisely, too.

Your Income

Income is the money you earn. You might have income from an allowance, gifts, babysitting, or doing odd jobs for neighbors. Some of your income, such as an allowance, may be regular. You may receive other income, such as money for your birthday or a holiday, which comes only once a year.

Receiving a Paycheck

A paycheck is the main source of income for most people. Some teens might receive a paycheck for a part-time job. When you receive your first paycheck, you may notice the amount is not as large as you expect it to be.

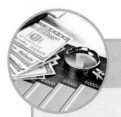

Deductions are amounts of money that an employer subtracts from your paycheck before you receive it. The most common deductions are for federal and state income taxes, Social Security, and Medicare. If you receive health benefits, you may have a deduction for that as well, **6-5**.

The income you earn before these deductions is your **gross income**. After the deductions, the amount of money you earn is your **net income**. This is the actual amount of money you will be managing.

Budgeting Your Money

Basic money management involves using a budget. A **budget** is a written plan for spending your money wisely. It helps you see how much money you have and how you spend it.

Your **expenses** are the ways you spend your money. You may spend money to go to a ballgame or to buy a gift for a friend. You might also spend money to buy lunch and school supplies.

Gross income   Deductions   Net income

Town Department Store

Employee	Kristy A. James	**SSN**	987-65-4321
Pay Period	3/8/XX to 3/21/XX		
Pay Date	3/27/XX	**Net Pay**	$827.70
Check No.	12341234		

Earnings	Hrs.	Current	YTD	Deductions	Current	YTD
REGULAR	80.00	1113.73	5923.12	FICA	69.06	494.17
OVERTIME			1872.99	MEDICARE	16.15	115.58
				FED. TAX	116.17	880.89
				STATE TAX	52.40	347.68
				HEALTH	32.25	225.75
TOTALS	80.00	1113.73	7796.11		286.03	2064.07

6-5 A paycheck stub shows how much gross income you earn and how much is taken out for deductions, which then equals your net pay.

Your expenses may be fixed or flexible. **Fixed expenses** are the regular expenses you cannot avoid. They do not vary much from one time to another. School lunches, dues to a club, and monthly savings may be examples of some of your fixed expenses. As you grow older, you will begin to become more responsible for yourself financially. You will have many more expenses that fall into this category, such as a car or rent payment and insurance costs.

Most of your expenses now are probably flexible expenses. **Flexible expenses** are costs that can vary from time to time, and do not occur regularly. Snacks, gifts, clothing, and magazines are flexible expenses for many teens. Your flexible expenses will not be the same each month. You can figure out how much they are on the average, however. You might also want to allot some money to a category of flexible expenses called *other expenses*. Then you will always have some money on hand for the unexpected.

Creating a Budget

To put a budget into action, you can write all the details or use a computer spreadsheet, **6-6**. List your sources of income and how much money you take in from each of these sources. Add those numbers together to determine your total income.

Then list each of your fixed and flexible expenses. Prioritize your expenses by listing the most important ones first. This will help you determine which expenses are needs and which ones might be wants.

My Monthly Budget		
Income		
Allowance	$40	
Babysitting	$50	
Gifts	$5	
Total income		$95
Expenses		
Fixed expenses		
Lunch	$30	
Savings	$10	
Flexible expenses		
Magazines	$5	
Snacks and Eating out	$10	
Clothing and accessories	$20	
Transportation	$10	
Other flexible expenses	$10	
Total expenses		$95

6-6 It is much easier to stick to a spending plan when you have put it in writing.

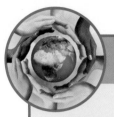

Global Connections

Money

Money is the currency used to pay for goods and services. You are familiar with the U.S. dollar and coins. Money looks very different around the world, however, and has different names. For instance, paper money in Great Britain is called *pounds*, while in most other European countries, the currency is *euros*. Many Latin American countries use *pesos*. In Arabic countries, *dinars* are used, and India uses the *rupee*.

Paper money and coins come in many sizes, colors, and shapes. Coins can be made from silver, aluminum, nickel, copper, brass, bronze, or (rarely) gold. They can be any shape or even have holes in the middle. Other countries' paper money is often very colorful. Most countries will only accept their own currency, traveler's checks, or credit cards. Before travelling, learn the value of a U.S. dollar in that country to know how much you are really paying.

Add your fixed and flexible expenses to come up with a total amount of expenses. Then compare it with your total income. These figures should be the same.

If your expenses are greater than your income, you will need to find a way to reduce your expenses or to increase your income. If your income is greater than your expenses, you can afford to spend a little more in one area or another. You can also add extra income to your savings.

Following a Budget

After you create a budget, keep track of all the money you spend. Try to stick to the budget, but remember that a budget should be flexible. Sometimes you will spend more than you have planned, and sometimes you will spend less. Record the actual amount you spend. Then compare it with the amount you had budgeted.

Evaluate your budget regularly. When you notice you are spending more in one area, revise your budget by reducing expenses in another area. If you know you are going to have to spend more money one month, you can try to save extra another month. With practice, you will be able to budget your money to best meet your needs and reach your goals.

Using Financial Services

As you manage your money, you may benefit from the services of financial institutions. Types of financial institutions you might use include banks, savings institutions, and credit unions. Many financial institutions offer similar services, such as savings accounts, checking accounts, and online banking, **6-7**.

Savings Accounts

Many people choose to save money in a savings account. People save money based on their needs and wants. Some people may open savings accounts to save money for a college education, a car, or a house. Other people open savings accounts to have money available for any unforeseen expenses.

A savings account pays you interest. **Interest** is an amount of money paid to you for the use of your money. Interest is computed as a percentage of the amount of money in your account. It is paid on a regular basis.

Types of Financial Services

- Savings and checking accounts
- Debit cards
- Online banking
- Automated teller machines
- Direct electronic paycheck deposit and funds transfer
- Overdraft protection
- Credit card accounts
- Automatic bill payment plans
- Personal and business loans
- Home mortgages

- Retirement accounts
- Financial counseling
- U.S. savings bonds
- Money market accounts
- Certificates of deposit
- Cashier's checks, money orders, traveler's checks, and certified checks
- Trust, investment, and estate management
- Safe-deposit boxes

6-7 The services each type of financial institution provides may vary in order to meet the needs of its customers.

Financial institutions use your money to make investments or loans to other people. These people must then pay interest to the financial institution. If you have a savings account, you receive a portion of that interest. The interest rate for a savings account is usually fairly low.

Before opening an account, be sure you clearly understand the services the financial institution offers. Some financial institutions may require you to maintain a minimum balance in your savings account. Other financial institutions may not require any minimum balance at all. Financial institutions may charge you fees to open an account. Interest rates also vary among financial institutions. It is important to shop around and choose the financial institution that best meets your needs.

Other Ways to Save and Invest Money

In addition to savings accounts, many financial institutions offer other services to help you save and invest your money.

- A **money market account** is a type of savings account that offers a higher rate of interest, but the rate changes daily. A large minimum deposit is often necessary to open a money market account. Limited check writing and money transfer privileges are typically available with this type of account.

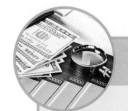

Financial Literacy Connections

Saving Your Money

Savings goals are an important part of budgeting money. A good way for you to save money is to put aside a set amount each month for savings. You could also put aside the change you get each day and add it to your savings. When you receive gifts of money, you might want to add this money to your savings as well. Getting in the habit of saving money will help you now and in the future.

- **U.S. savings bonds** are a type of savings in which you loan the government money for at least a year. When the loan is due, the government will repay you the full amount of the bond, plus interest. The U.S. Treasury issues U.S. savings bonds in amounts varying from $25 to $5,000. They are available for purchase at most financial institutions.
- A **certificate of deposit (CD)** is a savings tool that requires you to deposit a certain amount of money for a specified period of time. When you purchase a CD, you earn interest for the length of time you have the CD. In order to receive the highest amount of interest, you cannot withdraw money before the specified time. There is also a penalty for withdrawing money early.
- An **individual retirement account (IRA)** is an investment option providing tax benefits to those workers saving money for retirement. There are several different types of IRAs available. One common type is a traditional IRA. With a *traditional IRA*, taxpayers do not have to pay taxes on earnings until they withdraw the money when they retire. Another common type of IRA is the *Roth IRA*, which taxes contributions, but withdrawals are tax free.

Checking Accounts

Checking accounts allow you to pay bills and purchase items by writing checks on your account, **6-8**. When you write a check, you are authorizing your financial institution to deduct the money from your account to pay the person or business indicated on the check.

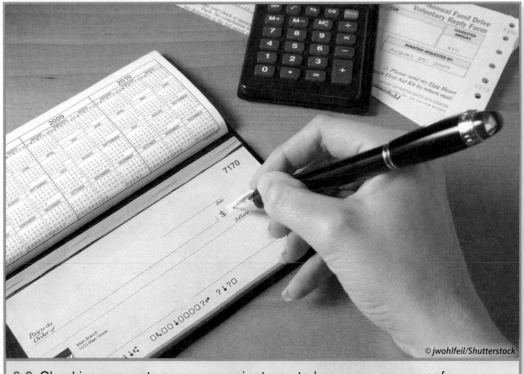

© jwohlfeil/Shutterstock

6-8 Checking accounts are a convenient way to keep your money safe.

Financial institutions often offer several types of checking accounts. Some accounts let you earn interest when you maintain your account balance at a certain level. Other types of accounts may charge you for the checks you write. Still other accounts may require you to keep a minimum balance. Compare services at several financial institutions before deciding which place offers the best services for you.

Opening a Checking Account

Financial institutions often require you to be at least 18 years of age to open your own checking account. You can open a *joint account*, however, with a parent or legal guardian before you are 18 years of age. You and anyone else listed on the account needs to sign a signature card. The signature you use on this card should match the signature you use for any financial or legal papers you need to sign.

After you open a checking account, you will have temporary checks with your account number. You will use these until your personal checks arrive from the financial institution. When you receive your checks, you will also get a check register. This helps you keep track of all your transactions.

Writing a Check

When you write a check, you need to fill out all the information correctly, **6-9**. Carefully enter the following information on your check using blue or black ink. If you make a mistake when filling out a check, destroy it.

- **Date**—should be the day you write the check.
- **Pay to the order of**—record the name of the person or business receiving the check.
- **Payment amount in numbers**—write the amount close to the dollar sign and list the cents as a fraction of 100.

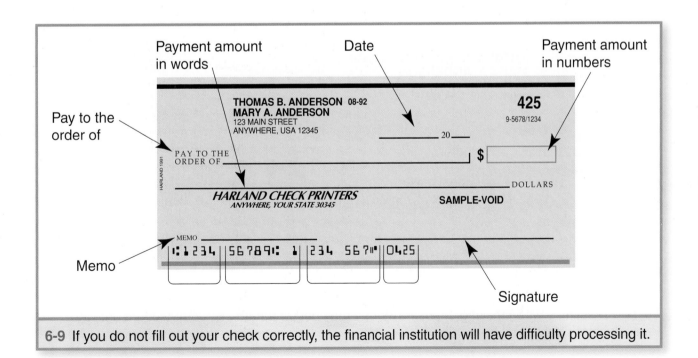

6-9 If you do not fill out your check correctly, the financial institution will have difficulty processing it.

- **Payment amount in words**—write the amount of dollars and the word *and*, followed by the cents as a fraction of 100. Fill remaining space with a line.
- **Memo**—state the reason for writing the check.
- **Signature**—should be the same as the one on the signature card at the financial institution.

After you write a check, immediately record the transaction in your check register. You will need to list the check number, the date, the person receiving the check, and the amount. If you had to destroy a check, record the check number and write the word *void*. Keep accurate records of how much money you have in your account. Also, never write a check for more money than you have in your account. This can cause your account to be *overdrawn*.

Endorsing a Check

In order to cash or deposit a check, you must endorse it. To **endorse** a check is to sign your name on the back of the check in the space provided for a signature. Once you endorse the check, anyone can cash it. Therefore, do not endorse a check until just before you are going to cash it. You can also write *for deposit only* when endorsing a check. This guarantees that the money will go directly into your account, regardless of who cashes the check.

Making a Deposit

When you want to deposit money in your account, you need to fill out a *deposit slip*, **6-10**. Follow these steps to correctly fill out a deposit slip:

1. Date and sign the deposit slip.
2. List all the currency, coins, and checks you are depositing. There is space on the back of the deposit slip to list more checks, if necessary.
3. Add the total amount you are depositing and record it after the word *Subtotal*.

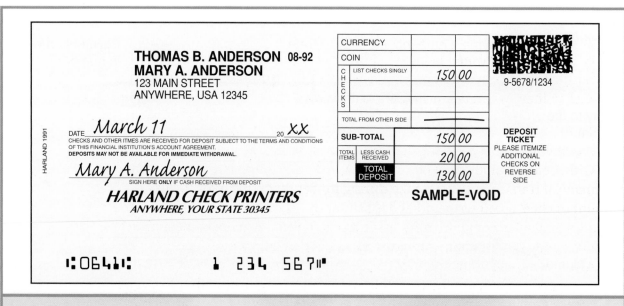

6-10 Sometimes when making deposits, money may not be added into your account until the next business day.

4. Record any withdrawals after the words *Less cash received*.

5. Subtract withdrawals from the subtotal and write this amount after the words *Total deposit*.

6. Write the transaction in your check register. Also, keep any receipts to help you balance your checkbook.

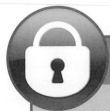

Safety Connections

Entering Your PIN

Whenever you use your debit card and enter your personal identification number, make sure to always cover the keypad or computer screen with your hand. This ensures that other people cannot look over your shoulder and memorize your PIN. If at any point you suspect that someone else may know your PIN, request a new number from your bank.

Using ATM and Debit Cards

Many financial institutions have automated teller machines (ATMs). An *automated teller machine (ATM)* is a computer terminal that allows customers to complete transactions with their financial institutions. An **ATM card** enables customers to use an ATM to make deposits, withdraw money, or transfer money from one account to another.

Your financial institution issues you an ATM card with a *personal identification number (PIN)*. Keep your PIN in a safe place where no one else can see it. This card gives you access to the machine at any time of the day or night.

To use an ATM, put your card into a slot in the machine and enter your PIN. You then have access to a menu of choices. Simply follow the prompts to complete your transaction.

A **debit card** enables customers to perform transactions at ATMs or make purchases at stores. You can use a debit card instead of checks or cash. Your financial institution issues you the card with a PIN. Whenever you use a debit card, the amount is immediately deducted from your checking account. Always make sure you have enough money in your account before using a debit card. If you do not have sufficient funds, your financial institution will charge additional fees for overdrawing your account.

When you are finished using an ATM or debit card, immediately record the transaction in your check register. Save your receipts in a safe place so you can refer to them when balancing your checkbook.

Balancing Your Checkbook

When you open a checking account, your financial institution will provide you with a bank statement every month. A **bank statement** is a record of all the financial transactions you make during the month. It includes the total amount of checks you wrote, total deposits and withdrawals, any charges, and an ending balance. Some financial institutions send statements in the mail and others provide online statements for you to view at your convenience.

After reviewing your statement, you should *balance your checkbook*. To do this, you need to compare the transactions on your statement with the ones in your check register. Sometimes your statement may show additional charges, such as a fee for using an ATM. When these appear on your statement, you need to subtract them from the balance in your check register. Contact the customer service division of your financial institution if you have any questions about fees or items on your statement.

The next step in balancing your checkbook is to account for any transactions in your check register that do not yet appear on the statement. To do this, you can use the balancing worksheet that often appears on the back of your statement, **6-11**.

Online Banking

Many financial institutions offer online banking services to their customers. The financial institution assigns user identification numbers and security codes. This enables customers to access their accounts at any time of the day or night. To prevent someone else from accessing your account, keep identification numbers and security codes in a safe place.

Common online banking features and services include
- viewing statement and account balances
- setting up online payments or direct deposit
- making deposits and transferring funds
- reordering checks
- managing CDs and IRAs

Using a Balancing Worksheet

1. Write the balance as it appears on your bank statement.
2. List any deposits that are not on the statement.
3. Add the balance and deposit amounts and write the total.
4. List any checks and withdrawals that are not on the statement. Add these amounts together and record the total.
5. Subtract the total amount in step 4 from the total in step 3. This amount should match the current balance in your checkbook. If it does not, repeat the process and check your math carefully. If the amounts still do not agree, you might want to contact your financial institution for help.

6-11 The following steps will help you complete a balancing worksheet.

Reading Review

1. What is the difference between gross income and net income?
2. What is the difference between fixed expenses and flexible expenses? List two examples of each type of expense.
3. In addition to savings accounts, list four ways to save or invest money.
4. What is a bank statement?
5. List two common online banking features and services.

Managing Credit

Objectives

After studying this section, you will be able to
- **define** the term *credit*.
- **identify** various types of credit.
- **list** the advantages and disadvantages of credit cards.
- **give examples** of ways to establish credit.
- **describe** factors that make a person a good credit risk.
- **explain** how to use credit wisely.

Key Terms

credit	finance charge	revolving credit
installment credit	noninstallment credit	

People can use credit to buy almost anything they might need or want. There are many types of credit available. There are also advantages and disadvantages to consider before using credit. Learning how to manage credit wisely can help you enjoy your purchases without creating financial worries.

Understanding Credit

Credit allows people to charge goods and services or to borrow money. When you use **credit**, you are buying or borrowing now and paying later. Credit is more costly than using cash because you have to pay interest on the money you borrow. You should also remember that when you use credit, you are spending your future earnings, **6-12**.

Using credit wisely can help people buy items they need now. For instance, some people might use credit to buy a house or a car. If a washing machine breaks unexpectedly, a person can use credit to buy a new one right away. A person might also use credit to purchase a

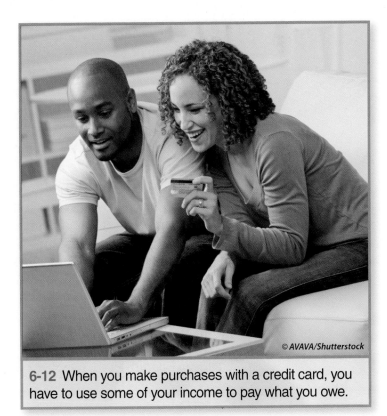

© AVAVA/Shutterstock

6-12 When you make purchases with a credit card, you have to use some of your income to pay what you owe.

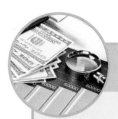

Financial Literacy Connections

Costs of Credit

Finance charge is an umbrella term, which includes other fees that the creditor may issue to the consumer. Examples include transaction fees, services charges, and interest rates.

The annual percentage rate may or may not include finance charges, depending on the type of loan. For installment credit, finance charges are included in the APR. The APR is determined by the amount of money borrowed and the time it takes for the consumer to return the loan. For revolving credit, the APR does not include finance charges, but is fixed per year. When first opening a credit account, the APR may be zero, but will go up the next year. Always read the fine print before agreeing to any contract.

new suit for a job interview. Misuse of credit, however, can lead to financial disaster. If you would not be able to save the money to make a purchase, then you probably cannot afford to buy it using credit.

Types of Credit

People are able to choose from several different types of credit depending on their needs. One type of credit is a *cash loan*. Financial institutions, finance companies, and credit card agencies all grant loans to people. When you are approved for a loan, you sign a contract agreeing to the terms and conditions of the loan. This includes the amount of the loan, the interest rate, and the number of loan payments.

Installment credit is a cash loan you repay with interest in regular payments. People typically use this type of credit for personal loans and large purchases such as a car or furniture. Student loans are another example of installment credit. Payment plans for installment credit are set up to cover the cost of the purchase and finance charges. A **finance charge** is the dollar amount you pay for credit. Finance charges consist of interest and fees. The interest you pay depends on the *annual percentage rate (APR)*, which is the yearly credit cost the lender charges.

Another type of credit is **noninstallment credit**, which is an amount you repay in one payment. Single payment loans and 30-day charge accounts are examples of noninstallment credit. Another example is the credit extended for services, such as those received from doctors or dentists. Depending on the type of credit you receive, you may or may not have to pay interest.

Revolving credit is a specified amount of money that is repeatedly available as long as you make regular payments each month. With revolving credit, you can pay the full amount you owe each month, or you can spread payments over time. When you do not pay the full amount, a minimum payment amount is set. This amount is usually a percentage of the total balance you owe. You must also pay a finance charge.

Retailers and credit cards typically offer revolving credit. People can use these cards to purchases goods and services wherever businesses accept them, **6-13**.

Credit Cards

Credit cards allow people to purchase goods and services as well as borrow money. Some credit cards are noninstallment, 30-day charge accounts. Other types of credit cards offer revolving credit. There are both advantages and disadvantages to using credit cards.

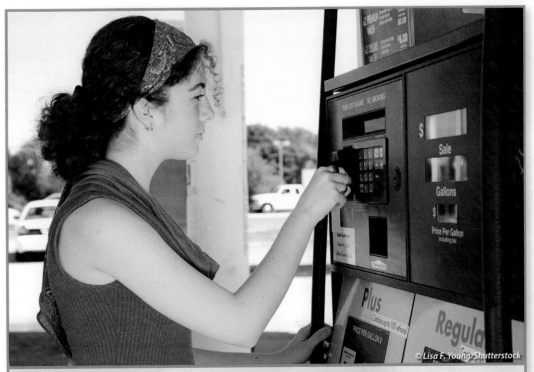

6-13 Gas stations, grocery stores, and restaurants are just a few examples of businesses that usually accept credit.

Advantages

When used wisely, credit cards offer several advantages.

- **Convenience.** Credit cards are convenient to use. They make it easy to buy items. You also do not have to carry large amounts of money.
- **Establish good credit.** You can establish good credit by making payments on time and paying the full amount you owe each month. This will help when you are applying for loans or credit cards. It can also be useful when completing rental applications or even applying for some jobs.
- **Emergencies.** Credit cards can be useful when emergencies occur. If your car breaks down, a credit card can help you take care of the situation right away.
- **Record of purchases.** Credit cards provide a good record of purchases. If you lose a receipt and you need to return something, your credit card statement provides a record of the purchase.

Disadvantages

You need to be aware of the disadvantages of using credit cards in order to be able to use credit wisely.

- **Overspending.** The convenience of using credit cards can cause overspending to occur rather easily. You wind up spending money you do not have. This reduces your future income and you do not have as much to spend later.

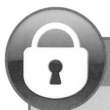

Safety Connections

Fraud

Credit cards can be lost or stolen. A person could also steal your credit card number without even taking your card. If theft occurs, someone may use your card or number to make a lot of purchases and rack up debt. You might be responsible for paying part of the cost. Many companies will only charge a small fee or not charge you at all for unauthorized purchases, however. If you realize your card is lost or stolen, report it to the company right away.

- **Expenses.** Interest rates for credit cards are usually very high. You could pay around 20–25 percent interest on the amount you owe. If you spend more than you can pay, you must pay a finance charge on the balance you owe.
- **Serious debt.** The more you continue to spend without paying off the balance, the more finance charges you must pay. This brings you into debt. If you cannot pay the minimum balance due or you miss a payment, you will be charged late fees and additional finance charges. The inability to pay your debt affects your credit rating, which makes it difficult to obtain credit in the future.

Establishing Credit

You may have difficulty getting credit at first. This is because companies want to make sure you are a good credit risk. Following are several ways to establish credit:

- Hold a job and earn your own money.
- Open a savings account and save money regularly. This shows financial responsibility.
- Open a checking account and manage it properly. Follow the guidelines for your account and do not let it become overdrawn.
- Apply for a credit card from a local company, such as a department store or gas station. If you are accepted, use the card responsibly and pay off what you owe every month.

Your Credit Rating

When you apply for credit, the company (creditor) decides whether you are a good credit risk based on your credit rating. A *credit rating* is an assessment of your ability to repay a debt. Three factors, called *the three Cs* determine your credit rating.

- **Character.** Creditors consider your financial history and determine your honesty and reliability to pay a debt. If you have a history of paying bills on time or using credit responsibly, you are more likely to achieve a higher character rating.
- **Capacity.** Creditors look at your ability to earn money and repay debt. Your rating depends on your employment history and current salary and debts.
- **Capital.** Creditors check your assets. If you have a savings account, a car, a house, or other personal property, then you have capital. The more capital you have, the better your rating will be.

Using Credit Wisely

Managing credit wisely can be difficult. The convenience of credit can easily lead to overspending and financial worries. Following are some tips to help you stay in control of credit use:

- Consider your options carefully before making a purchase. If you do not think you can save money for an item, then you probably should not buy it.
- Try to be selective when obtaining a credit card. Find the card with the lowest interest that best meets your needs. Also, limit the number of credit cards you have.
- Keep track of all the purchases you charge so you are less likely to overspend.
- Try to pay off balances in full each month. This helps you avoid interest charges.
- Stop using a credit card for a while if you are only able to make the minimum payment each month. This is a warning sign that you are headed for trouble.

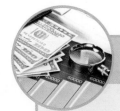

Financial Literacy Connections

Your Credit Report

A *credit bureau* is an agency that collects information on a person's credit practices and makes it available to businesses. A credit bureau is also called a *credit reporting agency*. The three major credit bureaus are Experian, Equifax, and TransUnion LLC.

A credit bureau establishes a report for you when you begin to use credit. This account of your credit history and financial practices is a *credit report*. It includes any credit you have ever had. If you miss payments or make late payments, it includes that information, too.

Creditors use credit reports to help them determine whether people are good credit risks. Therefore, it is important to check your credit report for accuracy. By law, you can receive a free credit report yearly. If you find errors, you can contact the agency to dispute them.

Reading Review

1. What is credit?
2. List four advantages of credit.
3. List three disadvantages of credit.
4. What are four ways you can establish credit?
5. Name *the three Cs* that determine your credit rating.

Section 6-4

Managing Technology

Objectives

After studying this section, you will be able to

- **compare and contrast** the benefits and drawbacks of technology.
- **give examples** of proper cell phone etiquette and netiquette.
- **identify** ways you can protect yourself when using the Internet.
- **demonstrate** how to use technology responsibly.

Key Terms

technology	blog	etiquette
hybrids	obsolete	netiquette
webcams	identity theft	cyberbullying

Technology is an important nonhuman resource. Learning how to manage technology can help you organize and maintain many aspects of your life. Understanding the benefits and drawbacks of technology can also help you to better handle other resources. For instance, you can use technology to help you organize your time by using scheduling programs on your cell phone or computer. Washing dishes in a dishwasher instead of by hand can save you both time and energy. Setting strong passwords when shopping online can help prevent someone from stealing your money. Effective use of technology can help you reach your goals now and in the future.

Life Connections

Managing with Technology

Human and nonhuman resources can be managed using technology. People are able to save time and energy by shopping and paying bills from home through the Internet. Many people use *smart phones*, or cell phones that also function as handheld computers, to manage their daily schedules, addresses, telephone numbers, and shopping lists. Budgeting software can manage a family's money. Technological innovations are constantly changing people's abilities to manage their resources and lives more effectively. Many things people thought were impossible in the past are now considered necessities.

Research Activity

Conduct research on the Internet to discover what the next advances in technology might be. Write a paragraph about how one or two of them could influence people's abilities to manage their resources.

Impact of Technology

Technology is the use of scientific knowledge to improve the quality of life. As in the past few decades, technology continues to grow at an amazing rate. Think about how much time you spend on the computer or cell phone each day. How often do you watch TV or stream movies instantly?

What electric appliances do you use in the kitchen to make cooking and cleanup easier? Try to imagine how a life without technology would affect you.

Benefits

Technology today benefits people in many ways. With the help of technology, chores take much less time than they used to. This allows more free time for family and leisure activities. Technology advances in health care provide better treatments and even cures for diseases. Advances in technology allow people to communicate instantly with others from around the world.

The Internet is also a valuable resource, **6-14**. Websites contain information and services such as maps, insurance costs, airline reservation information, and computer games. People can use online banking and shopping to check account balances and buy items at any time of the day or night. Technology helps people perform many time-consuming tasks more easily and efficiently.

Technology in the Home

Technology in the home includes everything from microwave ovens to computers. Appliances such as dishwashers and washing machines help people complete chores more quickly. Families can choose from a wide variety of computer programs to assist them with everything from budgeting to scheduling. Home security systems can help prevent break-ins. Fire alarms and carbon monoxide detectors help keep family members safe. Climate control systems help monitor energy usage in the home by allowing people to adjust temperatures remotely. Home technology is advancing at remarkable rates.

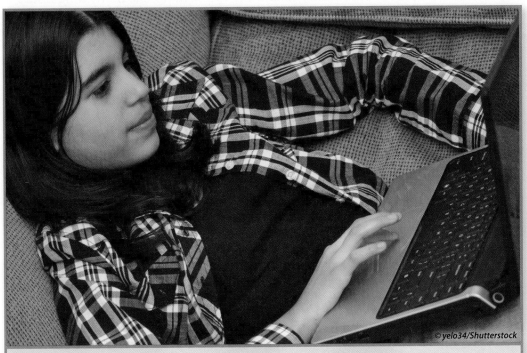

© yelo34/Shutterstock

6-14 The Internet allows people to research topics quickly and conveniently without leaving home or work.

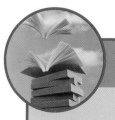

Electronic Readers

Electronic books were first being developed in the 1970s, when the first document was transferred into a digital format. This laid the foundation for future texts to become digitalized. It was not until the 1990s, however, that the first electronic reader, or *e-reader*, was introduced to the public. Today, e-readers are becoming more prevalent. E-readers have the ability to hold thousands of books, magazines, and newspapers in one lightweight device, and are environmentally friendly because they do not use paper. While there are positive aspects to e-readers, many people still prefer printed books to e-books. Find and read articles to research the growing trend of e-readers along with the pros and cons of going wireless. How do you feel about e-readers?

Home Entertainment Technology

Home entertainment technology gives people many more choices than ever before. People can read books and newspapers online or by using electronic readers. Satellite TV and radio let people choose from over hundreds of different stations. Cable companies offer technology that allows people to tailor their own viewing experiences. Televisions have improved screens to enhance viewing. People can watch movies on their televisions or on their computers through the Internet. Video games are more realistic and have better graphics. Some gaming systems incorporate motion-controlled technology that gives users the chance to be more physically active. Ongoing technological advances provide many hours of enjoyment for people without ever leaving home.

Technology in Society

Technology benefits society in many ways. Technological advances continue to provide new and efficient modes of transportation from airplanes to automobiles. Flying from one part of the country to another can save people many long hours of travel. Today's cars offer many modern conveniences that older vehicles did not have. For instance, some cars have navigational technology that provides you with directions when you need them. Safety features such as airbags are common. Automobiles produced with newer technologies, called **hybrids**, have a gasoline engine and an electric motor, **6-15**.

Benefits of technology in education have created a completely new learning environment. Using the computer to complete your assignments allows you to work more quickly and accurately. The use of the Internet means you can research a homework assignment by performing a few simple keystrokes.

© Christian Delbert/Shutterstock

6-15 Plug-in hybrids benefit the environment by using less fuel and reducing pollution.

Many colleges offer online courses. Electronic learning programs often let students set their own goals for learning. They can work at a pace that is appropriate for them.

Technology is also an important part of daily life in workplaces everywhere. For instance, most retail stores use computers to read product codes and add your total bill. Libraries use computers to track the books. Many teachers use computers to record students' grades. Weather centers have technology that helps predict storms and natural disasters and send warnings to communities. Healthcare facilities rely on machines that make it easier to diagnose diseases. Factories use automated machines to complete repetitive tasks.

Communicating with Technology

Technology has improved the way people are able to communicate with one another, **6-16**. For instance, most cell phones provide text messaging and Internet capabilities. This lets friends and family communicate with one another more frequently.

Computer technology allows people to instantly interact with others from all over the world through e-mail, instant messages, or voice conferencing. Video calling programs provide an opportunity for people to call one another through the Internet. They use **webcams**, or small video cameras, to show live images of the callers.

Social networking sites provide a platform for people to share daily activities and interests with others. When joining a site, you must create a profile that includes personal information you are willing to share with others. Members can search for other friends and family to invite them to join their personal network. People then communicate using a blog-like format, e-mail, or instant messaging. A **blog** is an online journal or diary.

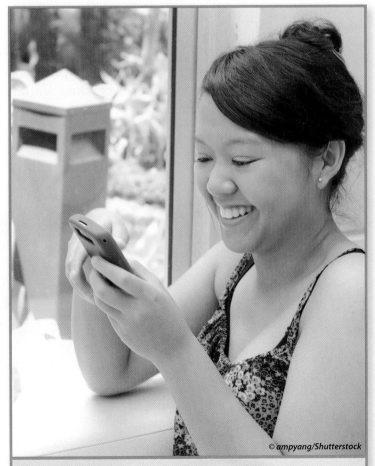

© ampyang/Shutterstock

6-16 Newer technologies make communication much quicker and easier.

Drawbacks

In addition to the benefits of technology, there are also some serious drawbacks. Companies may eliminate jobs because automated machines can do a task once performed by a person. Workers may be required to learn new career skills if technology in their workplace is updated.

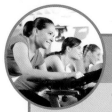

Health Connections

Technology Affects Health

Although technology is a prevalent part of modern life, too much time spent playing video games, using the computer, or texting can negatively affect your health. Frequently texting or clicking can cause *repetitive stress injury*, an irritation caused by overwhelming the joints with too much of the same motion. Sitting still for extensive periods of time while using technology can also cause poor vision, poor posture, and is linked to weight gain. Limit the amount of time allotted for use with technology per week. When not using digital products, incorporate plenty of exercise and stretching into your daily routine.

Because technology changes rapidly, devices may become **obsolete**, or no longer useful, after just a few years. Trying to keep up with the latest advances in technology can put a strain on a person's budget. Using some of the newer technologies may also be difficult for someone who has never used them before. This can cause a person to feel frustrated and stressed.

There are also negative aspects of using the Internet. People can spend hours browsing the Internet or communicating with friends instead of spending time with their families. Parents must be concerned with safety when their children are online, **6-17**.

Children are not the only people who need to be concerned about safety when using the Internet. Not everyone on the Internet is honest. Posting personal information and photos on social networking sites can draw attention from strangers who could be dangerous. Identity theft is another potential hazard of using the Internet. **Identity theft** is the illegal use of someone's personal information to obtain money or credit. Anyone can become a victim when using the Internet. Learning to use technology responsibly, however, is one way you can protect yourself from letting it happen to you.

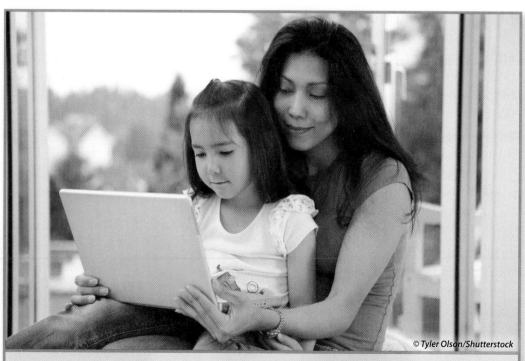

© Tyler Olson/Shutterstock

6-17 Adults may want to restrict children from certain websites.

Using Technology Responsibly

The purpose of technology is to improve the way you live. To achieve that objective, technology research is constantly moving forward. You can keep up with the latest technology by reading books, taking courses, or talking with other people. Think about whether you really need the most current technological device as soon as it hits the store shelves. Check reviews of products before buying them. Sometimes it might be better to wait until a product becomes more affordable. Another device with better features might be available in a few months.

It is also important to remember that although technology may be convenient, it should not replace personal interactions with family and friends. Balance your time wisely. Try not to spend too much time watching TV, talking on the phone, or playing computer games. Meet a friend and go for a walk instead of texting each other. Have a family night instead of sitting at the computer. Learning how to control technology will help you to receive the most benefits from it.

Cell Phone Etiquette

How many times have you been in a public place and have heard someone else's phone conversation? How does it make you feel when you are with a friend and he or she is talking on the phone or texting someone else? **Etiquette** refers to proper and polite ways to behave, **6-18**.

Cell Phone Etiquette Guidelines

- Turn your cell phone off or silence the ringer while in public places such as restaurants, stores, hallways, or buses. Loud conversations and ringtones are often disruptive to others. Let any calls transfer to voice mail until you are in a private area and can talk freely. If you must take a call, talk quietly and keep your conversation brief.
- Keep your phone turned off in movie theaters, plays, or other darkened public events. Do not text or check the time. Ringtones and lighted screens can be annoying to other people who are trying to enjoy the show.
- Avoid gossiping, arguing, or discussing personal matters in public places.
- Do not remain too close to others while talking on the phone. Be sure to keep your voice low.
- Do not call or text someone when you are spending time with another person. This is inconsiderate to those around you.
- Be mindful of your cell phone plan, and the plan of the person you are calling or texting. Consider the possible costs involved in making or receiving calls and texts.
- Do not talk on a handheld phone or try to text while driving. Also, do not check messages or surf the Internet. It is very unsafe and can cause an accident. In some states, this behavior is against the law.

6-18 When using a cell phone, there are certain guidelines of common courtesy you should follow.

Netiquette

The term netiquette refers to proper behavior when using the Internet. Although e-mail and instant messaging is not a personal form of communication, you need to be mindful of what you say to other people. This also includes any messages or posts you write in response to blogs, on social networking sites, or in chat rooms. Your correspondence should be polite and considerate of other people's feelings. It is important to remember that the people who read your message cannot see your facial expressions or other body language. This can cause a message to be misunderstood.

The following tips can help you to communicate better with others when using the Internet:

- Keep your message brief and to the point. Include a short, but meaningful, subject line.
- Do not use all capital letters when sending a message. People might think you are shouting at them.
- Always use correct grammar, spelling, and punctuation in your correspondence.
- Avoid using text abbreviations or emoticons. You might include them in messages to some of your closest friends. They are not appropriate, however, in messages to other people or in business correspondence.
- Read your messages carefully before sending or posting them. Remember that you do not always know who will be reading them. Some e-mail messages might be forwarded to others. Also, even if you try to delete a post online, versions can still exist on another person's computer.
- Do not send messages immediately when you are angry or upset, **6-19**. Instead, take time to calm down and think about what you want to say.
- Accept responsibility for what you write. Do not post or e-mail anything you would not be willing to say to the person face-to-face.
- Do not send or forward chain letters.

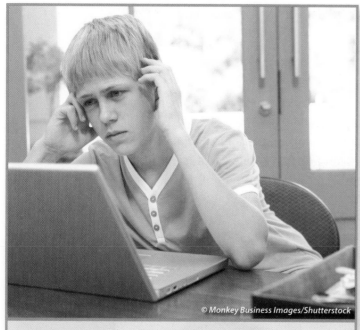

© Monkey Business Images/Shutterstock

6-19 Sending a message when you are angry could just make a situation worse.

Internet Safety

People worldwide use the Internet every day. The Internet is a useful tool to help you research topics for school projects, keep in touch with your friends, and hear about the latest news locally and globally. You can easily spend hours surfing websites, watching videos, and playing games. The Internet is a place where you can look for jobs and meet new friends. The amount of information you can obtain from the Internet is endless.

The Internet is just like any other community, except much larger. Within this community, there are people who may pretend to be someone they are not. These people can be dangerous. They may obtain information about you and try to steal from you or harm you physically. Always use caution when spending time online. The following tips can help protect you when using the Internet:

- Never reveal private information. This includes your name, address, phone number, social security number, passwords, or names of family members, schools, and workplaces.
- Never reveal personal information about someone else.
- Learn about privacy rules for social networking sites before joining. Try to only create a personal profile that friends or family can access.

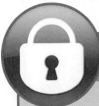

Safety Connections

Evaluating Websites

Because there is a surplus of information on the Internet, look for these indicators in the web address to make sure you are looking at a safe, reliable Internet source.

- *https.* Websites beginning with *https:* instead of *http:* are secure. If you must send or view personal information, make sure the website begins with *https.*
- *.gov.* These websites are a government resource containing accurate national and international information.
- *.edu.* These websites are for particular schools and universities. Information is educational and reliable.
- *.org.* Information from these websites comes from a recognized nonprofit organization and is safe.
- *.com.* This is the most common website. Information may not always be reliable. Check information against other reference materials for validation.

- Select e-mail addresses and screen names that keep you anonymous. Try using letters and numbers. Do not give away gender or any other personal information.
- Do not send photos of yourself to anyone you meet online. The person could alter the photos or use them in a way you would not want them to.
- Avoid meeting online friends in person. These meetings can be risky because people can pretend to be something they are not. If you really want to meet, get a parent's permission first.
- Immediately tell your parents or another trusted adult about anyone you meet online who makes you feel uncomfortable or threatened.
- Report any cases of **cyberbullying**, or cruel and hurtful messages you receive or witness online, to your parents or a trusted adult. Do not join others who are bullying. Keep a record of any messages you might receive, but do not respond to them. Many times a bully is seeking attention. If you ignore it, he or she might stop. In the event the bullying continues, report it to the Internet service provider or the authorities.

Reading Review

1. Give three examples of the benefits of technology.
2. How has technology improved the way people are able to communicate with one another?
3. Give three examples of the drawbacks of technology.
4. List four examples of cell phone etiquette.
5. What is netiquette?

Chapter Summary

Section 6-1. Managing the resources of time and energy will help you throughout life. You can manage time by planning your use of it. This involves preparing a daily schedule, avoiding wasting time, and improving your study habits. You can manage your energy by eating nutritious foods, getting enough sleep, and participating in regular physical activity.

Section 6-2. To reach your goals, it is important to manage your money wisely. To manage money, you must be able to prepare a budget to balance your income and fixed and flexible expenses. As you manage your money, various financial services can help you to save and invest your money.

Section 6-3. You can use credit to charge goods and services or to borrow money and then pay later. There are various types of credit available. Using credit involves both advantages and disadvantages. There are several ways to establish credit. Several factors determine whether a person will be a good credit risk. Once you have established credit, it must be managed wisely to avoid overspending and financial worries.

Section 6-4. Technology can help you organize and maintain many aspects of your life. There are many benefits as well as drawbacks of technology. Using technology involves responsibility. Using cell phone etiquette and netiquette will help you to communicate properly using technology. Following certain precautions can help you to use the Internet safely.

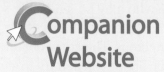

Companion Website
www.g-wlearning.com

Check your understanding of the main concepts for Chapter 6 at the website.

Critical Thinking

1. **Draw conclusions.** How might the information you learned in this chapter help you to manage your resources?
2. **Determine.** Should there be laws censoring information on the Internet?
3. **Analyze behavior.** Why is cyberbullying a problem? What might cause someone to be a cyberbully? How can victims of cyberbullying overcome this situation?

Common Core

College and Career Readiness

4. **Math.** Make two schedules for your own use—one for a weekday and one for a Saturday. First make to-do lists for each day and decide which activities are most important. Estimate the amount of time it will take to perform each task. Prepare schedules that will

allow you to complete the activities you need to do and want to do.

5. **Reading.** Look through a magazine and select one advertisement. Read the ad and analyze how it attempts to influence you to buy the product. How much does advertising influence how you spend your money?

6. **Speaking.** As a class, discuss the advantages and disadvantages of using credit. Then break into two groups and debate the pros and cons of using credit.

7. **Math.** Prepare a budget for yourself. Include your income, fixed expenses, and flexible expenses. Try to follow the budget for a week. Evaluate the budget and make adjustments as necessary.

Technology

8. **Investigate new technologies.** Research the newest technologies used for communication. Consider the advantages as well as the drawbacks of these technologies. Present your findings to the class.

Journal Writing

9. Think about all the resources you have. Make a list of them. Now write a paragraph beginning with the statement, "If I could donate any resource to benefit someone in need or my community, it would be…" Then explain why you would donate that resource.

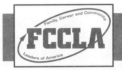 FCCLA

10. Teach others in your school or community how to make, save, and spend money wisely through the *FCCLA Financial Fitness* program. Possible project topics may include understanding banking (accounts, credit, and investments), tracking your spending and creating a personal spending budget, or becoming a savvy spender. Use the *FCCLA Planning Process* to guide your project planning. See your adviser for information as needed.

Chapter 7
Being a Responsible Consumer

Sections

Reading Prep

College and Career Readiness

After reading each section, answer this question: If you explained the information to a friend who is not taking this class, what would you tell him or her?

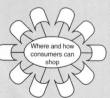

Concept Organizer

Where and how consumers can shop

Use a diagram like the one shown to indicate where and how consumers can shop for goods and services.

Companion Website

Print out the concept organizer for Chapter 7 at the website.

Companion Website
www.g-wlearning.com

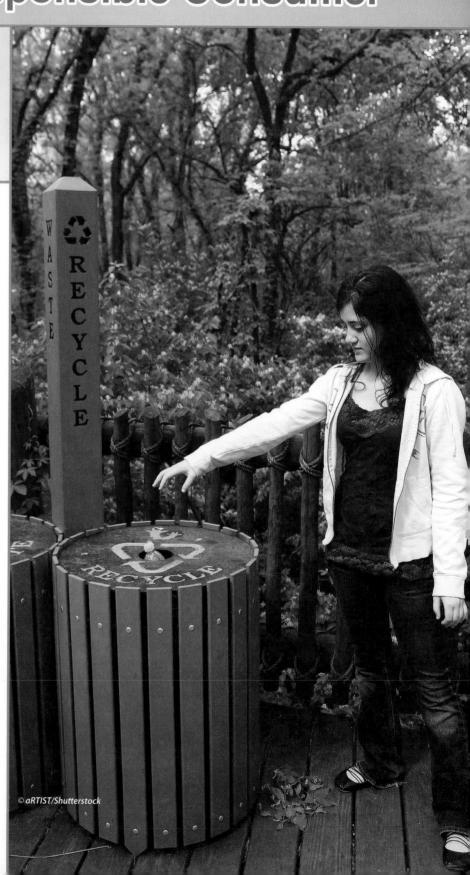

© aRTIST/Shutterstock

Section 7-1

Consumer Basics

Objectives

After studying this section, you will be able to
- **identify** decisions you need to make in order to be an informed and responsible consumer.
- **evaluate** advertisements using smart consumer buying techniques.
- **describe** consumer rights and responsibilities.
- **demonstrate** how to write a letter of complaint.

Key Terms

consumer	endorse	impulse buying
E-commerce	bait and switch	redress
T-commerce	comparison shopping	exchange
advertisement	warranty	refund

In today's marketplace, shoppers are fortunate because they are able to choose from a wide variety of goods and services. There are many places to shop and spend money. This can also be a problem, however. You may have so many choices that you become confused. For this reason, you need to be informed and responsible when buying goods and services. Then you will get the most value for the money you spend.

Consumer Decisions

A **consumer** is a person who buys or uses goods and services, **7-1**. As a consumer, you make decisions all the time. Some decisions you make out of *habit*. You may not even be aware of these decisions. For instance, you may always go to the same salon whenever you need a haircut. Other decisions, however, are more important. They involve a lot of planning.

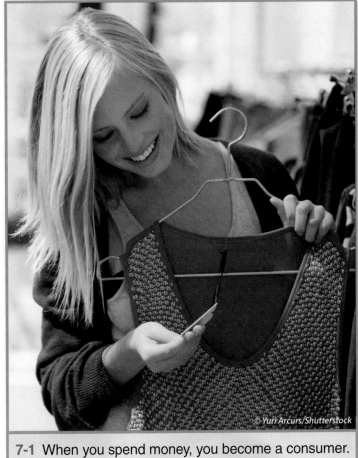

© Yuri Arcurs/Shutterstock

7-1 When you spend money, you become a consumer.

Needs, Wants, Values, and Goals

To be a smart consumer, you should develop a shopping plan that reflects your needs, wants, values, and goals. You should also consider your resources, such as how much money you have available to spend.

When developing your plan, you must first meet your needs. For instance, all people need to eat, so they buy food. People also need clothing and shelter. After you meet your needs, your wants, values, and goals will most likely determine your course of action. For instance, your goal might be to save money because you really want a car. You may then spend less on other purchases while you are saving for the car. Using the decision-making process can help you determine what purchases are most important.

Where to Shop

Informed consumers are aware of the types of places where they can shop, **7-2**. Getting to know the types of stores in your area provides options for you. Following are several types of places people often shop.

Department stores offer a wide variety of products and services under one roof. Products of different qualities and in a wide variety of price ranges are often available. They frequently have special sales and coupons. Department stores may offer many services. They often issue their own credit cards. Other services might include delivery, gift wrapping, clothing alterations, bridal consulting, interior decorating, and wardrobe planning.

Discount stores carry national brands at lower prices than department stores. They generally have fewer salespeople and offer fewer services than department stores. Their return policies may be more limited. Discount stores can offer lower prices because you do not have to pay for extra services.

Superstores are very large retail stores that offer a wide variety of merchandise. They may carry groceries, clothing, automotive supplies, fitness equipment, electronics, jewelry, furniture, appliances, and toys, **7-3**. Prices are often lower because the store is able

© liza1979/Shutterstock

7-2 You will probably choose to shop at different stores for different items.

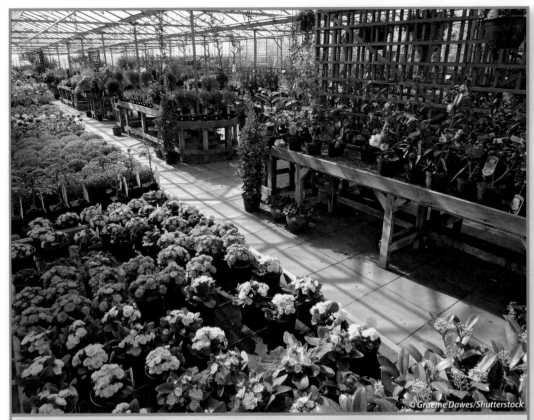

© Graeme Dawes/Shutterstock

7-3 Some superstores may have garden and tire centers, while others might offer prescription services.

to buy large volumes of products, which allows them to pass their savings to consumers. They also offer limited services.

Warehouse clubs offer a wide variety of products at wholesale prices. Products are usually available for purchase in *bulk*, or larger quantities. Consumers must pay an annual membership fee to be able to shop at these stores.

Factory outlet stores are operated by manufacturers to sell only their products to consumers. Prices are lower in factory outlet stores because you are buying directly from the manufacturer. There is no retail store owner. Factory outlet stores have fewer employees than department stores and offer few, if any, services.

Items for sale at factory outlet stores come directly from the factory. Some of these goods are from past seasons. Some of them may be *irregulars*. This means the items have slight defects. If you are thinking about buying an irregular item, look for the defect. Then decide if the defect will affect the item's use.

Off-price discount stores sell brand name merchandise at significantly discounted prices. They purchase overstock clothing and accessories from manufacturers at lower prices. They may also purchase items from other retail stores that have excessive inventory. Off-price discount stores then pass these savings to consumers. They usually provide limited services.

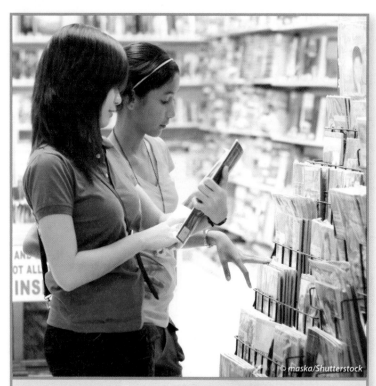

7-4 Bookstores, music shops, and barbershops are all specialty shops.

Specialty shops sell only one type of product or service, **7-4**. These shops offer a wide selection of the type of product or service. Prices may vary from low to high depending on quality of the merchandise and services the shop offers.

Mail-order shopping through catalogs is a convenient way to shop. You can either mail, phone, or fax your order to the company. Placing an order online is also possible. Many people like to shop by mail order because they do not have to spend the time and energy looking in stores. You may also find a wider selection of colors and sizes using mail-order catalogs.

A disadvantage of shopping by mail is that you have to wait for your purchase to arrive. Then it may not perform as you had expected. You will have to reorder if your selection is not available. You should know the company's return policy in case you need to return an item. In most cases, you are responsible for paying the postage.

Yard sales, thrift shops, and consignment stores offer used merchandise. Variety, prices, and quality of items varies from place to place. Yard sales, or garage sales, are held at people's homes for a limited time, such as a weekend. Thrift shops sell clothing and other items people donate to raise funds for a charitable organization. Consignment stores sell items for a person and then pay the owner a portion of the sale price.

Electronic Shopping

E-commerce means shopping online. The Internet is a popular way to shop because of the convenience it provides consumers. People can purchase just about anything online from books to automobiles. People can order airline tickets and make hotel reservations. Many retail stores offer online shopping services. Consumers usually need to use a credit card to place an order.

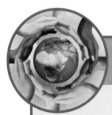

Global Connections

M-Commerce

The term *M-commerce* refers to the capability of buying and selling goods and services through wireless handheld mobile devices. With more smart phones in use worldwide, global commerce has increased tremendously. If you want to buy a pashmina scarf from India or a tribal mask from Kenya, your smart phone makes it easy for you to get one from anywhere you happen to be. Mobile applications (apps) are the new marketing tool for retailers. Retailers can use apps to track customers' interests in certain products, make reordering easy, and redeem coupons or discounts. The apps can even turn a mobile device into a scanner to authenticate and purchase products. M-commerce is the future of consumerism.

T-commerce refers to shopping using television. Shopping networks offer products people can buy at any time of the day or night. Items have an order number and the consumer phones in to place orders using a credit card. *Infomercials* are extended length commercials that provide information about a product and a toll-free number for ordering. *Interactive television* allows you to buy goods or services instantly with your remote control.

Advertising

Advertising has a big influence on how you spend your money. An **advertisement** is a paid public announcement about goods, services, or ideas for sale. People who produce and sell products and services spend a great deal of time and money on advertisements, **7-5**.

Companies use many different types of advertising media to convince you to buy their products and services. You hear advertisements on the radio. You see advertisements in stores, on TV, in magazines and newspapers, and on billboards and posters. You receive advertisements by direct mail. The Internet is also a common place to see advertisements. Companies advertise their products or services online through websites, social networking sites, banner ads, and pop-up ads.

Careful consumers can find useful information in many advertisements. You can learn about clothing, food, personal care items, or movies from advertisements. You can also learn about changes and improvements in products.

Do not be convinced, however, that a product is good or you must have it just because of an advertisement. Advertisers may lead you to believe a product will do more than it will really do. For instance, using a certain brand of toothpaste will not really help you get a boyfriend or a girlfriend.

Advertisements often include special offers and slogans to attract your attention. Sometimes well-known people endorse products and services. **Endorse** means to publicly express support or approval. Famous people often receive a lot of

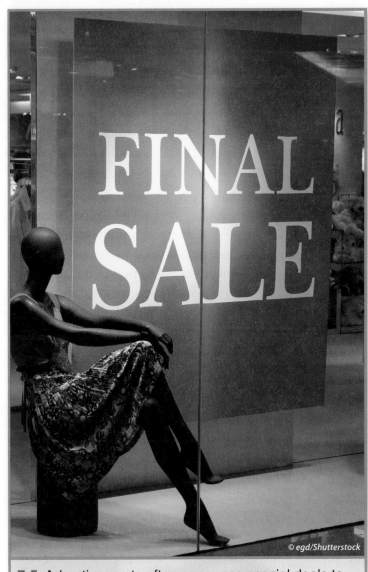

© egd/Shutterstock

7-5 Advertisements often announce special deals to convince you to buy the product or service.

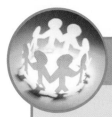

Evaluating Advertising Claims

Look at advertisements critically and be realistic about their claims. Ask yourself if the ads offer any fact-based information, or do they only present persuasion tactics. You may need to find another way to get *unbiased*, or fair, information about the product. There are a number of options to learn what people who are *not* paid by the company really think about the product's quality and usefulness. The easiest way is to talk with people you know who use the product.

The Internet is another great tool for learning the truth about a product or service before purchase. Use a search engine to enter the name of the product along with the word *review*. Unbiased consumer magazines, such as *Consumer Reports*, also provide this service by field testing products and rating them. The Federal Trade Commission (FTC) has a Bureau of Consumer Protection to protect consumers from fraudulent claims by companies. That website is at www.ftc.gov/bcp.

Financial Literacy Activity

Choose a product or service you want to purchase and practice finding available information about the prices and the product options. How does the information you find compare with the product's advertising claims? Remember that the most expensive option is not always rated the highest. Discuss which option you would purchase based on reviews, other information, and pricing.

money to endorse products. Advertisers want you to think that a product must be good if a famous person uses it and likes it.

Advertisers may even use a bait and switch tactic. **Bait and switch** means advertisers promote a product at a low price to get your attention, but then try to persuade you to buy a more expensive item.

Always ask yourself if you really need a product, or if you just want it because of its advertising. Use the decision-making process to make a purchasing decision. List the product's pros and cons. This will help you avoid purchasing a product based on advertising alone.

Guidelines for Shopping

- Have plenty of time to comparison shop.
- Make a shopping list before you leave home.
- Follow your shopping list and resist impulse buying.
- Check for good quality.
- Be sure instructions and care directions are included.
- Ask about return and exchange policies.

7-6 Following these guidelines for shopping will help you make wise purchasing decisions.

Consumer Buying Techniques

Smart consumers practice **comparison shopping**, which means looking at competing brands and models of a product in several stores, **7-6**. You compare quality, features, and prices before buying. By doing this, you can determine the product that best suits your needs.

Learn as much as you can about any product before you buy it. Read hangtags, labels, and care instructions. Warranties and use and care manuals are other sources of accurate information. A **warranty** is a written statement provided by a manufacturer that guarantees a product is in good condition. If the product breaks within a certain time after purchase, the manufacturer will often repair or replace it. People can also give you information about goods and services from their practical experience.

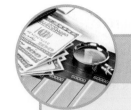

Financial Literacy Connections

Smart Shopping

In addition to avoiding impulse shopping, resist the temptation to purchase a product under pressure. The pressure may come from a sales associate, a friend, or a *limited time only* sale date. Take the time to evaluate the product to make sure it is something you need. Using the comparison shopping strategy, you can verify that the product is of good quality, a reasonable price, and right for you. Comparison shopping will also eliminate the possibility of buying on impulse, buying out of habit, or buying products just because they are on sale. Overall, you will have the satisfaction of purchasing the best option for you while saving money.

Impulse buying is the opposite of comparison shopping. It is not a good way to shop. **Impulse buying** is an unplanned or spur-of-the-moment purchase. Impulse buying often leads people to buy items they do not really need. Some of these items may not be returnable. You will regret buying a sale item if you never use it. By following a shopping plan, you can avoid impulse buying.

Consumer Rights and Responsibilities

President John F. Kennedy created the *Consumer Bill of Rights* in 1962. The basic consumer rights he listed include the right to safety, the right to be informed, the right to choose, and the right to be heard. Two additional basic consumer rights were added later. These include the right to redress and the right to consumer education. **Redress** means to correct something that is wrong. See Figure **7-7** for a description of these rights.

To deserve these basic rights, consumers must be willing to accept certain responsibilities. Following are ways to be a responsible consumer:

- **Use products properly.** Always read and follow the operating and care instructions for products you buy. You may ruin an electric popcorn popper by immersing it in water. This would be your fault, not a fault of the company that made it. If you read the operating instructions, you will know how to care for and use a product properly.
- **Become an informed consumer.** Making careful use of consumer information can help you make decisions about the products and services you need. Many sources of consumer information are available to you. Newspapers and magazines often evaluate products and services. You can also look at labels and tags directly on a product for information.
- **Make careful choices.** Practice comparison shopping to choose among various products and services. Deal with companies you can trust. Then select the products and services you need and can afford.

Consumer Rights

The Right to Safety	You have the right to know the goods and services you purchase will be safe. To assure you of this right, government agencies inspect much of what you buy. They keep track of complaints about products and do their best to keep unsafe products off the market.
The Right to Be Informed	You have the right to know the facts about goods and services before you buy so you can make the right choices.
The Right to Choose	You have the right to choose from a variety of goods and services. When several companies offer a product, they are more likely to compete by lowering prices or improving quality.
The Right to Be Heard	You have the right to speak out if you are not satisfied with a product or service.
The Right to Redress	You have the right to redress. This is an extension of the right to be heard. This means you can expect action to be taken upon your complaints.
The Right to Consumer Education	You have the right to become educated about your consumer rights. Various consumer education programs are available to help you.

7-7 As a consumer, you have the following rights.

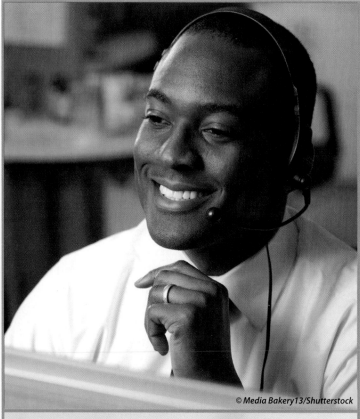

© Media Bakery13/Shutterstock

7-8 Many companies employ customer service representatives to listen to your feedback about their product or service.

- **Express likes and dislikes.** Tell producers and sellers what you like and dislike about their products and services, **7-8**. If you do not make an effort to do this, you cannot expect companies to produce the quality goods and services you need and want. Many companies have websites that will give you an opportunity to contact them. Sending your thoughts helps them to know what customers like or dislike.
- **Take action to have a wrong corrected.** Express your problem to a seller in a polite and fair manner. You may need to write a letter to the manufacturer. Do not be afraid to ask for what you believe to be a fair response to your request.

- **Become educated about your consumer rights.** Many agencies offer help through publications and seminars on consumer education topics. You also have the opportunity to become an educated consumer by attending consumer education classes at school and in your community.

Complaining

Complaining is a very important consumer right and responsibility. By knowing the right way to complain about a product or service, you will more easily solve your consumer problems.

Suppose you purchased a sweater at your favorite clothing store. The first time you washed it, half the sweater unraveled even though you followed the care instructions. You have the right and responsibility to file a complaint about this situation.

Plan to return to the store as soon as possible. Before you go, you will need to decide what action you want to take. If you really want the same style of sweater, you might try to exchange it. **Exchange** means to substitute one item for another. If you do not want another sweater in return, you can ask for a refund. A **refund** is repayment of a product's purchase price.

Be sure to take tags and receipts to prove you bought the sweater at that store. State your problem clearly and briefly to a salesperson or customer service representative. Also, explain how you would like to solve the problem. Always be calm and polite when expressing your complaint. Most stores want their customers to be happy so they will return in the future. If you happen to be dealing with someone who is unable to help with the situation, ask to see the manager. Then restate your complaint.

You may not always be able to reach a solution to your problem at the store. The store might refuse to exchange your sweater or refund your money. In such a case, you should write a letter of complaint to the manufacturer. The store manager will most likely have the name and address of the supplier. If not, you can always check online. Libraries also have reference books that list addresses for many companies.

Writing a Complaint Letter

Complaint letters follow the form of other business letters, **7-9**. List your address and the date at the top. Then list the name, title, and address of the person to whom you are writing.

In the body of the letter, you should describe the product or service about which you are complaining. Include where and when you purchased it and how much you paid. Enclose a copy of your receipt and mention this in the letter.

Writing Connections

A Complaint Letter

When you write a complaint letter, it is actually beneficial to both you and the company. For you, the letter is communicating your consumer right to express dissatisfaction with the potential of getting a refund, exchange, or making a better product. For the company, the letter notifies them of fixable errors. It also communicates that the customer enjoys the company's merchandise enough to express dissatisfaction. This gives the company an opportunity to work on the consumer/business relationship. You should not feel guilty about writing a complaint letter, as long as you keep a positive tone.

8599 North Orchard Lane
Lexington, IN 46315
January 15, 20XX

Mr. Carlos Gonzalez
Director of Customer Service
Funwear Clothing Company
480 Monroe Street
Decatur, IL 61658

Dear Mr. Gonzalez:

On January 5, I purchased a red, blue, yellow, and green striped
cotton pullover from the Teen Boutique in Lexington, Indiana.
The style number is 5231. I paid $17 for this shirt, and I have
enclosed a copy of my receipt.

I washed the shirt in cold water on gentle cycle as the care label
suggested. When I took it out of the washer, I was surprised to
find that the colors had run together in many places. My pullover
now has blotches of color all over it. A copy of the care label
and a photo of the shirt after it was washed are enclosed.

I attempted to return the shirt to the Teen Boutique and get
another one like it. There were no shirts left in my size, however,
and the store manager refused to refund my money. Therefore, I
would like to have my money refunded. I am willing to send you the
shirt if your company needs it to research this problem.

Thank you for your attention to this problem.

Sincerely,

Amy Jackson

Amy Jackson

Enclosures

7-9 Complaint letters should be clear and complete in explaining a problem.

Then state the problem you are having and how it happened. This is the reason for your complaint. Maybe an item was defective, or never delivered.

Finally, you should state the action that is necessary to solve the problem. This is important. The company must understand what you want in order to solve your complaint. You might want an exchange, a refund, or to have the product repaired. Be firm about what you want, but try to give your letter a positive tone. Letters that are positive and clearly written are likely to get a better response than letters that are angry and provide little information about the problem.

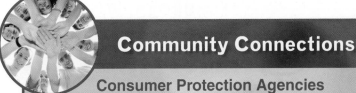

Community Connections

Consumer Protection Agencies

In some serious cases, you may need to contact a consumer protection agency to help solve your consumer problems. These agencies work to represent and protect the consumer and consumer rights. The Federal Trade Commission's *Bureau of Consumer Protection* is the nation's consumer protection agency, but there are also state, regional, county, and city agencies. These agencies would investigate the claim, file a report, and initiate any legal procedures. This action should be used as a last resort, or if the product poses a serious threat to the consumer population.

Keep a copy of the complaint letters you write. If you do not get a response from a letter, you may need to write another one. Enclose a copy of the first letter with your next letter, and give a date by which you expect action.

Other Ways to Solve Consumer Problems

You may need to look for other sources of help if your letters do not solve the problem. Better Business Bureaus, trade associations, and governmental consumer offices can help. They may be able to put pressure on businesses to act on your complaint. They may also be able to suggest alternate methods of solving your problem.

If all these methods of solving your problem fail, you may decide to take it to court. You should only use this method if the problem is very serious and the other methods have not solved the problem.

Reading Review

1. To be a smart consumer, what should your shopping plan reflect?
2. List six places you can shop for items.
3. What does e-commerce mean?
4. List six consumer rights.
5. List six consumer responsibilities.

Section 7-2

Environmental Responsibility

Objectives

After studying this section, you will be able to

- **identify** renewable and nonrenewable natural resources.
- **apply** ways to conserve energy and resources.
- **explain** how to use energy efficiently.
- **discuss** the importance of minimizing waste.
- **propose** strategies to reduce, reuse, and recycle waste.

Key Terms

natural resources	conserve	mass transit
renewable resources	ecosystem	landfills
nonrenewable resources	photosynthesis	recycled
	climate change	composting

Social Studies Connections

Conserving Public Lands

As the country expanded in the 1800s, people became increasingly aware of the need to protect the natural environment. The government started setting aside land, and in 1872, Yellowstone National Park became the country's first national park. Today, there are 58 national parks in the United States that are used for human recreation, animal and plant species protection, and the conservation of natural resources. They can never be sold or developed.

Shortly after the turn of the 20th century, President Theodore Roosevelt made conservation a high priority. An avid sportsman, naturalist, and conservationist, he established the U.S. Forest Service and designated 190 million acres for forest preserves, parks, and monuments. He also created 50 wildlife refuges, expanded the national park system, and helped pass laws protecting our natural resources and critical soil erosion issues. He is considered one of the *greenest* presidents in history.

You live in many environments. The closest to you are your home, school, and community. Everybody lives on the same planet Earth, however, and the global environment is everyone's concern. If the planet, or portions of it, is unclean, the health and safety of every living being is affected. Scientists are continually researching and finding ways to best protect local and global environments. Every person can be a part of the solution by simply becoming aware of environmental problems and taking steps in their own lives to solve them.

Natural Resources

Natural resources are those materials found in nature and shared by everyone. Natural resources are undisturbed by humans, but every manufactured product is composed of natural resources in some form.

These include air, water, soil, plants, animals, and minerals. The energy people use in their daily lives comes from natural resources.

Natural resources are categorized in two ways. **Renewable resources** simply exist or rebuild themselves fairly quickly after use, such as sunlight and fast-growing plants. **Nonrenewable resources** are those that have formed very slowly and are limited in supply, such as minerals and *fossil fuels*. Fossil fuels were formed by the decomposition of animals many millions of years ago and contain large amounts of carbon. They include coal, petroleum (oil), and natural gas.

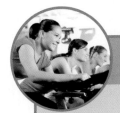

Health Connections

Air Pollution

Air pollution can affect your health. Children, older adults, and people with respiratory conditions, such as asthma, are the most vulnerable to the effects of poor air quality. There are short- and long-term effects on health. Short-term effects include irritation to the respiratory system, which can restrict the ease of breathing and increase the chances of catching a cough. Over a longer period of time, lungs can become permanently damaged and it becomes more difficult for your body to fight against lung diseases.

The Environmental Protection Agency regulates pollutants that are released into the air. To caution people of current air quality, many weather reports include an *Air Quality Index Rate*. To learn more, visit www.epa.gov.

Most countries' governments are attempting to conserve nonrenewable natural resources, and protect the natural environment from harm by human activities. To **conserve** means to use carefully in order to prevent loss or waste of resources. Because most natural resources are limited, the United States has federal laws to help keep the air and water clean. The Environmental Protection Agency (EPA) was created to enforce these laws for the good of the environment.

Consequences of Pollution

An **ecosystem** includes all of the living and nonliving things existing in that particular environment. Some ecosystems are delicate, and some are hardy. Pollution upsets the natural balance of all healthy ecosystems. Burning fossil fuels for energy produces massive amounts of carbon emissions every year, **7-10**.

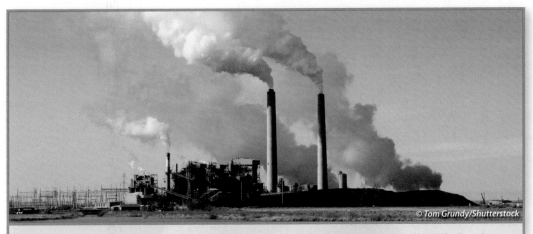

© Tom Grundy/Shutterstock

7-10 Coal burned at power plants is the biggest contributor to air pollution in the U.S.

It is estimated that ecosystems' natural processes, such as photosynthesis, can only cleanse about half of it, however. **Photosynthesis** is how plants turn carbon dioxide into oxygen. The remaining carbon dioxide contributes greatly to *air pollution*, making it unclean and unhealthy. The EPA has conducted extensive research about the effects of pollution on the environment and consequently people's health.

Climate Change

Climate change is any significant change in measures—such as temperatures, precipitation, and wind—of the Earth's climate lasting for an extended period of time. The EPA, along with other federal agencies, monitors extreme weather conditions and determines how air pollution has contributed to this situation. For instance, they have documented that the decade 2000–2009 was the warmest in recorded history. This is at least partially due to the overabundance of carbon dioxide, which is one of the greenhouse gases. *Greenhouse gases* trap the Earth's heat in the atmosphere and contribute to warmer temperatures throughout the world. Scientists have shown that the increase in temperatures is related to the increase in dangerous storms, **7-11**.

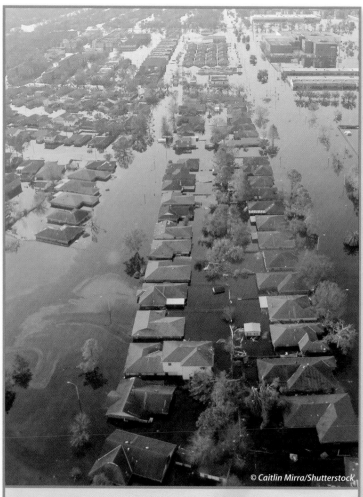

7-11 In 2005, Hurricane Katrina caused severe destruction along the Gulf Coast. Most of New Orleans, LA became flooded and there was significant loss of life.

© Caitlin Mirra/Shutterstock

Health and Well-Being

In addition to dangerous extreme weather conditions, air, water, and soil pollution increases many diseases and directly affects the quality of the food people eat. Industrial waste and sewage from manufacturing plants and chemicals used in farming enter the air, water supplies, and surrounding soil. These substances are toxic, causing great harm to all plant, animal, and human life. While there are now laws that limit this type of pollution, it still exists and is a subject of great concern to many people.

Conserving Energy and Resources

Imagine you do not have energy supplied to your home for 24 hours. How would this affect your daily routines? Your cooling and heating systems, appliances, lighting, and entertainment systems would all be affected. Americans depend on energy sources for comfort, convenience, and fun. Experts are finding ways to increase energy conservation to protect nonrenewable natural resources and reduce pollution.

Most of the energy used to run homes and businesses is electrical, which must be generated in power plants. Natural gas is a nonrenewable resource used in many homes as a heat source. Natural gas can be used in furnaces, ranges, water heaters, and clothes dryers. Unfortunately, using and producing necessary energy in the traditional ways is depleting limited fossil fuels and polluting both air and water in the process.

Alternative Sources of Energy

Engineers are working on solutions to environmental problems caused by traditional energy production methods. The obvious answer is to turn continually renewable resources, such as sun, wind, or water into effective power sources. Some alternatives are currently used, but not yet on the major scale to end the dependence on nonrenewable natural resources for energy needs.

Wind Energy

Wind energy was one of the first natural resources people used for power by creating sails to move boats and windmills to grind grains. Wind occurs because the sun cannot heat the Earth's surface evenly due to physical differences in land areas, such as mountains, valleys, and lakes. As hot air rises from the ground, cooler air moves in to fill that space forming wind. That energy can be harnessed to generate electrical power. While this form of energy production is still not widely used, it has the greatest potential for growth. Experts predict that by the mid-21st century, one third of the world's electricity will be wind generated.

Solar Energy

Solar energy creates electricity by harnessing the sun's heat in special solar panels connected to the local power grid, **7-12**. That energy powers

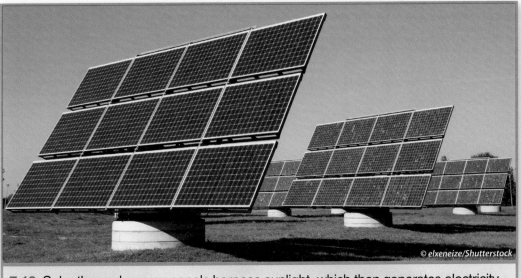

© elxeneize/Shutterstock

7-12 Solar thermal energy panels harness sunlight, which then generates electricity.

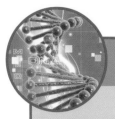

Science Connections

Wind Turbines

Most wind energy comes from using turbines that can be from 100- to 500-feet tall. A *turbine* is an engine that has a part with blades caused to spin from pressure. Wind turbines have two or three 200-foot-long blades—making them resemble a very large pinwheel when spinning. As wind pressure spins the blades, a pole connected to a generator in a nearby plant spins to create electricity. The largest wind turbines can generate enough electricity to supply up to 600 U.S. homes a year. Wind farms often have hundreds of these turbines in particularly windy areas, such as ridge tops. Smaller turbines placed in a backyard can produce enough electricity for a single home or small business.

the building where it was generated. Any unused energy is sold back to the community for the needs of others. Solar energy is already being used to run many homes and offices. On a much larger scale, solar energy power plants use several ways to concentrate the sun's energy as a heat source. The heat then boils water to drive a steam turbine that creates electricity in much the same way as other power plants, supplying electricity for thousands of people.

Water Energy

Water energy is also called *hydroelectricity*. Power is generated through the force of falling or flowing water. It is the most widely used form of renewable energy, **7-13**. Hydropower is the least expensive source of renewable energy in the United States, but it cannot be used on a smaller scale like solar power.

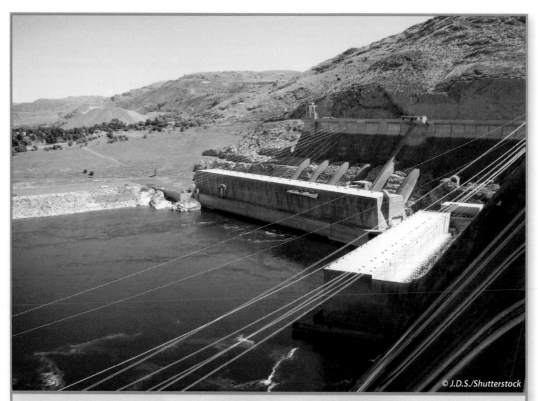

© J.D.S./Shutterstock

7-13 Almost one-fifth of the world's electricity is produced by hydroelectric power.

Geothermal Energy

Geothermal energy is created when cooler water seeps into Earth's extremely hot magma layer under the crust. The water is heated by the magma's high temperature and rises to the surface. When heated water is forced to the surface, geothermal energy plants can capture that steam and use it to create electricity. There are a number of geothermal plants in the United States, mainly near areas with volcanic activity.

Using Energy Efficiently

In addition to finding renewable energy sources, efficiency is increased through energy conservation. Using less energy means using fewer resources. Think carefully about how you use items that need power. Often, the same job can be done without using as much power. By taking some simple steps, you can conserve energy, save money, and protect the environment, **7-14**.

Ways to Conserve Energy and Reduce Pollution

- Keep the thermostat set at 65°F in the winter and 78°F in the summer.
- Securely shut doors and windows when the heat or air conditioning is on.
- Turn off lights, computers, and other appliances when not in use.
- Use compact fluorescent bulb (CFLs) in place of incandescent bulbs.
- Use a microwave oven whenever possible instead of a conventional oven or cooktop.
- Keep both the refrigerator and oven clean. Avoid leaving the doors open for any length of time, and close tightly.
- Run dishwashers and washing machines with full loads. Air dry dishes and clothes when possible.
- Clean the lint filter in your dryer after every use.
- Use cold water instead of warm or hot when possible.
- Shut off water faucets completely. Fix any drips or leaks.
- Water grass and plants early in the morning.
- Arrange drapes and furniture so they do not cover vents or registers.
- When not using the fireplace, keep the damper closed.
- *Weatherstrip* (place narrow plastic, fiber, or metal strips around exterior doors and windows) to prevent air leaks.
- Use recycled paper and products. Use discarded paper for scrap paper or use the opposite sides in printers and copiers.
- Reuse plastic bags and containers. Use them instead of plastic wrap or aluminum foil.
- Use cloth napkins and towels instead of paper ones.
- Use rechargeable batteries for devices used frequently.
- Maintain and repair durable products instead of discarding and buying new ones.
- Buy used furniture—there is a surplus of it and it is much less expensive than new.

7-14 A few simple steps can help you save energy at home.

In the Home

Appliances are now designed to use much less energy than they did in the past. Refrigerators and home furnaces/air conditioners are just two appliances that have been redesigned. EnergyGuide labels are required on many appliances, **7-15**. These labels give consumers information about the energy- and cost-efficiency of an appliance. You can use these labels to comparison shop for appliances that are environmentally friendly.

How Computers Can Save Energy

Computer technology is increasingly being used to help conserve energy. Computers are added to many appliances and heating/cooling systems to save energy in various ways. For instance, some irons have an automatic shut-off feature. These irons are programmed to shut off when not in use for a set amount of time. Other appliances, such as lighting systems and coffee makers, can be programmed to start and stop working at specific times.

Programmable thermostats help to save energy and money by preventing the unnecessary use of central heating or cooling systems when no one is in the home. The homeowner programs the exact times and temperatures into the controlling thermostat based on their working and

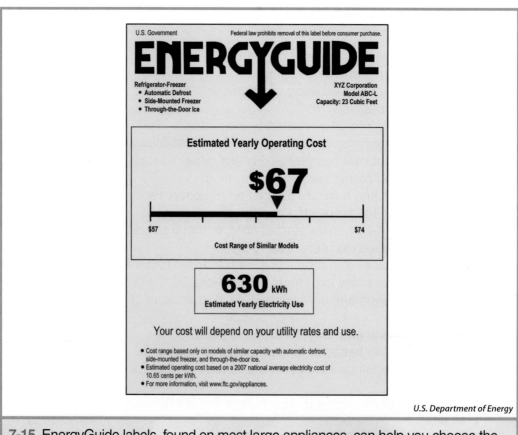

U.S. Department of Energy

7-15 EnergyGuide labels, found on most large appliances, can help you choose the most energy-efficient model.

daily schedules. The furnace or central air conditioner then turns off or on when the home's temperature reaches the desired temperature at the chosen times.

Using Transportation

Because most transportation methods use petroleum-based products for fuel, they are a primary source of both pollution and nonrenewable natural resources. More energy-efficient cars and trucks are now available. These vehicles have redesigned engines to increase the amount of miles driven on one gallon of gas, or *mpg*. Hybrid and electric vehicles' power comes from various combinations of gasoline and/or electric batteries, which mean they use less gas. More fully electric-engine cars are anticipated in the future to further decrease the use of fossil fuels. Carpooling also reduces gasoline usage.

Mass transit is the system that is used for moving large numbers of people on buses, trains, or subways. Fuel consumption is reduced because fewer single-driver cars are on the roads. The more people take mass transit, the more efficient it becomes. Mass transit options also save money because the fares are much less expensive than gas and toll fees.

Go Green

Biomass and the Benefits of Biofuels

Biomass energy is the energy made from plants and their byproducts. It has been used since people discovered they could burn wood to cook food and keep themselves warm. Wood is still the largest biomass energy resource today. Other sources of biomass energy have been developed more recently, however, because trees are one of the slowest renewable resources. One benefit of biomass as an energy source is that it can be converted directly into liquid fuels, called *biofuels*, to help meet transportation fuel needs.

The most common biomass sources for biofuels are corn grain (for ethanol) and soybeans (for biodiesel). The carbon emissions of biofuels are lower than gasoline, making biofuels a less polluting fuel option. In the near future, agricultural by-products, such as the stalks, leaves, and husks of corn plants and wheat straw will also be used for biofuel production.

Minimize Waste

Most of our solid waste, or garbage, goes to landfills. **Landfills** are places where trash is compacted and buried underground. There are many problems associated with the operation of landfills, however. Burying trash contributes to pollution. As garbage decomposes, it contaminates the ground, water, and air. In newer landfills, special linings are used to prevent this from happening.

Space is another problem. Many landfills are full or soon will be full. Also, some waste materials do not break down quickly. Other materials, such as metal, do not decompose at all. Since landfills are bad for the environment, most communities do not want to create more of them. Many cities now pay huge fees to have their garbage taken to landfills far away. Therefore, the expense of landfills is another issue. Consider other ways to dispose of or reuse products to minimize landfills.

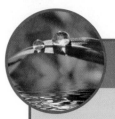

Go Green

Repurposing

Repurposing is another form of recycling. Old items are turned into something else useful instead of being thrown away. Examples of repurposing include the following:

- use worn out clothing as dusting or cleaning cloths
- turn plastic product containers into a kitchen herb garden
- use an old tire as a child's sandbox in the backyard
- turn old ripped jeans into shorts by cutting off the legs, and make a purse out of the leftover material

Repurposing is a creative and fun exercise. You are only limited by your imagination in what you can save from the landfill.

Reduce, Reuse, and Recycle

You can reduce the amount of waste created by buying products with less packaging or those made from recycled materials. **Recycled** materials are reprocessed resources that are reused in a different form. Using materials over again conserves primary natural resources and keeps potential garbage from ending up in landfills. Many products, such as shoes, bags, tires, furniture, crafts, and plastic products, are now made with some or 100% recycled materials.

Buying in bulk versus single packages automatically saves on wasted packaging materials. Think about all of the disposable *convenience* products that are used once and then thrown in landfills. Paper towels, disposable diapers, Styrofoam® cups, or plastic plates and utensils could all be replaced with reusable items. If every person reused even a portion of items seen as disposable, landfills would be greatly reduced. Ask yourself if convenience should be at the expense of a healthful environment.

How to Recycle

Most household waste is recyclable. Items that are often recycled include those listed in **7-16**. You can recycle old newspapers, cardboard, aluminum cans, glass bottles, and most plastic bottles and containers. When buying products, you may want to buy items that can be recycled or that come in recyclable containers. Look for the recycle symbol on

---

What Is Recyclable?

- *Aluminum, corrugated cardboard, glass, paper, plastics, and tin cans.* These items can be taken to recycling centers and made into new items.
- *Clothing.* Service and religious organizations will pick up used clothing.
- *Yard waste.* Cut grass, leaves, and other yard waste is about 20 percent of all landfill waste. Check online or at your local library to learn how to build a backyard compost.
- *Old oil, batteries, and tires.* Most service stations will accept these items for safe disposal.

7-16 Pollution can be reduced by recycling household items.

the product. Curbside recycling programs or centers exist in many communities. Some cities and counties require trash to be separated into paper products, bottles, and cans.

Consider composting as an alternative to tossing leftovers in the garbage or waste disposal. **Composting** is the natural breakdown of organic, or *biodegradable*, material. If done properly, composting will not cause pollution. Instead, as natural materials break down, they add oxygen back to the air and become a good fertilizer for soil. Many people compost grass clippings and leaves by letting them decompose in their own yards.

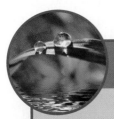

Go Green

Composting

Composting is the collection of biodegradable materials in a container that over time decompose through a chemical reaction. It is a natural way to dispose of waste, create fertilizer, and reduce the contribution to landfills. The chemical reaction ultimately produces an environmentally friendly, dirt-like material. This final product is rich in nutrients for soil and is used for gardening or cultivating fields.

Think of a composting pile as you would a houseplant. Both need food, water, oxygen, and temperature control. For the compost pile, brown and green materials are needed. Brown materials include dead leaves, dried grass, and wood chips or sawdust. Green materials include fruit and vegetable parts, green plant matter, and if possible, farm manure. Ideally, the compost pile will have an equal amount of brown and green materials. The compost pile is ready to be used when the bottom turns a dark brown and looks similar to dirt.

Reading Review

1. Distinguish between renewable resources and nonrenewable resources.
2. What upsets the natural balance of all healthy ecosystems?
3. List four alternative sources of energy.
4. List four ways of using energy efficiently.
5. What is composting?

Chapter Summary

Section 7-1. There are many decisions you need to make to be an informed, responsible consumer. Informed consumers are aware of the types of stores where they can shop. As a consumer, it is important that you evaluate advertisements and use smart consumer buying techniques. As a consumer, you also have certain rights and responsibilities. By knowing the right way to complain, you will more easily solve your consumer problems.

Section 7-2. Caring for the environment is everyone's responsibility. It is important to conserve energy and resources. Natural resources are categorized in two ways—renewable resources and nonrenewable resources, such as minerals and fossil fuels. Engineers are working on solutions to environmental problems caused by traditional energy production methods. By using energy efficiently and minimizing waste, resources can be conserved. You can help to do this by reducing, reusing, and recycling waste.

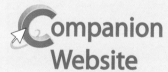

Companion Website

www.g-wlearning.com

Check your understanding of the main concepts for Chapter 7 at the website.

Critical Thinking

1. **Evaluate.** Think about an item you want to buy. Develop a shopping plan that would reflect your needs, wants, values, and goals.
2. **Compare and contrast.** If you were given $1,000 to spend in only one store, where would you go shopping? What would you buy?
3. **Determine.** What can be done about recycling resources in your home? in your community? in the world?

Common Core

College and Career Readiness

4. **Math.** Choose an item you would like to purchase. Compare the price of the item at four types of stores or online sources. Which store or source offered the best price?
5. **Speaking.** Divide into small groups. Within your group, think of situations in which you or your parents have had problems with products or services. Choose one of these situations. Role-play for the class the way the situation was handled or the way you think it should have been handled. Then discuss how to complain to get the best response.

6. **Writing.** Think of a product or service you purchased that was not what you expected it to be. Following the guidelines described in the chapter, write a letter of complaint.

7. **Reading.** Using current online or print sources, research your community's current recycling efforts. Present your findings to the class. Then using the decision-making process, plan a group recycling or cleanup project. Ideas might include painting over graffiti, cleaning roadsides, collecting discarded paper and aluminum cans, or helping raise money for a local environmental improvement organization.

Technology

8. **Internet research.** Locate a website for an online retailer and find an item that interests you. Which factors can you easily evaluate online and which are more difficult? Share your findings with the class.

Journal Writing

9. Evaluate yourself as a consumer. Write three paragraphs. In the first paragraph, write about what you believe are your rights as a consumer. In the second paragraph, write about what you believe are your responsibilities as a consumer. In the third paragraph, write about your environmental responsibilities.

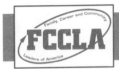

FCCLA

10. Dynamic leaders demonstrate good character and moral courage. They also model good character, solve problems, foster positive relationships, manage conflict, build teams, and educate peers. Conduct an *FCCLA Dynamic Leadership* campaign to influence your peers in positive ways about environmental responsibility. Choose one aspect of environmental responsibility and then use the *FCCLA Planning Process* to help guide the strategies you use to educate your peers. You might use a digital presentation, public-service announcement, or run a special event for your school community. See your adviser for information as needed.

Unit 3
Managing Your Career

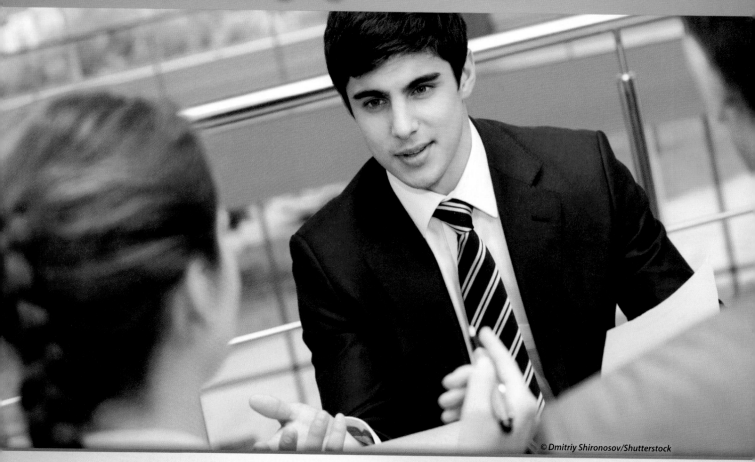

© Dmitriy Shironosov/Shutterstock

Unit Essential Question

How can you take responsibility for your own life in relation to your goals and aspirations?

Exploring Career Pathways

Human Resources Careers

Are you good with details? Do you like to help people in the workplace? Perhaps a career in human resources is for you. Here are some careers in this pathway many people enjoy.

Human Resources Assistant

Human resources assistants often work with a human resources director. They help maintain a company's employee personnel records. They update information, create reports for managers, and assist with getting information from job applicants. Many answer employee questions about wages and benefits. Attention to details, good organizational skills, strong computer skills, and ability to keep information private are essential. Most of these positions require training beyond high school. Some require an associate's degree.

Human Resources Director

With exceptional interpersonal skills, human resources directors are involved in many aspects of employee relations. They interview and hire employees according to a company's policies. These workers also help employees improve their skills through training and professional development activities. They work with compensation, benefits, and labor relations. Human resources directors may also provide programs to improve employee safety, wellness, and ability to balance home and work life. A bachelor's degree is required to enter this career. Courses in management principles, accounting and finance, labor law, and collective bargaining provide valuable background. Integrity, fair-mindedness, and strong ethical standards are key personal traits for human resources directors.

Industrial-Organizational Psychologist

Psychologists study human behavior through observation, interpretation, and recording interactions between people and their environments. *Industrial-organizational psychologists* use these skills in the workplace. They apply their skills to improving the workplace and quality of work life. They often screen, train, and counsel people who are job applicants for an employer. Many work with company managers to improve the work setting and worker productivity. Many positions require a master's degree. Some require a doctorate. Personal traits necessary for psychologists include compassion, sensitivity, and excellent communication skills. Leadership ability, patience, and perseverance are key qualities.

Is this career path for you? Pursue one or both of the following activities to determine if you are suitable for a career in human resources.

- Interview a worker in human resources from an employer in your area. Ask about the education and training this person needed to perform this work. What career path has the person followed? What aspects about the work are personally satisfying? What aspects would he or she like to change? Write a summary of your findings to share with the class.
- Use the *CareerOneStop* and *Bureau of Labor Statistics* websites to research additional careers related to human resources. Give an oral report to the class about one career of interest to you.

Chapter 8
Learning About Work

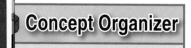

● Reading Prep

College and Career Readiness

After reading the material under each of the main headings, stop and write a three- to four-sentence summary of what you just read. Be sure to paraphrase and use your own words. Is this activity helpful in understanding the material?

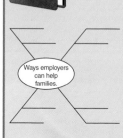

Concept Organizer

Ways employers can help families.

Use a diagram like the one shown to list four ways employers can help families. Then list two benefits of each one.

Companion Website

Print out the concept organizer for Chapter 8 at the website.

Companion Website
www.g-wlearning.com

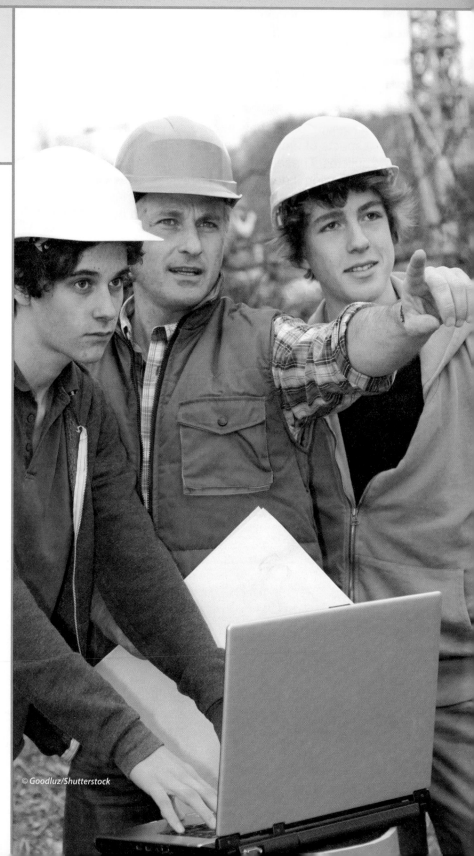

© Goodluz/Shutterstock

184

Section 8-1

Reasons People Work

Objectives

After studying this section, you will be able to
- **identify** reasons people work.
- **distinguish** between an occupation and a career.
- **explain** how your career could affect your lifestyle.

Key Terms		
ambition occupation	tasks	career

Work is effort required to accomplish an activity. When you do laundry or clean the house, you are working. Babysitting, delivering papers, or other part-time jobs are also types of work you might do. Your schoolwork, however, is probably the most important work you do right now.

Everyone does some kind of work. In this chapter, the term *work* often describes paid jobs. Most adults have a job of some sort, **8-1**. Soon you will be choosing the type of work you will do as an adult.

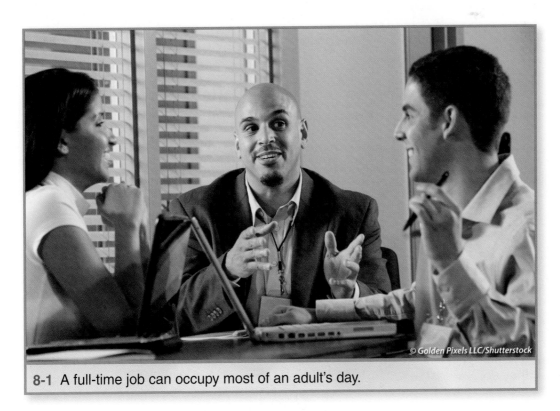

© Golden Pixels LLC/Shutterstock

8-1 A full-time job can occupy most of an adult's day.

Why People Work

Money is probably the most important reason people work. Everyone must work in order to pay for his or her needs. Some people must also pay for the needs of family members who are dependent on them, such as their children. These people must choose a job in which they will earn enough money for food, shelter, and clothing for the entire family.

Most people wish to have money for wants as well as needs. For instance, one person may be happy with enough extra money to go out of town for a weekend. Another person might want to buy an expensive car.

Many people work for reasons other than needing money. Doing a job they enjoy is one reason people work, **8-2**. For instance, a person who enjoys working with animals might become a veterinarian. On the other hand, becoming a teacher when you do not like working with people would not be a wise choice. You probably would not enjoy the work. You might not do the job well, either.

Many people work so they can be independent. Right now, you are probably dependent on other people for your needs. When you get a full-time job, you will find it easier to be less dependent on others. Being able to provide for your own wants and needs is an important step in the development process.

Ambition often plays an important role in a person's work. **Ambition** is a desire or drive to achieve and succeed. When you are motivated to succeed, you often find your work more satisfying.

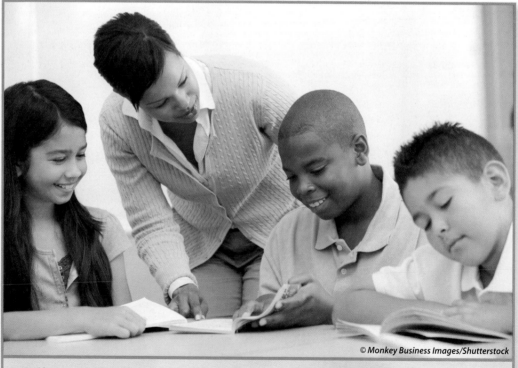

© Monkey Business Images/Shutterstock

8-2 If people like their work, they often find fulfillment and satisfaction in the job they do.

An Occupation or a Career?

As you begin thinking more about what you want to do for a living, you will come across the terms *occupation* and *career*. These terms can be easily confused. What is an occupation and what is a career? How are these two ideas different?

Whatever you do for a living is your occupation, or job. Being an administrative assistant, customer service representative, mechanic, or graphic designer are just a few examples of occupations, **8-3**.

A job often consists of several different tasks. Tasks include all the smaller duties you perform throughout the day. For instance, you might have a summer occupation as a sales associate at a local retail store. Your tasks might include answering customers' questions, processing sales, folding clothes, stocking shelves, arranging for deliveries, and assisting with the displays.

Your summer occupation as a sales associate is not your career. A career is a broader concept than that. Your career is the sequence of jobs you have over a period of years. A career requires planning. During your career, your occupation may change several times. As your career progresses and you gain more experience, your responsibilities at work often increase.

While you are still in school, you might make plans for a career in the foodservice industry. Perhaps your ultimate goal is to become a franchise owner. During your career in foodservice, you may have many occupations. You may start out as a dishwasher or a busperson. You might then work as a line cook at a fast-food restaurant and become a shift supervisor or even a manager. You might then take a job as an assistant cook at a fine dining restaurant. If you work hard, you are likely to reach your goal of becoming a franchise owner. Each of your jobs in the foodservice industry can help prepare you for your career goal.

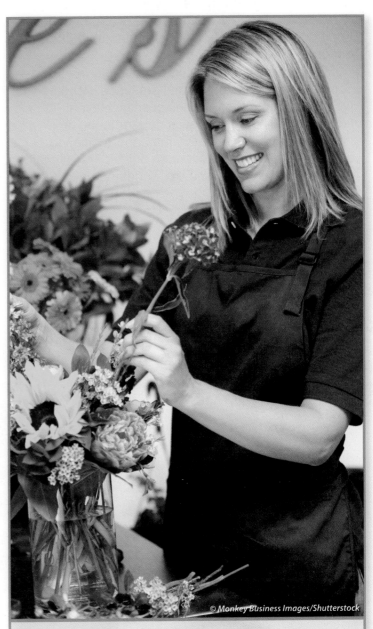

© Monkey Business Images/Shutterstock

8-3 People with the same occupation often do very similar work.

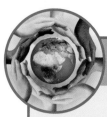

Global Connections

Travel for Work

People in many types of jobs have to travel occasionally. Some business travel involves daylong trips for brief meetings in nearby locations. Much business travel, however, requires overnight or extended stays in distant cities or even other countries.

If learning about different cultures and exploring other countries is one of your values, think about a career in the travel industry. Some careers may require foreign travel, such as travel agents, airline pilots or flight attendants, cruise directors, or tour guides.

Other possibilities include working for a company with an international presence. People working in international sales positions, event coordination, corporate travel departments, or corporate training may have the opportunities to travel to their company's foreign offices. Travelling for work is a good way to see the world and have it paid for by your business.

Careers Affect Lifestyles

The career you choose will affect your *lifestyle*—the way you and your family live. Your career may determine where you live. Some jobs are easier to get in certain parts of the country. Some jobs are more available in cities than in small towns. Suppose you want to work for a national organization that focuses on healthcare. To have more job opportunities, you may have to live near the organization's headquarters. If you want to teach high school calculus, however, you may be able to find a position almost anywhere, 8-4.

The location of your job can affect your lifestyle in many ways. Where you work and live will affect the types of recreational activities you and your family can enjoy. In a rural area,

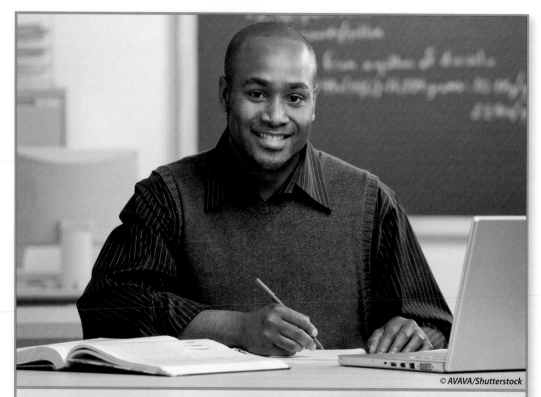

© AVAVA/Shutterstock

8-4 A career in teaching allows you more freedom when choosing where you want to live and work.

there may be limited opportunities to attend professional sporting events or museums. This same area, however, might provide you with the chance to enjoy outdoor activities such as horseback riding or dirt bike riding.

The area in which you live might also affect the types of schools available for children to attend. An urban area might offer more programs for children with special needs. Some parents, however, might not wish to raise their children in a city. Therefore, these parents might look for jobs in suburban or rural areas.

Your career will provide opportunities for you to make new and different friends. You are likely to develop friendships with people you meet at work. Your family and your friends' families may have common interests. You may enjoy getting together for group activities.

Your career choice will affect how much money you have and the way you can spend it. When your salary is low, you must spend your money carefully. If you have a high-paying job, however, you may be able to spend your money more freely.

Different careers have different working hours. Retail is one business known for long hours. In some careers, your job does not end when you go home at night. Teachers must prepare for class the next day. People who work for utility companies may be called in to work following a major storm with downed power lines.

Your work schedule and travel requirements will affect the amount of time you have to spend with your family. Many married workers feel it is important to work the same schedule as their spouses. This gives them more free time to spend together. Others enjoy spending the time their spouses are working or traveling to pursue individual activities or goals. Some parents find it worthwhile to work different schedules so there is always an adult available to care for the children.

Vacation policies are another point when considering the career path you choose. In some jobs, employees may be able to take paid vacations whenever they want. People who do seasonal work, however, may be limited to taking vacations during the off-season. Parents may be limited to taking vacations when school is not in session.

When choosing a career, you must consider your values as they relate to family and work. Think about all the ways in which your family and work can affect each other. Decide which values are most important to you. Then choose a type of work that will allow you to keep your values in order.

Reading Review

1. List two reasons people work.
2. _____ is the desire or drive to achieve and succeed.
3. Differentiate between an occupation and a career.
4. _____ include all the smaller duties you perform throughout the day.
5. How can your choice of career affect your lifestyle?

Balancing Family and Work

Objectives

After studying this section, you will be able to
- **summarize** the effects of personal life on work performance.
- **explain** how work influences the family.
- **describe** how company policies can assist families.
- **suggest** ways families can balance family and work demands.

Key Terms

dual-career family
children in self-care
family-friendly policies

fringe benefits
flextime
job sharing

telecommuting
support system

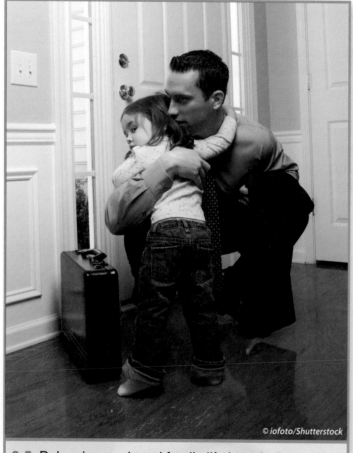

8-5 Balancing work and family life is a challenge for many people.

© iofoto/Shutterstock

Many people work. They also have personal lives. Most people have families with whom they like to spend time. They have family members who need help and attention from them. People who work must balance the time they spend at work with the amount of time they spend with their families, **8-5**.

Effects of Personal Life on Work

One factor that can affect an employee's work performance is his or her personal life. Unexpected circumstances may conflict with work. Car trouble or a household emergency can cause an employee to be late for work. An extended illness, accident, or death in the family can result in an employee missing work for several days. Other family situations that might arise include a child's music recital, a parent-teacher conference, or the birth of a baby.

Working parents often face challenges when balancing work and child care responsibilities. A child may be sick or need to see the doctor. Parents must still go to work, however. They may have to arrive at work late. If parents are worried about their children, they may have trouble concentrating at work. This can affect their job performance.

Reading Connections

Learn About FMLA

Find out more about the federal government's FMLA, or *Family and Medical Leave Act*. The law provides certain employees with up to 12 weeks of unpaid, job-protected leave per year. It also requires that their group health benefits be maintained during the leave. Use the Department of Labor website at www.dol.gov to learn about why the law was created and how it applies to both employees and employers.

In most cases, employers have policies that permit employees to take time off when needed. Sometimes, only a few hours are necessary, such as for a parent-teacher conference. In other cases, such as the birth or adoption of a new baby, employers may provide a leave of absence for a much longer period of time.

Some companies may expect employees to make up the time they take off from work, **8-6**. Other companies may deduct employees' wages if they come in late or miss work. In this case, time missed for emergencies can affect the amount of money a person earns in a pay period.

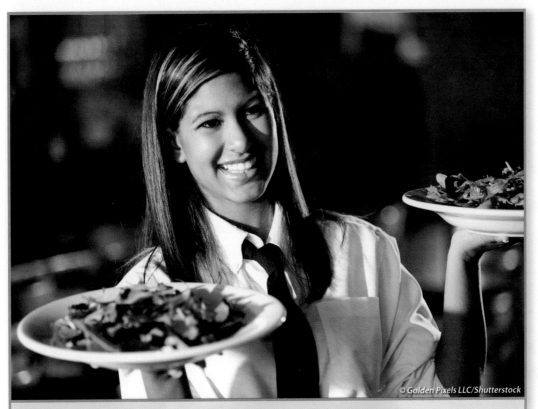

© Golden Pixels LLC/Shutterstock

8-6 Employees might be able to arrange with an employer to make up time by coming to work early, staying late, or taking shorter breaks.

Taking time off can affect your work performance. You are not able to accomplish as much when you work for a shorter amount of time. Even if you make up the time, you interrupt your normal work routine. You may not be available when other people need you. Then your absence might affect the job performance of a coworker.

Most employers realize that employees cannot always avoid difficulties at home. If an employee allows home life to interfere with work too much, however, his or her job could be in jeopardy.

Demands of Work on Families

A person's job should be a high priority in his or her life. This can put certain strains on the family, however. Making sure family life remains important is sometimes difficult. Job obligations and long commutes may force employees to spend time away from their families.

Working parents may be concerned with the amount of time they miss spending with their children. There may be older family members who require care. Responsibilities concerning the home must still be fulfilled.

Concerns of Working Parents

In many families, both parents need to work for financial reasons. When both parents work, they are a **dual-career family**. These families need to plan carefully to meet all responsibilities. Meals need to be prepared. Caring for and maintaining the home takes time. School activities, grocery shopping, and other errands can pose scheduling challenges. Managing resources, such as time and energy, becomes very important.

Single-parent families have many of the same concerns as dual-career families. They have similar responsibilities to fulfill. They must often manage everything by themselves, however. They may not have another adult in the home to help.

Relationships with Children

Most parents are concerned about having enough time to build and maintain healthy relationships with their children, **8-7**. This may be especially hard when they must also meet the demands of a job. Parents may miss parts of their children's development, such as their first steps, because they are working away from home.

© forestpath/Shutterstock

8-7 A parent may try to spend as much free time as possible with a child.

Depending on work schedules, some couples work different shifts. One adult may work during the day and the other at night. In some single-parent families, the adult may need to sleep while children are in school and then work in the evenings. In cases such as these, there is often little time between shifts to share meals or family time with children.

Unplanned work schedules can also affect the family's plans. For instance, a meeting at work may last longer than its scheduled time. A parent is then unable to attend a child's after-school activity. Having to work additional time on the weekend may mean a parent misses planned family activities.

Child Care

When the single parent or both parents work during the day, they may have to find other options for child care. Younger children may have to attend a child care program. This is a difficult decision for many parents. They may evaluate several programs before choosing the best one for their children.

The safety and well-being of their children are a major concern to parents. They want to make sure child care providers are skilled and qualified with appropriate licenses and certifications. Parents will want to get to know the child care employees.

Parents may consider other matters, too. The number and ages of children attending the program is often a factor. Parents may also wish to know what activities their children will be doing, if they will be fed during the day, and how much rest time they will be given.

Children in Self-Care

Children in self-care are those children who stay home by themselves while parents work. They usually have limited or no adult supervision during these times. Many states have laws against leaving children home alone under a certain age. Most parents, however, will not leave children home alone, regardless of their age, until the children are old enough to assume responsibility for any unforeseen situations.

Working parents may be anxious about leaving children home alone. The safety of the unsupervised children is a major concern. Parents often worry about the activities and friends their children are involved with during those hours. They have to trust the children to make wise choices.

Other Situations

Some child care situations involve problems parents must solve. If a child is sick, the parent might not be able to stay home with the child. Parents might ask a relative, neighbor, or friend to take the child to the doctor or to stay with the child. Some communities have special centers at hospitals where sick children can stay

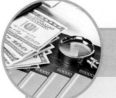

Financial Literacy Connections

Costs of Child Care

The cost of child care can be a major concern to many parents. Extra meetings, overtime work hours, or work-related travel means parents have to make special arrangements with a child care center, which often cost more. Sometimes child care costs as much as a parent's salary. A parent may then consider it to be more cost efficient to stay home with the children.

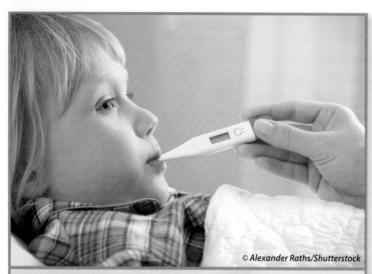

© Alexander Raths/Shutterstock

8-8 Making arrangements ahead of time can help parents minimize work absences when their children become sick.

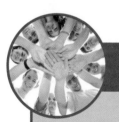

Community Connections

Adult Living Centers

Some communities have adult living centers for older people who need some assistance with everyday living skills. For these people, assisted living facilities or nursing homes may be an option. Assisted living facilities are communities with apartment-style or room living for those who have less chronic health concerns. These facilities have attendants who are on site and ready to help 24 hours a day. Nursing homes are for older adults who may need more frequent medical care and attention. Both types of centers may sponsor special activities. This gives them the opportunity to be around people their own age, while health issues can be monitored.

while their parents are at work. Many parents try to make arrangements before children get sick, **8-8**. Then there are some options from which to choose if a child becomes ill suddenly.

Sometimes children have days off from school, or school might be canceled because of bad weather. It is helpful if parents have planned ahead of time for these events. This way the children will know where to go if they find out they will be home alone.

Caring for Older Relatives

Some families have responsibility for the care of an older relative. An example of such a family might be a husband and wife, their children, and the husband's father. This means the husband is a member of the *sandwich generation*. He is responsible for the care of his parent and his children. He is in between these two groups.

The older person may live in the same home as the family. If the person is healthy and active, it may not be a concern for him or her to be home alone. If the older person is in poor health, however, he or she may not be able to stay alone. Someone may need to be with the person all the time. This can be a concern for a dual-career family.

People in this situation can consider several options. They can hire a caregiver or nurse to stay with the older person while no one is home. Assisted living facilities may also be an option in some communities.

Ways Employers Help Families

Many employers are finding their workers accomplish more when they are not worried about family matters. Therefore, more companies are developing family-friendly policies, services, and benefit plans. **Family-friendly policies** are company rules that affect the family positively. For instance, federal law requires companies to allow workers a certain amount of time off to have a baby or adopt a child. After their leave is over, they can return to their jobs.

Other examples of family-friendly services include child care services offered at work and seminars about work and family concerns. Fitness centers may be located within the building. Many companies have found such services increase productivity and reduce stress.

Employers usually offer fringe benefits to full-time employees. **Fringe benefits** include paid vacation and holiday time, sick leave, health and life insurance plans, and retirement benefits, **8-9**. Sometimes employees are able to choose the benefit plan they would like from a menu of options. Those with families may choose differently from those who do not have dependents.

Flextime

Flextime is the freedom to work hours that are convenient to an employee's personal situation. For instance, a single parent may need to take children to a child care center. The center may not open until after the employee is scheduled to work, however. The employer may then permit the employee to work a flexible schedule. The employee may be able to come to work a little later. He or she might skip a break or stay late to make up for this time. Flextime helps the employee manage family situations as well as the demands of the job.

Sometimes employers offer flextime for the entire staff. This might offer solutions for problems all employees encounter. For instance, people who might be late because of heavy traffic would not have to worry. He or she would just start work later in the day. On the other hand, employees might want to start work earlier and leave earlier.

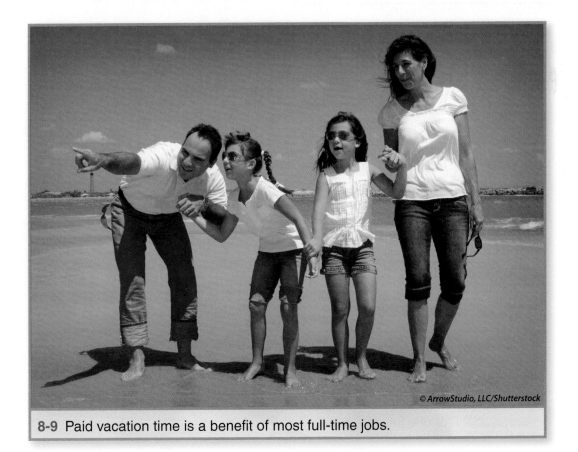

© ArrowStudio, LLC/Shutterstock

8-9 Paid vacation time is a benefit of most full-time jobs.

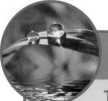

Go Green

Telecommuting Is Environmentally Friendly

Conserves Energy. Producing, maintaining, and repairing transportation equipment such as automobiles, buses, and trains takes a tremendous amount of energy—most often supplied by nonrenewable resources. Building highways also consumes much energy, not only in the operation of the construction and repair equipment, but also in the manufacture and transportation of the raw materials for production. More people telecommuting to work will decrease the need for expanded highways and associated road maintenance. From the business perspective, the potential for energy savings in the areas of on-site heating, cooling, and lighting could be significant.

Protects the Environment. Fewer vehicles on the roads mean less pollution-causing emissions and healthier air quality. In addition, with more people telecommuting, existing highways could be reduced in size and parking lots could be converted to more environmentally friendly uses, such as parks.

Job Sharing

Job sharing is when two people do the same job, but work at different times of the day or week, **8-10**. For instance, two accountants may share one job. One might work in the morning, while the other works in the afternoon. They are both responsible for all the demands of the position. Another example might be two administrative assistants who work for one person. Both might work two and a half days a week. They can arrange the hours that best suit their personal situations.

Telecommuting

Telecommuting is a work program in which an employee works at home by connecting electronically to a central office. The employee can send e-mail to coworkers and download files from shared space on the company server.

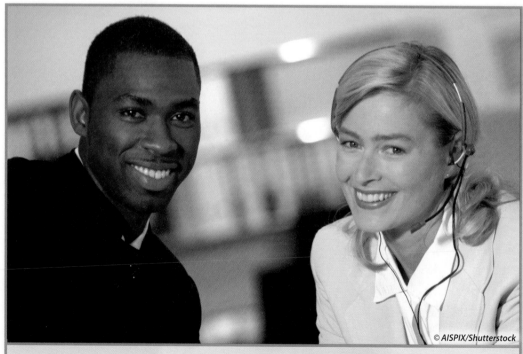

© AISPIX/Shutterstock

8-10 In some situations, two people who work part-time might share the responsibility for one full-time job.

Telecommuting is especially convenient for people with children or limited transportation. The work schedules for employees who telecommute are often the same as their coworkers. One disadvantage is that it may be difficult for some employees to concentrate on work in their own homes. To avoid distractions, the employee may need to work in an area of the home set up as an office. He or she may want to work away from children or other people in the home.

Balancing Family and Work Demands

Employees may sometimes feel as though they are being pulled in two directions. Work, of course, is important. As an employee, you have a commitment to your employer. You still have tasks at home that need your attention, however. Several steps can help people balance home and work demands.

Delegating Tasks and Making Schedules

All family members can share the responsibility of daily chores. If parents know they will not be able to do or complete a job, they can ask another family member to help.

A schedule can also be a helpful tool in delegating tasks. The schedule might include the times each family member has a commitment. It might also include a list of household chores. Family members can then check to see what they can do to help when they are home.

Chores may include hanging up clothes, putting dirty clothes in the hamper, emptying the dishwasher, and taking out the trash. Another important daily task of the home is meal planning and preparation, **8-11**.

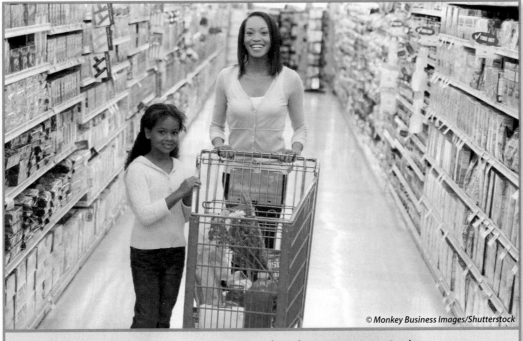

© Monkey Business Images/Shutterstock

8-11 Grocery shopping is a time-consuming, but necessary task.

Someone must make decisions regarding what the family will eat. Grocery shopping is a task teens can do. They might also prepare a meal so it is ready when parents arrive home. Eating together whenever possible is an important goal. It can be a time for family members to share feelings and events with one another.

Setting Priorities

Balancing the demands of family and work is often challenging. There never seems to be enough time to do everything. Sometimes children will expect parents to put their activities first. For instance, a teen may need a parent to drive him or her to play practice. If the parent has an evening meeting, however, he or she may not be able to provide the ride. Prioritizing work and home responsibilities can help you strengthen your family life. Being respectful of each family member's outside commitments can help the family maintain a healthy balance. Using a joint family calendar is also a good way to manage potential conflicts.

It is common for parents to feel work-related stress. At home, the parent can sort out the events of the day and regroup in order to be productive the next day. People often allow work concerns to bother them at home, however. This can put stress on the rest of the family. Children might feel neglected if a parent continues to think only about work. No matter how stressful work is, spending quality time with family members should be a high priority.

Support Systems

Regardless of whether parents work, all families need support systems. A family's **support system** consists of people who provide aid and assistance for individuals in the family. This support includes emotional and instrumental support.

People often need someone to talk to or share problems. They will seek someone who can give *emotional support*. This person is usually a good listener and, if requested, gives advice, **8-12**.

Other times, a person will ask someone to give *instrumental support*. This kind of support requires the giver to do or give something to the person in need. For instance, a parent may need someone to watch children while taking another child to

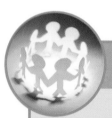

Life Connections

Balance

Working too much can put a strain on family members. Each person in the family has to set realistic standards for the work he or she can handle. For instance, your mother might do your laundry each week. If she is working outside the home, it may be difficult for her to accomplish this task. You could learn to do your own laundry, or even do laundry for the whole family. By volunteering to do household chores and assuming responsibilities, you are showing maturity. Learning to balance work and family concerns now can help you throughout the rest of your life.

Speaking Activity

Think about how you and other family members can help to balance the current work necessary to keep your household running smoothly. Do some family members have certain preferences or skills, such as cooking, outdoor maintenance, or home repair? Ask your parents if you can hold a family meeting to discuss how best to balance the work so that it is fair and efficient.

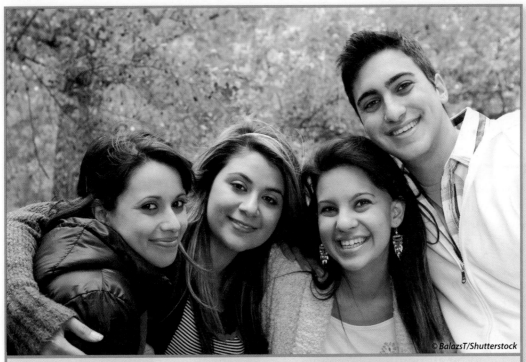

© BalazsT/Shutterstock

8-12 Support systems can include family members as well as good friends.

the doctor. Most families will face situations in which they need someone to help them. You might be able to identify times when you have given emotional or instrumental support to a friend or family member.

Reading Review

1. What may happen if an employee allows home life to interfere with work too much?
2. What are family-friendly policies?
3. What is flextime?
4. Name three ways that can help people balance home and work demands.
5. List one example of emotional support and one example of instrumental support.

Chapter Summary

Section 8-1. People work for many reasons. What you do for a living is your occupation. Your career is the sequence of jobs you have over a period of years. Your career could affect your lifestyle. This may include where you will live, who your friends are, how much money you will have, and your working hours. Consider your values as they relate to family and work.

Section 8-2. Balancing the demands of family and work is a challenge faced by all families. Working parents may be concerned about responsibilities at home, including care of children or older relatives. There are ways employers can help their employees balance family and work life. Employees may manage their resources by delegating tasks and making schedules. Setting priorities can help determine which tasks are most important. Support systems provide aid for all family members.

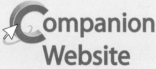

Companion Website

www.g-wlearning.com

Check your understanding of the main concepts for Chapter 8 at the website.

Critical Thinking

1. **Summarize.** Describe how each of the following would be affected by your career choice.
   A. where you live
   B. how much money you make
   C. who your friends are
   D. amount of time you have to spend with your family
2. **Analyze.** How might an employee's family responsibilities conflict with his or her work responsibilities?
3. **Predict.** Create an imaginary schedule for your family that balances work and family life. Use flextime, telecommunication, and job sharing if necessary. Predict how each family member will share responsibilities at home. Include examples of technology that can help family members complete tasks.

Common Core

College and Career Readiness

4. **Speaking.** As a class, develop a puppet show for children that helps them understand why their parents have to work. Perform the show at a local child care center.

5. **Listening.** Interview a working adult. Ask about his or her employer's family-friendly policies and benefits. Discuss why these policies are important to the employees. What other policies or benefits would they like their company to adopt?

6. **Writing.** Imagine you are the owner of a company. Write a family-friendly policy for your employees. What makes your policy a family-friendly one? How would the policy benefit both your company and employees? Share your policy with the class.

7. **Reading.** Read an article online or at the local library about family-friendly policies. How does this information relate to the information in the chapter?

Technology

8. **Telecommuting.** Interview someone who telecommutes. Ask the person what some of the advantages and disadvantages are to telecommuting. How does telecommuting affect his or her productivity? How does telecommuting affect his or her family life? Based on this interview, would you like to be a telecommuter?

Journal Writing

9. Write about your life 15 years from now. What career do you hope to have? Describe your lifestyle. Describe how you think you would balance your family/personal life with your work.

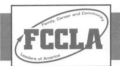 ## FCCLA

10. As an *FCCLA Community Service* project, examine ways families in your community find balance in their lives. Gather these tips and create a public-service campaign to share these tips with others. Use the *FCCLA Planning Process* to guide your actions. See your adviser for information as needed.

Chapter 9
Making Career Decisions

Sections

Reading Prep

College and Career Readiness

Look up this chapter in the table of contents. Use the detailed contents as an outline for taking notes as you read the chapter.

Concept Organizer

Family and Consumer Sciences Career Area	Occupation

Use a diagram like the one shown to list the seven family and consumer sciences career areas. Provide one occupation for each area.

Companion Website

Print out the concept organizer for Chapter 9 at the website.

Companion Website
www.g-wlearning.com

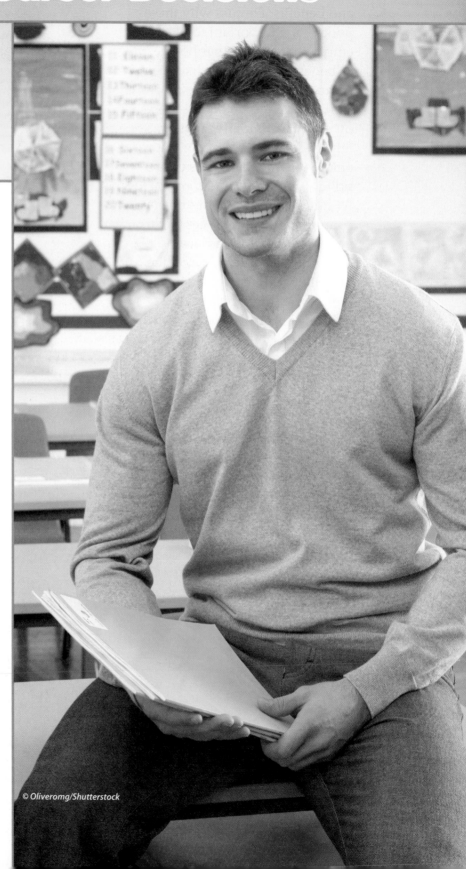

© Oliveromg/Shutterstock

Researching Careers

Objectives

After studying this section, you will be able to
- **describe** how interests, aptitudes, and abilities can help you choose a career.
- **identify** the career clusters.
- **list** sources of career information.

Key Terms

interests	postsecondary	certification
aptitudes	major	job trends
abilities	work-based learning	job shadowing
career clusters	internships	mentor

What do you want to do when you get older? People have probably asked you that question a number of times already. Whatever your answer is now, however, may not be anything of interest to you when you are older, **9-1**.

Interests, Aptitudes, and Abilities

Understanding yourself a little better will help you prepare for the future. What are your favorite activities? What are your natural talents? Do you have any skills that could help you earn some extra spending money? Answering these questions will help you decide which careers might be right for you.

Interests

Your **interests** are what you enjoy learning about or doing. Knowing your interests helps you identify careers you may enjoy. Do you enjoy working with people, objects, or ideas? Most jobs focus on one of these areas more than the other two. People

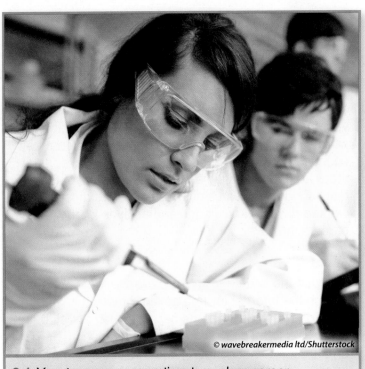
© wavebreakermedia ltd/Shutterstock

9-1 Your teen years are a time to explore career possibilities, discover new interests, and develop new skills.

who prefer a certain type of work often share some general characteristics. For instance, if you like personal interaction, you might do well as a social worker or a salesperson. If you enjoy working with objects—maybe building models or fixing small appliances—you might enjoy a career as an engineer.

Some jobs are routine while others involve constant change. Manufacturing assembly line jobs involve the same work each day. Computer technicians, human resource managers, and child care workers, however, face constant change. Which do you prefer? Also, ask yourself whether you prefer being outdoors or inside. The answer may help you choose a career. Many construction workers and farmers do most of their work outdoors. Air traffic controllers are usually inside. Real estate agents work both outside and indoors.

Aptitudes

Aptitudes are the natural talents with which you were born. Some people have artistic aptitude, so drawing is an easy and fun activity for them. Other people find science easy and stimulating. Everyone has aptitudes.

Sometimes your interests are clues to your aptitudes. You may excel at activities you have not yet tried. If you take a computer programming class, you may discover you have a natural aptitude for programming. Maybe you will discover a natural aptitude for management when you are the leader of a group project.

Every career requires certain aptitudes. If you know what your aptitudes are, you can identify careers that need those aptitudes. For instance, being an accountant requires an aptitude for math. Therefore, you would be more likely to enjoy success as an accountant if you have a math aptitude.

Abilities

Your **abilities** are skills developed through training or practice. Abilities may be either physical or mental. For instance, you might have the ability to run long distances without tiring. You might be able to quickly and easily add a long column of numbers or memorize lines for a play.

When you have an aptitude for something, it is easier to learn the necessary skills. Hard work and a sincere interest can overcome a low aptitude, however. Your ideal career is one that interests you while also making the best use of your aptitudes and abilities.

Life Connections

Discovering Your Aptitudes

If you are not sure about your aptitudes, taking an *aptitude test* is a good idea. These tests can reveal your innate personality traits and the activities in which you are most likely to succeed. Your guidance counselor will have aptitude tests you can take, and there are many available online. The results of those tests suggest careers you may enjoy. You must still work to develop knowledge and abilities for these careers, however.

Research Activity

Use the search term *free career aptitude test* to search the Internet for free aptitude tests. It is a good idea to take more than one because they are all quite different and may give you new career ideas. There are many websites offering aptitude tests. Some provide other types of interesting tests you may also find helpful.

Career Clusters

The **career clusters** are 16 groupings of careers based on common knowledge and skills, **9-2**. Within each cluster, a number of *career pathways* are identified to indicate more specific areas of expertise. For instance, the following is an example of the career pathways within the finance career cluster:

- Securities and investments
- Business finance
- Accounting
- Insurance
- Banking services

Having several career areas that interest you is good. The more you learn about each group of careers, the easier it will be to make a decision. As you read and collect data about a given career, your interest will either increase or decrease. The career clusters are designed to help you discover your interests and passions. They give you the information to choose an educational pathway for success in high school, college, and a career.

Education and Training

When choosing a career, look at the required amount of education and training. How long are you willing to go to school? How much time are you willing to spend learning specific skills? For instance, a medical career requires many years of education and training beyond high school.

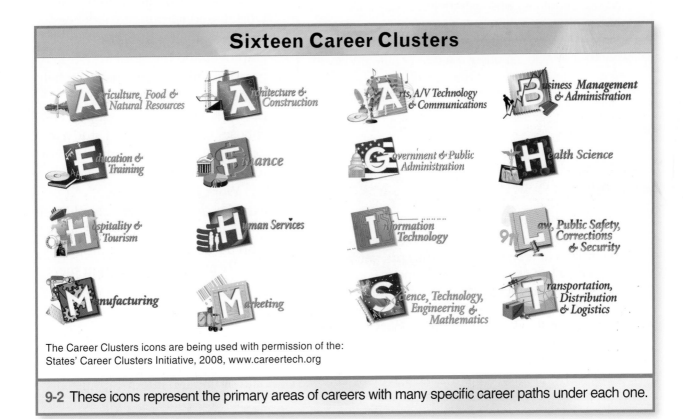

Sixteen Career Clusters

Agriculture, Food & Natural Resources

Architecture & Construction

Arts, A/V Technology & Communications

Business Management & Administration

Education & Training

Finance

Government & Public Administration

Health Science

Hospitality & Tourism

Human Services

Information Technology

Law, Public Safety, Corrections & Security

Manufacturing

Marketing

Science, Technology, Engineering & Mathematics

Transportation, Distribution & Logistics

The Career Clusters icons are being used with permission of the: States' Career Clusters Initiative, 2008, www.careertech.org

9-2 These icons represent the primary areas of careers with many specific career paths under each one.

For some sales positions, however, a high school diploma and on-the-job training is often sufficient.

Many jobs require **postsecondary** education and training, meaning additional schooling beyond high school. You might pursue a two-year *associate's degree* at a community college or a certificate from a trade school. Most professional positions require a four-year *bachelor's degree* from a college or university.

During the first several years of college, you will typically take basic courses required by the school for all degrees. During the final two years, classes are more concentrated on your **major**, the academic subject chosen as a field of specialization. You will then earn a bachelor's degree in this subject upon acceptable completion of all courses. Some higher-level positions require a *master's degree*, which means completion of specific courses beyond a bachelor's degree. A *doctorate degree* is the highest level of degree in a particular field of study. People who earn a doctorate degree are experts in their field.

Work-Based Learning

Work-based learning programs provide opportunities for students to learn about jobs through direct work experience as part of their school courses. School program coordinators monitor the work-based learning experience to make sure it is a success for the employer and the student. Work-based learning experiences can help students make career decisions, network with potential employers, choose further courses of study, and develop the job skills important for future employment.

Work-based learning experiences at the high school level are called *co-op programs*. Students who participate in co-op programs usually attend school part of the day and then work the remainder of the day.

Internships are supervised, practical job experiences at the postsecondary level. They are either paid or unpaid. Internships usually last several quarters or one semester.

Global Connections

Study Abroad

One great benefit of earning a college degree is the opportunity to take approved classes at a university in another country. These classes are approved by the institution and count toward your degree. Nearly every four-year college or university offers this choice—and usually at the same tuition cost. The extra costs involve travelling to the country and other expenses during the time spent abroad. There are many different types of programs that vary by institution. Depending on your major, some colleges only offer programs in certain European countries, while others have Asian and Latin American choices. When looking into colleges, also ask about the study abroad programs available. This is a wonderful way to experience a new culture and even learn a new language.

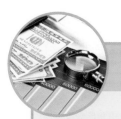

Financial Literacy Connections

Earning While Learning

Apprenticeship programs train employees to learn a skilled or technical trade. They are entry-level jobs that may last several months or many years, depending on the industry. An *apprentice* works closely with an experienced worker to learn their skills in preparation for doing a similar job. Classroom instruction may also be involved. A high school diploma is necessary to enter one of these programs. Apprenticeship programs are available in many career areas from culinary arts to auto mechanics.

An internship often counts as a class in your major. Many programs now require students to complete an internship to earn a degree.

Some companies offer training for newly hired employees to obtain the specific skills they need. Company training programs may involve formal classes, on-the-job training, or a combination of both.

Certification and Licensing

A **certification** is a special standing within a profession as a result of meeting certain educational and work requirements. Many careers have professional certifications, such as teachers, nurses, accountants, and project managers.

Licensing differs from certification because a government agency determines the regulations that must be met. Having a license gives a person or a business the permission to use or do something. For instance, a child care facility must be licensed by the state to remain open and provide its unique service. Both certificates and licenses are documents with expiration dates. Therefore, they must be renewed. They are usually on display to assure customers that the person or business is qualified to do the job.

Sources of Career Information

As a student, you have access to many valuable sources of information to investigate careers. Taking advantage of them can help you choose the career that is right for you.

School Guidance Counselors

School guidance counselors are good resources for career information. They can answer most questions about the education, training, and experience needed for certain careers. Counselors have catalogs from many colleges, universities, and career and trade schools. They can tell you about the admissions process, academic requirements, and tuition costs at schools that might interest you, **9-3**.

Part of a guidance counselor's job is to be aware of current career trends. **Job trends** are the general patterns of whether hiring is increasing or decreasing in certain job sectors. You can also ask your guidance counselors for help in finding a good aptitude test. They may be able to tell you about careers new to you that will fit your aptitudes and abilities. Talk with your counselors from time to time. They can help you set career goals and start moving in the right direction.

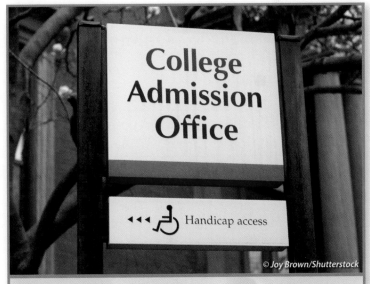

© Joy Brown/Shutterstock

9-3 The college admission process can be daunting if you are not prepared for what is expected. School guidance counselors can help students through the necessary steps of the process.

The Internet and Libraries

Using the Internet is an excellent way to explore careers and perform job analysis for specific occupations. Educational requirements, job trends, and salary ranges are the types of information you can find. Some websites match people's skills and aptitudes to relevant careers. Many job-search websites work like help-wanted ads in the newspaper, **9-4**. You can search by job title, company, and city. Information is usually up-to-date and easily available. Most offer the ability to apply for positions as well. Social media websites sometimes have exclusive listings.

Both your school library and the public library have many informational career resources. If you need help finding information on a specific career, ask a librarian. He or she will be familiar with the library's resources, which include articles in *periodicals*, or magazines.

One helpful book is the *Occupational Outlook Handbook*, which lists education and training requirements, job duties, and salary ranges for each occupation. It also includes potential for advancement,

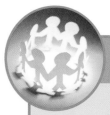

Life Connections

Making a Career Plan

When you start thinking about choosing a career, it is helpful to create a career plan. A *career plan* is a list of the steps you need to take to reach your career goals. First, determine your career goals, which are based on your lifestyle choices, aptitudes, and abilities. Find out if there is a growing demand for that career.

Then determine the necessary education and training for your chosen career at this point in time. Your career plan should also include any cocurricular and volunteer activities that might prepare you for that particular career. Finally, research the kinds of entry-level jobs to help you gain experience while you complete your education.

Writing Activity

Choose a career of interest to you now based on your goals. Write a one-page career plan taking all these considerations into account.

Online Career Resources

Source	Internet Address
USAJOBS, the official job site of the U.S. Federal Government	www.usajobs.gov
Occupational Outlook Handbook, U.S. Department of Labor (Bureau of Labor Statistics)	www.stats.bls.gov/oco
Occupational Outlook Quarterly, U.S. Department of Labor (Bureau of Labor Statistics)	www.bls.gov/opub/ooq
U.S. Department of Labor (Employment and Training Administration)	www.doleta.gov
The Occupational Information Network (O*NET™)	www.onetonline.org
CareerOneStop	www.careeronestop.org
Mapping Your Future	www.mappingyourfuture.org

9-4 Take advantage of the many resources available online for your career research.

job outlook, and job prospects. The U.S. Department of Labor revises this information every two years. It is also available online.

Another useful reference published by the U.S. Department of Labor is the *Occupational Outlook Quarterly*. The quarterly publication covers a wide variety of career and work-related topics. For instance, it lists unusual occupations, tips for jobseekers, salary trends, and results of new studies from the Bureau of Labor Statistics. It is also available online.

People

People you know can be a good source for finding out about different careers. Talk with friends, neighbors, relatives, and people in your community about their work. These people can provide you with realistic information about their careers and the education and training required. Ask about the career path leading to each person's current position. Find out what they like and dislike about their jobs. Also, ask about the working conditions and benefits such as insurance, retirement plans, and onsite child care.

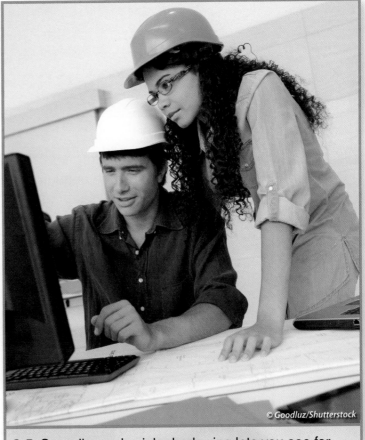

© Goodluz/Shutterstock

9-5 Spending a day job shadowing lets you see for yourself what that career is like and ask any questions.

You may even be able to have a job shadowing experience. **Job shadowing** involves spending time at work with someone whose career interests you, **9-5**. Job shadowing can be arranged through a counselor or teacher, but you can also choose to job shadow someone you know. Make sure you research the job you are shadowing so you can ask relevant questions and learn more.

Some people also decide to find a **mentor**, who is a trusted person to guide someone's career. Mentors are people who have already had success in their careers. They give helpful advice to others just starting out or rising in their own careers. A mentor can be someone inside your workplace or a trusted acquaintance who knows you and values your skills.

Reading Review

1. How do your interests and aptitudes affect your career success?
2. Your skills developed through training or practice are called your _____.
3. A bachelor's degree is earned through a(n) _____.
4. List four sources of career information.

Section 9-2

Career Options

Objectives

After studying this section, you will be able to
- **describe** family and consumer sciences career groups.
- **give examples** of jobs in each family and consumer sciences career group.
- **list** opportunities for entrepreneurship you could explore right now.

Key Terms		
cooperative extension agents	consumer advocates	buyers
consumerism	dietetics	entrepreneurs
	food science	

Many careers in the 16 career clusters involve using the family and consumer sciences (FCS) skills you learn in this course. This section focuses on those careers within the family and consumer sciences area. It also provides information on how you can develop your own business opportunities right now.

Family and Consumer Sciences

FCS careers are divided into smaller groups according to subject matter and include the following:
- Child and human development
- Family relations
- Education and communications
- Personal and family finance
- Food science, nutrition, and wellness
- Textiles and apparel
- Housing and interior design

By taking FCS courses now, you will learn many skills that are useful in a number of careers, as well as in your personal life, **9-6**. For instance, dietitians need food science, nutrition, and wellness skills to advise their patients on how to maintain their health. They also need child and human development skills to relate to people. Many careers in business require an understanding of personal and family finance. In almost any career that exists, you can find ways to use your family and consumer sciences skills.

Family and Consumer Sciences

Major Categories	Postsecondary Training and / or Associate's Degree	Bachelor's Degree or Higher
Child and human development	Child care teacher Parent's helper Professional nanny Scout leader Teacher's aide Youth counselor	Child care center or preschool administrator Designer of children's clothing, toys, or furniture Early childhood educator Parent educator Recreation director
Family relations	Counseling paraprofessional Home companion Homemaker services director Hot line counselor Older adult living facility aide	Crisis center counselor Family health counselor Family/marriage therapist Social worker
Education and communications	4-H leader Journalism intern Teacher's aide	Cooperative extension agent Family and consumer sciences teacher or college professor
Personal and family finance	Bank teller Collection agent Consumer product tester Consumer service representative Credit bureau clerk Loan officer assistant	Consumer affairs director Credit counselor Credit bureau researcher Financial planner Loan officer Money investment advisor Retail credit manager
Food science, nutrition, and wellness	Banquet manager Caterer Chef or chief cook Cook's helper Dietitian's aide Executive chef Laboratory assistant Pastry chef Personal trainer Restaurant hostess/host Short-order cook	Athletic trainer Dietitian Food service manager Sports nutritionist Food technologist Food chemist Product developer Quality control supervisor Restaurant owner/manager Sanitation supervisor
Textiles and apparel	Alterationist Color consultant Dry cleaner Fashion coordinator Fashion or textile designer Salesperson Stocker Tailor/reweaver Visual display artist	Apparel historian Apparel marketing specialist Fashion editor or writer Merchandise buyer or manager Store manager Textile market analyst Textile scientist Visual display manager
Housing and interior design	Appliance salesperson Carpet layer Carpet and upholstery cleaner Design assistant Drafter Drapery/slipcover maker Home furnishings salesperson Home lighting assistant Landscaper Plumber Upholsterer	Appliance designer/engineer Architect Facilities planner Home furnishings buyer Home furnishings writer/editor Home furnishings and lighting designer Interior designer Kitchen and bath designer Landscape architect Public housing consultant

9-6 This table lists some occupations at different education and training levels for careers in family and consumer sciences areas.

Careers in Child and Human Development

Child and human development careers are diverse. Some involve educating and caring for children, researching child behavior, planning children's entertainment, and designing or marketing children's products. Working in each of these areas requires an understanding of children's special needs for their growth and development. Babysitting is a good way to prepare for a career in early childhood education and services.

People who educate and care for young children may work at playgrounds, camps, child care centers, nursery schools, preschools, or kindergartens. Many programs provide care for children before and after school or while their parents are at work. Federal and state government agencies provide programs for educating young children, such as Head Start. All child care centers must follow state and federal laws to operate. Inspecting child care centers for safety features and practices is also a career option.

Some other career options in this field include

- researching how education or family lifestyles affect child development. People in education, health care, or business use this information.
- planning children's entertainment, writing children's books, or creating games to help children learn.
- designing educational programs for children at different levels of development.
- designing or marketing children's products, such as toys or clothes. Having a background in child development helps these people design items to suit the needs of children.
- helping people handle development issues beyond childhood.

People who enjoy successful careers in child and human development have certain traits, **9-7**. They get along well with children, and most children like them. They feel comfortable playing with children and caring for them. They are patient and enjoy working with people of all ages.

Traits for a Career in Child and Human Development

- Interested in children
- Understand children's needs
- Communicate well with children
- Enjoy being physically close to children
- Good physical and emotional health
- Ability to cope with children's noise
- Dependable and responsible
- Adaptable and flexible
- Have a sense of humor
- Cheerful and sympathetic
- Self-confident
- Imaginative and creative
- Empathetic and patient

9-7 Do you have the traits needed for a successful career in child and human development?

Careers in Family Relations

Family counselors, therapists, and psychologists help people and families become mentally, emotionally, or spiritually healthy. They help families cope with challenges related to social, personal, career, or educational development. Religious organizations, schools, counseling centers, and mental health clinics have these positions. You might begin a career in family counseling as a camp counselor. With a college degree, you may want to become a marriage and family counselor. Some jobs are in social work for child welfare or other family agencies working to resolve difficult family situations.

Working in family relations requires a genuine interest in people and a concern for their well-being, **9-8**. They must have excellent communications skills and keep personal facts about their clients confidential.

Traits for a Career in Family Relations

- Sincere interest in helping people
- Sensitive to the feelings of others
- Respect the confidence of others
- Enjoy guiding people to meet challenges
- Good communication and listening skills
- Ability to lead conversations
- Interested in self improvement
- Loyal to coworkers
- Willing to put in extra effort when needed to meet your responsibilities

9-8 Do you have the traits needed for a successful career in family relations?

Careers in Education and Communications

More FCS professionals work in education and communications than in any other area. Most careers in this area require a college degree. You could begin to prepare for a career in FCS education by working with children through babysitting or assisting in a child care center. After high school, you might become a teacher's aide.

People who teach family and consumer sciences may work in middle school, high school, college, or the community. They may teach in only one area of FCS or they may teach in all areas. Most FCS educators have a broad background in all areas of family and consumer sciences. They are friendly and enjoy working with people, **9-9**.

Family and consumer sciences educators may teach living skills for adults in a community. Topics could range from money management to nutrition. FCS professionals in education with advanced degrees may become curriculum specialists. They plan what will be taught in various family and consumer sciences courses.

FCS educators may also work for a county cooperative extension program. **Cooperative extension agents** provide practical and research-based information to agricultural producers, business owners, youth, consumers, and others in rural areas and communities of all sizes, **9-10**.

Traits for a Career in Education and Communication

- Interest in both family and consumer sciences and education
- Friendly and approachable
- Organized
- Good communication and listening skills
- Enjoy teaching new ideas to others
- Ability to lead a group
- Works well without supervision
- Sensitive to the needs of others
- Dependable and responsible

9-9 Do you have the traits needed for a successful career in education and communications?

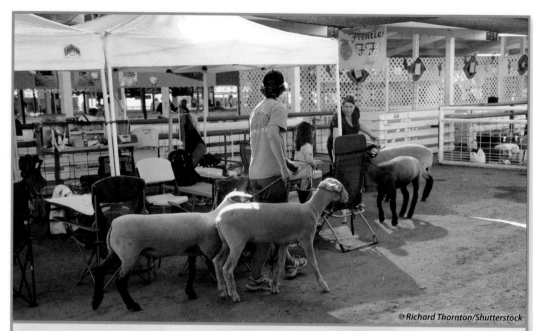

©Richard Thornton/Shutterstock

9-10 Cooperative extension agents also work with 4-H leaders to plan programs for youth.

Cooperative extension agents work at offices within the Cooperative Extension System of the U.S. Department of Agriculture (USDA).

Careers in Personal and Family Finance

Many people working in personal and family finance help people to become better managers and informed consumers. People who do well in personal and family finance careers are good with details and numbers. They are responsible and enjoy challenging work. You might break into this area by doing office work or being a consumer survey assistant. They usually have a business background and a college degree, **9-11**.

People in this area of FCS may help others set savings goals and plan for future expenses. Money managers and credit bureau employees advise people on how to invest their money, reduce certain expenses, and decrease what they owe (credit). They may work in collection or credit departments or help people apply for loans. They help others combine their bills and become debt free. They also investigate people who apply for credit.

Traits for a Career in Personal and Family Finance

- Enjoy working with numbers
- Detail oriented
- Like sharing new ideas and information with all types of people
- Organize and supervise people
- Work well without close supervision
- Take full responsibility for your own efforts and actions
- Prefer mentally challenging work
- Able to concentrate on work activities
- Enjoy being in a position of responsibility

9-11 Do you have the traits needed for a successful career in personal and family finance?

Consumerism is the promotion of the consumers' interests. Some companies employ customer service representatives. These people take complaints from customers and resolve problems related to the company's products or services.

Consumer advocates support the rights of the consumer to obtain safe goods and services at fair prices. They are often hired by government agencies, corporations, consumer protection organizations, and community groups to ensure that consumers' needs are met. For instance, the Food and Drug Administration, the Federal Trade Commission, Better Business Bureau, and Chambers of Commerce have positions in consumerism.

Careers in Food Science, Nutrition, and Wellness

There is more to health and wellness than just eating the right foods. Proper exercise and nutrition also play a large part in maintaining a healthful lifestyle. Food science, nutrition, and wellness is the broadest category of FCS careers. There are employment opportunities in hospitals and other care centers, any company working with or selling food, and sports and wellness facilities.

To work in this field, you must enjoy experimenting and solving problems with precision and thoroughness. An interest in science, personal health, and wellness is essential. High standards of cleanliness are important for people who work directly with food.

Some careers also involve the marketing of food, such as with advertising agencies, photographers, and demonstrators, **9-12**. Some of these FCS professionals create cookbooks or work for the mass media writing or editing food information.

Dietetics applies the principles of food, nutrition, business, social and basic sciences in different settings to promote nutritional health. *Dietitians* are professionals who provide nutritional services, perform research, and educate. Dietitians work in health care, public health, food industry, business, journalism, private practice, and corporate wellness settings. Dietitians must earn a four-year

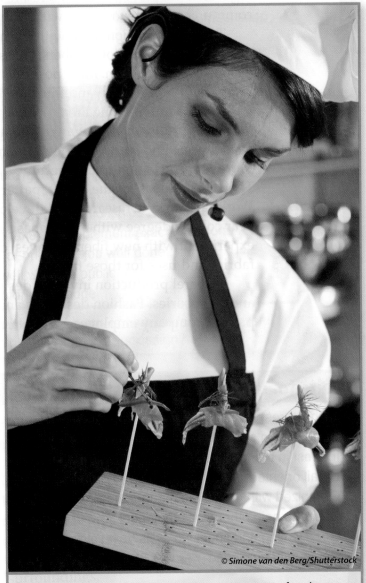

© Simone van den Berg/Shutterstock

9-12 Demonstrators show ways to prepare food or use appliances at exhibits, trade shows, and in stores.

Chapter 10
Getting the Job You Want

Sections

Reading Prep

College and Career Readiness

Imagine you are a business owner and have several employees working for you. As you read the chapter, think about what you would like your employees to know. When you finish reading, write a memo to your employees that includes key information from the chapter.

Concept Organizer

Use a diagram like the one shown to indicate what should be included in a good portfolio.

Companion Website

Print out the concept organizer for Chapter 10 at the website.

Companion Website
www.g-wlearning.com

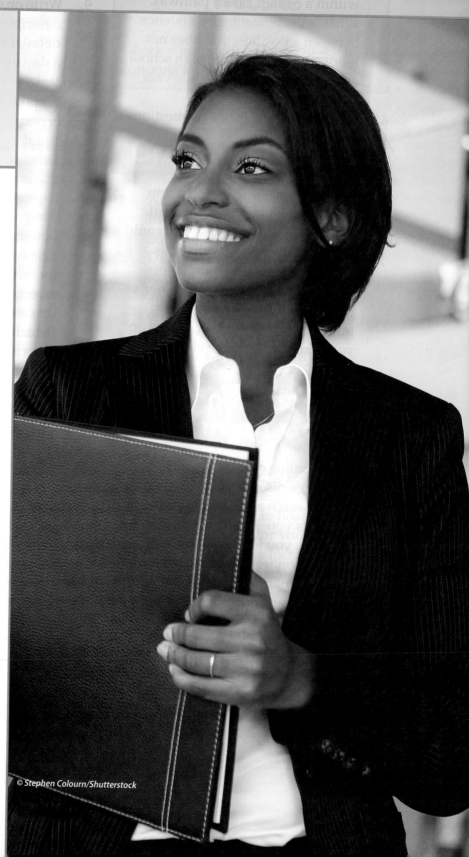

© Stephen Colourn/Shutterstock

Applying for Jobs

Objectives

After studying this section, you will be able to
- **explain** how to search for a job.
- **describe** how to apply for a job.
- **prepare** a résumé.
- **write** a letter of application.

Key Terms

networking	references	letter of application
professional organizations	letter of recommendation	portfolio
résumé		

Before you can be a successful employee, you need to know how to find a job. The first step in getting a job is to learn about job openings. Maybe you hear of a family who needs a babysitter. Perhaps you know a person who needs some help grocery shopping or running other errands. These are good job leads for work in your early teen years.

The Job Search

As you mature and look for jobs in the business community, job searching becomes more challenging. You may learn about jobs by reading the help-wanted ads in newspapers or on the Internet. You may even apply for a job when you have not heard about an opening. For some jobs, you may want to

Life Connections

Work Permits for Minors

To protect the safety of teen workers under a certain age, a *work permit* must be obtained for businesses to legally hire them. A work permit also ensures that teens do not neglect their education while they work. Restrictions vary by state on the ages of working teens, the hours they can work, and duties they can perform. If you are under your state's legal hiring age, first obtain a *Letter of Intent to Hire* from your prospective employer. The letter should list the hours you will be working and duties you will be performing. A parent's written consent may also be required. The next step is to bring the necessary information to your school's administration office. They will issue the work permit, sometimes called an *employment certificate*.

Research Activity

Work permits vary by state. Search the Internet for the restrictions and requirements in your state. Find the same information for several surrounding states and compare the requirements in a short paragraph.

apply in person. For instance, you might walk into a restaurant and ask if they need help, **10-1**.

When you hear of job openings that interest you, apply for them as soon as possible. Sometimes you may use the phone to do this. When calling about a job, always be polite to the person who speaks with you. Be sure to state your name clearly and mention the position that interests you. People who are friendly and courteous often make a better impression than those who are not.

Networking

Networking is making contacts with people who may be able to help you find a job. The easiest place to start networking is with adults you already know, especially those in careers of interest to you. Teachers, coaches, school guidance counselors, family members, and friends are excellent sources of job information. People who know you and your strengths are more willing to suggest possible jobs.

Other job networking resources include people at organizations where you volunteer and other activities you participate in outside of school. Think about organizations you belong to, such as FCCLA, city sports leagues, or clubs, as potential sources of career information.

Professional organizations are recognized associations that unite and inform people who work in the same occupation or industry. They exist to provide members with current industry information, sponsor

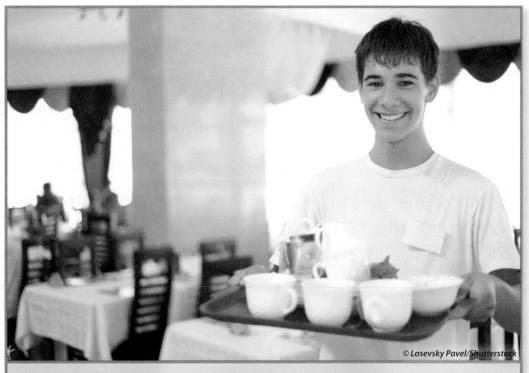

© Losevsky Pavel/Shutterstock

10-1 Sometimes dropping by a foodservice business to fill out a job application leads to a position because the job turnover is often high.

professional educational programs, and serve as a resource for updating skills. Depending on the profession, they sometimes issue professional certifications—indicating a person has specific qualifications in the subject area.

Some professional organizations accept junior members who are still in school or learning the trade. Joining a professional organization is a good way to meet people already in your chosen career. They often know about job openings before anyone else. They are also great places to find mentors.

Applying for the Job

When applying for most jobs, be prepared to complete a job application, **10-2**. A job application is a representation of you, so you want it to present the most positive image. Always give correct information and double check your spelling and grammar.

Most job applications ask for the same types of information, which includes your contact information, education, and work experience. It is a good idea to gather this information before applying. Filling out an application will be easier when you have all the necessary information with you.

Later in life, you may be applying for professional-level jobs. To express your interest in these jobs, letters written in a clear business style stating your interest and qualifications are often requested. Many jobs now require applicants to apply online through their websites.

A Résumé

The information needed for job applications is organized as a résumé. Your résumé is a short history of your education, qualifications, and work experience. Your résumé is the single most important document you need when searching for jobs. Sometimes, a prospective employer will determine whether to consider you for a position by only looking at your résumé.

Résumés include much of the information requested on job applications. Your résumé should include more information, however, about your qualifications, **10-3**. The essential categories for all résumés are *contact information*, *career objective statement*, *education*, *work experience*, and *honors and special skills*. Your résumé will change and evolve as you gain more experience and continue your education.

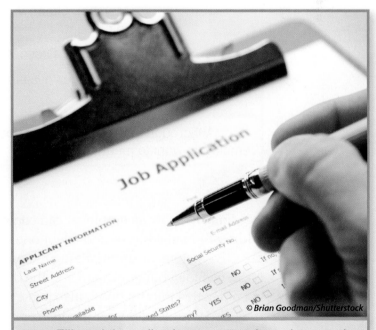

© Brian Goodman/Shutterstock

10-2 Fill out job applications accurately and as neatly as possible.

Parker Washington
150 South Station Street
Addison, Texas 77059
(555) 555-6543
pwashington@provider.com

Objective	Start my career in the foodservice business by assisting restaurant serving or kitchen personnel.
Education	Green Valley High School, Addison, Texas, 20XX to present. Focus on food science, nutrition, and wellness. Graduating in June, 20XX.
Experience	Volunteer, Addison Food Pantry, 20XX to present. Responsible for assisting with food drives as assigned and maintaining a running inventory of food in stock. Assistant stocker, Green Valley Convenience Mart, 20XX to present.
Computer skills	Proficient in keyboarding and Microsoft Word, Excel, and PowerPoint.
Honors and Activities	Green Valley High School honor roll, 20XX. Treasurer, Family, Career and Community Leaders of America (FCCLA), Green Valley High School chapter, 20XX to present. Member, Green Valley High School cooking club, 20XX to present. Co captain, Green Valley High School varsity baseball, 20XX. References available upon request.

10-3 A thorough résumé presents a positive, professional image and helps employers want to meet you.

First, list how an employer can contact you. This includes your name, address, e-mail address, and telephone number. After that, write a short career objective statement summarizing the type of position you are currently seeking. Next, include your education and the dates you attended each school. As you get older, this information will expand to possibly college or a trade school. You may also wish to add your grade average if it is high.

The work experience section lists any part-time work including volunteer positions. Take the time to think about your work experience.

You may realize you already have quite a bit of experience. For instance, volunteering at a hospital or having an internship qualifies as work experience. If you shovel snow, babysit, have a pet-sitting service, or even organize a bake sale, then that counts, too. Any experiences working with or helping others should be included.

Finally, make sure your résumé includes your special skills, honors, and activities. Be sure to include any skills that would be helpful in certain jobs, such as writing or drafting skills. Your honors and activities include any school or community groups in which you have been involved. Be sure to list any awards received and offices you have held.

References

Prospective employers want to know as much as possible about potential employees

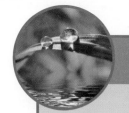

Go Green

The Paperless Résumé

Job hunters are moving away from hard-copy résumés because most employers want résumés submitted electronically or on their websites. Paperless résumés are easy to create and use while saving paper. Many websites are available to help you create and update electronic résumés for easy access and submission. If you must print a résumé, use recycled paper.

One benefit of submitting résumés electronically is the ability to use different industry *keywords* to get your résumé noticed. Because companies receive hundreds of résumés daily, they identify good candidates by filtering résumés with keywords matching the job requirements. Read the job description carefully and include the many important words throughout your résumé. For instance, if applying for an office manager position, likely job description keywords may be *management, efficient, computer skills, personable,* or *bachelor's.* Keeping track of different résumés written for different types of positions can be daunting. Separating your electronic résumés by job category helps you keep track of your work history and relevant experience.

before they are hired. **References** are people who know you and your work habits well, but are not relatives. They are able to discuss your personal qualities and job skills with potential employers. Teachers, coaches, and former employers make good references. They can give valid information on your work performance and reliability. Often employers will call your references to ask them specific questions about you and your suitability for the position.

You can also ask references to write a letter of recommendation for you. A **letter of recommendation** is a written document you can show to any prospective employer testifying to your abilities. It serves as a formal recommendation for an employer to hire you.

A résumé can include three or four references. Another option is to create a separate references document and write *references available upon request* at the end of the résumé. Always get permission first to list someone as a reference.

Letter of Application

A **letter of application** accompanies your résumé expressing interest in a position and providing more information about your qualifications, **10-4**.

150 South Station Street
Addison, Texas 77059
April 25, 20XX

Mr. Eric Carter
Manager
Valley Barbeque Restaurant
Addison, Texas 77059

Dear Mr. Carter:

I am interested in pursuing a career in the foodservice industry. Mrs. Sheffield, my Green Valley High School guidance counselor, suggested I contact you about any entry-level positions that may be available in your restaurant. I would be happy to assist your serving staff or kitchen personnel. I am currently a junior and have already taken food science and nutrition classes, with more planned for my senior year.

I live close to Valley Barbeque and it has long been one of my family's favorite places to eat. So I am very familiar with your restaurant and I enjoy the friendly employees. I love to cook and helped start the cooking club at Green Valley High, which meets monthly to prepare different meals chosen by the members. As a volunteer at the Addison Food Pantry, my responsibilities include assisting with food drives and maintaining a running inventory of food in stock. I am also an assistant stocker at Green Valley Convenience Mart, a position I have held for the past two years. My long-term career goal is to eventually open my own restaurant after attending culinary college and gaining enough experience in all aspects of the business.

My résumé is enclosed and I would appreciate the opportunity to discuss how I could be of service to Valley Barbeque. Please contact me at (555) 555-6543 or at pwashington@provider.com. Thank you for your time and consideration.

Sincerely,

Parker Washington

Parker Washington

10-4 A letter of application explains how your relevant skills and qualifications can benefit the company that hires you.

Consider a letter of application as a personal representation of you. Although a résumé is straightforward, your letter of application can be more personal and express a high level of interest.

Letters of application are business documents that should be well written and error free. It is a good idea to have someone proofread your letters for spelling and grammar before sending. Letters of application should be professional, but can also be creative to let your personality shine and help distinguish you from others.

Portfolio

Depending on the company and the position, some employers ask to see an applicant's portfolio. A **portfolio** is an organized collection of your work showcasing your talent and skills. Include samples of your written materials, photographs, and artwork relevant to the job for which you are applying. Place the samples neatly in a folder or binder for protection and easy viewing. You may also choose to create an electronic portfolio. Be able to discuss your work in detail including the goals, implementation process, and outcomes of the projects. Other documents to keep in your portfolio are

- a current copy of your résumé
- letters of recommendation
- list of references
- documentation of awards and honors
- certifications, if any

Make sure your portfolio is organized and up-to-date by adding new materials over time. Consider your education and career goals as you create a portfolio. It may also be required for college admissions.

Reading Review

1. List three sources of information you can use to learn about job openings.
2. What are the five main categories of information that must be on a résumé?
3. People who can discuss your personal qualities and job skills with potential employers are your _____.
4. Why would an employer want letters of application from job applicants?
5. What are the two primary functions of a portfolio?

The Interview Process

Objectives

After studying this section, you will be able to
- **demonstrate** how to interview for a job.
- **compare and contrast** the advantages and disadvantages of a part-time job.

Key Terms		
interview	follow-up letter	part-time job

When your résumé and letter of application attract the attention of an employer, they will want to talk to you. Sometimes the initial discussions take place on the telephone, other times you will be asked to a formal meeting. Almost every company wants to meet the job candidates in person at some time. The company learns more about you and decides whether you are a good fit for the job. You learn more about the duties and responsibilities of the position and meet people you might work with. This also helps you decide if the job and company are right for you.

The Job Interview

An **interview** is a meeting between an employer and a job applicant. If you apply for a job in person, you may have an interview at that time. If you apply online or by telephone, you may be asked to set up a time for a face-to-face interview.

Being well-prepared for the interview is crucial to your success. Most companies have websites providing all public information. Study the website before your interview. This shows the prospective

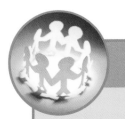

Life Connections

Interview Questions

There are some commonly asked questions in interviews that you should be prepared to answer. An interviewer often begins by asking you to state something about yourself. Other typical questions can include
- What are your strengths and weaknesses?
- Where do you see yourself in five years? in ten years?
- What are your favorite subjects in school? your least favorite subjects? Why?
- Why do you want to work here?
- What types of work do you dislike doing?
- Describe your computer skills.
- Give specific examples of your experience working on a team project. What do you like or dislike about working on team projects?

Speaking Activity

Practice interviewing with adult family members or friends. Tell them the job you are interviewing for and have them play the roles of the interviewers. Ask for their honest feedback after the interview and work on the questions that were difficult for you to answer.

employer you know about their business and can explain why they should hire you. The interviewer is more likely to be interested in you when you are interested in and knowledgeable about the company.

Understand that you are making a *first impression* in your interview, which is the one most people remember. Plan to arrive at the interview 10 minutes before your appointment to show you are reliable.

Dress appropriately for an interview. For men, a blazer, tie, and dress pants are always appropriate. Women should wear a suit, conservative dress, skirt or dressy pants, and a nice top. Never wear jeans, shorts, T-shirts, skimpy clothing, or those with rips or tears. Be sure your clothes are clean and well pressed and your shoes are polished.

Be well groomed for your interview. Interviewers know that people who care about how they present themselves are also likely to care about their work. Make sure your hair and nails are clean and trimmed. Women should wear light makeup and very little jewelry. Obvious body piercings and tattoos may prevent you from getting some jobs.

Greet the interviewer with a firm handshake, and display a positive attitude throughout the meeting, **10-5**. Be friendly and sit up straight. Look the interviewer in the eye and show confidence in yourself. Listen carefully to any questions the interviewer asks you. Answer the questions truthfully and with enthusiasm.

Be prepared to ask the interviewer insightful questions that indicate you understand the business and the position. You may wish to ask about anything you have not already discussed. It is acceptable to ask when you can expect the interviewer's decision and if they need any further information. Thank the person for their time.

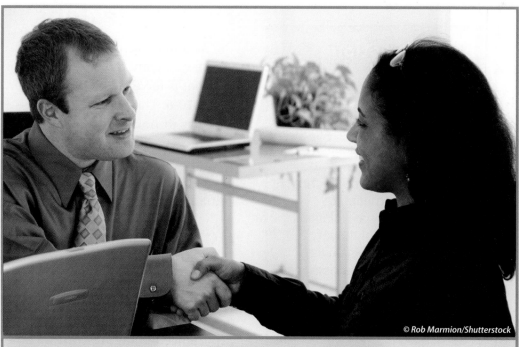

© Rob Marmion/Shutterstock

10-5 During an interview, you demonstrate your personal interaction and speaking skills. Make sure the interviewer remembers you in a positive light.

Send a professional **follow-up letter** to your interviewers thanking them for the interview opportunity and expressing continued interest in the job. This should be sent within three days of the interview. Follow-up e-mails are also acceptable, especially if the interviewers give you their business cards. Follow the same rules of writing a business letter for follow-up e-mails.

Making a Decision

Before making a hiring decision, all the job candidates will be interviewed. You will probably receive a letter, e-mail, or phone call regarding the interviewer's decision.

You may either accept or reject a job offer. If you receive more than one offer, take some time to evaluate and compare them. Consider each position's location, travel requirements, income and benefits, work schedule, duties and responsibilities, and potential for advancement. Then decide which position is the most appealing to you and where you might be the most comfortable working.

Let the employer know your decision as soon as possible. If you decide to accept the job, find out when and where you need to report to work. If you reject it, do so professionally and positively via the telephone.

People may not receive job offers for a number of reasons. Making a poor first impression is one common reason. If you are punctual, well groomed, and have a good attitude, you should not be rejected for this reason. Another common reason is the company hired a more qualified person. People often apply for several jobs before receiving a job offer. Do not be discouraged if this happens to you. You will eventually find a position that benefits both you and your employer.

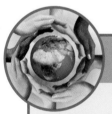

Global Connections

International Work

With the increase of global trade, some jobs pay you to conduct work in foreign countries. When considering your career goals and the education needed to attain them, think about whether international travel is one of them. If so, you might want to consider majors such as International Business, Global Marketing, International Relations, or others that lead to careers with foreign travel.

While the interviewing process may remain the same for global positions, sometimes the qualifications include passing foreign language tests. For those who want to work for the U.S. government in a diplomatic career, the process is more intensive. You must pass the written and oral Foreign Service Exams, receive medical and security clearances, and face a final review panel.

Part-Time Jobs

You may have reached a point where you want a **part-time job**, or one that is fewer than 40 hours per week, **10-6**. The interview process is just as important for obtaining part-time work as it is for full-time jobs. Any part-time jobs you have now will provide you with valuable work experience.

Advantages

Having a part-time job helps you earn extra money while learning about job responsibilities. You also gain experience managing your income and expenses. Part-time jobs

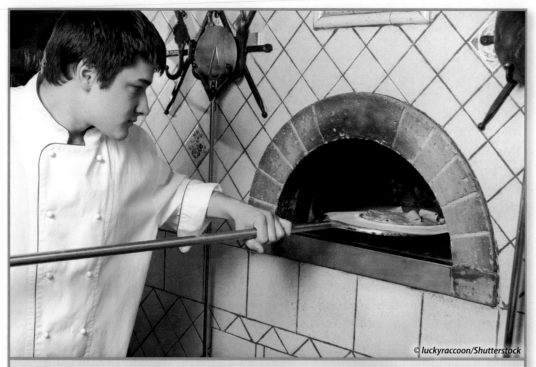
© luckyraccoon/Shutterstock

10-6 Part-time jobs are usually entry-level positions providing your first experience working for a company with rules, responsibilities, and certain expectations.

will teach you how to get along with others, especially those who are very different from you. You learn useful job skills that will help you succeed in the future. Many times, part-time positions also lead to full-time jobs. At the very least, your employers are good references.

Disadvantages

Working while in school does have some disadvantages, however. You have less time to devote to schoolwork, which may affect your grades. Time with your friends is reduced. Depending on how many hours you work, there may be less time for fun activities.

Reading Review

1. Why is it important to dress appropriately and be well groomed for job interviews?
2. What are the two functions of a follow-up letter?
3. True or false. You can take as much time as you want to decide about accepting or rejecting a job offer.
4. Name two advantages and disadvantages of having a part-time job while you are still in school.

Chapter Summary

Section 10-1. You must make an effort to find job openings. Networking and joining professional organizations may help you find suitable job openings. Create a solid résumé that includes your contact information, career objective statement, education, work experience, and honors and special skills. Résumé information can also be used to fill out job applications. Find people who know you and your work habits to serve as your job references. Develop a letter of application to accompany your résumé. Create a portfolio to showcase your skills using your best work samples to show prospective employers.

Section 10-2. You must interview with employers to be considered for jobs. Prepare for your interviews by researching the company, which indicates your desire to work there. Dress appropriately, be well groomed, and show a positive attitude throughout the interview. Send a follow-up letter to thank the interviewers for their time and express continued interest in the position. You may receive a job offer. Whether or not you decide to accept a particular offer depends on you and your career goals. Teens often decide to work part time while in school. Consider the advantages and disadvantages of working when in school before accepting a part-time job.

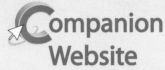

Companion Website
www.g-wlearning.com

Check your understanding of the main concepts for Chapter 10 at the website.

Critical Thinking

1. **Prepare.** Write a list of 10 questions you think an employer might ask you if you were applying for a job. Prepare responses to these questions. Then, working with a partner, take turns asking each other your lists of questions. Evaluate one another's responses to see how you would handle these questions in a job interview.

2. **Analyze.** How can parents help teens develop skills they will need in the workplace?

3. **Organize.** Interview a local employer in your community. Ask the person what qualities he or she looks for in an employee. Review the application process. What does the employer look for when reviewing applications? Gather any other information that would be useful for someone looking for a job. Compile your results with those of your classmates into a *Job Hunters Guide*. Include the answers to frequently asked questions, as well as several sample job applications. Distribute these to other students.

Common Core

College and Career Readiness

4. **Speaking.** Interview an employer about what qualities he or she looks for when interviewing a job applicant. Prepare a list of questions prior to the interview. Present your findings to the class.

5. **Writing.** Make a list of four people you could use as references. Given your experiences with them, what positive things would each person say about you and your work habits? Obtain their permission to use them as references. Create your references document with their complete contact information including e-mail addresses.

6. **Reading.** Find and read at least two books in the library that give advice on searching for jobs and how to interview well. Write the best advice in a notebook to use when you are preparing for interviews.

7. **Writing.** Practice writing letters of application for actual part-time jobs that interest you. Be sure to check your letters for correct spelling, grammar, and punctuation. Send the best ones along with your current résumé.

Technology

8. **Research and application.** Search the Internet for résumé-creating websites. Practice creating several different résumés for various careers of interest to you. Use as much of your own information as possible. Save them for future reference when searching for professional careers after college or trade school.

Journal Writing

9. Start a career section of your journal to document your job searching activities over time. Record both your positive and negative interview experiences to help you learn from the past and improve your interviewing skills.

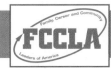 ## FCCLA

10. Prepare for the *Job Interview STAR Event* through a career portfolio that includes a résumé, letter of application, two letters of recommendation, educational experiences, and career-related education. Practice mock interviews with peers or local community members. See your adviser for information as needed.

Chapter 11
Preparing for Job Success

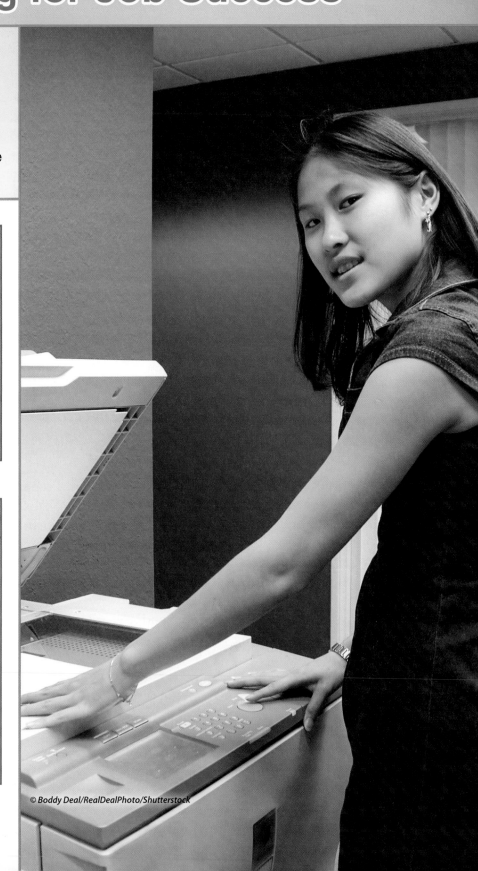

Sections

Reading Prep

College and Career Readiness

As you read the chapter, write a letter to yourself. Imagine that you will receive this letter in a few years when you are working at your future job. What would you like to remember from this chapter? In the letter, list key points from the chapter that will be useful in your future career.

Concept Organizer

Qualities of good employees

Use a diagram like the one shown to list five qualities of a good employee.

Companion Website

Print out the concept organizer for Chapter 11 at the website.

Companion Website
www.g-wlearning.com

© Boddy Deal/RealDealPhoto/Shutterstock

Employability Skills

Objectives

After studying this section, you will be able to
- **describe** skills needed for employment.
- **appraise** your academic, technology, communication, and thinking skills.

Key Terms

employability skills	scientific principles	critical thinking
superior	CAD programs	

Although you may not realize it, you are developing job skills daily. These personal qualities and skills follow you into the workplace. Most successful employees have certain qualities and skills in common. You learn many of these skills throughout your education and then develop them further when working. They help you to be successful on the job and in your personal life as well.

Skills Needed for Employment

Employability skills are the basic skills you need to get, keep, and succeed on a job. They are sometimes called *transferable skills* because they are helpful in any part- or full-time job. Employers assume their employees have basic skills in reading, writing, math, and science. Most jobs require workers to know how to use a computer and access the Internet, **11-1**. Good communication and highly developed thinking skills are also important.

Academic Skills

Every day in school, you use learned academic skills to study and complete assignments. People use these same skills in work environments.

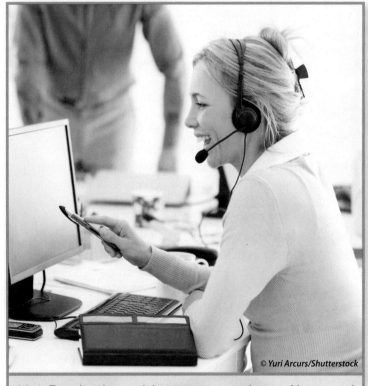

© Yuri Arcurs/Shutterstock

11-1 People who work in customer service positions need good computer and communication skills to be successful.

An employee's **superior**, or boss, evaluates his or her work just like your teacher evaluates your tests and homework. The only difference is that in school, you receive passing or failing grades. At work, an employee may earn a promotion or a raise. If work performance is poor, an employee might lose his or her job.

The ability to read and comprehend material is required in most jobs. For instance, employees in any business must be able to read and respond to the communications they receive. You must read and understand directions to follow them properly.

Writing papers, essays, reports, and other assignments in school can help improve writing skills. In the workplace, excellent writing skills make you a valuable employee. Business letters and e-mails, proposals, evaluations, presentations, and articles must all be written clearly, concisely, and without errors. Many companies reward good writers because they are crucial to gaining new business.

Math is a basic part of everyday life. Every time you balance a checkbook, measure a room, or calculate mileage, you use math skills. For instance, cashiers and bank tellers must be able to count money and make correct change. Other jobs require advanced math and science skills. Engineers, chemists, and airline pilots must perform difficult calculations accurately to do their jobs—and in some cases, save lives. Laboratory researchers use **scientific principles** to examine a problem, research possible solutions, and analyze potential outcomes. New products are developed in this way.

Technology

Most jobs require some degree of computer skills. The Internet is a useful research and marketing tool for businesses. Word processing software makes writing letters and reports easier. Spreadsheet software helps track income and expenses for budgeting purposes. Many people use electronic presentation software to make business presentations.

Jobs with artistic elements use creative software for drafting, design, illustration, and photographic manipulation. They are called **CAD programs**, or computer aided design. These programs save hours of time previously spent drawing and designing by hand.

Communication

One of the most important job skills is the ability to communicate well. Any job requires some degree of personal interaction. Therefore, you must be able to communicate

Global Connections

Technology and the Global Economy

Before computers were common in companies and homes, the ability to do business with other countries was expensive and limited. All communications had to be mailed and people attended meetings in person, which was costly when flying internationally. Only very large corporations were able to afford the high cost of doing business in other countries.

By the 1990s, entrepreneurs, companies, and their employees were dependent on computers to conduct business, allowing faster and more economical trade. Information was instantaneous, and the global economy was greatly expanded. Anyone with a computer now can develop a product, create a website to market it, and make sales electronically. Conducting business across country borders is now viewed as necessary to many people's job success.

by speaking and listening. How you communicate may influence whether you get a job or a promotion. It also affects how you get along with your coworkers.

You are learning communication skills in school right now. You make speeches, give oral reports, debate issues, work on team projects, and solve challenges. Listening to teachers, coaches, parents, and friends help you to develop good listening skills.

For many jobs, communication is vital to success. For instance, salespeople need to make convincing presentations to clients. Babysitters need to listen to children to effectively care for their needs, 11-2. Potential employers will evaluate your communication skills during interviews. By learning to communicate well now, you will be a step ahead when looking for a job.

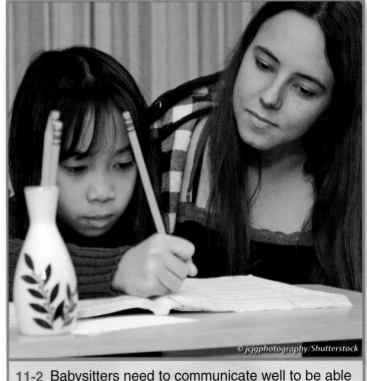
© jcjgphotography/Shutterstock

11-2 Babysitters need to communicate well to be able to help children when necessary.

Thinking

The ability to think and make good decisions based on presented information and your own research is needed in any job. **Critical thinking** is looking at all sides of an issue to analyze the situation and solve problems. This is especially important in management positions and in marketing or advertising where decisions impact a company's sales and profits. Critical thinkers look for creative ways to meet challenges and solve problems. With the highly competitive nature of most industries, companies need people with strong critical thinking skills.

Organizational skills are higher-level thinking skills and apply to every type of job. You need to be able to organize your time, tasks, and belongings. When you plan ahead, you are giving yourself enough time to get all your work done. Breaking large tasks into a series of smaller tasks will make jobs seem easier.

Reading Review

1. What are employability skills?
2. How do new product developers use scientific principles in their work?
3. Give three examples of how teachers use communication skills in their work.
4. What is the meaning of critical thinking?

Leadership and Teamwork

After studying this section, you will be able to
- **list** the qualities and characteristics of a good leader.
- **identify** your opportunities for leadership.
- **describe** roles, responsibilities, and characteristics of effective team members.

Key Terms		
leader	career and	teamwork
natural leaders	technical student	cooperate
motivation	organizations	
committee	(CTSOs)	
agenda		

Have you ever worked in a group at school or in your community? Many academic classes require group projects. Most school and community functions are organized through group efforts. Group members divide responsibilities according to their talents and strengths.

Learning how to lead and work in a group is important to your success in a career, as well as in a family and your community. Each person brings different skills to a group. Working as a group, you can accomplish more than when working alone.

Being an Effective Leader

A **leader** is the person who guides a group toward a common goal. Sometimes, a leader is the person who formed the group. Other times, the group elects a leader. Sometimes, leaders of groups emerge even though they are not chosen to lead. Groups can also have more than one leader. Various group members may lead specific tasks that relate to their strengths and abilities. For instance, one group member may have artistic ability and can lead others in making posters or flyers. Another group member may have excellent writing skills and can work with others to develop any communications the group needs to send.

You may know people who are **natural leaders** because they can get group members to easily follow their lead and do what they ask. These people have certain traits and skills. They show confidence in their abilities and can assert their views positively. They also know how to be good team players.

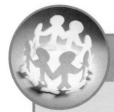

Life Connections

Parliamentary Procedure

Many organizations and most governments follow the same pattern for their business meetings. *Parliamentary procedure* is a fair and orderly way for leaders to conduct meetings. Understanding it will help you take a more active role in meetings. The book *Robert's Rules of Order* gives detailed information on this procedure.

A meeting is called to order by the president or leader of the group. Only one person may speak at any given time. First, the leader asks the secretary to read the minutes from the last meeting. *Minutes* are a record of what takes place at a meeting. The group then approves the minutes or recommends changes to them.

Next are the *officers' reports*. The treasurer reports on the group's income and expenses. Other officers may give reports on special projects.

The chairperson for each standing, or permanent, committee gives a status report. Special committees form for one purpose only and then disband, but they also report.

Unfinished business and new business are the final agenda items. Unfinished business is the topics discussed at the last meeting that still need a group decision. After that, any new business is discussed.

To end the meeting, a member of the group will *move to adjourn*. Another member will *second the motion*, or agree to adjourn. This signals the meeting is over.

Speaking and Listening Activity

As a class, practice using parliamentary procedure to run a pretend meeting. Using *Robert's Rules of Order*, hold short meetings about different topics. Rotate the roles so everyone has the opportunity to be a leader, officer, and member.

You may be a leader already. Do you feel at ease leading a class discussion? Have you conducted meetings as an officer in a club? Have you been involved in a community project? These are leadership roles. Developing your leadership skills now can help you at home, at school, in your community, and in the workplace.

Not everyone has an aptitude for leadership. You can, however, develop some skills needed to become an effective leader, **11-3**. Practicing these skills will help you fill leadership roles and meet the responsibilities you are given.

Effective Leadership Qualities

- Positive outlook
- Ability to motivate others
- Show responsibility by completing tasks
- Keeping promises
- Accepting blame
- Does not take advantage of others
- Explains positions and reasons with others
- Listens to other group members ideas
- Develops support among team members
- Encourages participation of all team members
- Makes sound decisions
- Works to resolve conflicts
- Maintains open communication with all group members

11-3 Effective leaders often possess similar qualities.

Motivate Members

Motivating group members is a big part of being an effective leader. **Motivation** is feeling the need or desire to do something. It creates action and produces results. An enthusiastic leader is excited and positive about the group's work. Your excitement about a project transfers to the rest of the team. An eager, motivated group is a productive one.

Everyone likes to be recognized and praised by a group or team for their efforts, **11-4**. Praise makes people feel special. Effective leaders give praise in front of the group as a motivating tool. When members need instruction for improvement, however, have this discussion in private.

Successful teams and groups are more motivated by reason and persuasion than by commands. Instead of telling group members what to do, ask them for help. Get the group's input when making big decisions.

To get more people involved, ask new people to join your group. Motivate new members by helping them feel welcome. Be friendly and formally introduce them to the other members. Encourage them to take part in activities.

Work with Committees

Group leaders are usually responsible for appointing committees and then directing their efforts. A **committee** is a group of people working together for a special purpose. Committees have many functions, depending on the needs of the organization or business. If committees are not organized and well managed, however, they are ineffective.

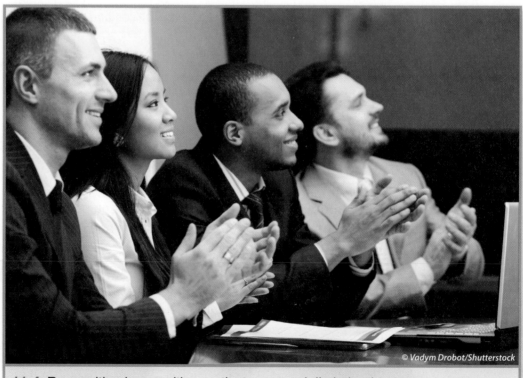

© Vadym Drobot/Shutterstock

11-4 Recognition is a positive motivator, especially in business teams.

When selecting a committee, make sure the members understand the committee's purpose and their duties. The leader of a committee is called a *chairperson*, or the chair. Everyone on a committee can express his or her opinions and help make decisions. Committee chairs give reports about their committees' progress at full group meetings. A meeting's **agenda**, or outline of items to consider or do, includes committee reports as an order of business.

Solve Problems

No group is without problems and challenges. For instance, your group may have trouble completing a project on time. In this case, ask the group for their suggestions about different ways to complete the project. Do not make all the decisions yourself. Group members want to be part of the solution to a problem.

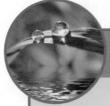

Go Green

Green Committees

A growing number of businesses have *Green Committees*. They consist of dedicated employees who volunteer to make their companies more sustainable. Often, the recommendations coming from an office's Green Committee become policy followed by the entire company. Every business is different, so Green Committees face different challenges and issues to increase environmentally friendly business practices. The recycling of recyclable products may seem an obvious solution. Some Green Committees, however, spend much time just getting basic green practices put in effect.

For instance, businesses such as architecture and design firms and book publishers use a tremendous amount of paper. Their Green Committees might suggest numerous ways to decrease paper consumption. Such policies could include always using the double-sided printing option, never printing e-mails, or turning scrap paper into notepads. There are many other environmental business practices to utilize. If you work at a business with a Green Committee, consider joining it to make a difference.

The decision-making process helps solve group problems. Suppose you are the chair of your school's dance committee. You learn that the band the committee wanted for the homecoming dance is already booked that night. As a leader, help the group list alternatives. One group member might suggest another band. Another might think a DJ is a better option. The committee discusses each option and chooses the best alternative, which most likely includes a vote. Each member should have the opportunity to make his or her opinion count.

Some issues may concern only a few group members. Perhaps several members disagree on an issue and this prevents them from getting along. Address such problems as soon as possible so the entire group is not affected. In this situation, only discuss the issue with those concerned. Ask for their ideas about how to resolve the issue so it does not negatively affect the group. Then make sure the parties honor their agreements.

Encourage Cooperation

Cooperation means working together as a team to reach your goals. As a leader, set a good example to encourage cooperation among group members. Help members accomplish their tasks whenever you can. Do not sit back, boss around other people, and wait for others to do the work. You cannot expect group members to cooperate with one another if you cannot cooperate with them.

Many people do not cooperate with a leader who orders others around. Build group members' confidence by saying, "I know I can depend on you." You will get a better result than if you say, "Do it this way." Keep your members involved by making them feel needed and important. If a member has a new idea, be willing to try it, **11-5**.

Manage Group Resources

In addition to funds, a group's resources include the ideas, talents, and skills of the members. Each person brings a unique skill set to the group. To manage these resources effectively, match tasks to the members' skills. Avoid discouragement by ensuring projects and activities can be done easily.

You may need to guide the group to make the best use of the resources. Some members try to dominate a group or insist they serve on every committee. Remind these people to give others a chance to get involved. Other group members may be shy and hesitate to volunteer. Encourage these people to help with an activity or serve on a committee they would enjoy.

Opportunities for Leadership

Take advantage of leadership opportunities now to develop your leadership skills. Teen leaders are needed in a wide range of groups at school and in the community. Become active in organizations and clubs that interest you. Attend meetings and participate in activities. Volunteer to serve on committees, and let the group know you want to be considered for leadership roles.

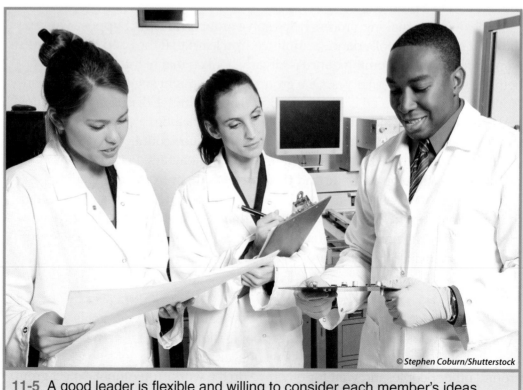

© Stephen Coburn/Shutterstock

11-5 A good leader is flexible and willing to consider each member's ideas.

Leadership Opportunities at School

Your school may have career and technical student organizations (CTSOs). CTSOs help students develop leadership skills and prepare to work in certain jobs. Most schools offer CTSOs in a number of areas.

FCCLA

The only CTSO with family as its primary focus is Family, Career, and Community Leaders of America (FCCLA). FCCLA helps young people become leaders at home and in the community through a variety of programs. Members learn skills, such as planning, goal setting, problem solving, and decision making.

Leadership opportunities are available at local, district, state, and national levels. Members can attend meetings at each of these levels. At the meetings, members visit exciting places, meet new people, and hear motivational speakers.

FCCLA also gives students the opportunity to compete in STAR Events. STAR stands for *Students Taking Action with Recognition*, **11-6**. Participants are judged against a set of criteria that stresses teamwork and personal development.

Other Organizations

There are many ways to become a leader in school. You could become active in the student government, which provides excellent leadership experience. Consider running for a class officer position or become a member of the student council.

Maybe you are in a club or on a team at school, **11-7**. You can practice leadership skills in these types of groups, too. You can be a leader when you work on group projects or on committees at school. You can also be a

---

FCCLA STAR Events

- Advocacy
- Applied Technology
- Career Investigation
- Chapter Service Project
- Chapter Showcase Display
- Culinary Arts
- Early Childhood
- Entrepreneurship
- Environmental Ambassador
- Fashion Construction
- Fashion Design
- Focus on Children
- Good Innovations
- Hospitality, Tourism, and Recreation
- Illustrated Talk
- Interior Design
- Interpersonal Communications
- Job Interview
- Leadership
- Life Event Planning
- National Programs in Action
- Nutrition and Wellness
- Parliamentary Procedure
- Promote and Publicize FCCLA!
- Recycle and Redesign
- Teach and Train

11-6 STAR competition includes individual and team events in many areas of leadership, social issues, and community service.

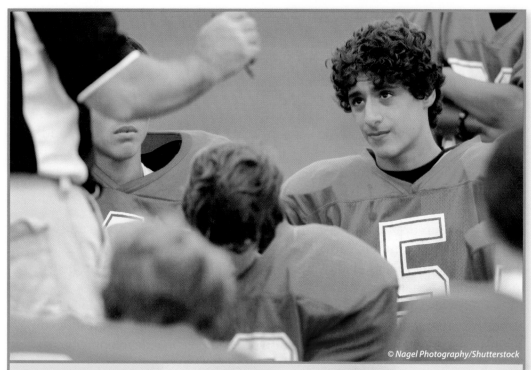

© Nagel Photography/Shutterstock

11-7 How you and your team handle both victory and defeat is on display for everyone to see. Take a leadership role and handle them both positively.

leader by identifying something that needs to be done in your school and then volunteering to do it. What ways can you think of to practice your leadership skills in school?

Leadership Opportunities Outside School

Scout troops and other youth groups, such as 4-H, offer leadership opportunities. In addition, they encourage community service work. These organizations offer many chances to be a leader.

A religious organization is another good place to take a leadership role. Becoming involved in a youth group is a good way to start. Adult leaders value good ideas and the opinions of highly involved teens. Recognized youth leaders can serve on certain adult committees in some religious organizations.

Teamwork

In any team or group, the number of members is always larger than the number of leaders. Group members are just as important to a successful group as the leader. Teamwork is the effort of a group of people acting together to do something or to reach a goal. In the workplace, people working in the same department consider themselves a team. The work they do jointly and alone contributes to reaching their department's goals. This leads to the company's overall success.

Groups need team members to fill many important roles and responsibilities. Team members need to actively listen and participate during group meetings. They need to analyze ideas and information presented. Team members also need to be able to brainstorm new ideas, **11-8**. They need to evaluate results of decisions. Effective group members complete their assignments and stay focused on the goal.

Like leaders, a team needs a positive attitude. Group members must **cooperate**, which means work well with others. When people work together, their single accomplishments become part of a larger effort. Team members need to be respectful of others' ideas. They also need to be receptive to new ideas.

Being a member of a group can help develop both your decision-making and problem-solving skills. Effective team members help make good decisions. They make suggestions about how to overcome challenges and solve group problems.

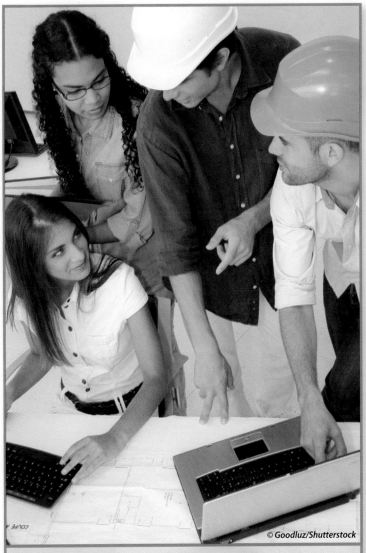

© Goodluz/Shutterstock

11-8 Leaders appreciate good suggestions from their team members.

Reading Review

1. How can developing leadership skills during the teen years help people as adults?
2. Give examples of five people who are considered good leaders.
3. List four leadership opportunities teens have in school.
4. What are three characteristics of effective team members?

Being a Successful Employee

Objectives

After studying this section, you will be able to
* **summarize** the qualities of a good employee.
* **recognize and evaluate** a person's work ethic.

Key Terms		
dependable	trustworthy	work ethic
punctual	tactful	

When your employer pays you to do a job, he or she expects it to be done to a certain standard. Otherwise, someone more capable will be hired. Think about the job as if you were the owner of the company. How effectively and efficiently do you want your employees to work? What qualities do you want them to have?

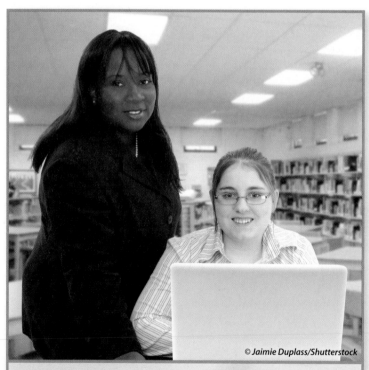
© Jaimie Duplass/Shutterstock

11-9 Teachers, just like employers, appreciate all your good qualities and work habits in school that will make you successful throughout your life.

Qualities of a Good Employee

As a student, you are much like an employee. Your schoolwork is the job and your teacher is your boss. The qualities of a good employee are very similar to the qualities of a good student.

Consider your work habits at school. Do you use time wisely or waste it? Can you finish a task without parents or teachers closely supervising you? Are you dependable and reliable? Can you make a schedule for what you need to do and follow it? Are you on time for your classes? Do you have a good attendance record? The answers to these questions tell you if you have the qualities of a good employee, **11-9**.

Works Well with Others

Good workers cooperate with their bosses and coworkers. They are flexible enough to realize that all people are different and have different ideas. They are willing to try new ways of doing things. Cooperative employees do not always expect to get their own way. They are willing to work for the good of the overall group.

In school, if you follow directions, study, and do your work, you cooperate with your teachers. If you do your share of the work on a group project, you cooperate with your classmates.

Hard Working

You do not have to be the smartest employee to get ahead in a career. Most people succeed by being willing to learn and working hard to do their best. In school, put the time and effort needed into every school assignment. This includes your favorite and least-favorite classes. Try to be neat and make as few errors as possible. If you follow these guidelines, you will be doing your best in school.

In your family, be willing to help with chores around the house. Keep your room neat and clean. Help with the shopping and take your turn preparing meals. Doing assigned tasks shows you are hard working and dedicated. Employers value an employee's willingness to work hard.

Dependable

Employees are more likely to succeed when they are **dependable**, or trusted to do or provide what is needed. Your boss depends on you to get your work done correctly and on time. Do not take a lot of breaks or do activities at work that are unrelated to your job. Complete your own work and do not expect others to do it for you. When you are on time to your classes, you are **punctual**. Punctual students are likely to be punctual employees with good attendance records.

Before you are hired, most employers want to know your background. What you have done in the past is a good indication of what you will do in the future. Make sure your references can say you are dependable and reliable.

You exhibit dependability through your daily living. You are dependable at school when you complete your assignments on time. Your parents know you are dependable when you arrive home at the time you said you would.

Honest

Trustworthy people are honest. Honesty is an important quality for every employee. Employers want to know that you are truthful and will not steal, **11-10**. People feel comfortable trusting you with money and materials when they know you are an honest person.

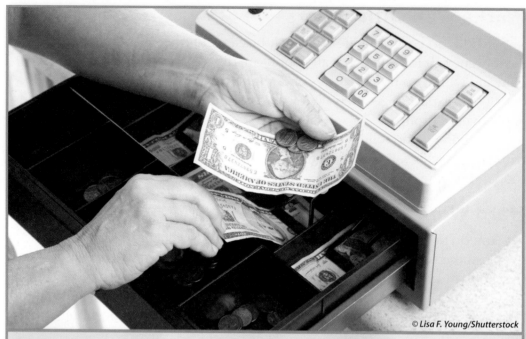

© Lisa F. Young/Shutterstock

11-10 Cashiers must be trusted with the money in the cash register by their employers.

Honest students become honest employees. Avoid cheating on tests or other schoolwork and you have a greater sense of achievement. Honesty helps you enjoy this same success on the job.

Positive Attitude

Everyone prefers to be around people with positive attitudes because they make others feel positive, too. This is particularly true in the workplace. When you spend eight or more hours around the same people daily, unpleasant coworkers can make a job unbearable. People with negative attitudes are rarely rewarded.

Positive people are enthusiastic and confident. Employees who enjoy their work perform better than those who do not care—and it shows. Whatever your job, you can learn to care about it and develop enthusiasm for it. Self-confidence is critical to developing a positive attitude. When you know you can do a job well, you are more likely to be enthusiastic about it.

Make a conscious effort to be positive. Begin by complimenting people about their ideas and good performance at school. Also, avoid complaining and arguing. Having a positive attitude can help you achieve success at work and in all areas of life.

Respect Others

Most successful employees understand it is important to respect others. Respect involves simple common courtesy. It means staying within certain boundaries and following the directions you are given. It also means knowing the rights of your coworkers.

The respect you owe your boss is much the same as the respect you owe your teachers. They are to be respected for their experience, knowledge, and assistance.

You need to respect the people who make the rules even when you do not agree with them. This may be frustrating at times, but respect is essential. Doing the opposite of what your teacher or boss asks you to do would be disrespectful. It could also lead to your dismissal.

Coworkers and customers deserve your respect in the workplace, too. When you show respect for your coworkers, they will enjoy working with you. When you show respect for customers, they will want you to serve them again in the future.

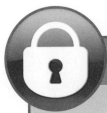

Safety Connections

Sexual Harassment

Sexual harassment includes unwelcome sexual comments, gestures, advances, and requests for sexual favors. Certain remarks about a person's body is one example. Sexual harassment interferes with your ability to feel safe and do your best. It can even make going to work or school frightening and unpleasant.

Sexual harassment is a serious issue, and is also against the law. If it happens to you, firmly tell the person making you uncomfortable to stop. If the person continues, ask for help from someone you trust. Talk to a parent, teacher, or guidance counselor. If it happens in the workplace, explain the situation to your boss and ask for help ending it. Always keep a written record of what happens.

Can Learn from Criticism

You may receive criticism from your boss, your coworkers, and customers. Criticism is not always negative, though it is often perceived that way. Constructive criticism is information given by someone to help you improve your work or learn new tasks. Understanding the true nature of criticism makes learning from it easier.

After receiving any criticism, make sure you fully understand it and the changes you are expected to make in your work. Do not become defensive or blame others because this reflects poorly on you. Ask questions if you need something clarified. Then let your employer know the steps you are taking to improve. If you need any help along the way, ask for it.

Knowing how to give criticism kindly is also helpful in the workplace. For instance, you may need to help an employee learn a new job. Be **tactful**, or careful not to offend or upset other people, when instructing others or giving criticism. You want your comments to help your coworker do a better job. You do not want to hurt his or her feelings. Say something positive before you explain how he or she needs to improve.

Well Groomed

Well-groomed workers look more professional, **11-11**. They have a high standard of personal cleanliness and wear neat, clean clothes suitable for the job. For instance, working in an office requires different clothing from assisting at a day camp. Casual workout clothes are not suitable for office work. Those clothes might be fine for the day camp job, however.

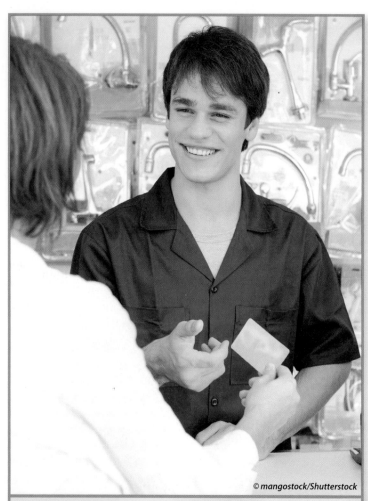

© mangostock/Shutterstock

11-11 You do not have to wear fancy or expensive clothes to be well groomed and appear professional at work.

Being well groomed also helps you feel better about yourself. Successful employees choose to look and act their best to represent their companies in a positive manner.

Work Ethic

A **work ethic** is a person's belief about work based on his or her values. Not everyone has the same work ethic. Some people think simply showing up and doing the minimal amount of work is acceptable. Others believe that always doing the best job you can is extremely important. Someone who comes to work on time and is prepared to do the job has a positive work ethic. Someone who takes frequent breaks, misses more days than allowed, or is unreliable may have a negative work ethic.

A good work ethic is an asset in not only the workplace, but in every situation where you are expected to perform tasks. People who are consistently willing to do what is asked (and more) are likely to be rewarded and promoted.

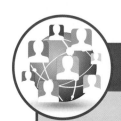

Social Studies Connections

Workplace Discrimination

All employees have rights protected by the government. Employers cannot *discriminate*, or unfairly treat a person or groups of people differently from others. The following laws address specific employee groups that have been discriminated against in the past:

- The *Equal Pay Act of 1963* protects men and women performing equal work from sex-based wage discrimination.
- *Civil Rights Act of 1964* prohibits employment discrimination based on race, color, religion, sex, or national origin.
- The *Age Discrimination in Employment Act of 1967* protects individuals who are 40 years of age or older.
- The amended *Americans with Disabilities Act of 1990* prohibits employment discrimination against qualified individuals with disabilities in the private sector and government positions.

Your employer wants to know they are paying you for being an efficient employee working to the best of your abilities. This is true even if the job is something you do not particularly like. If you really dislike the work, you should consider doing something else. Otherwise, you may do substandard work and lose your job.

Leaving a Job

When you choose to leave a job, do so in a professional manner. It is standard practice to give your employer at least two week's notice of your last day, **11-12**. Make sure you leave on a positive note. You want to use your employer as a good reference and include the experience on your résumé. Put your resignation in writing and thank your employer for the opportunity to work with the company. Even if you did not enjoy the work, you still gained valuable experience in the workplace.

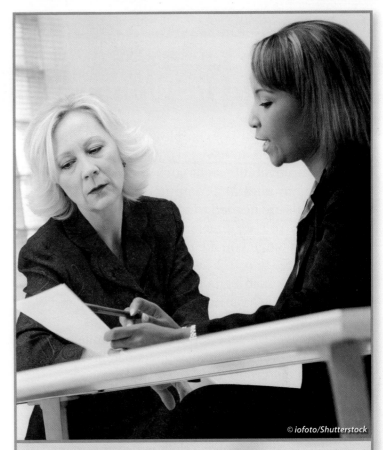

© iofoto/Shutterstock

11-12 Giving at least a two-week notice before leaving a job gives the employer a chance to hire someone to fill your position.

Reading Review

1. How can you show you are a dependable person at school?
2. Name five qualities of a good employee.
3. Give two guidelines for providing helpful criticism to a fellow employee.
4. Why is a good work ethic a valuable asset to have in life?

Chapter Summary

Section 11-1. Employers want their employees to have certain job skills. Employability skills such as academic, communication, computer, and thinking skills are needed to some extent in most jobs. You are developing all these skills now while you are in school.

Section 11-2. Learning how to lead and work in a group is important to your success in a career, as well as in a family and your community. Leaders must set goals, motivate members, work with committees, solve problems, encourage cooperation, and manage group resources. Team members are expected to complete their assignments, stay focused on the group goals, and be cooperative. Having good decision-making and problem-solving skills is also important for an effective group member.

Section 11-3. Many of these are the same qualities you need to succeed in school are also valued in the workplace. Employers want people who work well with others, are hard working, cooperative, dependable, and honest. They also want positive, well-groomed workers who respect others and can learn from constructive criticism. A good work ethic is also important for success in any field. When you choose to leave a job, do so professionally and give your employer at least two week's notice.

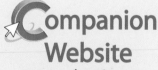

Companion Website
www.g-wlearning.com

Check your understanding of the main concepts for Chapter 11 at the website.

Critical Thinking

1. **Discuss.** In small groups, hold a discussion about why critical thinking skills are necessary for success in a career. How do employers recognize employees with outstanding critical thinking skills? Discuss how you can develop these skills now.

2. **Propose.** As a leader, what would you do to motivate group members who are doing their fair share?

3. **Summarize.** Interview an adult who is a leader. Consider talking to the president of a civic group or a school PTA, a sports coach, or a religious leader. Ask this person what skills they think a good leader should have. Report your findings to the class.

Common Core

College and Career Readiness

4. **Speaking and listening.** Choose a TV program or movie featuring characters struggling with their communication skills. Determine the communication problems and how they affect the characters' relationships at home or work. Decide how the problems could be best solved. Give a short report to the class citing specific examples.

5. **Writing.** Write a one-page paper about a leadership problem you have witnessed. It may be something you personally experienced as either a group leader or a member. It could also be a larger, current issue that is being discussed in the news. Use the problem-solving method to find solutions and then choose the one you think is best. Explain why.

6. **Math.** Assume you are the leader of a committee formed to manage distributing bake sale proceeds of $1,000 to four charities. The amounts going to each one are to be determined by your committee. It has already been decided that some charities are more deserving than others. How would you lead your committee to decide the amounts to give to each charity? Show your work.

7. **Speaking.** Break into groups. Develop role-plays in which an employee's behavior indicates a poor work ethic. Then role-play a situation that shows an employee has a good work ethic. What are the differences? Do you think they are visible to the employer?

Technology

8. **Online research.** Choose a leader you admire from history. Conduct research online to determine which qualities this person possessed that made him or her a great leader. Write a short report about the person's leadership qualities and how they contributed to the important decisions he or she made.

Journal Writing

9. Write a journal entry about the kind of employee you envision yourself to be in ten years. What career did you choose and what do you think are your boss's expectations? Did your work ethic in school influence your success in your chosen career? If so, how?

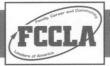

FCCLA

10. Learning to use parliamentary procedure takes training and practice. Volunteer to lead a meeting for your FCCLA chapter (or other student organization in your school) in learning how to conduct a successful meeting through parliamentary procedure. This is an orderly system of conducting business that protects the rights of group members.
    - Discuss the impact of following or not following this procedure on the effectiveness of an organization. How might failure to use parliamentary procedure impact decision making?
    - Use the information in the *FCCLA Chapter Handbook* to guide your training. See your adviser for information as needed.
    - After you gain confidence in using parliamentary procedure, have your adviser or an officer from a community group evaluate your ability to conduct a business meeting.

Unit 4
Understanding Children and Parenting

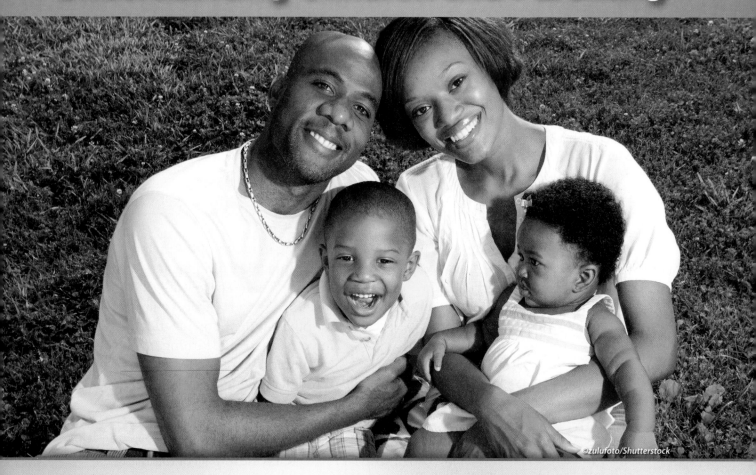

©zulufoto/Shutterstock

Chapter 12   Taking Care of Children
Chapter 13   The Business of Babysitting
Chapter 14   Parenting

Unit Essential Question

How can understanding the development and care of children enhance the quality of life for all people?

Exploring Career Pathways

Child Care and Education Careers

People who educate and care for children have great passion for nurturing and seeing children grow and develop. Here is a possible career path some may find rewarding.

Child Care Worker

Child care workers are warm and nurturing. They perform a combination of basic child care and some teaching duties. Many child care workers care for children in their homes, which are generally licensed through a state agency. In a preschool or child care facility (also regulated by a state agency), they may assist the preschool teacher with educational activities. Some workers are nannies who provide care and nurturing activities in the child's home. At a minimum, child care workers need a high school diploma. Some have a Child Development Associate (CDA) credential. Child care workers should be mature, enthusiastic, and capable of communicating well with children and parents. They must anticipate and prevent problems and know how to deal effectively with disruptions.

Preschool Teacher

Preschool teachers work with children ages three to five. They are responsible for using curriculum that enhances children's physical, intellectual, social, and emotional development. Preschool teachers introduce children to reading and writing, creative arts, social studies, and science. They use music, games, art, videos, books, computers, and other tools to teach concepts and skills. The minimum requirement for working as a preschool teacher is a CDA credential or an associate's degree. Preschool teachers are organized, dependable, patient, and creative. They communicate effectively with children, parents, and staff.

Preschool Administrator

Preschool administrators are responsible for the successful operation of preschools. They manage day-to-day activities, train staff, monitor children's progress, and maintain record keeping. Preschool administrators, often called *directors*, must have at least a bachelor's degree. Their diverse skills include strong interpersonal skills, financial competency, creative ability in motivating others, and effective organizational skills.

Is this career path for you? Pursue one or both of the following activities to determine if you are suitable for a career in child care and education.

- Select a child care and education activity that interests you. Make arrangements for a job shadowing experience with someone in your community who works in this career. While shadowing, note the foundational workplace skills, education, and training required for performing this job.
- One of the best ways to learn about a career is through firsthand experience. Consider volunteering regularly at a child care facility, preschool, or family child care provider's home.

Chapter 12
Taking Care of Children

Sections

Reading Prep

College and Career Readiness

Predict what you think will be covered in this chapter. Make a list of your predictions. After reading the chapter, decide if your predictions were correct.

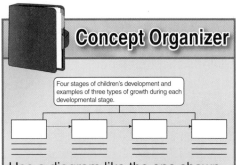

Concept Organizer

Four stages of children's development and examples of three types of growth during each developmental stage.

Use a diagram like the one shown to list the four stages of children's development. Under each stage, give one example of each of the three types of growth for the developmental stages.

Companion Website

Print out the concept organizer for Chapter 12 at the website.

Companion Website
www.g-wlearning.com

© S. Borisov/Shutterstock

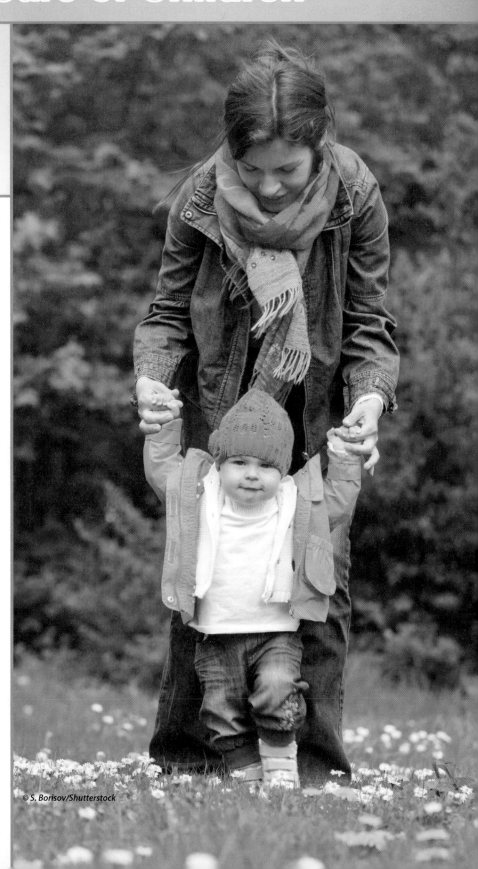

Section 12-1

Child Growth and Development

Objectives

After studying this section, you will be able to

- **summarize** the four types of development.
- **explain** why early brain development is the most critical period in human development.
- **describe** the characteristics of a newborn.
- **describe** the physical, intellectual, social, and emotional development of infants.
- **describe** the physical, intellectual, social, and emotional development of toddlers.
- **describe** the physical, intellectual, social, and emotional development of preschoolers.

Key Terms

physical development	early brain	infant
intellectual	development	babbling
development	newborn	toddlers
social development	reflexes	preschoolers
emotional		
development		

Understanding and getting along with children is important for many reasons. You may have younger relatives with whom you spend time. You may be interested in babysitting. Even if you do not plan to be around children much, you can learn more about yourself by studying children.

Children grow and change very quickly. Just six months can make a big difference in what a child can do and think. At eight months, a baby may be starting to crawl. A couple of months later, the same child may be walking. To help understand how children differ, this chapter will present three main age groups. These are infants, toddlers, and preschoolers. While studying each group, you will learn how they grow and develop and how to care for them.

How Children Grow and Develop

Growth and development take place in all children all the time. You may not notice the changes, but they are always taking place. The four different types of growth and development are physical, intellectual, social, and emotional, **12-1**.

Physical development is the growth or change in body size and ability. It includes growth of bones, muscles, and internal organs. Growing taller, gaining weight, and building stronger muscles are types of physical development you can see. As children gain coordination, physical development is also visible. Other physical changes are not as easy to see, such as the maturing of internal organs. For instance, as the stomach matures, foods digest more easily. As the heart and lungs mature, children can run longer without tiring.

Intellectual development refers to the development of the mind. It involves the ability to think, reason, use language, and form ideas. Children of all ages use their senses to learn about the world. They smell, listen to, look at, taste, and feel different objects and persons as they increase their intellectual growth and development.

Social development involves learning to communicate and get along with others. Part of this involves learning to adapt to new people. Social development also includes learning and following rules. For instance, children learn quickly that it is wrong to hit other children.

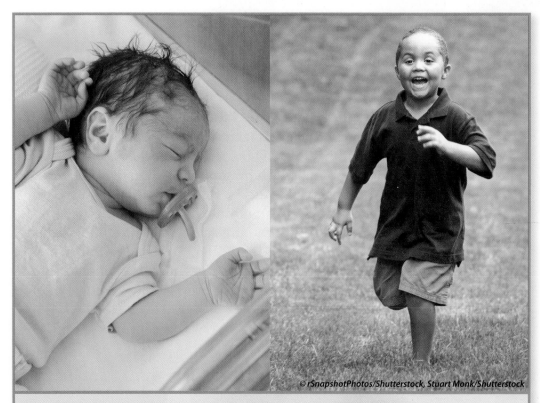

© rSnapshotPhotos/Shutterstock, Stuart Monk/Shutterstock

12-1 From birth to five years of age, the physical, intellectual, social, and emotional development of infants is dramatic.

Emotional development is the way in which a person develops and expresses emotions. Such emotions include love, happiness, fear, and anger. Emotional development involves learning to recognize and accept these emotions. It also involves finding ways to express emotions that other people accept. For instance, very young children may express anger through a temper tantrum. As these children develop, they learn more acceptable ways to express their anger.

Each of these four types of development is dependent on *early brain development*. **Early brain development** is the most critical period of human development. It occurs from conception until around the third birthday. The first year is the most important for brain growth and development. Because the brain is not fully developed at birth, it is important to stimulate its growth by providing many different experiences. Positive experiences, such as the act of a parent cuddling his or her baby, are necessary to promote brain growth. During this time, children learn to do many things.

No two children develop in exactly the same way. Many factors affect children as they grow and develop. Such factors determine whether children will be ahead of or behind normal growth and development patterns for their age. Some factors relate to heredity and some to environment. For this reason, not all children may fit the norms of development this chapter addresses. The norms are simply guidelines for how many children typically develop at a certain age.

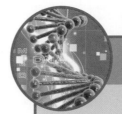

Science Connections

Windows of Opportunity

During early brain development, there are *windows of opportunity*, or limited time frames to develop critical skills. If these windows are missed, it is difficult for the child to develop these abilities at a later time. Following are five major developmental tasks and their approximate windows:
- *Vision.* Birth to six months.
- *Vocabulary/speech.* Birth to three months.
- *Emotional control.* Birth to three months.
- *Math/logic.* Birth to four years.
- *Small and large muscle development.* Birth to eight years.

It is crucial for caretakers to stimulate and encourage all types of development. Having interesting objects, lights, sounds, and people will aid in early brain development and help reach goals within these windows of opportunity.

Growth and Development

Infants grow and change quickly during the first year. If you do not see an infant for one month, when you see him or her again the changes will be amazing. **Newborn** describes the infant for the first month after birth.

Newborns

Have you ever seen a newborn? This baby may not have been as cute as you expected. He or she probably had wrinkled skin. Newborns often have colored marks on their skin. Their noses may be flat.

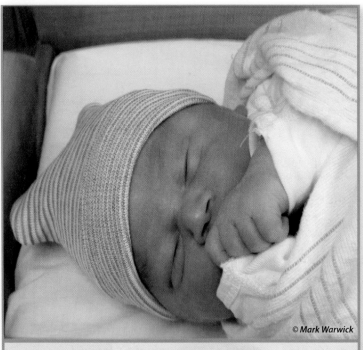

12-2 A newborn's appearance is different from that of an older infant.

Their eyes may be squinted and smoky in color. A newborn's head may look squashed, **12-2**.

In the first month, the newborn adapts to a whole new world. There are bright lights and loud noises. Newborns breathe and learn to eat to survive. Before birth, these issues were not problems for infants. The mother's body provided a safe, comfortable environment.

Newborns are born with many reflexes to help them survive. **Reflexes** are reactions that happen automatically. If you touch a newborn's cheek, the head turns toward your hand and the newborn begins sucking. This reflex helps the infant find food.

Physically, a newborn is quite different from an adult. A newborn has a short neck and sloping shoulders. The abdomen protrudes and the chest is narrow. The legs and arms have soft bones that do not yet support the body. Because of this, infant bones do not break as easily as adult bones. The infant's heart rate and breathing rate are faster than that of an adult.

Newborns respond to touch and warmth. Sometimes they stop crying if a person just picks them up. Newborns also respond to human voices. In fact, after a few weeks, they can detect their parents' voices from those of others. Newborns can see colors and shapes. They pay more attention to new objects than to old objects. These actions show that newborns are already learning about their world.

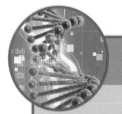

Science Connections

A Newborn's Senses

In many ways, newborns are helpless. Newborns, however, are much more aware of their surroundings than people once thought. Their eyes, ears, noses, skin, and tongues all function as sense organs from birth. In other words, they send information to the brain about how things look, sound, smell, feel, and taste. As a result, even newborns can begin developing intellectually, socially, and emotionally, as well as physically.

Infants

From the time a baby is born until he or she is twelve months old, a baby is called an **infant**. As infants grow, they change from almost full helplessness to having ability to move and communicate on their own.

Physical Growth

Infants grow very quickly. They grow one and one-half times in length and triple in weight from birth to the first year. Infant weights change so much because organs and muscles are growing. The heart, lungs, stomach, and muscles become bigger and stronger. The brain is developing a great deal, too.

Because organs are growing quickly, most of the infant's growth is in the abdomen. The head and abdomen look large in comparison to the rest of the body.

As muscles grow, infants can do more and more. At one month of age, infants try to hold their heads up. By two months, they can hold their heads up for a short time. As they lie on their stomachs, they usually can turn their heads from side to side.

By three months, infants have some control of the movements of their arms and legs. When lying on their stomachs, they can hold up their heads and chests by supporting themselves with their arms. Infants also have better control of the muscles in their hands at this age. They can grasp objects and often drop them.

Between six and nine months, babies can sit up without support. They begin *crawling*, or pulling themselves along with their arms while their abdomens stay on the floor. Eventually, infants begin to *creep* on their hands and knees by lifting their tummies and knees off the floor in an alternating motion. These infants can pull themselves to a standing position. They may walk along the edge of a support such as a sofa, or they may walk with the help of a person, **12-3**. Infants at this age can grasp small objects with their thumbs and forefingers. They can pick up objects and place them where they want with ease. Preference for the left or right hand may show by twelve months.

Intellectual Growth

Infants learn quickly about their world. At first, infants cry when they have needs. They may be hungry or require a diaper change. Infants soon learn that when they cry, someone picks them up. When they want someone near, they may begin to cry as a call. This is the infant's first form of communication. Between six and eight weeks, babies begin to coo, or make a light, happy noise. If you touch, talk to, or smile at an infant, the infant will coo in response.

By the fourth or fifth month, infants begin *babbling*. **Babbling** involves repeating a string of one-syllable sounds such as *da-da-da* or *be-be-be*. If you talk to

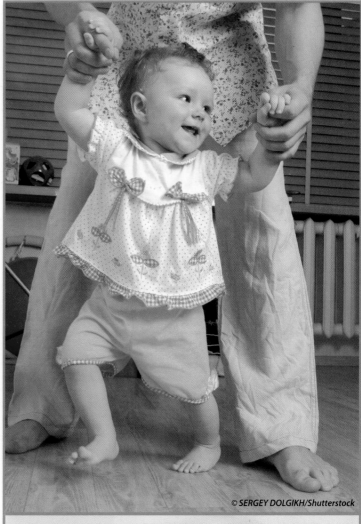

© SERGEY DOLGIKH/Shutterstock

12-3 Improved muscle strength and control allow older infants to walk with assistance.

the infant, he or she begins babbling in response. The infant may even imitate sounds you make.

As early as nine months, some infants may say simple words. Other infants may not begin to talk until after their first birthday. Remember, it is normal for the rate of development to differ for each child.

Besides learning language, infants learn about objects in their world. Learning about objects is the basis of science and math learning. Infants start to learn about object characteristics. Objects may be hard, soft, sticky, rough, or smooth. They come in different colors and shapes. Infants may explore objects by touching them, moving them, or even putting them in their mouths, **12-4**.

Social and Emotional Growth

Infants are born with certain personality traits. As infants build on their basic personalities, they grow socially and emotionally. Infants respond to the adults around them. They begin to form attachments to those who touch, feed, talk to, and play with them.

Learning to communicate is part of the infants' social development, too. For social development to begin, infants need to recognize that there are other people around them. Additionally, infants need to understand that they are separate people from their parents. This sense of self begins at five to seven months. Once infants understand the idea of *self*, they learn that others care for them. At this point, they can attach to others. Infants may form attachments to special objects as well as to people.

For infants to grow socially and emotionally, they need to develop a sense of trust. Trust grows when infants can depend on their parents or other adults to meet their needs.

Infants show emotions early in life. They show happiness through smiling, laughing, and cooing. They show anger by crying loudly and moving their arms and legs.

At about six months, infants begin to show love. They may do this through hugging, kissing, or following a person. Infants tend to feel love for their parents and others who spend much time around them. They do not seem to care much about strangers or children with whom they do not spend much time.

By the tenth or eleventh month, infants begin to show *separation anxiety*.

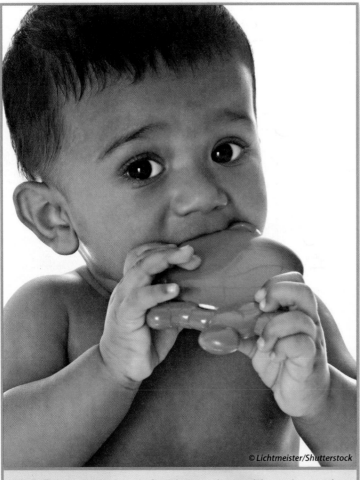

© Lichtmeister/Shutterstock

12-4 Because babies often learn about objects by putting them in their mouths, always keep babies' toys clean.

Infants may feel this anxiety because they fear caregivers who leave them will not return. They may cry or scream when a parent leaves the house or day care. Separation anxiety relates to attachment. Anxiety may also cause children to have more fear of strangers, or develop *stranger anxiety*.

Toddlers

As infants grow, they become more and more able to act on their own. Sometime after the first birthday, most children begin to walk. This marks the beginning of the toddler years. Children between the ages of one and three years are called **toddlers**. This is because their walk is so unsteady, especially when they first start walking, **12-5**.

Ability to get around more easily allows toddlers all kinds of new experiences. Each new experience helps toddlers grow and develop even more.

Physical Growth

Toddlers continue to grow taller and heavier. There are other physical changes, too. Their bones and muscles become much stronger. The spine becomes more erect. Toddlers also lose some of the baby fat they had as infants. All these changes make moving much easier for toddlers.

Children begin to walk at different ages. Some may start before their first birthday. Others may not walk until they are fifteen or sixteen months old. Neither case is abnormal. By the second birthday, most toddlers learn to run. At their third birthday, toddlers walk steady and upright.

Toddlers may start climbing sometime around their first birthday. They may climb furniture and steps. Toddlers typically learn to climb up more quickly than they learn to climb down. They also begin to operate wheel toys.

As toddlers gain more hand coordination, they are able to throw balls. They are not yet good at catching, however. They begin eating with a spoon and drinking from a cup, though they may miss their mouths at times. Toddlers can stack building blocks and put pegs in a Peg-Board™.

Intellectual Growth

Some toddlers begin to talk soon after their first birthdays. Others may take much more time. These words are usually one or two syllables. Toddlers may also have trouble pronouncing certain words, and may substitute their own sounds. As toddlers grow, their speech usually improves.

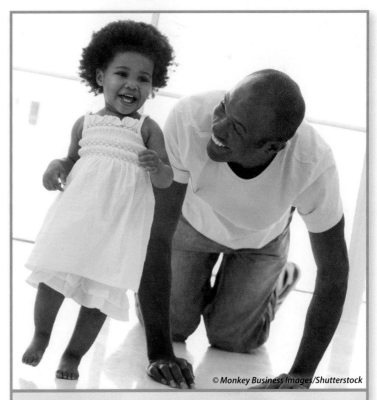
© Monkey Business Images/Shutterstock

12-5 Because a toddler's walk is unsteady, adults should be close by to help if needed.

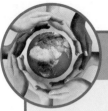

Global Connections

Language Learning

Across the globe, the process of learning a language is the same for all infants, regardless of language and culture. The language acquisition process begins at birth. Newborns are familiar with their caregiver's voice and show a preference for the language spoken. Within the first six months, even before infants' first words, they are able to distinguish the patterns of the language spoken in their environment and are aware when another language is spoken.

At the toddler stage, language learning continues through interaction with adults and other children. This person-to-person interaction is vital. Toddlers who spend time only watching television will have difficulties speaking the language. Regardless of location, all infants and toddlers need language encouragement and guidance.

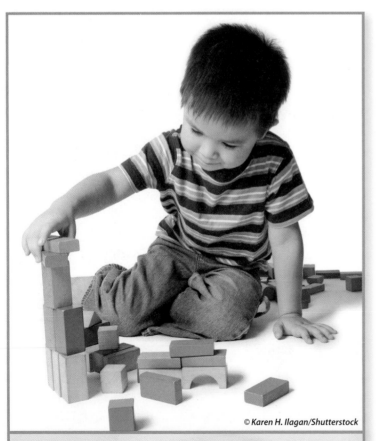

© Karen H. Ilagan/Shutterstock

12-6 Toddlers learn to use blocks for building instead of banging together as they develop.

Toddlers understand more words than they can say. They can point to their heads, feet, and toes when you ask them. They may not be able to say all these words, however. Toddlers learn to say words by listening and imitating what they hear. By eighteen months of age, many toddlers may use one- or two-word sentences. After the second birthday, toddlers may begin to use sentences with three or more words.

As toddlers learn more about how things work, they begin to apply what they know to meet a goal. For instance, the toddler may want a toy that is on a blanket. He or she may know that pulling a string attached to a toy makes the toy come closer. This may allow the toddler to realize that pulling on the blanket will bring the toy closer.

Toddlers also start to compare objects. For instance, toddlers can tell when two objects are the same color or different colors. They understand how round objects are similar because they can roll them. Understanding concepts about objects helps toddlers make sense of the world around them, **12-6**.

Social and Emotional Growth

As with infants, toddlers care most about their parents and other close caregivers. Toddlers, however, begin to enjoy playing with other children their age. Improved language and physical skills make playing with other children more fun.

Toddlers are building stronger self-concepts. They are beginning to realize that they can make things happen. Toddlers are proud of their own accomplishments. These might include feeding or dressing themselves. Toddlers may also enjoy saying *no* to many things even when they do not mean no. These toddlers are learning that they can control what happens by saying a word.

As toddlers build their self-concepts, their emotions may be strong. They are happy and proud when they can do what they want. In contrast, toddlers get frustrated easily when they do not get their own way. Sometimes anger leads to temper tantrums. Toddlers will scream, cry, and jump around. In most situations, toddlers are not angry with any one person. Toddlers are just angry because things are not working the way they want them to.

Toddlers continue to love the people around them, and they need much love from others. If others do not show toddlers love, they begin to feel unwanted. If parents and caregivers show toddlers love even when they throw temper tantrums, they will be able to get past their angry stages. Toddlers become more confident and learn to accept themselves as they are.

Preschoolers

Preschoolers are children ages three, four, and five. As these children leave the toddler stage, they become more confident. Their physical, intellectual, social, and emotional changes prepare them to handle more tasks and responsibilities.

Physical Growth

As preschoolers grow, their arms and legs become longer in relationship to the trunk. Their proportions are more similar to those of an adult. Preschoolers look thinner than toddlers, but they are much stronger.

Stronger bodies help preschoolers run faster, climb higher, and jump farther than toddlers. As coordination improves, preschoolers learn new skills. They can hop, skip, and ride swings. They can also balance on one foot or balance while walking a line. Preschoolers become much better at throwing and catching. This is because they can bend and shift their weight more than toddlers can.

Hand muscles continue to improve. Preschoolers can feed themselves with forks and spoons. They are able to work large buttons, zippers, and laces. Five-year-olds may even be able to tie shoelaces. Preschoolers draw and color better than they did as toddlers. They can cut out shapes using scissors. Younger preschoolers can build towers from blocks, but the towers will most likely be crooked. Five-year-olds can build straight, high towers from blocks.

Intellectual Growth

Preschoolers are very eager learners. They ask many questions about the world around them. They also spend much time observing objects and actions, **12-7**.

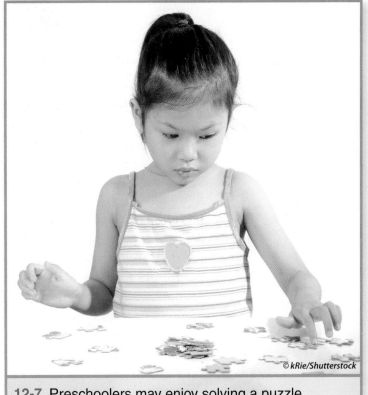
© kRie/Shutterstock

12-7 Preschoolers may enjoy solving a puzzle.

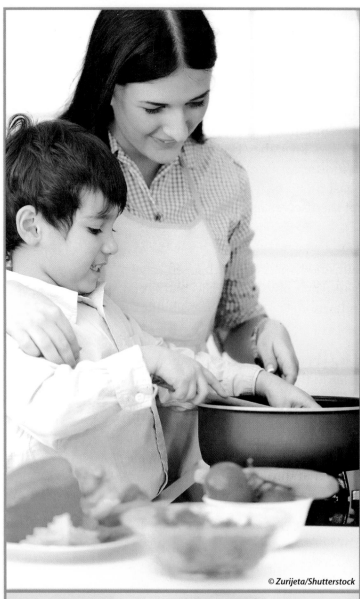

© Zurijeta/Shutterstock

12-8 Preschoolers are eager to help with tasks like helping in the kitchen.

Because they have longer attention spans than toddlers, preschoolers take the time to learn many new facts and solve new problems.

The language ability of preschoolers improves quickly. Besides learning new words, preschoolers begin to learn about grammar. They start to learn rules for making words plural or singular and speaking in past or present tense.

In the preschool years, children begin to use their imaginations. They may pretend to be other people, animals, or objects. They enjoy imagining they are in different places, such as in an airplane or a jungle. Sometimes preschoolers have trouble separating what is real from what is imaginary. The children may believe what they have dreamed really happened.

Preschoolers begin to grasp more abstract concepts than they could as toddlers. They begin to understand time concepts and start to understand amounts and numbers of objects. They also begin to comprehend ideas about space, such as *up*, *down*, *over*, and *under*. Because these ideas are new to preschoolers, though, they may become confused. For instance, they may say "My birthday was yesterday," even though the birthday was a week ago.

Social and Emotional Growth

As preschoolers leave the toddler years, they become eager to please adults. Because they can do more, they do not get as frustrated about an inability to do things. Preschoolers are proud to be helpful. They may want to help with household tasks such as setting the table or feeding a pet, **12-8**.

Preschoolers begin to spend more time with peers and away from parents. Unlike toddlers, preschoolers like to interact with other children as they play. Preschoolers may work together to build a castle out of blocks. These children are able to share and take turns. They accept adult rules when playing in a group.

Preschoolers control their emotions better than toddlers. This is partly because they can use language better. They can express frustrations and wants using words. They can understand spoken reasons when they cannot do something. Communication allows children to be more patient and cooperative.

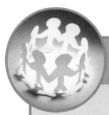

Life Connections

Preschoolers

Preschoolers require a lot of attention and interaction to stimulate their physical, intellectual, and social and emotional growth. All types of development are constantly being challenged. Preschoolers are surrounded by new ideas, concepts, and people. They need guidance in sorting and understanding the environment around them.

Science Activity

Try one of the following observation activity ideas to encourage a preschooler's intellectual development:

- *Alike and different.* Find pictures or objects that are exactly alike. Mix the objects together and ask preschoolers to sort the items into groups. This promotes observation skills.
- *Liquid comparison.* Gather liquids with differing colors, consistencies, and scents. Using an eyedropper, drop each type of liquid onto wax paper and have preschoolers compare the similarities and differences between liquids.
- *Shape sorting.* Find a *shape sorter*, which is a box with holes cut out at the top in the shape and size of wood blocks that accompany the box. Have preschoolers drop the wood shapes into the correct slot. Explain the shape names and ask the preschooler to describe shape differences during the experiment.

Reading Review

1. List four types of development.
2. Why are reflexes important to newborns?
3. How much do infants grow from birth to the first year?
4. What marks the beginning of the toddler years?
5. _____ are children ages three, four, and five.

Care Guidelines

Objectives

After studying this section, you will be able to
- **describe** how to safely hold a baby.
- **identify** differences in feeding infants, toddlers, and preschoolers.
- **explain** how to bathe infants, toddlers, and preschoolers.
- **explain** key guidelines for dressing infants, toddlers, and preschoolers.
- **describe** the importance of appropriate sleep and rest for young children.

Key Terms

formula	self-dressing	toilet learning
burping	features	

As children grow and develop, the amount and kind of care they require changes, too. As you care for children, you need to keep these differences in mind. Infants require a great deal of care. Caring for toddlers can present challenges. Because their skills are improving, toddlers like to try new activities. You may find caring for preschoolers much easier than caring for younger children. This is because preschoolers have more self-care ability and are eager to help you. Some care tasks may seem awkward or difficult for you at first. The following guidelines may help make these tasks a little easier. With practice, caring for children of any age will feel more natural to you.

Holding a Baby

When picking up a baby, you need to place your hands to support the head and back, **12-9**. Put one hand under the head and shoulders. Let your wrist and arm support the upper back. Place your other arm around the baby and slide the hand under the lower back. Pick up the baby slowly. Quick movements startle young babies. When startled, they may throw out their arms. This makes them more difficult to pick up and may cause them to cry.

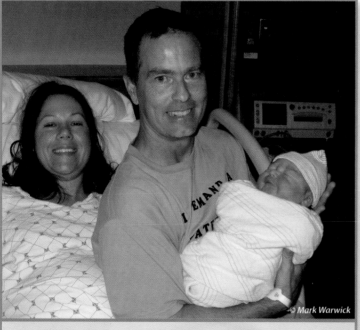

© Mark Warwick

12-9 When holding a baby, support the head and back.

Hold a baby securely, but not too tightly. You should not feel that you might drop the baby easily as you hold him or her. If you sit down, you can lower the baby onto your lap. Then you can remove the hand from under the lower back and move your other arm so that the baby's head and neck rest on it.

Feeding Children

Mealtime should be a calm, enjoyable experience for children of any age. As children get older, they want to be more involved in their meals. It is important for the caregiver to keep the child's level of physical growth in mind.

Feeding a Baby

When parents expect you to feed a baby, they should write detailed instructions for you. A parent may also go over the directions with you verbally. These instructions should tell you what, when, and how much to feed the infant. If you need to warm food, parents need to explain or write the directions for you. Parents should also prepare foods that require mixing ahead of time.

You may likely need to feed an infant a bottle of breast milk or *formula*. **Formula** is a special milk mixture designed to meet the nutritional needs of infants. Filled bottles are refrigerated. You will need to warm them according to the directions the parents leave for you. After warming the milk and before feeding the infant, test the temperature of the milk or formula. Do this by shaking a drop or two on the inside of your wrist. It should feel only slightly warm.

Hold the baby in a half-lying, half-sitting position for feeding. Cuddle the baby to give him or her feelings of security and love during feeding. As you feed, keep the bottle nipple full of milk so the baby will not suck too much air, **12-10**.

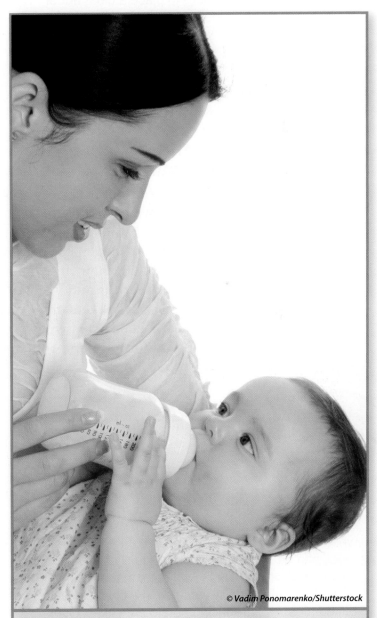

© Vadim Ponomarenko/Shutterstock

12-10 When feeding a baby, tilt the bottle so air does not reach the nipple.

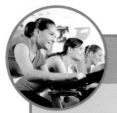

Health Connections

Burping a Baby

To burp a baby, move him or her to a sitting position on your lap. Lean the baby forward slightly and gently pat or rub the back. Be sure to support the baby's head and arms. Another way to burp is to hold the baby firmly against your shoulder. Let the baby look over your shoulder as you pat the back. After patting the baby a few times, you should hear a burp. With either method, be sure to place a cloth under the baby's face and mouth each time. A little milk or formula may come up with the burp.

No matter how careful you are, the baby will always swallow a little air with the milk. This air, or gas, can hurt the baby's stomach and cause the baby to fret or cry later. You can help the baby get rid of this air by burping. **Burping** involves gently patting or rubbing a baby's back to help expel excess air from feeding. Burp the baby at the midpoint and end of a feeding.

You may also need to spoon-feed a baby. Follow the adults' directions about what, when, and how much to feed. Use a small baby spoon and put only a little food on it each time. Babies are messy eaters. Their reflexes may cause them to push food out of their mouths after you feed it to them. Therefore, you should put a bib or feeding cape on the baby before feeding.

Mealtime for Toddlers

Toddlers are just learning to feed themselves. They enjoy the ability to eat on their own, but do not have very good eating skills.

If you are caring for a toddler, the child's parents should let you know what to feed him or her. You may need to get the food ready. When you feed a toddler, keep his or her level of coordination in mind. Most toddlers can eat with their fingers fairly well. They have more trouble with spoons. Raw fruits and vegetables cut into bite-size pieces are easy for toddlers to eat. Crackers and small pieces of bread are also easy for toddlers to eat. Foods eaten with a spoon, such as soup or applesauce, may be difficult for toddlers. Younger toddlers may give up and just try eating with their fingers.

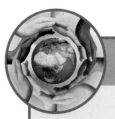

Global Connections

Cultural Foods

Introducing cultural foods to children is a good way to broaden their tastes and food experiences while promoting cultural awareness. Integrating new foods can be done subtly and gradually. Try matching the child's favorite dishes with ones that are similar from other cultures. For instance, if a child enjoys baked fries, try introducing potato pancakes. Over time, other types of dishes can be introduced, which will expand mealtime options.

Your attitude sets the tone for the meal. Be pleasant, understanding, and patient. When toddlers do a good job with self-feeding, give them some praise. For them, it is tough work learning to get the spoon to their mouths without spilling the food. Help with feeding if a toddler becomes too tired before finishing the meal.

Meals for Preschoolers

You can be more creative when feeding preschoolers than when feeding younger children. Although you still need to provide nutritious meals, you do not have to worry as much about safety or mess. As with meals for other children, follow any guidelines parents leave when you are caring for preschoolers. Preschoolers can feed themselves fairly skillfully. They may like to join in preparing foods, **12-11**. These factors can make mealtime more enjoyable and less frustrating for you.

By the time children reach the preschool years, they have some definite ideas about which foods they like and dislike. You can avoid problems by understanding a preschooler's tastes. Most preschoolers do not like foods with very strong flavors. Their taste buds are not ready to handle these foods. Spicy sauces and strong vegetables such as spinach are examples of strong foods. You can avoid problems with spicy foods by not adding many seasonings to foods. Also, serve stronger vegetables raw or slightly cooked. They tend to have a milder flavor than fully cooked or overcooked vegetables.

Most preschoolers will watch you while you eat. A preschooler takes cues about food preferences from parents and caregivers. If you refuse to eat tomatoes, a preschooler may do the same. It is important not to bias a child's perception of a food with your preference.

Keep mealtime conversation fun and happy. Praise preschoolers for good eating habits. When preschoolers feel they have pleased you, they often do the same thing again. In this way, you can help the child form good food choices.

Bath Time

Most parents do not leave bathing to babysitters, but you may need to bathe a child at some time. Understanding some basics will help you give the child a safe, comfortable bath.

Bathing a Baby

Newborns are usually given sponge baths. This is because their navels (where the umbilical cord was) have not yet fully healed. During the sponge bath, gently clean the baby with mild soap and water while the baby is lying on a towel. Begin with the head and work to the feet, washing the diaper area last.

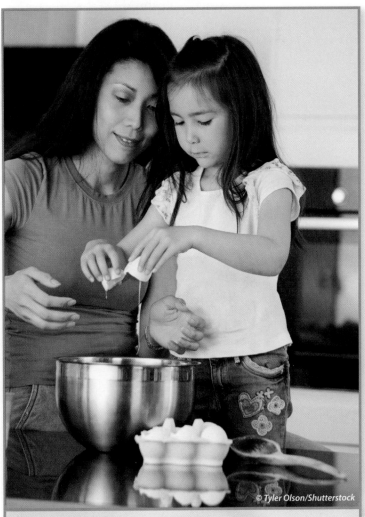

© Tyler Olson/Shutterstock

12-11 Preschoolers are able to help prepare simple food items.

After a few weeks, babies are ready for tub baths. When you give a tub bath, be sure to gather all your supplies before starting. This includes washcloth, towel, mild soap, clean clothes, and diapers. You may also use oil or lotion as a parent or caregiver instructs you. Remember that older infants can pick up small objects easily. You also know they like to learn about objects by putting them in their mouths. Therefore, if you are bathing an infant, do not keep cotton swabs or other small objects within the infant's reach. The infant could put such an object in his or her mouth and choke on it. *Never leave a baby alone in a tub.*

Bath Time for Toddlers

Most toddlers find bath time fun. They like to splash water and play with toys. Do not let the playing fool you. Helping toddlers with bath time is a serious responsibility.

If toddlers try to stand or walk in a bathtub, they can slip and hurt themselves. For this reason, you need to stay with them the whole time they are in the tub. You can use a smaller tub made for toddlers with a nonskid bottom. Even then, it is important to stay with the toddler.

When you fill the tub for toddlers, the water should only be a few inches deep. It should be warm, but not too hot. Help the toddler soap up and rinse off. Begin with the head and work down to the feet. Be careful when washing around the eyes, nose, and mouth. Getting soap in these areas may bother the toddler. During the bath, allow time and toys for play. Toddlers like toys that float and toys that squirt water, **12-12**. When you play with toddlers as you bathe them, they learn more about water and safety.

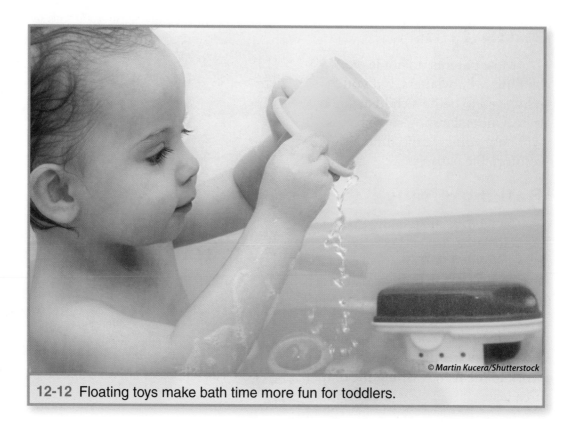

© Martin Kucera/Shutterstock

12-12 Floating toys make bath time more fun for toddlers.

Bath Time for Preschoolers

Preschoolers require less help to bathe themselves than toddlers, but may still need some assistance such as with hair washing. You should still stay nearby to keep an eye on the child's safety and remind the preschooler to wash certain spots such as the neck and ears.

Some preschoolers may not want to take a bath. To avoid problems, let the preschooler know about bath time 15 minutes in advance. The child can use that time to finish what he or she is doing.

Dressing Children

Children's clothing should be practical, safe, and washable. As children grow, they may want to express themselves through their clothing choices. The amount of help children need from you changes as they grow.

Clothing a Baby

Safety and comfort are major concerns in clothing infants. Stretchy, one-piece outfits are popular for these reasons. Check clothes for loose buttons, thread, or other items before putting an outfit on an infant. The infant may pull off and swallow these items. Infants do not know to help when you are dressing them. Therefore, gently push the arms and legs through sleeves and pant legs when clothing infants.

Diapers are the most important articles of clothing for babies. A small baby needs seven to ten diapers a day. Do not leave wet diapers on a baby for long periods of time. Doing so can cause the baby to get a rash.

Families may choose to use cloth or disposable diapers. Changing diapers requires the same basic steps with either kind. First, place the baby on a flat, firm surface. Remove the soiled diaper while holding the child to prevent a fall. Next, clean and dry the baby's skin, always wiping from front to back. Finally, put on and fasten a fresh diaper. If using cloth diapers, most no longer require pinning. Simply place the folded diaper in a diaper wrap (outer covering) and fasten it with the hook-and-loop tape tabs, **12-13**. Before changing a diaper on your own, you may want to practice with guidance from an adult.

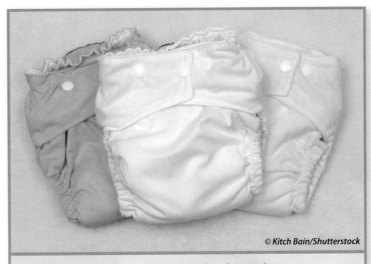

© Kitch Bain/Shutterstock

12-13 Cloth diapers have similar fastenings as disposable diapers.

Clothing a Toddler

Because toddlers move around so much, their clothes should fit comfortably. If clothes are too tight, movement is uncomfortable. Tight clothes can irritate the skin. If clothes are too loose, however, toddlers can trip over or get tangled in their clothes.

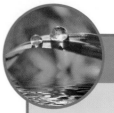

Go Green

Cloth Diapers

Although disposable diapers are convenient to use, cloth diapers are both environmentally friendly and financial savers. Each year, billions of disposable diapers are thrown away into landfills and require decades to decompose. Made of cotton, cloth diapers are washable and reusable and contain less resources and chemicals than disposable diapers. By using cloth diapers, caregivers can minimize the impact on the environment and financially save on the amount of expenses that diapers require.

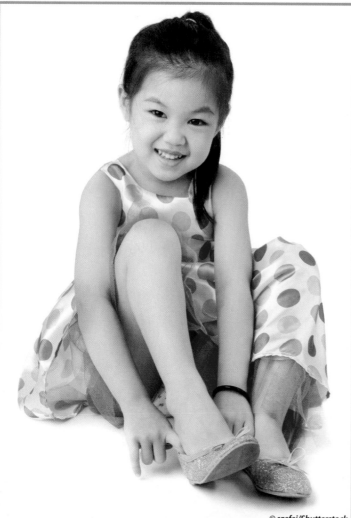

© szefei/Shutterstock

12-14 Young preschoolers may still need help with small buttons and zippers.

Toddlers develop likes and dislikes in clothes. They might like a certain color. You can help toddlers develop self-help skills by letting them choose between a few outfits.

As with eating, toddlers like to dress and undress as much as they can on their own. Many self-help skills are still a little beyond them. For instance, toddlers cannot yet tie shoes or button small buttons. You can make them feel good about their dressing skills by asking them to help you. Toddlers do not need as much help when they remove clothes.

Clothing Preschoolers

As preschoolers grow, they become more skillful in dressing themselves. Young preschoolers may still need much help, but older preschoolers may need hardly any help, **12-14**. These children may still make mistakes such as putting a sweater on backward or inside out.

You can help preschoolers by choosing clothes for them with self-dressing features. Self-dressing features are clothing characteristics that make dressing easier for children. They include zippers with large pull tabs and elastic waistbands. Designs that make it easy to tell the front from the back are also a self-dressing feature.

Preschoolers form stronger ideas about clothing likes and dislikes. Keep the preschooler's tastes in mind as you choose outfits for him or her. As with toddlers, let preschoolers make some of their own clothing choices.

Toilet Learning

For most children, *toilet learning* takes place during the toddler years. Toilet learning is the process by which children develop bladder and bowel control and successfully learn how and when to use the toilet. Once children finish this process, they do not need to wear diapers. Some children, however, may still need assistance with their toileting.

You may care for toddlers at different stages of independent toileting. In early stages, children may have many accidents. Children will feel bad about having an accident. You should help them clean up and change clothes without making a fuss. Some parents will put diapers on these children as a convenience to you. If these children tell you they need to use the bathroom, you should help them do so. If you do not, they may become confused about their toileting.

As toddlers grow older, they get better about letting you know when they need to use the toilet. They may need your help with their clothes. If a toddler asks for your help, go with him or her to the bathroom right away. These children have not gained much control over their elimination. Making them wait even a couple minutes could lead to an accident.

Even when children have finished toilet learning, they may need reminders. You might remind them shortly after a meal, before going outside to play, and just before bedtime or nap time. This will help children avoid embarrassing accidents.

Although preschoolers have mastered toileting fairly well, they may still have problems at night. Check with their parents about any bedwetting problems. Limit preschoolers' fluids just before bedtime and remind them to use the toilet before climbing into bed. Leave a light on in the bathroom so children can easily find the bathroom at night.

Sleep and Rest

Sleep is a need for good health and growth. During sleep, the body repairs tissue and makes cells. Sleep also helps you feel better. When you do not get enough sleep, you can feel tired, weak, and grumpy.

Infants

Lack of sleep can have the same effect on infants. Because infants are growing so quickly, they need much sleep, **12-15**. They spend more hours asleep than awake each day. Throughout the whole day, they may sleep a few hours and then wake up. Babies often cry as a call to an adult when they awaken. They may also be hungry or need a diaper change.

To get the baby to sleep throughout the night, parents may need to adjust the baby's daytime sleep. They may awaken the baby

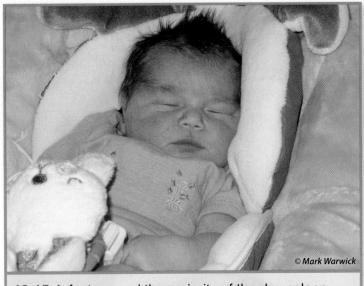

© Mark Warwick

12-15 Infants spend the majority of the day asleep.

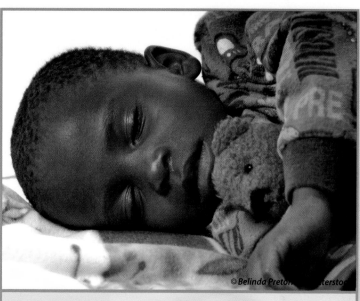

12-16 Toddlers need a sufficient amount of sleep each night.

after four hours of afternoon napping. If you are babysitting, the parent may ask you to awaken the baby by a certain time if the baby does not wake up on his or her own. Follow these directions to help parents avoid an unnecessary sleepless night.

Toddlers

Toddlers may need from 10 to 12 hours of sleep each night, **12-16**. They may also need an afternoon nap. The nap may last from one to three hours. In addition, younger toddlers may also take a short morning nap.

Naps should be at the same time every day, usually right after lunch. If a nap is too late in the afternoon, it could interfere with night sleep. Time for bed should be the same every night. When you are caring for a toddler, the parents should let you know times for naps or night sleep. Follow these times as closely as possible. Having a fixed sleep routine helps children know what to expect. Also, this consistency gives children a feeling of security.

Preschoolers

Preschoolers need about 10 hours of sleep each night. Most preschoolers still take a short afternoon nap, about an hour long.

Preschoolers are usually better than toddlers at accepting bedtime. They may still need quiet time before bed, however. Let them know when bedtime is coming. Help them relax by reading them a story or doing another quiet activity. Letting preschoolers sleep with a favorite toy can provide comfort when going to sleep.

Reading Review

1. Describe how to safely pick up a baby.
2. What is burping?
3. Why are newborns usually given sponge baths?
4. What are the most important considerations in children's clothing?
5. What is toilet learning?

Section 12-3

Safety and Health Concerns

Objectives

After studying this section, you will be able to
- **explain** how to avoid situations that might threaten a child's safety.
- **describe** how to help children stay healthy and how to care for them when they are sick.
- **identify** ways to help meet the special needs of children with disabilities and gifted children.

Key Terms		
childproofing	disability	gifted children

Children can be very active and curious. They often move from place to place as they explore. They may try to learn how objects are made and how they work. Children do not understand how they can be hurt or become sick. They may want to find out what happens when they put objects in their mouths. Children do not realize they can choke on some objects.

Caregivers need to help create an environment in which a child can be active and safe at the same time. If an accident happens, you may need to take some steps to treat an injury. Preventing children from becoming sick is another caregiver responsibility. You may also care for children who are sick or have special needs. Understanding more about children's safety and health gives you the tools to handle each of these situations in the best way possible.

Safety

As children grow and try new things, accidents are bound to happen. Scrapes and bruises seem to be a natural part of childhood. You cannot keep a child from harm all the time. In fact, minor bumps and falls are good learning experiences for children. These experiences help children learn they can be hurt. They start to see that they need to act safely.

Some accidents involving children can result in serious injury or death. They might include falls from high places, drownings, burns, or poisonings. These types of accidents are usually preventable, **12-17**. When you care for children, you are responsible for accident prevention. You need to know what types of accidents are likely to happen with young children. Alert yourself to unsafe situations and objects, and correct dangers before they result in accidents whenever possible.

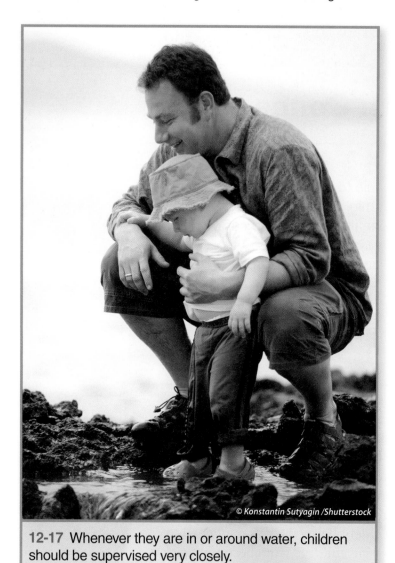

© Konstantin Sutyagin /Shutterstock

12-17 Whenever they are in or around water, children should be supervised very closely.

Childproofing a Home

Parents do much to make their homes safe for their children. They take steps to childproof their homes. **Childproofing** a home is making the home safe for children by keeping potential dangers away from them. It involves putting unsafe items where children cannot reach them. For children who can climb, putting items on a high shelf may not be enough. Place unsafe items behind locked doors. Other childproofing steps may involve preventing falls, bumps, and cuts. For instance, placing soft pads on sharp edges and corners of low tables can help prevent injuries like these. Childproofing also involves checking toys and clothes for child safety.

Poisons are a major danger to children. Many household items are poisonous. Because you know how to use these items safely, you may not think of them as dangers. For instance, using shaving lotion on your skin is harmless. If a small child drinks a full bottle of this lotion, however, a serious poisoning could result. Keep all poisonous products out of the reach of children. Figure **12-18** lists some of these products.

When you are caring for a child, you need to respect the childproofing measures the parents take. For instance, you may need to use a product such as a cleanser to remove a spot on the floor. As soon as you finish, return the cleanser to its storage place. Do not leave the cleanser on the floor or on a table the child can reach.

Changing Safety Needs

To prevent accidents, predicting what situations and objects might be dangerous for a child is important to safety. As children grow and develop, the types of dangers to them change. An open stairway is not a danger to a newborn because the baby cannot get to the stairs. Older infants and toddlers, however, are able to get to stairways. Because these children cannot yet climb up and down stairs well, the stairway is a danger. To protect these children, place a child safety gate at the top of a stairway.

Dangerous and Poisonous Home Products Checklist

Kitchen
- drain cleaners
- furniture polish
- oven cleaner
- dishwasher detergent
- cleansing and scouring powders
- metal cleaners
- ammonia
- rust remover
- carpet and upholstery cleaners
- bleach

Bathroom
- all drugs, medications, and vitamins
- shampoo
- hair dyes and permanent solutions
- hair spray
- creams and lotions
- nail polish and remover
- suntan lotion
- deodorant
- shaving lotion
- toilet bowl cleaner
- hair remover
- bath oil
- rubbing alcohol
- room deodorizer

Storage Areas
- rat poison
- insecticides
- mothballs

Bedroom
- all drugs, medications, and vitamins
- jewelry cleaner
- cosmetics
- perfumes and colognes
- aftershave

Laundry
- bleaches
- soaps and detergents
- disinfectants
- bluing and dyes
- dry cleaning fluids

Garage/Basement
- lye
- kerosene
- gasoline
- lighter fluid
- turpentine
- paint remover and thinner
- antifreeze
- paint
- weed killer
- fertilizer
- plant spray
- ice-melting products

General
- flaking paint
- repainted toys
- broken plaster
- plants

12-18 Many products that seem harmless to you can be dangerous to children.

When you care for a child, awareness of typical dangers for the child's age group is important. Then you can more effectively prevent accidents.

Safety for Infants

Babies do not have strong muscles, so they cannot control their movements well. This means you cannot leave them alone on any high places from where they might fall. Infants can get to the edges of sofas, beds, or tables by crawling or rolling. They cannot always catch themselves if they

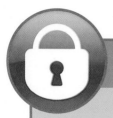

See Figure **12-19** for other steps for keeping infants safe.

Safety Connections

Bathing Infants

Infants do not understand that they cannot breathe under water. They can drown in a few inches of water. Therefore, you should never leave an infant alone in a tub of water. If you must leave the bathing area, carry the baby with you.

start to fall. The safest place to leave a baby alone is in a crib or playyard.

Infants put many objects in their mouths. If these objects are too small, infants may choke on them. Therefore, check for small objects in areas that infants can reach. Also, do not try to feed infants small foods such as nuts, popcorn, or hard candies. See Figure **12-19** for other steps for keeping infants safe.

Safety for Toddlers

Toddlers are adventurous, curious, fearless, and fast. They want to find out about objects and will try just about anything to get to them. This makes keeping items out of their reach a little tricky. You have to think more about what children might get into when they are toddlers than when they are infants. For instance, older toddlers may be able to reach pans on the cooktop to see what is in them. Keep handles turned to the center of the cooktop so toddlers do not spill hot food on themselves.

Encouraging Infant Safety

Safety Precautions	Hazards to Prevent
• **Support** infants when set in high places, such as a sofa or a dressing table.	• Infants rolling or crawling, resulting in a fall and injury.
• **Secure** infants in cribs, high chairs, or strollers by using side railings or safety straps.	• Infants climbing out of cribs, high chairs, or strollers, resulting in a fall or injury.
• **Supervise** and support infants in bathtubs.	• Infants lacking control of their own movements and drowning in a couple inches of water.
• **Block** infants from dangerous areas, such as stairs, storage rooms, or garages.	• Infants rolling or crawling, resulting in a fall and injury in an unprotected area.
• **Keep** small objects, such as paper clips, buttons, or hard candy away from infants.	• Infants putting small objects in their mouths and choking.
• **Check** the intended area before setting an infant down.	• Infants receiving injuries from objects that are in the way or left within reach.
• **Examine** all toys before giving them to an infant.	• Infants choking on small, detachable parts or injuring themselves on sharp edges or broken toys.
• **Carry** the child with you if interrupted while caring for the infant. Attend to infants at all times.	• Infants receiving injuries in a number of ways when left unattended.

12-19 When caring for infants, you must constantly watch for potential hazards.

Toddlers often try actions they cannot yet do. They may not be strong enough or coordinated enough. Therefore, you need to watch toddlers closely as they play and move around. For instance, a toddler may try to run downstairs as he or she has seen older children do. If the toddler loses concentration, he or she may trip or fall. This is why caregivers should escort toddlers up and down stairs. See Figure **12-20** for other safety tips.

Safety for Preschoolers

Preschoolers are more independent and able than toddlers. Their new abilities extend their areas of play. As they try new activities and explore new areas, they often take new risks. Because preschoolers can think and communicate fairly well, you need to help teach them to look out for their own safety.

Preschoolers do not need to be in your sight every second. They do need to let you know, however, what and where they are playing. Check on children often as they play. Be sure to remind children to play safely. If children are going outside, remind them to put on shoes to protect them from stepping on objects that may cut them.

Some play is more risky. You should watch children at all times when there is a higher chance of an accident happening. This includes playing in pools (even wading pools), near a busy street, or on large play equipment such as slides.

Encouraging Toddler Safety	
Safety Precautions	**Hazards to Prevent**
• **Select** a safe place for the toddler's high chair, such as away from electrical cords and appliances.	• Toddlers pulling or grabbing objects which can fall on top of them or disrupt the high chair.
• **Keep** unused doors and windows shut and locked.	• Toddlers closing doors or windows on their hands or feet or finding an unsafe place to play.
• **Use** safety plugs in electrical outlets.	• Toddlers poking their fingers or small objects into the outlet and causing electrical shock or a fire.
• **Turn** pot and pan handles toward the center of the cooktop, out of a toddler's reach, when cooking.	• Toddlers disrupting a pot or pan may result in burning the toddler or starting a fire.
• **Escort** toddlers up and down the stairs and encourage them to use the handrail, if possible.	• Toddlers losing their balance, resulting in a fall and injury from lack of strength or coordination to climb up or down the stairs by themselves.
• **Use** safety latches on cabinets, such as a medicine cabinet or a cleaning supply cabinet. Keep harmful products out of the reach of all children.	• Toddlers pulling open cabinet doors and exposing themselves to lethal products. (*Note:* Medicines and cleaning products can be fatal when used incorrectly.)

12-20 Care must be taken to keep active toddlers safe from harm.

By preschool age, you can begin teaching children to be more responsible for their own safety. You can help by explaining safety rules and following them yourself. State and use the rules as they apply. For instance, you may take a preschooler for a walk. When you come to a street corner, tell the child to stop and look both ways. You should also stop and look both ways. See Figure 12-21 for other safety tips for preschoolers.

Car Safety

Using proper restraints is vital to keeping children safe in cars. These restraints, such as car seats and safety belts, help prevent serious injury or even death from a car accident. All states have laws that require children of certain ages and weights to be in approved child restraints whenever

Encouraging Preschooler Safety	
Safety Precautions	**Hazards to Prevent**
• **Keep** unprotected play areas locked and secure from preschoolers.	• Preschoolers becoming trapped in unsafe areas or injured from hazardous objects.
• **Remove** doors of unused or vacant cabinets and appliances.	• Preschoolers playing near storage areas in which they could become trapped and suffocate.
• **Instruct** preschoolers to play together in a designated area when playing outside.	• Preschoolers wandering off when playing alone and getting lost or encountering a stranger.
• **Discourage** preschoolers from approaching stray or nondomestic animals.	• Preschoolers exciting an unknown animal and causing it to attack without warning.
• **Check** outside play areas for broken glass and other sharp objects.	• Preschoolers lacking awareness of harmful objects in their way when they are busy playing.
• **Teach** preschoolers traffic safety, but also supervise when they are going to cross the street by themselves.	• Preschoolers chasing a toy into the street, lacking awareness of an approaching car.
• **Supervise** water activities.	• Preschoolers diving for something too deep to reach or hitting their heads on hazardous objects because they are not strong swimmers.
• **Use** safety plugs in electrical outlets.	• Preschoolers poking their fingers or small objects into an outlet, causing electrical shock or a fire.
• **Turn** pot and pan handles toward the center of the cooktop, out of a preschooler's reach, when cooking.	• Preschoolers disrupting a pot or pan may result in burning a preschooler or starting a fire.
• **Use** safety latches on cabinets such as a medicine cabinet or cleaning supply cabinet. Keep harmful products out of the reach of all children.	• Preschoolers pulling open cabinet doors and exposing themselves to lethal products. (*Note:* Medicines and cleaning products can be fatal when incorrectly used.)

12-21 These precautions are necessary for the preschooler's safety.

riding in a car. See the *National Highway Safety and Transportation Administration* website for the latest information on child safety restraints.

Adult seat belts are not safe for babies and small children. Each child needs a car seat or safety restraint that is the right size for him or her. Do not hold a child on your lap in a motor vehicle. In a crash or a sudden stop, the child will be thrown from your arms. Also, do not put your seat belt around you and a child. Your weight may crush the child if you are thrown forward.

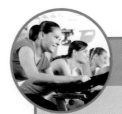

Health Connections

Nosebleeds

Nosebleeds are common among young children. Although they may look bad, most nosebleeds are not serious. You can help stop the bleeding with a few simple steps. Have the child sit quietly with the head tilted forward. Put a cold, wet washcloth over the nose. Be sure the child can breathe through the mouth. Press toward the center of the nose on the nostril that is bleeding for 10 minutes. If the bleeding does not stop, try again. Call the child's doctor or other health professional for help if the bleeding does not stop in 15 minutes.

When Accidents Happen

When a child is hurt, you need to stay calm and provide help. Some accidents cause fairly minor injuries, such as a scraped knee. You can treat these injuries yourself. In many cases, little more than a good cleaning, bandage, and hug are needed to make things better.

Some injuries are more serious and need immediate medical attention. These include severe bleeding, head injuries, poisonings, sprains, and broken bones. When you are caring for a child, be sure emergency numbers are near the phone. Make certain you have the parents' cell phone number or other number at which you can reach the parents. When a serious injury occurs, call the parents right away and explain the situation. They will let you know what steps to take next.

If a child swallows a poison, keep the container and try to find out how much was swallowed. Check the container for steps to take in case of a poisoning. If steps are given, follow these right away. Get in touch with the parents, a doctor, or a poison control center. These people will give you further instructions for how to help. Have the container handy while calling. Give as much information as possible to the person helping you.

Health

Young children are not able to take care of their own health. Most children do not understand that how they take care of themselves affects their health. When they become sick, they may have a hard time understanding what is wrong with them.

It is up to adults to see that children stay healthy. Adults must also take care of children when they become sick. Whenever you take care of a child, you take some responsibility for the child's health. Even if you are watching a child for one evening, your actions affect the child's health. If a child is sick, you may need to provide special care.

When Children Are Sick

From time to time, parents may ask you to care for children who are sick. Sick children need special care and attention. Feeling sick may make a child feel uncomfortable, sad, or even a little scared. You may need to give extra attention to emotional needs as well as physical needs when caring for sick children.

Discuss a child's illness with a parent before the parent leaves you alone with the child. Check on any special instructions carefully and write them down. You may need to give medications at a certain time. The child may need to stay in bed. Certain foods may be off limits. Follow any instructions carefully.

You may need to help children with problems related to illness. A very young child may not know how to blow his or her nose. You may have to help. A child might vomit. Such a mess may be difficult for you to handle, but you need to stay calm and clean up the mess in a matter-of-fact way. The child will already feel bad. If the child thinks you are angry or upset about the mess, he or she will feel worse.

Children who are sick may want you to stay nearby. You might read stories or play quiet games with them. Keep conversation cheery, but do not get children too excited. Such forms of special attention help comfort children and keep them from becoming bored or cranky. If you see that a child is getting tired, allow the child to rest alone for a while.

Children with Special Needs

All children are different. That is what makes each child unique and special. Some children with certain differences require assistance and treatment. Children with physical or *cognitive disabilities* (or intellectual disabilities) have special needs, as do children who are gifted.

You may spend time with children who have special needs. Their needs may cause you to treat them differently in some ways. You should always remember that children with special needs are just like other children in most ways. You may need to use sign language with a child who has a hearing impairment. That child will like to run, play, laugh, and eat just as much as any other child. Treat children with special needs just like other children in as many ways as possible.

When you care for children with special needs, discuss the needs with a parent. Find out if the children require any particular medications, equipment, or actions. Write down these instructions for your reference. The more you understand about a child's special needs, the better you can care for the child.

Physical Disabilities

A **disability** is a functional limitation that interferes with a person's ability. A physical disability affects a part of the body. People who are deaf, blind, or paralyzed are examples of people with physical disabilities.

Children with disabilities may need special tools to adapt to their surroundings. A child who is paralyzed may need to use a wheelchair to get around. A child with vision loss may need to use a cane or guide dog. With some support, however, most children with disabilities can help themselves as much as other children their age. As with all children, doing things on their own helps children with disabilities develop positive self-esteem and self-confidence, **12-22**.

Many children with physical disabilities do not have other types of disabilities. Children with physical disabilities are often as brilliant and talented as their peers who do not have noticeable physical disabilities. Like other children, some children with disabilities may have a low self-concept. This may or may not have anything to do with their physical disabilities. You can help by praising these children for what they can do well.

Cognitive Disabilities

Children with cognitive disabilities cannot learn as well as other children their age. Cognitive disabilities may affect intellectual, social, and emotional development. In some ways, they may affect physical development because coordination may be poor.

There is a wide range of cognitive disabilities. The mildest may hardly be evident during early childhood.

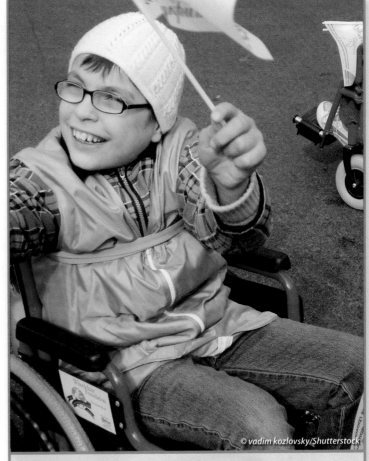

© vadim kozlovsky/Shutterstock

12-22 Participating in activities can help children with disabilities build self-esteem.

Children with cognitive disabilities may not learn to talk or read as well as other children.

Other children with cognitive disabilities are significantly behind their peers. They may think more like toddlers even though they are almost ready to start school. Some children with cognitive disabilities can learn more simple concepts in reading, math, and science. They may require special teaching methods in the learning process. Other children may only learn, say, and understand a few simple words. They can, however, be taught to care for themselves. Children with the most severe cognitive disabilities may require care around the clock.

As with all children, those with cognitive disabilities need to have good self-concepts, **12-23**. Allow children with such disabilities to do as much as they can on their own. Cognitive disabilities do not always affect other abilities. These children may be just as physically strong and able as any other child.

It may help you to think of children with cognitive disabilities as being younger than they really are. For instance, a preschooler may think and act like a toddler. This child may throw a temper tantrum. This action may surprise you because the child looks too old for this behavior. For a child who thinks at a toddler's level, however, this behavior may be natural. In many ways, you may need to treat this preschooler just as you would treat a toddler.

Gifted Children

Some children develop more quickly than other children. **Gifted children** are those who show outward signs of high achievement or potential for high achievement in skill or intelligence. There are a variety of ways a child shows giftedness. He or she may excel at math or English skills. Art, music, sports, and leadership are other areas in which children may be gifted. Children may also be gifted in more than one way.

Children who are gifted intellectually may

- talk before other children of the same age
- have more words in their vocabularies
- be able to explain ideas much better than other children their age
- have better memories than other children
- have intense curiosity and long attention spans
- stay with one task or problem three or four times longer than other children their age

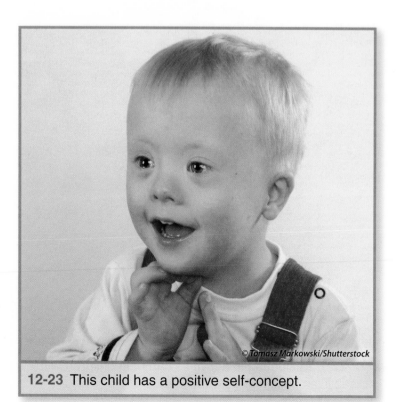

© Tomasz Markowski/Shutterstock

12-23 This child has a positive self-concept.

Gifted children need special attention to develop their gifts to the full potential, **12-24**. Special schooling is generally available for gifted children through either public or private school programs.

As with other children with special needs, gifted children are more like others than different. They need to grow and develop physically, intellectually, socially, and emotionally, as do other children.

Just because children excel in one area, parents, teachers, and other caregivers cannot expect them to behave like adults. These children like to play with other children. They make mistakes and may get angry at times. You should treat these actions as you would with any other child their age. Otherwise, these children may feel pressure to excel in areas where they are not gifted. If they fail, they may develop poor self-concepts.

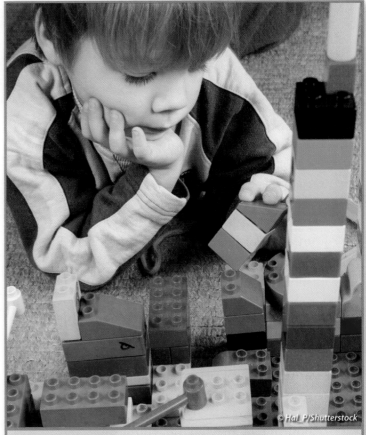

© Hal P/Shutterstock

12-24 Gifted children may display boredom in toys and games that are below their level of learning.

Reading Review

1. What does childproofing a home involve?
2. Why is using proper restraints vital to keeping children safe in cars?
3. If a child swallows a poison, what should you do?
4. What is a disability?
5. Why do children who are gifted need special attention?

Chapter Summary

Section 12-1. Children develop physically, intellectually, socially, and emotionally. Conception to three years of age is a critical time for early brain development. Growth and development happen rapidly when children are infants. Children start life as helpless newborns. By the end of 12 months, an infant is able to move and communicate on its own. Toddlers, children from one to three years of age, become more able to do things for themselves. Three- to five-year olds (preschoolers) develop more adultlike proportions and are able to grasp more abstract concepts.

Section 12-2. Care guidelines for children change as the child grows and develops. Infants require special care. Toddlers are more independent than infants, but still need much attention from caregivers. Preschoolers begin to take more responsibility in caring for themselves, but still require guidance. When caring for children, make sure they are properly fed, bathed, and dressed. Children should also get enough sleep and rest.

Section 12-3. When caring for children, you are responsible for keeping them safe. Be aware of unsafe situations and realize that dangerous situations vary for children of different ages. Take precautions to prevent these dangers from harming children. Know what steps to take when accidents happen to provide help quickly. You are responsible for protecting the health of children in your care. When children are sick, you need to give them the extra care and attention they require to help them feel better. When you are caring for children with special needs, try to remember they are more like other children than different. Children with physical and mental disabilities may need some help to function. Children who are gifted may need encouragement to develop and use their special gifts.

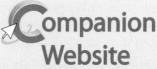

Companion Website
www.g-wlearning.com

Check your understanding of the main concepts for Chapter 12 at the website.

Critical Thinking

1. **Draw conclusions.** All children develop physically, intellectually, socially, and emotionally. Draw conclusions about ways you can contribute to the development of children you know.

2. **Make inferences.** What can parents do to encourage a toddler when he or she is reluctant to walk? What credible sources of information support your inferences?

3. **Analyze.** Observe the environment around you—at school, in the community, or at home. What behaviors do you see that could negatively influence the health and safety of children? What changes could be made to correct such behaviors?

Common Core

College and Career Readiness

4. **Listening.** Interview a parent who has a baby less than one year old. Ask the parent what changes in the infant's physical, intellectual, social, and emotional development have been most notable. Compare your findings with those of your classmates.

5. **Speaking.** Observe a toddler at play. Take notes on the child's physical, intellectual, social, and emotional characteristics. Discuss your observations with your classmates.

6. **Writing.** Work in small groups to write safety brochures parents can use to help them childproof their homes.

7. **Listening.** Invite a physical therapist or a child psychologist to speak to your class about caring for children with special needs.

Technology

8. **Internet research.** Use online sources to research the causes of accidental deaths of children in the United States. What can be done to prevent these deaths?

Journal Writing

9. Think about when you were a young child. If you could go back in time and eliminate one of your childhood illnesses or injuries, what would it be? Write about the experience.

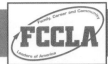 ## FCCLA

10. Plan a child development project that will positively impact your community for the *STAR Event Focus on Children*. Use the FCCLA Planning Process to create a project plan that addresses a current child development issue, a concern or a need—such as collecting shoes or coats, art supplies, or children's books—and donate them to a local Headstart organization or other early childhood program. Develop and give an oral presentation that shares your project with school administrators and community members. Step up to the challenge and present your presentation at your local and state FCCLA competitions. See your adviser for information as needed.

Chapter 13
The Business of Babysitting

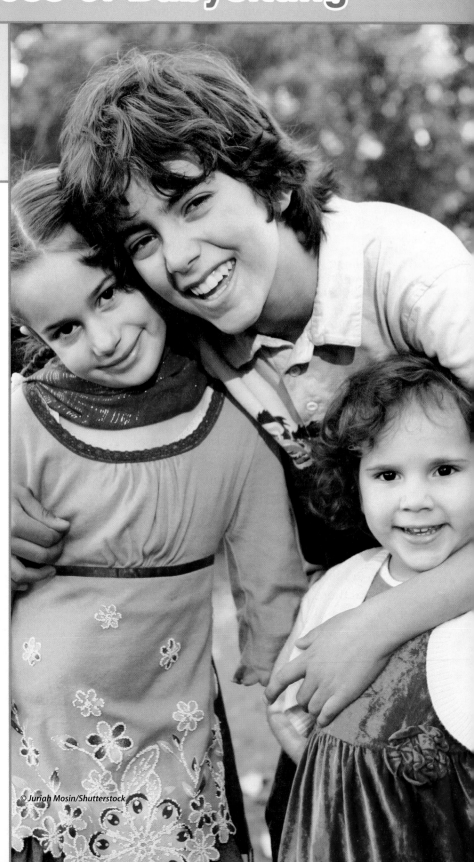
© Juriah Mosin/Shutterstock

Sections

Reading Prep

College and Career Readiness

As you read the chapter, take time to reread sentences or paragraphs that cause confusion or raise questions. Rereading will clarify content and strengthen your understanding of key concepts.

Concept Organizer

	Babies	Toddlers	Preschoolers
P			
L			
A			
Y			
T			
I			
M			
E			

Use a diagram like the one shown to find appropriate toys or activities for each of the three stages of young children. They should begin with the letters in the word PLAYTIME.

Companion Website
Print out the concept organizer for Chapter 13 at the website.

Companion Website
www.g-wlearning.com

Responsible Babysitting

Objectives

After studying this section, you will be able to
- **list** ways to prepare yourself for babysitting.
- **identify** ways to find babysitting jobs.
- **explain** the responsibilities babysitters have to the parents and children for whom they work.

Key Terms	
house rules	privileges

Babysitting, as in many businesses, involves providing a service in return for payment. You care for and protect children for a certain amount of time. In return, you receive payment. Remember that accepting babysitting jobs is a serious responsibility. The people who hire you trust you to keep their most valuable possessions—their children—safe and happy, **13-1**.

The key to success in almost any business is customer satisfaction. With babysitting, your customers are parents and children. Parents and children may have different ideas about what makes a good babysitter. Satisfying both may seem hard at times. You can satisfy parents if you are a responsible sitter. You can make children happy by doing special, fun activities with them. If you make efforts to improve your abilities as a sitter, you can take pride in your work and have a successful business you enjoy.

Finding a Job

You may have interest in babysitting, but you may not be sure how to start. Before beginning a job search, you need to look at yourself.

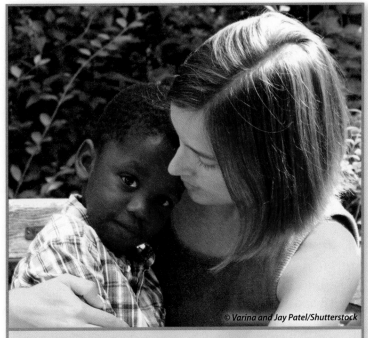

© Varina and Jay Patel/Shutterstock

13-1 Many teens enjoy the two main benefits of babysitting: having fun with children and receiving payment for doing so.

How do you feel about children? Have you spent much time around them? Do you feel confident in your ability to care for children? Are you responsible and able to follow directions without adult supervision? Your answers to these questions affect your readiness to start babysitting.

Before You Begin

Obtaining any job is easier if you have experience. If you spend much time around younger relatives, you may already have some knowledge of and experience in caring for children. Reading about child care, growth, and development can also offer background on how to work with children. Taking an *American Red Cross* babysitting class is another way to prepare yourself and let parents know you are serious about babysitting. Finding volunteer opportunities to be with children helps you get practice caring for and playing with them.

When you begin to care for children, make sure an adult you know is nearby to help if needed. You might volunteer for nursery services provided at community events or places of worship. Spending time with a neighbor and his or her children is another way to learn child care tasks. These experiences give you the chance to try care tasks such as feeding, diaper changing, and playing with children. Be sure to ask the adults questions about the best ways to handle various situations. You can try handling some tasks on your own knowing that an adult can help if you have questions or run into problems.

Early experiences with children help give you the confidence and skill to care for children on your own. They also help you find out whether babysitting is something you might do well. You may find that you enjoy the challenging responsibility of caring for children.

Searching for Jobs

Searching for your first babysitting job can be a job in itself. The best way to start is by talking with neighbors, friends, and relatives about your readiness to find babysitting jobs. They may want to hire you as a babysitter, or they may give your name to someone else. It is wise to take your first jobs from families you know, **13-2**. You will feel more comfortable asking questions and seeking help.

If you do not know anyone who needs a babysitter, try other sources. Some people may place ads in community newsletters. You might also find ads in newspapers or on a supermarket bulletin board, but be cautious when answering them.

Before taking a babysitting job with a family you do not know, talk with them on the phone. Be courteous

Community Connections

Babysitter's Training Course

If you have never babysat before or are looking for tips to help sharpen your child care skills, the *American Red Cross* offers a class on babysitter training and preparation. Created for students between the ages of 12 and 15, the class teaches how to be a caregiver to children and infants and how to be a good role model. It also covers safety issues, decision making and problem solving, sicknesses, emergencies, and résumé writing for future use. Visit www.redcross.org to find the nearest location in your area.

and businesslike. Answer any questions they have about your ability and experience. Following are some items about which you should ask the parents. Depending on the answers you receive, decide whether you have interest in working for the family.

- Ask the number and ages of the children who would be in your care. Do not take a job if the number or ages of children are more responsibility than you are ready to handle.
- Check on the location of the home to yours and the closeness to neighbors.
- Ask if you are expected to give baths or prepare meals.
- Discuss the hours the family will need you, the rate of pay, and arrangements for transportation.
- Ask for references from other babysitters.

If you do have interest in this job, arrange for a visit to the home before the actual babysitting experience. Have a parent or other adult go with you to meet the person requesting the sitter. You can become familiar with the family and discuss more details of the babysitting job. Discussion before the job can prevent misunderstandings later. If you do not feel comfortable with the family or with the babysitting arrangements, do not take the job. Take great care to avoid getting yourself into uncomfortable or unsafe situations.

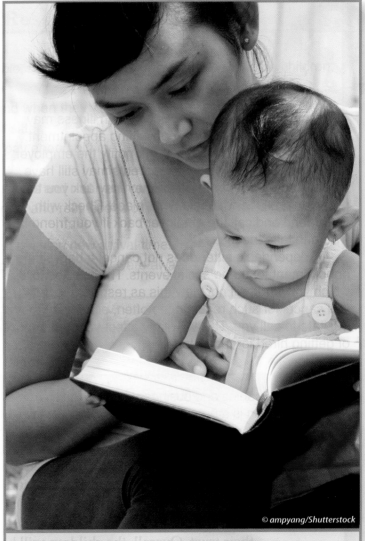

© ampyang/Shutterstock

13-2 Spending time with younger family members helps you gain experience for babysitting.

Being a Responsible Sitter

Parents want to hire dependable, trustworthy babysitters. If they know their sitter is responsible, parents do not have to worry while they are away from home. Follow all directions from parents. Think about safety at all times. You need to be mature enough to respect a family's privacy and to accept privileges without taking advantage of them. When parents see you are responsible, they are likely to think of you first for future babysitting jobs.

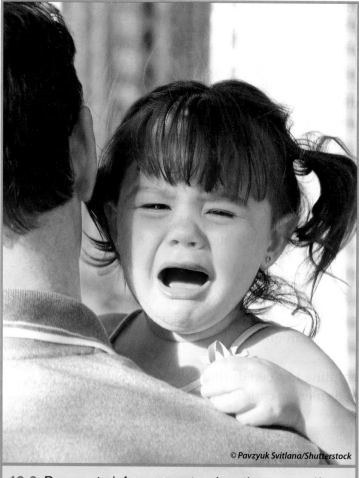

© Pavzyuk Svitlana/Shutterstock

13-6 Be sure to inform parents when they return if their child was unusually fussy or difficult.

- Discuss any problems with the children that concern you, **13-6**. For instance, you may have had trouble getting one child to eat dinner, or another may have had a nightmare. A parent may want to follow up on some items of concern. The parent may also be able to give you advice on how to handle the issue in the future.
- Give any phone messages a family member may have received. If a parent instructs you to answer the phone, give the messages in writing. Include the name of the family member called, the caller's name, and the time of the call. If the family member is to return the call, list the phone number.
- Thank the parent for payment. If you want to babysit for the family again, be sure to let the parent know. Even if you did not enjoy the job, be polite and cheery. It is important to leave all employers with a good

impression of who you are and your ability. The family may recommend you to someone for whom you would enjoy babysitting.

Reading Review

1. Name two ways you can prepare yourself for the business of babysitting.
2. What actions show parents you are a responsible babysitter?
3. What is your most important task as a babysitter?
4. Name two ways to show respect for the family's privacy and any privileges parents give you.
5. List three items to discuss with parents at the end of a babysitting experience.

Caring for Children

Objectives

After studying this section, you will be able to
- **describe** how to handle special child care concerns of babysitters.
- **use** age-appropriate toys and activities when playing with infants, toddlers, and preschoolers.
- **identify** items to collect for your babysitter's activity box.

Key Terms

developmentally appropriate activities	parallel play	cooperative play

Basic care needs are different for children of varying ages. Infants require much physical care. Preschoolers do not require as much care, but they may still want you to play with them. Before taking a babysitting job, learn how to care for children of various ages. With experience comes a better understanding of each age group, making caregiver tasks easier.

Keeping children happy can be one of the biggest challenges of babysitting. If you succeed, a smile and a hug may be your reward. Learning some special skills can help make your job more rewarding.

Meeting Children for the First Time

Children react in many ways when you meet them for the first time. Some children may take your hand and ask you to play

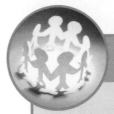

Life Connections

Babysitting Contract

When you babysit, you agree to an unwritten contract to care for children on your own. In this contract with the parents, you are agreeing to take responsibility for any issues that may occur when caring for the children. This includes the child's safety and happiness.

You need to prepare for any care needs or problems that may arise. You also need to keep children content. They may want you to entertain or play games with them. Sometimes children need comfort or guidance. Meeting these needs and wants increases the enjoyment children have in you as a sitter. Likewise, you will also find your work more pleasant and rewarding as you fulfill your role as a babysitter.

Writing Activity

Prepare a written contract for all the tasks you agree to do as a babysitter. Using *I-statements*, explain to parents how you will take responsibility when potential issues arise. Remember to sign your name at the bottom or your contract.

with them right away, **13-7**. Others may act shy and hide behind parents or furniture. Still others may take one look at you and start crying.

Try not to take negative reactions personally. Some children are just naturally shy or unsure around strangers. Say hello in a soft, friendly voice. Try getting on your knees so you are closer to the child's level. (Think how you would feel looking up at a person who was twice your size!) If the child resists these attempts, do not try to get too close. This may frighten the child even more.

You might try to take the child's mind off the meeting by asking a question. You might ask, "Who's that on your shirt?" The child may forget fear or shyness in an effort to answer the question.

Consider using new objects or games to gain a child's interest. You might show the child an interesting object, such as a seashell. Throwing a foam rubber ball into a small basket is a simple game idea. Try throwing the ball near the child. The child may bring the ball to you or throw the ball into the basket.

Sometimes a child may not warm up to you right away. It might be best just to leave the child alone for a while. You cannot force a child to like you. If you give a child time to warm up to you, he or she will figure out that you are friendly and trustworthy.

Caring for More Than One Child

It is easy to decide where to focus your attention when you babysit for one child. You may have trouble dividing your attention, however, when you care for more than one child. If you spend too much time with one child, another may get jealous. When children are different ages, they may not enjoy the same activities.

Safety and basic care needs come first. This means you will need to spend more time with younger children when they are awake. This does not mean, however, you should ignore older children during this time. If older children want your attention, ask them to be your helpers. You might have a toddler carry an infant's new diaper to the

© Kenishirotie/Shutterstock

13-7 A child's facial expression will let you know if he or she is comfortable with you.

changing table. A preschooler could help you get a toddler's lunch ready. This helps children feel needed.

When children are playing, you may spend some time with each child. You might also suggest games all the children will enjoy playing together. Children of all ages tend to enjoy music and stories. If you try games that require skill, older children will tend to do better. Older children are also better at catching and throwing balls. You might ask an older child to help the younger child by rolling the ball instead of throwing it. When they feel they are teaching younger children a new skill, older children often have feelings of delight.

When children are playing together, they are likely to have arguments. You may be able to ignore many of these. Children often settle their own arguments without the help of a sitter or adult.

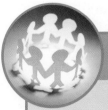

Life Connections

Disagreements

When children are having a disagreement, be sure to watch them closely. If an argument looks like it is turning into a fight, you may have to step in and do the following:

- Separate the children.
- Ask the children what is wrong.
- Try to find a solution without favoring a certain child. If the children want to play with the same toy, help each child to find another toy with which to play or help them in taking turns playing with the toy in question.
- Take the toy away for a while if the children still insist on the same toy.
- Try to get each child interested in something else. Most children forget about fights and start playing together again within a short time period.

Research Activity

Prepare for your role as a potential mediator by creating specific activities to diffuse an argument. Research activities that will be new experiences for the children, making sure both younger and older children are engaged in the new activity.

Serving as a Role Model

Young children often look up to their babysitters. They may follow you around or try to be like you. Having such devoted admirers is a big responsibility. When children admire you so much that they imitate your behavior, you become a role model for them.

Role models can affect people's attitudes and actions in many ways. Think about some of your role models. For instance, if you admire a sports figure, you may take up that sport. You might dress like an admired sibling or cousin. If you look up to a musician who is involved in helping world hunger, you may donate time or money to that cause.

Role models do not just cause positive changes in people. A child who looks up to you may also copy your negative actions. For this reason, you must be careful to set a good example. Use good manners around children, **13-8**. Refrain from using swear words or slang. Talk with children as courteously as you talk with adults. For instance, ask, "Talia, will you please bring me that spoon?" This teaches children more polite manners than saying, "Talia, get me that spoon."

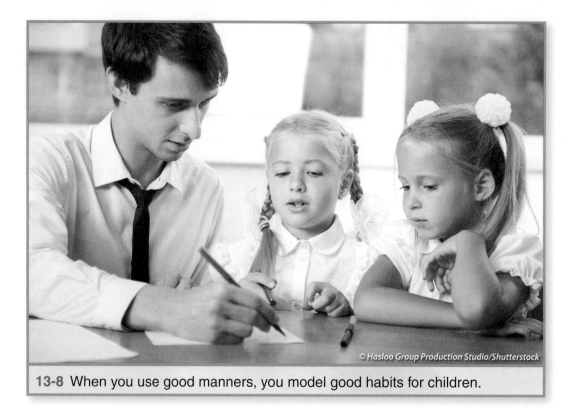

© Hasloo Group Production Studio/Shutterstock

13-8 When you use good manners, you model good habits for children.

Other actions model good ways to get along with others. Talk about others in positive ways. Admit to children when you make a mistake. Apologize if you let them down.

Serving as a good role model may take some extra effort from you at times. You can take pride, however, in seeing a child learn from you.

Helping Children's Self-Concepts

Children may take your opinion of them very seriously. Because of this, the way you treat children affects their self-concepts. If children think you do not like them, they may start to dislike themselves. Be careful to talk with children in positive ways. Answer questions, even if they seem silly, without sounding annoyed. Listen to children's problems and take them seriously.

When you must scold a child, talk only about the child's action. If Jenny is throwing her food, you might say, "Jenny, please stop throwing your food. Someone could slip on the floor and get hurt." This lets Jenny know you disapprove of her actions without criticizing her. It is better for Jenny's self-concept than saying, "Jenny, you're a bad girl for making such a mess."

Playtime

Play helps all children grow physically, intellectually, socially, and emotionally. The types of play activities and toys you offer to a child should suit his or her age. Understanding the development of children helps you to figure out developmentally appropriate activities.

Developmentally appropriate activities are activities that take into account the level of physical, social, emotional, and intellectual development of children at certain ages.

Choosing Play Activities and Toys for Babies

Infants exercise their muscles as they play with people and toys. They learn about what they can do and what objects are like. They also learn to spend happy times with others as they are sharing love and laughter.

When you play with babies, choose activities they will enjoy. Babies like to watch you make funny faces. They may reach for your face as you change expressions. Sounds can also be play for infants. You can entertain an infant just by talking or singing to him or her. Infants also love to watch movement. Hand games and rhymes such as *pat-a-cake* combine action and sound.

You can also move the infant in play. When you move the infant, the movements should not be too sudden or rough. The infant should feel secure the entire time. Do not bounce an infant in your lap as you hold him or her. You should not throw an infant. You can also move the infant's arms or legs while the infant is lying down.

Toys for infants should be fairly simple. Infants mainly like to look at, hold, touch, and mouth objects. Here are some tips to remember about toys for young infants.

- Choose washable toys and keep them clean.
- Make sure toys have no small parts an infant can remove. For instance, some stuffed toys have small plastic eyes attached with glue or thread. If these become loose, the infant may swallow or choke on them.
- Choose toys with bright colors because young infants prefer them.

Older infants enjoy activity games, such as blocks, balls, and large beads. You can move and place these toys in different ways that improve the infant's coordination. Boxes that fit inside each other, called *nesting toys*, are also good for this reason. See **13-9** for some toy suggestions for infants.

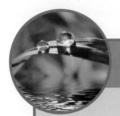

Go Green

Cleaning with Vinegar

Vinegar, which is inexpensive and found in most kitchens, can be used as an environmentally friendly cleaning product. Because vinegar is made from natural materials, it contains less toxic chemicals than cleaning products found at most stores. It is safe to use for cleaning children's toys and is environmentally friendly. Vinegar contains a natural acid that both disinfects and deodorizes materials. When mixed with water, vinegar serves as an easy, inexpensive, green cleaning solution.

Toys for Babies

- Crib mobiles
- Strings of large beads
- Rattles
- Squeak toys
- Nesting bowls or boxes
- Stacking toys
- Musical toys
- Small, soft toy animals
- Soft rubber squeeze toys
- Plastic framed steel mirror

13-9 Simple toys that are easy to hold are best for infants.

Choosing Play Activities and Toys for Toddlers

Toddlers love active play. They are interested in most everything and move around constantly. They enjoy walking and running. All this activity helps build muscles and improve coordination.

When playing with a toy or game, toddlers are mainly interested in themselves. After about two years of age, however, they become interested being around other small children. Through **parallel play**, toddlers show they like to play near each other, but not with each other. Parallel play is important because it marks the start of relating to peers. It is an important part of social and emotional development.

At this age, toddlers do not understand what it means to share or take turns. This is because toddlers do not realize people can own objects. They quickly take what they want from another child. Then toddlers may yell and scream if the owner wants it returned. You can explain the need to return the toy because it belongs to another child. The toddler, however, may or may not accept this. It may help to show the child another toy. If the toddler shows an interest, he or she will forget about the first toy.

You can also have fun with sounds. You might sing songs or think of animal noises to make. You can make rhythms with your hands and have the children repeat them or dance to them. You could hide, make a noise, and have children find you by sound. Toddlers enjoy chasing adults and having adults chase them. You can also have the child try other movements such as jumping up and down. These simple movements are fun for toddlers because the movements are still new to them. It is best to do activities such as these outside or in designated play areas.

Language can be a bigger part of play with toddlers than it is with infants. As you play with objects, talk with the toddler about the objects' sizes, shapes, and colors. Also, consider making sounds. For instance, you can roll a ball back and forth with a toddler. As you roll the ball, make the sound of a dog, cat, plane, or other object. Let the child repeat the sound when he or she rolls the ball.

Looking at books with toddlers is fun for them. Toddlers like to turn the pages for you while you read to them. For toddlers, make sure there is only a short sentence or two on each page. You could also let the child tell you what the objects are on each page.

Global Connections

Games and Toys for Toddlers

Although there are many different toys for children, toddlers from all over the world enjoy playing with similar types of toys and games. Board books, dolls, and circle games are examples of toys and activities that can be found internationally. Board books and dolls have bright colors, are durable, and are easy for toddlers to grasp. Circle games, which usually involve music, singing, and clapping, help toddlers improve listening and muscle coordination skills. All toys can be used to introduce cultural concepts and promote international awareness. For instance, you can integrate board books with multicultural nursery rhymes, introduce international dolls, or sing songs from other countries.

Safety is the most important factor in choosing toys and activities for toddlers. Toddlers are less likely to choke on small items, but they may still put things in their mouths. Because of this, toddler toys should not have small parts that can easily break. Their toys should be flame-resistant and free of sharp or rough edges. Toys that make noise should not be loud enough to damage hearing.

Toddlers often use riding toys with wheels. Such toys need to be the right size and skill level for the toddler. Otherwise, the toddler may lose control of the toy and fall or crash. Also, make sure that wheel toys do not easily catch on clothes.

Toddlers can have fun with many objects not even designed to be toys. See **13-10** for some toy suggestions for toddlers.

Preschoolers and Play

Improved language and thinking ability adds new dimensions to play for preschoolers. Preschoolers get along better with playmates than they did as toddlers. These children are learning cooperative play.

Cooperative play is a form of play in which preschoolers join together to play a group activity. Children who take part in cooperative play are able to share toys and take turns with play equipment. Preschoolers tend to prefer cooperative play in small groups, such as two or four children. With adult leadership, however, they will often try games in larger groups.

Preschoolers like to play with adults, especially on a one-to-one basis. Because preschoolers have fun with imagining things, you can stretch your imagination as you play with them. You can keep children entertained just by making funny faces. Children will try to make the faces themselves. You can also spend more time playing with preschoolers because they have longer attention spans.

Toys for Toddlers

- Floating tub toys
- Push/pull toys
- Blocks
- Toys with large pieces that can be taken apart and put back together
- Cartons and boxes
- Nonbreakable kitchen tools that do not have sharp edges (such as wooden spoons, pie pans, plastic cups)
- Riding toys
- Rocking chairs
- Picture books
- Sandbox and sand toys
- Bouncing balls

13-10 Toys that allow children to be active are fun for toddlers.

Toys for Preschoolers

- Books
- Crayons
- Finger paints
- Clay and modeling dough
- Puzzles with large pieces
- Board games designed for preschoolers
- Dolls
- Toy trains, cars, trucks
- Kitchen utensils and dish sets
- Dress-up costumes
- Hand puppets
- Tricycles and other riding toys
- Sandboxes
- Jungle gyms, slides, swings
- Balls
- Jump ropes

13-11 Preschoolers enjoy many types of toys.

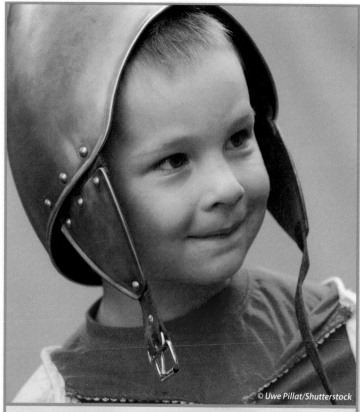

© Uwe Pillat/Shutterstock

13-12 Children can use their imaginations when playing dress up.

Preschoolers also enjoy active play. They like practicing new skills such as skipping, hopping, throwing, and catching. Many other games involve only simple movements. *Leap Frog* and *Simon Says* are examples. Watch preschoolers closely when they are active. They may overestimate their abilities. Accidents may happen when they try to imitate older children. If they see an older child on a high slide, they may try climbing the slide themselves.

Preschoolers enjoy toys they can use for creating, such as clays and doughs, paints, and paper and glue. Some of these items are messy, so be sure to protect the area with newspapers when children use them. Many other toys are safe and fun for preschoolers. See **13-11** for some ideas.

A Babysitter's Activity Box

Children love their own toys, but new ones are always exciting. You can collect items and keep them in a box at home. You can select a few items to take with you when you go on a job. Be sure to keep children's ages in mind as you choose items.

Lacing cards are fun for older toddlers and preschoolers. You can make them by drawing pictures on pieces of cardboard. Color the pictures and punch holes along the outlines with a paper punch. Let children use shoestrings with plastic tips to lace the cards.

Many children enjoy playing dress up, **13-12**. Look through your family's old clothes for items no longer in use. If family members agree, keep the clothing to take on your babysitting jobs. The children will be excited about their *new* clothes.

Many other items can be made or found. You might get new ideas in children's or craft magazines or search reliable websites on the Internet. You can add new items to your box a little at a time. You may get ideas for new games as you play with children, **13-13**. They may show you new games. As you gather ideas, you will look forward to babysitting jobs. Children will look forward to seeing you, too.

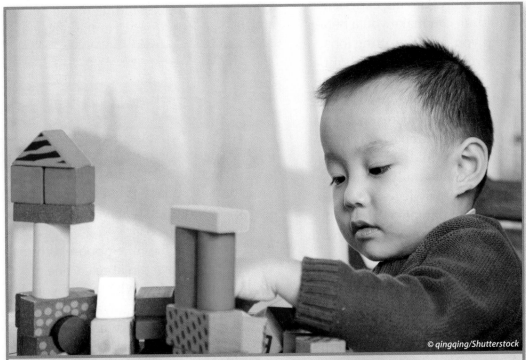

© qingqing/Shutterstock

13-13 You can find out what types of activities a child enjoys by watching him play.

Reading Review

1. Name a technique you might use when meeting a child who is shy or fearful around a new babysitter.
2. Why is it important to be a good role model as a babysitter?
3. Give an example of a developmentally appropriate toy or activity for each of the following: an infant, toddler, and preschooler.
4. What is the difference between parallel play and cooperative play?
5. List three toys or activity ideas a babysitter might keep in his or her activity box for babysitting jobs.

Chapter Summary

Section 13-1. Getting paid to watch children is an appealing job that requires serious responsibility. Having experience caring for children can make you a better sitter and help you get babysitting jobs.

Find out everything you can about a family before accepting a babysitting job. Ask any questions you have about caring for the children. When you are on the job, be sure to follow parents' directions closely and keep the children safe and happy. Respecting the family's privacy and not abusing the privileges extended to you is key. When parents return home, let them know how everything went with the children.

Section 13-2. If you are a good babysitter, children will enjoy having you care for them and parents will hire you again. Ability to put children at ease when you first meet them and skill in caring for more than one child well is valuable. Setting a good example for children by serving as a good role model shows responsibility.

Plan to choose toys, games, and activities that are appropriate for children's stage of development and growth. When playing with infants, you can help them discover what they can do. Toddlers enjoy parallel play while more mature preschoolers enjoy cooperative play.

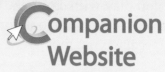

Companion Website
www.g-wlearning.com

Check your understanding of the main concepts for Chapter 13 at the website.

Critical Thinking

1. **Recognize values.** What values do you think are most important for babysitters? What role might these values play in your choice of babysitting jobs?

2. **Analyze behavior.** Suppose a child you are babysitting breaks one of the house rules. What might you do to guide the child toward positive behavior? Analyze what behaviors are appropriate for you as a sitter. When should you call the parent(s)?

3. **Identify reliable sources.** If you could choose one toy that every infant in the world should have, what would that toy be? Why is this toy a good choice? Use reliable Internet resources to document why such toys are good choices for infants of all cultures.

Common Core

College and Career Readiness

4. **Writing.** Write a one-page essay titled *What I Would Expect of a Babysitter If I Were a Parent.*

5. **Speaking.** Work with another student to role-play a parent interviewing a teen for a babysitting job. Write a list of questions a responsible parent would ask. Prepare a list of answers a reliable sitter would give.

6. **Math.** Use reliable Internet resources to investigate ways to calculate fees for babysitting. What factors are involved in setting babysitting fees? Should you add in the cost of travel to the job locations? Choose a method and calculate the rate you would charge for each of the following: one infant in your neighborhood; two preschoolers in your neighborhood; an infant, toddler, and preschooler five miles from your home.

7. **Reading.** Take a trip to your local library. In the children's section, select and read three books for the following: infants, toddlers, preschoolers. On separate index cards or in a file on your computer, record the name of each book, the author, date of publication, appropriate age level, and a brief summary about the book. Keep this list in your babysitter's activity box.

Technology

8. **Internet research.** Use the Internet to check out the babysitting course materials from the *American Red Cross.* How can taking such a course benefit you as a babysitter? Write a summary of your findings to share with the class.

Journal Writing

9. Think about your interest in babysitting. Why are you interested in becoming a babysitter? What traits or characteristics do you feel make you a reliable babysitter? Write about your thoughts.

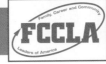 # FCCLA

10. Develop a babysitting business plan that incorporates developmentally appropriate activities for children at various stages of development. Demonstrate your knowledge through a portfolio and presentation that describes the business, describes the use of space and an emergency plan, includes an inventory list, outlines job roles and responsibilities, describes health and safety plans, and outlines marketing plans. Enter your project in your local and state *Entrepreneurship STAR Event.* See your adviser for information as needed.

Chapter 14
Parenting

Reading Prep

College and Career Readiness

Think of a movie you have seen that relates to this chapter. Sketch a scene from the movie or write a brief description. As you read the chapter, visualize the characters in the movie. How would the scene be different if the characters had read this chapter?

Concept Organizer

Pluses	Minuses	Implications

Use a diagram like the one shown to list some pluses (positives), minuses (negatives), and implications (interesting things that can happen) of being a parent.

Companion Website
Print out the concept organizer for Chapter 14 at the website.

Companion Website
www.g-wlearning.com

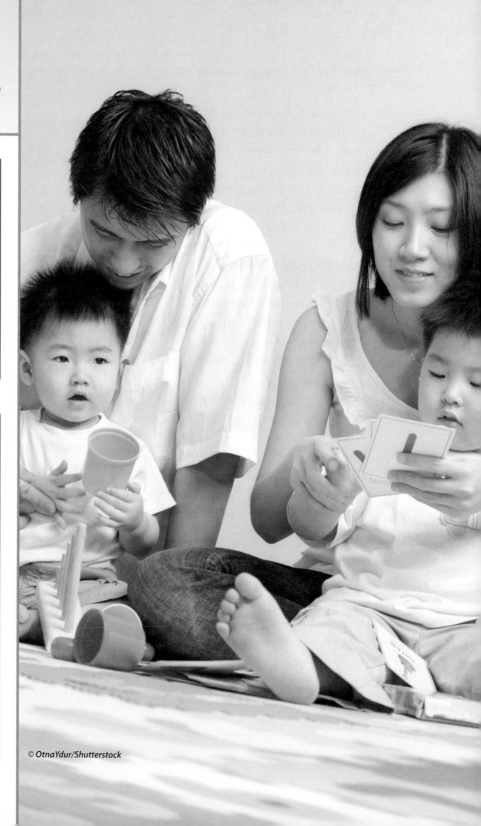

© OtnaYdur/Shutterstock

Understanding Parents

Objectives

After studying this section, you will be able to
- **explain** the reasons to choose parenting.
- **identify** the responsibilities of parenting.
- **describe** the impact having a child can have on a parent's time, energy, finances, and career.

Key Terms		
sacrifice	unconditional love	affirm

Have you ever seen a cute little baby and hoped that someday you would have a baby of your own? Before that day comes, you may want to explore some of the reasons to choose parenting and its responsibilities. If you see how parenthood will change your life, it will be easier to prepare for those changes. Understanding how certain factors affect your relationship with a child is also helpful.

Reasons to Choose Parenting

Parenting is a full-time job. Changing diapers, nursing illnesses, and soothing tears are just a few of a parent's duties. Although parents do not get a paycheck, they may have other rewards for their efforts. These rewards are the reason many couples choose to become parents.

Love

When parents show love for their children, the children respond, **14-1**. Love gives children a sense of security, belonging, and support. When children feel loved, they enjoy trying new experiences. They show love and caring for others.

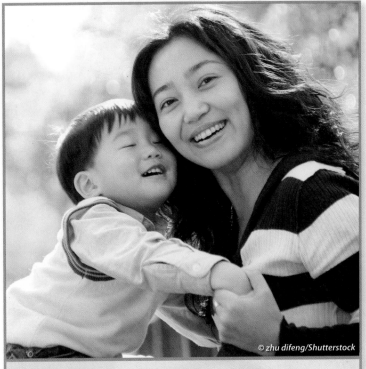

© zhu difeng/Shutterstock

14-1 Parents can see the results of their love as children smile, laugh, and play.

A parent knows that loving care helps a child grow and learn. As a child grows, he or she expresses love for the parent. This is a wonderful experience for a parent. To love a child and receive love in return from the child is one of the greatest aspects of parenthood.

Although love is part of parenting, a person should not have a child expecting to simply receive love. There are times when a parent seems to give more love than he or she receives. A child does not understand how to put the feelings of others before his or her own. A parent needs to keep giving love even when a child cries or argues. Loving support from others can help a parent get through these times.

New Experiences

Every age and stage of a child's life gives a parent many new experiences. A parent finds new feelings of closeness when he or she holds and cuddles a newborn. As the child grows and develops, the parent has many more new experiences, **14-2**. The parent may teach new words, play new games, and go to new places.

Life is more fun when people have adventures in work and play. With a child, a parent may enjoy birthday parties, scouting events, or school plays.

A parent feels great pride and joy through the child's experiences, too. A baby's first word or first step thrills a parent. A parent may treasure these moments even years later.

New Viewpoints

Children are naturally enthusiastic. They can be excited over finding a wildflower or seeing a train. They also love to laugh. They may find humor in a funny face or in looking at things upside down. This excitement and humor easily transmits to parents.

Adults may sometimes take everyday events for granted. Children, however, can help parents see life from a different viewpoint. This view helps parents renew their passion for the wonders in everyday life. For instance, a child may not believe a huge tree can come from a tiny seed. In explaining this to a child, a parent may have a renewed realization about how amazing this fact is.

© Rob Hainer/Shutterstock

14-2 Parents often feel excitement and even a little nervous on a child's first day of school.

Responsibilities of Parenting

Having a child is a big responsibility. A parent needs to provide a child security by offering love and attention. Parents do everything they can to meet their children's physical, intellectual, social, and emotional needs. Parents also serve as full-time role models for children.

The decision to have a child is not a simple one. People need to take it seriously. Having a child changes the parent's lives in many ways forever. Before having a child, adults need to look closely at the responsibilities of parenting. Deciding whether they are ready to make a lifetime commitment to care for a child is also important.

Preparing for Parenting

Having a child means sharing time, space, money, and other belongings with another family member. Deciding how a couple will share these items before having a child is crucial. Both partners may need to give up some activities to spend time with their child. Other lifestyle adjustments may also be necessary for parents to make, **14-3.** For instance, waiting to buy a new car allows parents to have money to buy baby furniture.

If people are ready for children, they are willing to sacrifice, or lovingly give up some of their time and belongings to benefit their children. If people are not ready, they may resent making such adjustments. Without readiness, caring for a child may cause tension and arguments.

Meeting a Child's Needs

Meeting a child's needs is a parent's primary responsibility. This includes meeting physical, intellectual, emotional, and social needs. Babysitters know what it is like to meet these needs for a few hours. Imagine what it is like to have this responsibility day after day for years.

Social Studies Connections

Parents' Attitudes Affect Children

Children can sense the attitudes of parents. They absorb the joys as well as the anxieties they feel in their homes. These feelings affect a child's security. Parents need to willingly make room for a child without making the child feel resented or insecure.

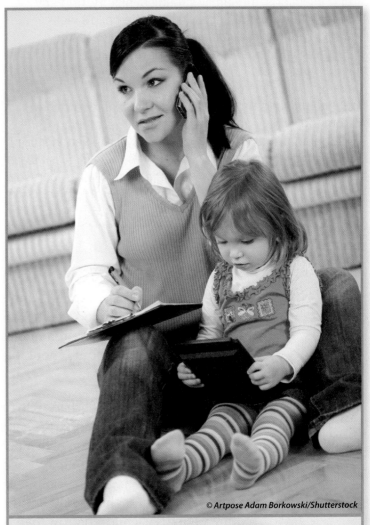

© Artpose Adam Borkowski/Shutterstock

14-3 Parents may have to adjust their schedules around the needs of their children.

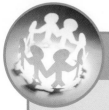

Life Connections

Medical History

Providing adequate medical care is one of the most important physical needs parents must meet for their children. Keeping a record of each child's medical history can help. Medical records contain essential information about each child's current state of health. They also show the history of treatment the child may have received.

Medical records often include any allergies the child may have. For instance, a child might be allergic to plants, animals, foods, or medicines. Medical records also list conditions or ailments the child may have and any medicines the child may be taking. The child's primary medical caregivers are listed as well. Medical records should also include any surgeries and injections, the family's medical history, and any other information that can impact the child's well-being. Medical records should be up to date and copies given to caregivers at home and at school.

Research and Writing Activity

Obtain a sample of a blank medical record form from the school nurse or your primary physician. Gather information about your family's medical history and fill out the form as accurately as possible. Ask a parent or guardian to review your form to make sure it is free of errors. Make copies of the form to give to caregivers as needed.

Physical Needs

Meeting physical needs requires providing shelter, food, clothing, and medical care. A parent needs to find the best ways to meet a child's needs and prepare to meet them. For instance, this might involve taking classes, reading, budgeting carefully, and asking questions. A parent might take a class at the hospital on how to diaper, bathe, and hold an infant. Learning how to make nutritious meals a child will eat is another way to prepare for parenthood.

Meeting physical needs takes time and financial resources. Grocery shopping, laundry, and doctor appointments are just a few tasks that take up a parent's time. Feeding and dressing a child takes additional time. All tasks are necessary to help a child grow healthy and strong.

Intellectual Needs

Parents need to help children learn. They are their children's first teachers. Young children learn through play. Therefore, providing toys and other objects that interest children is a major parental responsibility. Parents also need to provide challenging activities, such as cooking, playing with toys, and going to the zoo.

Parental involvement in learning changes as children begin school. Taking an active part in schooling and monitoring their children's progress can be challenging. Parents need to make sure their children get to school on time. They need to help children find time to study. Parents also affect their children's enthusiasm about school, **14-4**.

Social Needs

Providing children with chances to fulfill their social needs is another parent responsibility. As babies, children are happy to be around only their parents. As they grow, children need interaction with others. By interacting with other children and adults, children learn to communicate and share with others.

Helping children grow socially takes giving from the parents. Giving up some time alone with a child and trusting other adults to care for a child require giving. As children grow, parents may need to take children to social events. They may also host their children's guests as children play in the afternoon, have a birthday party, or stay overnight.

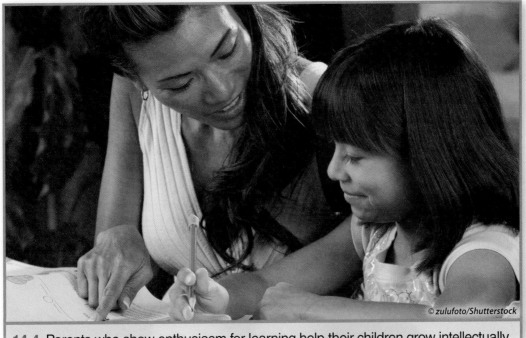

© zulufoto/Shutterstock

14-4 Parents who show enthusiasm for learning help their children grow intellectually.

Children may have disagreements or problems with their friends. During such times, parents need to provide comfort, understanding, and helpful suggestions for resolving problems. They may need to encourage children to patch friendships or make new friends. Parents can help children learn from problems in past friendships. In this way, children can feel secure enough to meet new people and grow socially.

Emotional Needs

To develop healthy emotions, children need to feel secure in their parents' love and care. This requires parents to make special efforts to show love to their children. Parents should offer **unconditional love**, or love given freely without conditions or limits. In other words, the parent must show love for a child at all times. This includes times when a child's behavior is inappropriate.

Parents need to openly express love to their children. This means parents should hug and verbally **affirm**, or positively validate their young children, **14-5**. Even when children feel they are too old for hugs, parents can say "I love you" through words and actions.

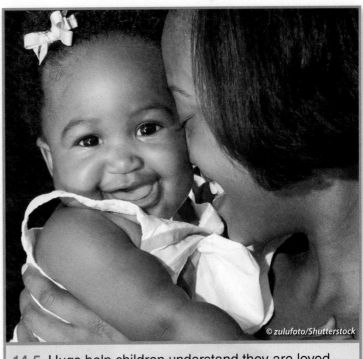

© zulufoto/Shutterstock

14-5 Hugs help children understand they are loved.

Parents as Role Models

Becoming a role model is also a parenting responsibility. Parents need to think about their actions and words when around children. Children are very likely to imitate both negative and positive aspects of their parents' speech and actions.

Teaching Values

Parents teach their children values. *Values* are the beliefs, feelings, and experiences parents hold that guide actions, attitudes, and judgments. Values define what a person thinks is good or important. Some values include honesty, respect, caring, truthfulness, and love.

Children accept the values by which they see their parents live. They consider values parents do not live by as less important. For instance, a mother may defend her friend when someone speaks untruthfully about that friend. Children who see this learn that truthfulness is an important value. A father may say "Tell them I'm not home" when a caller asks for him. Children who see this type of action may not think truthfulness is important.

Modeling Self-Esteem

A parent is the primary person to encourage healthy self-esteem in a child. As you recall, *self-esteem* involves liking yourself and feeling that you are a good and worthwhile person. A parent serves as a role model for self-esteem in many ways.

Parental actions can help a child feel important, building the child's self-esteem. For instance, parents build self-esteem when they show respect to children. They need to use polite language such as *please* and *thank you*. Listening carefully while children are talking shows children that parents value their opinions and take them seriously.

Parents need to model positive self-esteem for children. They should be careful not to put themselves down in front of children. If parents show they like themselves, children learn that self-esteem is natural. Suppose a parent shows pride in planting a beautiful garden. The children then learn to take pride in their achievements and know they are capable and worthy.

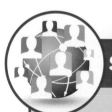

Social Studies Connections

Building Self-Esteem

Providing encouragement and affirmation builds self-esteem in children. When children do something well, parents need to tell them they are proud of their accomplishments. They should encourage their children to be proud of their new abilities. There may be times when children feel they cannot do anything right. It is up to parents to remind children of what they do well.

Impact of Parenthood

Parenthood has a powerful impact on a couple. Except in rare cases, becoming a parent is a lifetime commitment. A parent cannot change his or her mind about wanting a child after the child is born. Before having children, adults need to understand how parenthood will change their lives. They need to accept the reality of those changes and be ready to adapt to them.

Parenthood changes a couple's life in many ways. Parents use their time and energy differently. They need to make changes in the way they spend their money. Parenthood can affect careers, too.

Time and Energy Changes

Children bring a new commitment of time and energy, leaving parents with less time for themselves. They may not be able to spend as much time in leisure activities. A couple may travel, visit friends, or shop whenever they please. As parents, their activities may need to change depending on their child's needs. For instance, they may need to make arrangements in advance for babysitters. If a child becomes sick, they may have to cancel their plans.

Parenting requires much energy in caring for children. Feeding, dressing, and chasing after children demands extra energy, **14-6**. A parent may lose sleep as he or she gets up many times at night to care for a baby. Children can be messy, so parents may need to put extra effort into laundry and cleaning.

New time and energy demands can strain a couple's physical and emotional health. Parents need to support each other to prevent health problems. They need to share in care tasks.

Financial Impact

The cost of having and raising a baby shocks many new parents. Parents may spend much money on clothes, supplies, and equipment before the baby is born. This is just the beginning of such expenses.

Food supplies, medical bills, new clothes, and new toys all add to the expense. Child care is also an expense. The need for more new clothes, toys, and foods continues as babies grow and develop. For nights out, a babysitter becomes an expense.

As children grow older, expenses also grow. Instead of simple toys, children may need sports equipment and uniforms. School supplies, books, and events add to costs. Food and clothing costs increase. Transportation costs may increase as children take part in more events away from home.

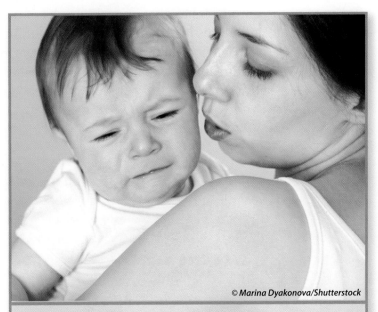

© Marina Dyakonova/Shutterstock

14-6 A parent may need to devote more time, energy, and patience to the care of a fussy baby.

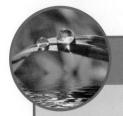

Go Green

Clothing Swap

One way caregivers can reduce some of the clothing costs is to attend or host a clothing swap. At clothing swaps, caregivers bring gently used clothing that their children or infants have outgrown and trade for clothing that is a better fit. In some areas, there are also stores that will trade for gently used clothing or offer cash. While reducing financial costs, clothing swaps are also environmentally friendly by reusing and recycling older materials.

Other expenses may result from having children. For instance, a larger home or car may become a necessity. Vacations are more expensive with children.

These new expenses may mean parents cannot buy things for themselves at times. When couples are ready for parenting, they do not mind cutting back for themselves to give more to their children.

Career Effects

Parenthood can impact a person's career. If a parent decides to stay home to care for a child, he or she may miss chances to advance at work. A six-month leave may affect chances for a promotion. Many companies make balancing career and parenthood easier for parents. Many offer periods of paid or unpaid leave and promise that the worker's position will be there when he or she returns. Some companies offer onsite child care at work, **14-7**. For companies with 50 employees or more, the *Family and Medical Leave Act* requires employers to give up to 12 weeks of unpaid leave for certain situations. Such situations include the birth or adoption of a child.

Having children may affect careers in other ways. Once an adult has children, getting more schooling becomes a challenge. A parent may need more education to advance in a job, but he or she may not have the time or money.

Because of family responsibilities, a parent may not advance as quickly in a career. For instance, a person may think about starting his or her own business. Starting a business may be too risky if he or she is responsible for a family. If the business is not successful, the parent may not have the income to support the family. In another case, a parent may be offered a high-paying sales job. Taking the job, however, would mean spending time away from the family. A parent in this situation may choose a less successful career because he or she feels this is best for the family.

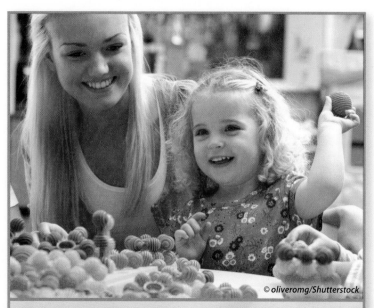

© oliveromg/Shutterstock

14-7 This mother is able to spend time with her daughter during the workday because her company offers on-site child care.

Reading Review

1. Name three reasons to choose to become a parent.
2. Why is it important to willingly make sacrifices in becoming a parent?
3. What needs are parents responsible for meeting? Give an example of each.
4. Give an example that shows unconditional love.
5. What are two changes parents can expect when children enter their lives?

The Parent-Child Relationship

Objectives

After studying this section, you will be able to
- **identify** factors that influence social readiness for parenthood.
- **explain** factors that affect the parent-child relationship, such as good health, financial security, and responsibility.
- **summarize** the differences between child abuse and neglect and identify sources of help.

Key Terms

sudden infant death syndrome (SIDS)	fetal alcohol syndrome (FAS)	child abuse
over-the-counter medications	guidance	child neglect
	positive discipline	Shaken Baby Syndrome (SBS)

Children need a secure, loving home environment. This means parents and children should have loving relationships that are free from major conflict. In such homes, children can grow to be happy, confident, and capable adults.

Many factors affect the kind of relationship a parent has with a child. Parents should be aware of these factors so they can have the best possible relationships. People who are ready for parenting are better able to have good relationships with their children. Learning parenting skills also helps improve relationships.

Readiness for Parenting

Certain qualities are necessary in order for a person to be a good parent. To relate well to a child, a parent needs to be in control of his or her life. The parent needs to take responsibility for his or her decisions and actions. A parent who has self-control is ready to devote time and effort to a relationship with a child.

Social Readiness

Before people can have any good relationships, they must like themselves. A parent with positive self-esteem can make decisions that are in the child's best interests. This parent also models positive self-esteem for the child.

Good relationships with other adults help strengthen a parent, **14-8**. When a parent has strong friendships, getting along with a child seems more natural. These people find it easier to show love and affection to children. They can also turn to friends or family members for support when caring for a child becomes rough.

A strong marriage benefits parents and their children. When a couple works at building a close marriage relationship, they are better able to give more love and warmth to children. When a couple is not getting along, the strain of caring for a child can be overwhelming. Parents who are angry with each other may take out some of their anger on their children.

Good Health

Good health is necessary to care for a child. The extra time and demands of child care may tax parental health. Establishing healthy habits before having children makes it easier to maintain those habits once children become part of the family. Nutritious eating habits, regular physical activity, and proper rest become even more important when caring for children. A parent who is not healthy cannot give a child enough attention physically, intellectually, or emotionally.

A Healthy Pregnancy

A mother's health is especially important during pregnancy. Good health lessens the mother's risk of having a child with poor health or birth defects. A mother's health may affect a child's physical and cognitive abilities.

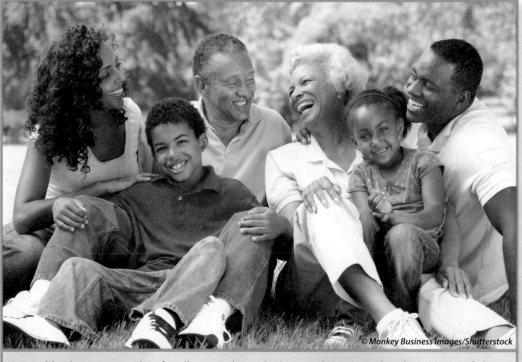

©Monkey Business Images/Shutterstock

14-8 Having supportive family members helps make parenting less stressful.

Many factors affect whether a mother is ready to have healthy children. Physical maturity is one factor. Studies show mothers between 20 and 32 years of age are most likely to have healthy children.

A woman's physical and mental health affects pregnancy, too. Women who feel much stress and tension may have more trouble and anxiety with birth. Their babies may be smaller and more fretful. Mothers who have enough relaxation time during pregnancy and get proper rest and sleep are more likely to have good mental health and healthy, content children.

Avoiding Harmful Substances

Using harmful substances during pregnancy can negatively impact the mother and her unborn child. Because harmful substances can cause physical and cognitive problems for children, pregnant women need to avoid substances such as drugs, alcohol, and tobacco products. For instance, if a woman uses drugs, alcohol, or tobacco products during pregnancy, she puts her child at greater risk for **sudden infant death syndrome (SIDS)**. With SIDS, an apparently healthy infant dies suddenly without warning or cause. Here are more facts about the use of drugs, alcohol, and tobacco products during pregnancy.

- **Drugs.** For good health during pregnancy, women should talk with their doctors before taking any prescription medications or over-the-counter medications. **Over-the-counter medications** are those sold legally without a prescription. Many medications can cause developmental problems for children. No one should take illegal drugs because they are dangerous and harmful to all people.

Health Connections

Physical Health Affects Pregnancy

A woman's weight and eating habits affect readiness for a healthy pregnancy. Women who eat healthful foods are most likely to have healthy children. An underweight or undernourished mother may not provide a child with enough nutrients for healthy growth and development. The child may be born with a low birthweight or other problems. You will learn more about nutrition during pregnancy in a later chapter.

Social Studies Connections

Fetal Alcohol Syndrome

When any amount of alcohol is consumed during pregnancy, the fetus is at risk for suffering fetal alcohol syndrome (FAS). The effects of FAS range from permanent physical and cognitive defects to death of the unborn child. Following are possible effects of FAS.

Physical:
- low birth weight
- smaller head, eyes, and lips
- diminished muscle coordination
- poor vision and hearing
- problems with the heart, liver, bones, and central nervous system

Cognitive:
- learning disabilities and possible retardation
- delays with speech development
- difficulties interacting in social situations
- hyperactive behavior

People with FAS require extra medical, educational, and therapeutic help. FAS, however, can be avoided altogether when no alcohol is consumed during pregnancy.

- **Alcohol.** Alcoholic beverages can pass through a woman's body quickly and affect not only her body, but also her unborn child. Therefore, a woman should avoid them during pregnancy. A woman who drinks steadily or excessively throughout pregnancy puts her child at risk for fetal alcohol syndrome. Fetal alcohol syndrome (FAS) is a condition that causes permanent physical and cognitive disabilities in children.
- **Tobacco products.** In any form, tobacco products are harmful to human health. This is especially true for pregnant women. If a woman uses tobacco products, she puts her unborn child at risk for low birthweight and other health problems. Even secondary smoke from others can cause such problems for children.

Financial Security

You have already read that raising children is costly. Lack of readiness to meet those costs can strain a parent's relationship with a child. A parent needs to be able to afford the child's needs. Otherwise, the parent may worry too much about money and fail to give a child the attention he or she needs.

People do not need to be rich to have children. Expensive toys and clothes are not necessary to give a child a happy home life. Parents, however, cannot avoid some expenses, **14-9**. When a child is sick, he or she may require the care of a doctor. Buying proper foods is necessary for a child to grow healthy and strong. If a parent works outside the home, child care is an additional expense.

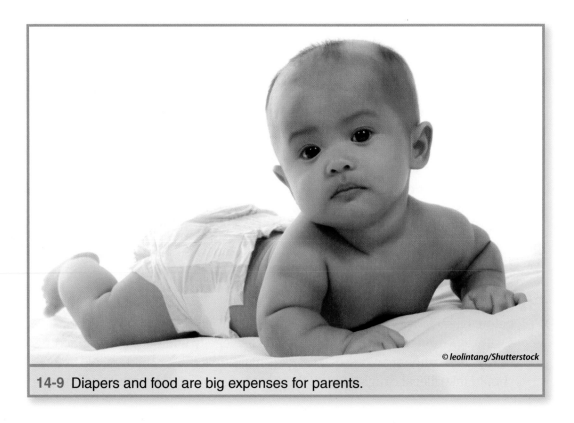

© leolintang/Shutterstock

14-9 Diapers and food are big expenses for parents.

Before having children, parents need to decide if they are ready to meet these expenses. If they are not ready, they may not be able to give the child proper care. Some parents may feel guilty about their inability to give enough to a child. Others may come to resent child care expenses. These negative feelings can harm a child's emotional, social, or intellectual growth.

Acting Responsibly

Before having children, parents need to be able to act responsibly. Caring for and shaping a child's life as well as consistently meeting a child's needs is a major responsibility for parents. Ability to follow through on promises and work to correct any mistakes they make is important, too.

Meeting a child's needs is important to growth and development. If a parent forgets to feed a child, the child may lack nutrients for healthy growth. Meeting needs is also important to the parent-child relationship. When the parent meets a child's needs consistently, the child learns to trust and love.

Following through on promises also builds a sense of trust and love. A mother may promise to take a child to the zoo. If she decides to visit her friends instead, the child will wonder whether the mother really cares. Parents may sometimes have good reasons for breaking promises. In these cases, they are still responsible for explaining things to their children.

Parents need to admit when they make mistakes. All parents make mistakes at times, no matter how hard they try to avoid them. A responsible parent works to avoid or correct these mistakes. For instance, to keep a child from falling down an open stairway, a parent can install a safety gate to prevent an accident.

Learning Parenting Skills

Parenting skills are important to having a good parent-child relationship. Some parenting skills are easy to learn. For instance, parents can ask someone to show them how to diaper a baby or read a pamphlet on planning meals for children. Improving these skills just takes a little practice.

Other parenting skills are harder to learn. Communication is an important skill that may not come easily to all parents. Parents are not always sure how much they can talk with children. A parent may not be sure how to speak at the child's level, **14-10**. Getting a child to understand why he or she cannot do something may be hard.

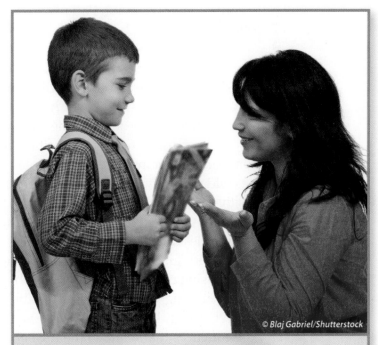

© Blaj Gabriel/Shutterstock

14-10 This mother understands the importance of communicating at her son's level.

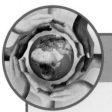

Global Connections

Parenting in Other Cultures

Parenting styles and expectations vary greatly by culture and often by country. For instance, it is common in the United States for infants and young children of working parents to attend daycare. This practice is unacceptable in many Latin American cultures. Babies are only cared for by family members because parents do not trust people outside the family group. Another example is that some Asian cultures are very demanding of children's progress in school. Some western cultures, however, do not hold their children to such high educational standards.

The more parents know about child development, the easier communication will be. Because each child is different, books and classes alone cannot help a parent communicate with a child. Watching other parents with their children is helpful. Parents also need to listen to and watch their children. They can learn what types of communication work best with each child. A child who resists a hug may prefer to talk. With love, patience, and time, parents can improve their skills.

Guidance and Positive Discipline

Guidance and discipline are important parenting skills. **Guidance** includes all the words and actions parents use that affect their children's behavior. **Positive discipline** includes intentional methods parents use to teach their children acceptable behavior. Positive discipline is a part of guidance. Both discipline and guidance help children learn acceptable forms of behavior.

The laws and rules that govern society help keep people safe. Certain behaviors, especially those that hurt other people, are not acceptable. Young children are not aware of rules to follow. It is up to parents to teach children to control their behavior. Parents need to set guidelines for their children to follow so they learn how to get along with others.

Guidance helps children learn *self-control*. For instance, children learn to control their tempers when they are angry. Parents also teach their children to respect the rights of others. Children can learn that they may hurt another child by snatching away his or her toy. Understanding these basics helps prepare children for obeying the rules of society.

Positive discipline involves setting limits for children with direct interaction from parents. For instance, a parent may tell a child that bedtime is 8:30 or say that the child may only play catch outside. Such limits are most effective when they are positive. A parent might say "Stay in the yard" rather than "Don't go in the street."

Positive discipline also involves enforcing the set limits. Parents may use many styles to enforce limits including

- encouraging children to follow limits by setting an example
- praising children for staying within limits
- discussing with older children the need for obeying limits

When a child does not follow the limits, the parent needs to set logical consequences that relate to the misbehavior. For instance, the child may have to sit in a chair for one minute per year of age after breaking a limit about running in the house.

The most important guideline is consistency. After a parent sets the limits, he or she should stick to them. A child should know exactly what the limits are. A child also needs to know the consequences for breaking the limits. When children receive consistent treatment, they can accept limits and know their parents love them, **14-11**.

Child Abuse and Neglect

Some actions lead to a poor relationship between parent and child. Poor parent-child relationships can harm all aspects of a child's growth and development. Two main types of harmful action are *child abuse* and *child neglect*.

Child abuse is harm to a child that is done on purpose. It may be physical, emotional, or sexual. **Child neglect** is failure to meet a child's needs. Neglect may be physical or emotional, or intentional or unintentional. Unintentional neglect occurs because a parent does not understand how to appropriately care for a child.

Physical Abuse and Neglect

Physical abuse is physical harm to a child that is intentional. Slapping, hitting, kicking, beating, or burning can be physical abuse.

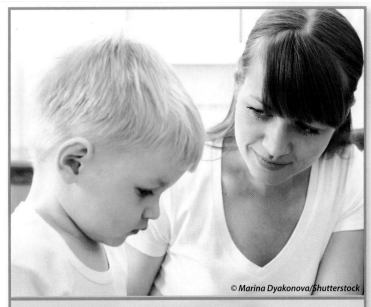

© Marina Dyakonova/Shutterstock

14-11 Discipline that is enforced consistently and with love helps a child understand his or her limits.

Health Connections

Shaken Baby Syndrome (SBS)

According to the Center for Disease Control and Prevention, about one in every four infants that suffer SBS dies from head injuries. An infant's brain is heavy in proportion to body size and is still developing. When an infant is violently shaken, the brain hits the sides of the skull, and the infant does not have enough muscle strength to control the shaking. The result is internal bleeding, bruising, and damage to brain tissue.

For survivors of SBS, the effects to the brain are severe and can last a lifetime. Consequences include cognitive disabilities, visual impairments, hearing difficulties, speech problems, and behavioral disorders. If you suspect a baby or toddler has been shaken, immediately alert a trusted adult.

This abuse often results in bruises, bleeding, or swelling of tissues. In severe cases, death may result. **Shaken Baby Syndrome (SBS)** is a form of physical abuse characterized by severe trauma to the brain. This can occur if a parent violently shakes a baby out of frustration for inconsolable crying.

Physical neglect is failure to provide proper food, clothing, housing, health care, or supervision for children. Parents who neglect children do not harm children through hitting or other physical acts. Instead, parents may not give children enough food or let them go outside in a snowstorm without a coat, gloves, or hat. Neglect also occurs when parents leave children who are too young to be home alone without supervision. These actions may expose children to illness or accidents.

Physical abuse and neglect can hurt a child's physical growth. Such acts also damage emotions. Many children who experience abuse and neglect develop fear as their main emotion. Some children become passive or withdrawn. Others become aggressive and hostile.

Emotional Abuse and Neglect

Parents abuse children emotionally when they belittle or harshly criticize. Calling children dull, stupid, or lazy, or demanding more than children are capable of doing can damage fragile emotions. For instance, expecting a one-year-old to have full toileting control and criticizing him or her for failure is unrealistic and abusive. Emotional abuse makes children feel worthless and unlovable, and may destroy self-esteem.

Emotional neglect involves failure to give children enough love or attention. Examples of emotional neglect include failure to
- show consistent interest in a child's achievements
- show consistent affection through hugging or touching a child

Like children who are emotionally abused, children who experience emotional neglect may feel unlovable. They may display poor self-esteem.

Children who are victims of emotional abuse or neglect may get good physical care. There may be no harm to their physical growth and development. Such children, however, may have trouble trusting or loving other people. They may experience harm to their social, emotional, and intellectual growth and development.

Sexual Abuse

Adults who abuse children sexually force children into sexual acts. Children are not ready in any way for these types of actions.

Sexual abuse can harm children physically and emotionally. The emotional damage often lasts a lifetime. When they become adults, these children may attach feelings of fear or hatred to physical relationships.

Causes of Abuse and Neglect

No one is sure why a parent abuses or neglects a child. Certain factors, however, seem to be risk factors for abuse and neglect. These include
- **Immaturity.** Immature parents may have poor self-esteem and unrealistic expectations of their children. Such parents may have little knowledge or understanding about child development. They may expect their children to make them feel loved. When the children do not, they may abuse the children. They may be so concerned about themselves that they neglect their children's needs.
- **Family stress.** Financial strain, loss of a job, substance abuse, marriage problems, and other forms of stress can impair a parent's ability to care

for a child. Some parents are better at dealing with stress than others. A misbehaving child can be too much stress for some parents. These parents may use hitting as a form of consequence for misbehavior and may not see when they have gone too far.

- **Victims becoming abusers.** A parent who was abused or neglected as a child may treat his or her child the same way. Some may know these actions are wrong, but lack knowledge about how to treat children differently. Others may think this is a *normal* way to treat children because this is the way they were treated as children. Abuse and neglect are not normal under any circumstances.
- **Limited parenting skills.** Some parents do not know how to meet children's physical, intellectual, emotional, or social needs. They may not realize that certain actions are harmful to children.

Sources of Help

Parents who abuse or neglect children need help. Children who are abused or neglected need protection. There are organizations and laws designed to deal with these serious problems.

As a requirement of law, certain people are required to report abuse and neglect. These include professionals who care for children, such as teachers and doctors. In some states, all people are required to report incidences of abuse and neglect. This way, agencies can take steps to correct problems. Other laws protect children from abusive or neglectful parents. If necessary, such agencies can place children in homes away from their parents if needed.

Many parents can receive help through counseling. Licensed counselors can help parents understand their problems, and can guide parents toward actions to correct them. Then they can give their children the loving home they deserve.

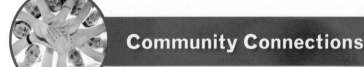

Community Connections

Help for Abuse and Neglect

There are state and local agencies designed to handle child abuse and neglect problems. Many states have child abuse centers or child protective services units. The *National Center on Child Abuse and Neglect* also provides help with these problems. These agencies can give education and psychological treatment to parents and children.

Reading Review

1. Name two factors that indicate a person is socially ready to have children.
2. What harmful substances should a woman avoid during pregnancy? Give a consequence of each.
3. What is the difference between guidance and positive discipline?
4. Failure to meet a child's needs for food, clothing, housing, and health care is _____. *(2 words)*
5. List two possible causes of child abuse and neglect.

Chapter Summary

Section 14-1. People who choose to have children look forward to enjoying parenthood. They want to share their love with a child. They want to have the experience of watching a child grow and learn under their care and guidance, and enjoy seeing life from their child's viewpoint.

Parenting responsibilities include willingness to share resources to help meet the physical, intellectual, social, and emotional needs of children. Parents serve as role models to teach their children important values and help build their self-esteem.

Parenthood has a strong impact on a couple's life. Adults must use their time and energy differently once children enter their lives. Changes in their spending habits and career adjustments are often necessary, too.

Section 14-2. Social, physical, and financial readiness for parenthood is important to strong parent-child relationships. Learning parenting skills such as guidance and positive discipline affects how parents relate to their children. Knowing the risks of child abuse and neglect can help parents avoid poor relationships with their children.

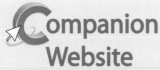

Website

www.g-wlearning.com

Check your understanding of the main concepts for Chapter 14 at the website.

Critical Thinking

1. **Draw conclusions.** Becoming a parent is a major life decision. Draw conclusions about how you will know when you are ready for parenting.
2. **Analyze decisions.** Suppose a couple you know is trying to decide whether they will both continue to work after children enter the family. What factors may influence whether the couple remains a two-income family or becomes a single-income family? How might either decision impact the family?
3. **Make inferences.** How can *all* parents benefit from good nutrition, regular physical activity, and proper rest? Make inferences regarding how these factors can directly and indirectly impact children.

Common Core

College and Career Readiness

4. **Speaking.** Read information about how finances impact children and families using reliable resources such as the *Kids Count® Data Book*. Give an oral report on your findings to the class.

5. **Reading.** Read one or more personal stories about fetal alcohol syndrome on a reliable organization website such the *National Organization on Fetal Alcohol Syndrome*. Share what you learn with the class.

6. **Writing.** Use reliable Internet resources to research Shaken Baby Syndrome (SBS). What are the causes? What can be done to prevent SBS? Write a report of your findings.

7. **Reading.** Use Internet or library resources to read the procedure for reporting child abuse and neglect in your state. Write a summary of the process in your own words.

Technology

8. **Online research.** Investigate parental-control software for protecting children from online sexual predators. What are the key features of parental-control software? Why should parents use such software? Locate a reliable video demonstration of this protective software to share with the class.

Journal Writing

9. Write a poem about what you think it means to be an ideal, responsible parent. Record your poem in your journal for later review.

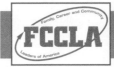 ## FCCLA

10. Develop an *FCCLA Families First* project related to learning how to nurture children. See your adviser about using the *Parent Practice* unit to provide a better understanding about effective parenting skills. Use the FCCLA Planning Process to develop the strategies related to your project. See your adviser about possibly submitting your project for the national *FCCLA Families First Program Award*.

Unit 5
Your Health and Nutrition

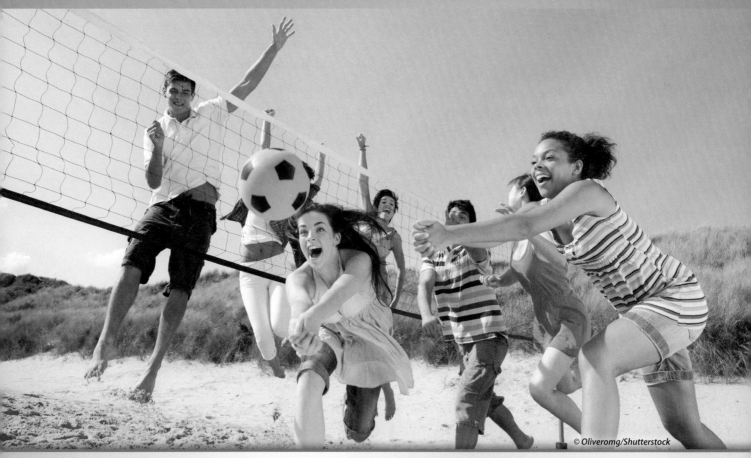

© Oliveromg/Shutterstock

Unit Essential Question

Do you have an obligation to take care of yourself by eating nutritious foods and maintaining your health?

Exploring Career Pathways

Food and Nutrition Careers

Do you like to work with food? Are you concerned with the nutritional health of others? Perhaps a career related to food and nutrition is for you. Here are some careers in this pathway many people enjoy.

Institutional Cook

Institutional cooks use a variety of commercial foodservice equipment. They prepare food for places such as hospitals and residential care centers. Keeping equipment clean and in good working order is essential. These cooks must accurately prepare menus and foods for special diets, and apportion food. Other skills include the ability to use a computer, manage time well, think critically, and solve problems. Communicating well is also key. Such employment requires a high school diploma. Many positions require working with an experienced mentor for a certain time. Apprenticeships are available for some jobs.

Foodservice Manager

Foodservice managers are responsible for the daily operations of places that prepare and serve food. They coordinate activities for the entire facility, such as the kitchen and dining areas. Their duties also include making sure customers are served appropriately and on time. Foodservice managers hire, train, and evaluate employees. An associate's or bachelor's degree is generally required for this career. Many people have additional experience working in food service. Personal traits such as flexibility, calmness, and strong leadership ability are assets to food service managers.

Dietitian

Dietitians are responsible for meal planning and supervision of food preparation and meal service. Teaching people to modify their eating habits to promote good health is also a requirement. Dietitians work in a variety of places, including hospitals, residential care centers, or in doctors' offices. Some choose a specialty, such as clinical dietitian, management dietitian, or consultant. A bachelor's degree is a requirement to become a dietitian. Certification and licensing vary by state. A supervised internship is required for certification. To receive the *Registered Dietitian* credential, individuals must pass an exam after completing their coursework and supervised internship. Some positions may require an advanced degree.

Is this career path for you? Pursue one or both of the following activities to determine if you are suitable for a food and nutrition career.

- Choose a food and nutrition career that interests you. Then contact a person in your community that works in this career to set up a job-shadowing experience. As you job shadow, note the workplace skills this person uses on the job. What education or training did this person need? What continuing education is required?
- Develop an FCCLA STAR Event project such as *Career Investigation* for a food or nutrition related career. As the foundation for your project, consider using another National FCCLA Program such as *Leaders at Work* or *Dynamic Leadership*. Share your project at local and state competitions.

Chapter 15
Promoting Good Health

Sections

Reading Prep

College and Career Readiness

Find a magazine article that relates to this chapter. Read the article and write four questions that you have about the article. Next, read the textbook chapter. Based on what you read in the chapter, see if you can answer any of the questions you had about the magazine article.

Concept Organizer

Health Hazards	
CAUSE	**EFFECTS**
	→
	→
	→

Use a diagram like the one shown to list the three health hazards from this chapter with several examples. Give three effects of each health hazard.

Companion Website

Print out the concept organizer for Chapter 15 at the website.

Companion Website
www.g-wlearning.com

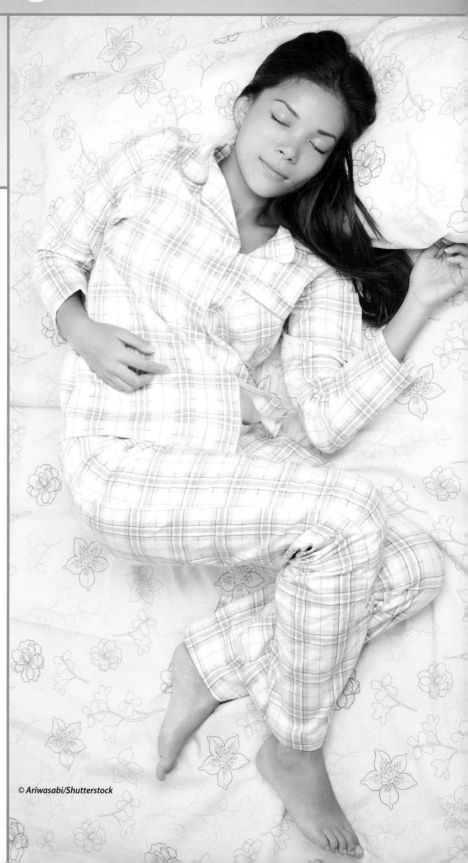

© Ariwasabi/Shutterstock

Health and Wellness

Objectives

After studying this section, you will be able to
- **discuss** factors that promote wellness.
- **identify** components of good grooming.
- **explain** how to clean and care for different parts of your body.
- **describe** how to manage the stress of everyday living.

Key Terms

wellness	acne	tartar
grooming	dermatologist	stress
deodorant	dandruff	
antiperspirant	plaque	

Your health is important to all areas of your life. If you are not healthy, you might have trouble functioning well physically, mentally, and socially. Learning the meaning of good health can help you act in a way to promote it.

The Wellness Revolution

Wellness is a term used more and more often to describe good health. Wellness is not simply absence of disease. Instead, **wellness** is related to your physical, mental, and social well-being. It means you take responsibility for keeping your mind and body in the best condition possible. You might say healthy people are in a "state of wellness." They have adopted a lifestyle that includes good health habits.

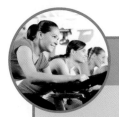

Health Connections

Interrelated Health

Your physical and mental health are related. For instance, having a headache (physical) can keep you from concentrating in class (mental). Likewise, worrying about passing an exam (mental) may cause an upset stomach (physical). This is because you are experiencing a negative or positive change. Your mental and physical health reflect these changes.

When a situation emotionally upsets you, evaluate your reaction. The evaluation will not only help you cope with the change that caused the reaction, but can also help you understand both the physical and mental response your body experiences. By taking care of one aspect of health, you are also positively affecting another aspect, and your entire well-being.

People who are physically healthy look and feel good. They have a high energy level and endurance for daily activities. Healthy people have enough strength to enjoy activities beyond their daily duties. They also look their best.

People who are in good health are usually sick less often than people who are not healthy. When healthy people *do* have an infection or an injury, they may heal more quickly than people who are less healthy.

Good mental health is a sign of a happy, well-adjusted person. Having a positive attitude makes each day more interesting. This positive attitude can also help you to face and solve problems easier.

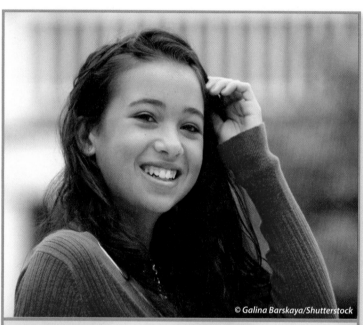

© Galina Barskaya/Shutterstock

15-1 Looking your best can also improve your self-concept and confidence.

Good Personal Health Habits

The way you look relates to the way you feel. If you feel your best, you also look your best. Good personal health habits send unspoken messages to others. You are communicating to people that you care about your appearance, **15-1**. You are more likely to have positive feelings about yourself when you know you look your best.

To promote good health, you will want to develop good grooming habits, eat healthful foods, be physically active, and get plenty of sleep. You will also want to have regular checkups and see your doctor whenever you are not feeling well.

Grooming

Good **grooming** means taking the best care of yourself and trying to always look your best. You do not need perfect features, expensive grooming aids, and high-fashion clothes to be well groomed. Simply keeping your body and hair clean and wearing clean, well-fitting clothing can give you a neat appearance, **15-2**. You will be giving others the impression that you care about yourself and feel you are a worthwhile person.

Science Connections

Perspiration

Bathing daily is even more important now than it was when you were younger. *Perspiration*, or sweat, is one of the reasons for this. Your sweat glands become more active as you mature. Perspiring is nature's method of cooling the body. Perspiration is odorless when it first appears. Bacteria, however, act upon perspiration and cause body odor. The odor remains on your skin if you do not bathe. Body odor will also remain in your clothes until you wash them. Taking a bath or shower will help you avoid the problem of body odor.

Caring for Your Skin

To keep your skin clean and your pores open, take a bath or shower each day. When bathing or showering, be sure to clean your whole body. A good bath soap and warm water dissolves and rinses away the dirt, oil, and perspiration from your skin.

After you bathe, use a deodorant or an antiperspirant to help control body odor. A **deodorant** controls odor by interfering with the growth of bacteria, but it does not stop the flow of perspiration. An **antiperspirant** reduces the flow of perspiration and controls odor.

Care for your skin properly to keep it looking healthy. Proper skin care involves following good health practices and keeping your face clean. Get plenty of fresh air, physical activity, and sleep. Eat healthful foods. Wash your face regularly. Avoid touching your face to keep any dirt on your hands from transferring to your face.

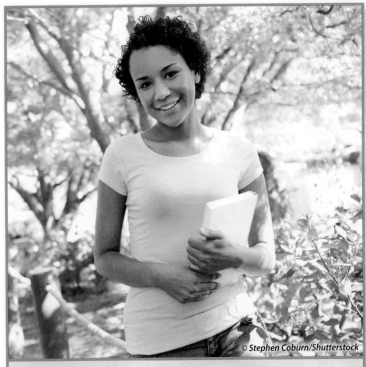

© Stephen Coburn/Shutterstock

15-2 People who are neat and clean have good grooming habits.

Acne

Acne is a skin disorder that results in the appearance of blemishes on the face, neck, scalp, upper chest, or back. Acne occurs when the opening of oil glands, or *pores*, plug up with dead skin cells. A *whitehead* forms when this plug traps a tiny bit of pus in the pore. As the plug enlarges, it pushes to the surface of the skin. When exposed to the air, it turns black and becomes a *blackhead*.

When whiteheads and blackheads become swollen and infected, they are called *pimples*. Keeping your hands away from whiteheads, blackheads, and pimples is important. Picking and squeezing usually cause more irritation and may create permanent scars.

If acne becomes a serious problem for you, see a dermatologist. A **dermatologist** is a skin specialist. He or she will be able to recommend a treatment for your acne.

The Sun and Your Skin

Most people enjoy being outside in warm, sunny weather. An unfortunate effect of being in the sun, however, is that it can cause permanent damage to the skin. The sun can dry the skin and cause premature wrinkling. It also gives off ultraviolet rays that can cause skin cancer.

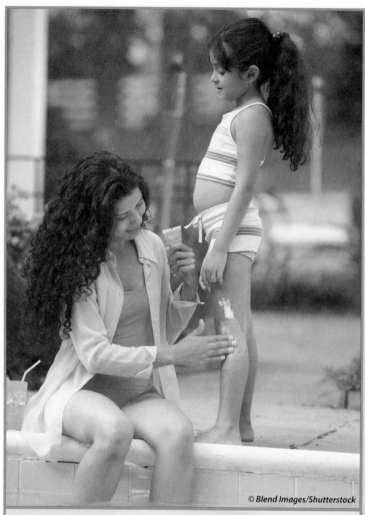

© Blend Images/Shutterstock

15-3 People should reapply sunscreen often when they are swimming.

Your best protection is to avoid exposure to the sun when the sun's rays are most direct. If you must be in the sun, keep your skin covered. Wear pants, long sleeves, and hats outdoors. Cover exposed areas of your skin with a good sunscreen. Sunscreens are rated by their degree of protection. This is known as the *Sun Protection Factor*, or *SPF*. The higher the SPF number, the more you will be protected. Look for products with an SPF rating of 15 or more.

Apply sunscreen even if you are sitting in the shade. The sun's rays can reflect off water, sand, and concrete. Reapply sunscreen after you wash, swim, or sweat heavily, **15-3**.

Caring for Your Hair

Before you can decide on the best care for your hair, you must know what type you have. Is it fine or coarse, thick or thin, curly or straight? Is it oily, dry, or normal? The terms *fine* and *coarse* refer to each strand of hair. The terms *thick* and *thin* refer to the whole head of hair.

How often you need to shampoo your hair depends on the type of hair you have. If you have oily hair, you may need to shampoo every day. If your hair is dry, you may shampoo it less often.

Dandruff, flakes of dead skin cells on the scalp, is a problem for many people. A certain amount of flaking on the scalp is normal. Regular brushing and shampooing usually removes the flakes. If they increase in size and quantity, however, you may have dandruff. There are many dandruff shampoos on the market to help with this problem.

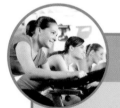

Health Connections

Lice

Lice are another hair problem that can affect anybody. These tiny insects live in clean or dirty hair. Although lice do not cause serious illness, they do cause severe itching.

Lice cannot fly or jump, but usually transfer from one person to another on items such as combs and hats. For this reason, avoid sharing items that touch your hair with other people.

You can detect lice by their eggs. These small white ovals attach to a strand of hair near the scalp. You cannot wash or brush them away. Special products available for purchase will help get rid of lice.

Caring for Your Hands and Feet

Having clean, well-shaped nails should be one of your good grooming habits. A weekly manicure will help keep your nails looking good and in shape. A *manicure* is a treatment for the care of your fingernails.

Pedicures are treatments for the feet. You should give yourself a pedicure about every two weeks. Trim your toenails straight across. This shape prevents painful ingrown toenails, which occur when the nail grows into the flesh. You may want to use lotion on your hands and feet to help keep them soft. Foot sprays and powders are available to reduce odor or infection.

Teeth Care

Properly caring for your teeth can remove plaque and help keep your teeth and gums healthy. **Plaque** is an invisible film of bacteria that forms on your teeth. It can cause cavities and gum disease. This problem usually starts between the teeth. If plaque remains on the teeth, it becomes a hard, crusty substance called **tartar**. A dentist or dental hygienist must remove tartar, **15-4**.

To remove plaque, brush your teeth after each meal. If you cannot brush your teeth after eating, swishing water in your mouth several times may help. It is better to use a soft toothbrush than one that is hard. The soft bristles are easier on the gums and do a better job of removing food particles caught between teeth. To prevent decay, use a toothpaste containing fluoride. Using dental floss each day can also help remove plaque and any food particles between your teeth.

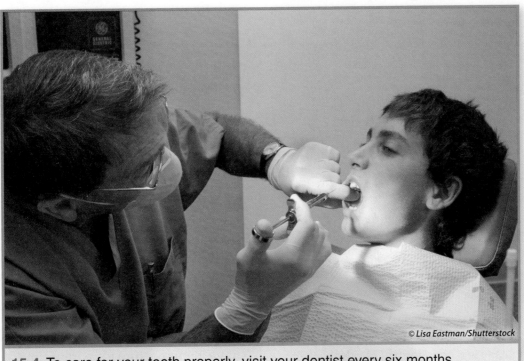

© Lisa Eastman/Shutterstock

15-4 To care for your teeth properly, visit your dentist every six months.

Eating Healthful Foods

Getting the right amounts of healthful foods can improve your appearance. Some foods are better for you. They contain substances that can affect the texture of your skin and hair in positive ways. Some affect the strength of your teeth.

Eating healthful foods gives your body the energy it needs to grow, develop, and work properly. Eat a wide variety of healthful foods. Select foods from each of the five basic food groups for meals throughout the day. (*Note:* You will learn more about eating a healthful, well-balanced diet later in this text.)

Being Physically Active

Physical activity benefits your body in many ways. When you are active, you are physically conditioning your body, **15-5**. Physical activity strengthens your muscles and makes them more flexible. This gives you better coordination. Your heart and lungs become stronger. When you are regularly active, you gain *endurance*. This means you are able to be active for a longer length of time without getting tired. Your blood circulation and digestion also improve with regular physical activity.

Regular physical activity improves your appearance and personality, too. Better circulation and plenty of fresh air contributes to healthier skin. You have better posture because your muscles are stronger. Being physically active also makes it easier for you to relax and feel more comfortable. Therefore, activity improves your personality. The decisions and problems you face each day seem less serious.

If you are not active regularly, your muscles lose their tone and become soft. A few hours of activity could leave you with sore, aching muscles for several days if you have been inactive for a long time.

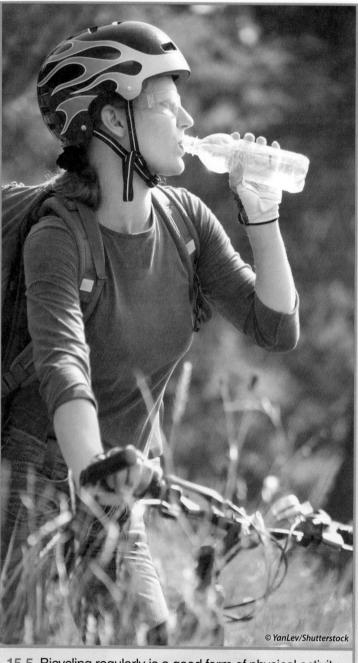

© YanLev/Shutterstock

15-5 Bicycling regularly is a good form of physical activity.

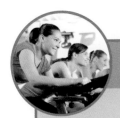

Health Connections

Physical Activities

Being physically active benefits you in many ways and is something you can do with or without a group of friends. You can also be physically active without being on a sports team at school. Any type of activity is helpful. Walking, jumping, jogging, bike riding, skating, aerobics, or swimming are all good physical activities you can do by yourself. Certain jobs you do at home, such as mowing the grass, shoveling snow, raking leaves, and doing some types of housework are also good activities. Most team sports you play for fun are also good ways of being physically active. Sports such as basketball, softball, or tennis give you the chance to be physically active as you share time with friends. With or without a social group, you can incorporate physical activity into any schedule.

Create a log of all the physical activity you do throughout one week. Analyze your log and look for parts of the day when you are less physically active. Try varying your fitness routine by adding new types of physical activities into your schedule.

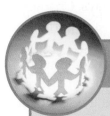

Life Connections

Regular Health Checkups

To remain healthy, it is important to see your family doctor for checkups on a regular basis. Most doctors recommend a yearly medical exam to make sure your physical health has not changed. It is also a good time to ask questions or talk with the doctor about any issues you are facing. Areas of concern can be a large weight loss or weight gain, frequent headaches, lumps, vision problems, or chronic fatigue. Sometimes a simple blood test provides answers. Your doctor knows what to look for and recommend for optimal health.

Cancer screening is part of a routine checkup. Ask your doctor about self-examination techniques and how to recognize unusual skin growths for early detection of some cancers. Males should examine their testicles and females their breasts for any lumps. In addition, females between the ages of 13 and 26 should receive the human papilloma virus (HPV) vaccine. This vaccine prevents infection of some human papillomavirus strains associated with cervical cancer. The Mayo Clinic advises that males between the ages of 9 and 26 receive the HPV vaccine to prevent genital warts.

Health Activity

Ask your doctor or older family member about self-examination techniques to spot cancer. There is also good step-by-step information about early breast, prostate, and skin cancer detection. Develop the habit of regular self examination to promote good health.

Getting Enough Sleep

Sleep is the most effective form of rest. Getting enough sleep is a very important health habit. As you sleep, more growth and repair takes place in your body than when you are awake. Getting the right amount of sleep also keeps your skin in better condition.

Your sleep needs may be different from the sleep needs of anyone else you know. Most young people, however, need 8 to 10 hours of sleep each night. Some teens require more sleep and some require less. Older people may need less sleep than teens because they are no longer growing and may be less active.

When you get the right amount of sleep, you look and feel better. You have more energy and are in a better mood. Getting enough sleep keeps you from becoming tired and drowsy during the day. You should not have a problem staying awake at school when you are getting enough sleep. Being sleepy in the daytime when you are getting plenty of sleep at night could indicate a physical problem.

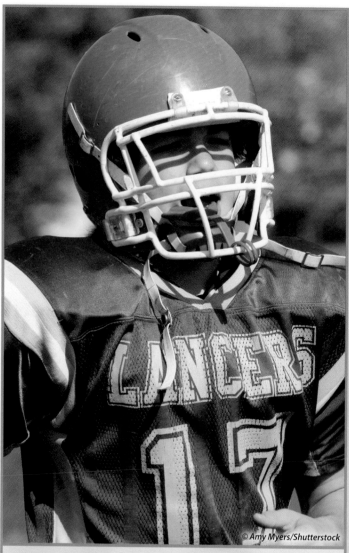

© Amy Myers/Shutterstock

15-6 The stress this athlete feels before a big game prepares him for the competition.

Stress

Stress is the mental or physical tension you feel when faced with change. It is a natural part of everyday living. Stress affects everyone at different times and in different ways. Change, however, is constant. It is important to know how to handle change.

Anxiety, fear, conflict, and worry can be signs of stress. These reactions might occur if you miss the school bus or if you have to make a presentation to the class. You might feel anxious when you visit the dentist. The more important the event is in your life, the more stress you will probably feel. Trying to meet a deadline can be stressful. Having your parents get a divorce would be more stressful, however, because this change would have a greater impact on your life.

Some stressful events are exciting and stimulating. You might get a good grade in a difficult class or be accepted into the college of your choice. The stress you feel before you compete in an event can make you rise to the challenge, **15-6**. This kind of stress is good for you. It makes your life interesting and challenging. It can help you become a better person.

The Body's Reaction to Stress

Because people are different, what may be stressful to one person may not be to another. Your best friend may find it easy to talk with anyone. For you, it may be much harder.

Your body reacts to stress in different ways. Many reactions you cannot control. Your heart may beat faster. You may breathe faster and perspire more. Your muscles may tense. Your mouth may feel dry. Your stomach may feel like it is in knots. Reminding yourself that you can control these feelings by relaxing helps you to deal with your body's reaction to stress.

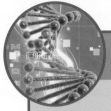

Science Connections

The Fight-or-Flight Response

The *fight-or-flight* response is a physical reaction during intense stress. It prepares the body for quick action. Whether you choose to fight or flee, your body thinks it needs all its resources. Perceived threats and stressful situations can also trigger the fight-or-flight response.

The fight-or-flight response causes your nervous system to release *adrenaline* and *cortisol*, which are hormones with long-term, negative physical effects. Adrenaline increases your heart rate, elevates your blood pressure, and boosts energy. Cortisol releases glucose, or sugar, in your blood stream to dull pain and increase immunity and energy. After the perceived threat or stress passes, your body then returns to normal and functions regularly.

Once the stressful event passes, your body returns to normal. If the stress or tension continues, it can cause physical problems that are more serious. Some of the most common ailments caused by stress in adults are headaches, stomach ulcers, heart disease, and high blood pressure. Taking a walk, deep breathing, or listening to music are just several ways you might find help to relieve stress.

How to Avoid Stress

To avoid stress, you may first want to learn to identify the events in your life that cause stress, 15-7. Take notice of any events that make you feel tense. Know your limits to avoid too much stress. Learn to say *no* to situations you cannot handle.

Because change often causes stress, try not to make too many changes at one time. You will not be able to avoid some changes, however. For instance, if a parent must move to a new city to keep his or her job, the family may have to move. On the other hand, you might be able to postpone some changes. Sharing your feelings with a parent may help everyone involved recognize how this decision is making you feel. You might be able to wait until the end of the school year to move.

Some stress can be prevented by planning ahead. For instance, planning can help you prepare for tests and complete assignments on time. If you have homework in all your classes, you can plan to start the work as soon as possible. If you wait until the last minute to start, you might cause yourself unnecessary stress.

Stress Rating Scale

Life Event	Point Value	Life Event	Point Value
Death of spouse	100	Trouble with in-laws	29
Divorce	73	Outstanding personal achievement	28
Marital separation	65	Begin or end school	26
Jail term	63	Change in living conditions (new house, remodeling, deterioration of home or neighborhood)	25
Death of close family member	63		
Personal injury or illness	53		
Marriage	50	Revision of personal habits (dress, manners, associations)	24
Fired from job	47	Trouble with boss	23
Marital reconciliation	45	Change in work hours or conditions	20
Retirement	45	Change in residence	20
Change in health of family member	44	Change in schools	20
Pregnancy	40	Change in recreation	19
Gain of new family member (birth, adoption, grandparent moving in, etc.)	39	Change in church activities	19
Change in financial state (better or worse off than usual)	38	Change in social activities (clubs, dancing, movies)	18
Death of a close friend	37	Change in sleeping habits	16
Change to a different line of work	36	Change in number of family get-togethers	15
Change in number of arguments with spouse	35	Change in eating habits (more or less food, different hours or surroundings)	15
Foreclosure of mortgage or loan	30	Vacation	13
Change in responsibilities at work (promotion or demotion)	29	Christmas	12
Son or daughter leaving home	29	Minor violations of the law (traffic ticket, disturbing the peace)	11

Research has shown that among people with more than 450 stress points within the past two years, about 90 percent will become ill in the near future. With 300 points, the illness rate is 60 percent, and with 150 points, only 33 percent.

Reprinted with permission from Journal of Psychosomatic Research, Vol. II, Holmes, T.H., and Rahe, R.H., The Social Readjustment Rating Scale, Elsevier Science Ltd., Pergamon Imprints, Oxford, England.

15-7 Check your stress level by adding the total points to every life event listed that has affected you within the past 24 months.

How to Handle Stress

You cannot always avoid stress, but knowing how to cope with it can help you feel better. The following suggestions may help you manage your stress.

Sometimes it helps to talk with someone about the situations you are facing. Talk with a trusted friend or someone you respect. You may be able to find some ways to improve your situation. Your family might see a solution that you cannot see. Your teachers, guidance counselors, or religious leaders are others you can talk with when you face situations that seem too difficult to handle.

It is okay to talk about how you feel. Get your feelings out in the open. Crying can be a way of relieving tension. Then you will be better able to deal with the problem.

When faced with a problem, try to find the cause. Decide how you might solve the problem. Facing your problem can reduce the stress. Then make plans to prevent the situation from occurring again, **15-8**.

Keeping your body healthy and fit can help you deal with everyday stress. Get plenty of rest and eat a balanced diet. Daily physical activity not only keeps you fit, but it can also relieve tension and help you relax. Go for a bike ride or swim laps in a pool. Call some friends for a game of basketball or tennis. Go shopping, run, paint. Doing something you enjoy can help you to see things differently when you focus on the stressful situation.

Learn to relax. Listening to soft music or taking a bubble bath can soothe your nerves and calm you. Reading can take your mind off your worries. Develop a hobby you enjoy. Try to find time for other forms of relaxation as well.

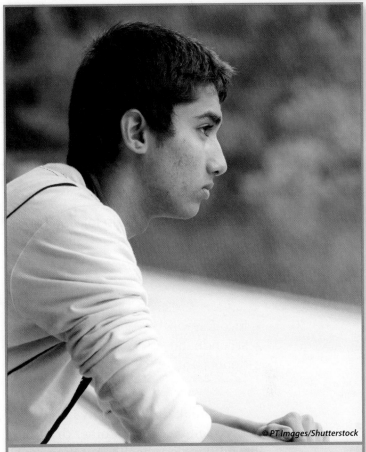
©PT Images/Shutterstock

15-8 Sometimes taking time to reflect on a situation can help you manage it.

Reading Review

1. _____ is related to your physical, mental, and social well-being.
2. What is the difference between a deodorant and an antiperspirant?
3. A skin disorder that results in the appearance of blemishes on the face, neck, scalp, upper chest, or back is called _____.
4. Name four physical problems or ailments related to stress.
5. Describe three ways to handle stress in your everyday life.

Health Hazards

Objectives

After studying this section, you will be able to

- **identify** health risks associated with the use of tobacco, alcohol, and other drugs.
- **list** sources of help for dealing with risks associated with tobacco, alcohol, and drugs.

Key Terms

nicotine	alcoholism	psychological
secondhand smoke	drug abuse	dependence
depressant	physical dependence	

Health hazards are any habits that could cause health problems. Using tobacco and alcohol or other drugs are health risks. Not only are these habits harmful to your health, but they are also often illegal. Purchasing tobacco and drinking alcohol are illegal for people under a certain age. Though age requirements vary from state to state, these activities are nearly always against the law for young teens. Many commonly abused drugs are completely illegal in the United States.

Sooner or later, you will have to make some decisions about these habits and your health. Knowing that many health risks are against the law and unhealthy for you may help you make these decisions.

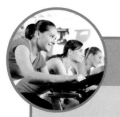

Health Connections

Smokeless Tobacco

Smokeless tobacco, which includes chewing tobacco and snuff, is also habit forming and harmful to health. Both types of smokeless tobacco irritate the insides of the mouth and may cause cancer of the mouth. Bad breath and discolored teeth are common problems. Putting snuff in the nose can also cause the membranes of the nose to become irritated. Users of smokeless tobacco may experience a loss of taste and smell.

Tobacco

People who use tobacco regularly become addicted to **nicotine**, a colorless and odorless drug found in tobacco. Nicotine gives the body a lift when tobacco products are used. The body quickly builds up a resistance to nicotine. More and more tobacco is then required to get the same feeling.

Cigarettes, chewing tobacco, and snuff are all forms of tobacco available in stores. Each form of tobacco is harmful.

Cigarettes

Cigarette smoking often begins in the early teen years. Teens who smoke may give the excuse that they were encouraged to smoke by friends who smoke. They may say they are following the examples of family members who smoke. Young people may also use the excuse that smoking is glamorous or that it will make them look more grown-up.

Teens who do not smoke have responses for these excuses. Some nonsmokers feel that true friends would not encourage you to do something unhealthy. They feel there are behaviors that are more positive you can model from family members. Many nonsmokers think there is nothing attractive about watching someone puff on a cigarette. They also believe that especially adults should be smart enough to know how unhealthy it is to smoke.

As a person inhales smoke, the linings of the nose, throat, and lungs become irritated. This happens to people who smoke pipes and cigars as well. A chronic cough often develops. Smoking begins to do its damage.

Smoking can cause coronary heart disease, which is the leading cause of death in the United States. Smokers are also more likely to suffer from various types of cancers and lung diseases. Pregnant women who smoke have a greater risk of having premature deliveries and low-birthweight babies. According to the Surgeon General, all cigarette packages and advertisements must include warnings of the dangers of smoking, **15-9**.

Studies show that stopping smoking is one of the best steps a smoker can take to improve his or her health. In a very short time, even days, breathing becomes easier and a cigarette cough may go away.

Cigarette smoke can be harmful to your health even if you do not actually smoke. When you are near people who are smoking, you breathe in smoke, which is called secondhand smoke. Because of the evidence of

Go Green

Secondhand Smoke Pollution

Breathing someone else's smoke is a type of air pollution that can be extremely dangerous to your health. According to the American Cancer Society, secondhand smoke has higher levels of cancer-causing agents, or *carcinogens*, than smoke inhaled directly. The cancer-causing particles in secondhand smoke are also smaller, so they are more easily absorbed into the blood system. The Center for Disease Control (CDC) asserts that over 3,000 people who never smoked die from lung cancer yearly.

Researchers determined that tobacco smoke contains at least 172 toxic substances. They include three regulated outdoor air pollutants, 33 hazardous air pollutants, 47 hazardous waste chemicals, and 67 known carcinogens. Ventilation, air cleaning, or separating smokers from nonsmokers does not control the pollution. Smoke-free buildings are the only remedy.

Surgeon General's Warnings

- Cigarette Smoke Contains Carbon Monoxide.
- Quitting Smoking Now Greatly Reduces Serious Risks to Your Health.
- Smoking Causes Lung Cancer, Heart Disease, Emphysema, and May Complicate Pregnancy.
- Smoking by Pregnant Women May Result in Fetal Injury, Premature Birth, and Low Birthweight.
- The Surgeon General Has Determined That Cigarette Smoking Is Dangerous to Your Health.

15-9 At least one of these Surgeon General's warnings must appear on every package of cigarettes and in all advertising.

secondhand smoke's harmful effects, many states and communities have passed laws to prevent smoking in public places. Many businesses have banned smoking in areas where people work or gather. Other businesses have both smoking and nonsmoking areas.

Alcohol

Alcohol is considered a drug. Most teens know the dangers associated with alcohol use. It is also illegal for minors to consume alcohol. For this and health reasons, teens should not drink beer, wine, or other liquors.

People who drink may give various excuses such as the following:

- *Peer pressure.* Those who use this excuse might try to become involved in group activities that do not include alcohol.
- *Problems and unhappy situations.* People who use alcohol to get away from problems with family, friends, or problems at work may only add to their problems. These people might want to seek solutions to their problems through improved communication and outside sources of help, such as peer counselors or therapy groups.
- *Media influence.* People who use this excuse often feel that drinking will cause them to be glamorous or successful like people in the media. Focusing on personal strengths, however, might be a more positive means to achieve desired success.
- *To relax and to like themselves better.* These people may find that reading and physical activity are more effective relaxation techniques than drinking. They may also find that being able to relax without alcohol gives their self-esteems the boost they need.
- *Boredom.* A few people say they drink because they are bored or have nothing better to do. Developing a hobby or contributing time to a worthy cause might be a more healthful alternative for these people.

Safety Connections

Drinking and Driving

Drinking and driving do not mix. In fact, it is illegal in every state to drive while under the influence of alcohol. Alcohol causes more traffic accidents and fatalities than any other single factor. Excessive drinking is a factor in nearly half of traffic deaths. Young people between the ages of 18 and 24 cause more of these deaths than any other age group.

The Effects of Alcohol

Alcohol acts as a **depressant**, which means it slows down activity in the brain and spinal cord. It can disrupt mental and physical activity and injure internal organs. Alcohol slows down a person's reflexes and causes a lack of muscle control. This causes people who have been drinking to have slurred speech and an unsteady walk. It also prevents them from responding to pain or danger as quickly as normal. For these reasons, use of alcohol increases the risk of being involved in all types of accidents.

Alcohol causes a lack of self-control and good judgment. People who have been drinking do not hold back any feelings or actions. They commonly become impulsive and aggressive.

The body feels the effects of alcohol quickly because it is absorbed into the bloodstream almost immediately. This happens even faster when a person is drinking on an empty stomach. People with a small body size feel the effects faster than larger people.

In addition to the immediate physical effects, alcohol has some lasting effects on health. Alcohol harms the tissues of the mouth and throat of heavy drinkers. The stomach and heart are also harmed. Although weight gain often occurs, the body is actually starving for nutrients because the person is drinking alcohol instead of eating food. Long-term use of alcohol harms the liver. Unborn babies can suffer from birth defects if the pregnant mothers are drinkers.

Drinking a large quantity of alcohol at one time can kill as it affects the ability to breathe properly. Combining alcohol with medications can also cause death.

Some people become addicted to alcohol. They have the disease called **alcoholism** and are unable to stop drinking. Alcoholism affects relationships with friends and family members as well as affecting the alcoholic's health. Recovering from this disease is very difficult.

Drugs

Drug abuse means using a drug for a purpose other than one for which it was intended. This use damages a person's health and keeps the person from functioning normally. Drug abuse creates an exaggerated sense of well-being and makes people unaware of reality.

People who abuse drugs use many of the same excuses used by people who use tobacco and alcohol, **15-10**. As with tobacco and alcohol, these excuses lack validity. Drug use adds to problems rather than solving them.

Excuses Some Teens Give for Using Drugs

- I want to be popular and accepted by friends.
- My best friends use drugs, and they got me to start.
- My parents or other family members use drugs.
- I have the money to buy drugs, and they are easy to obtain.
- Using drugs helps me escape from stress and other personal and family problems.
- I like the thrill I get from taking drugs.
- Using drugs gives me a good feeling and makes me happy.
- Using drugs makes me feel better when I am bored or lonely.
- Using drugs helps me overcome shyness and relax with people.
- Drug abuse appears glamorous on TV and movies, and using drugs makes me feel glamorous.

15-10 Teens use many excuses for using drugs, but drug abuse for any reason is damaging.

A number of activities could healthfully meet the needs expressed by people using these excuses.

Once a person starts abusing drugs, that person might develop a physical dependence on them. **Physical dependence** means the person is addicted to the drugs and his or her body begins to require the drug to function. People who smoke or drink may develop physical dependence, too.

A person can also develop a psychological dependence on drugs. **Psychological dependence** means the person craves the drug for the feeling it provides or because it provides an escape from reality. Once people are dependent on drugs, they often become ill if they stop taking the drugs.

Drug abuse is very damaging to all relationships, whether they be social, work, school, or family relationships. Drug abusers are likely to neglect their responsibilities. People who abuse drugs may do anything and harm anyone to get money to buy drugs.

Marijuana

Marijuana, also known as pot, is an illegal drug that is commonly abused. It is the product of the hemp plant and is ground and made into cigarettes. Using marijuana makes people feel they are on a "high."

Reactions to marijuana can be serious. The drug interferes with memory, learning, speech, and ability to think. It can cause existing emotional problems to increase. The lung tissue of marijuana smokers may be harmed. Smokers may also suffer panic attacks. Hospitalization may be required.

Many people believe they can use marijuana occasionally and not become addicted. This is not true. Marijuana causes physical and psychological dependencies that are difficult to break. Users will need more and more of the drug to get the same effect.

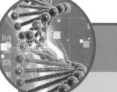

Science Connections

Anabolic Steroids

Anabolic steroids are drugs sometimes used illegally by athletes to help them become stronger, more muscular, and perform better. They also, however, have dangerous side effects, including cancer, high blood pressure, heart disease, fertility problems, and stroke. Anabolic steroids are made from *testosterone*, the male sex hormone. They are highly addictive and cause abnormal aggression. Unfortunately, the pressure for athletes to perform—even at the high school level—leads many to this illegal option. Many athletic associations ban their use. They include the National Football League (NFL), Major League Baseball (MLB), National Collegiate Athletic Association (NCAA), and the International Olympic Committee (IOC). Despite the dangers, the number of athletes who abuse anabolic steroids is unknown.

Cocaine

Cocaine is another illegal drug that is commonly abused. It is a white, powdery substance obtained from the coca plant.

People can become addicted to cocaine easily and quickly. After only a few days of being high, they become addicted and feel they must find a way to afford the drug. This can lead people to steal or even become drug dealers.

A concentrated form of cocaine that is often smoked is called *crack*. Crack is relatively inexpensive, which has led to its increased abuse. Crack is even more highly addictive, and therefore more harmful, than regular cocaine.

People who use cocaine often feel paranoia. They may abuse other drugs to calm down from the cocaine high. This combination of drugs can be deadly. Cocaine may cause seizures and damage to the heart, stomach, and liver. Because cocaine is often sniffed, it can also damage the nasal cavity.

Other Abused Drugs

People abuse many other illegal drugs. These include PCP, LSD, and heroin. These drugs are highly addictive and damage the blood vessels, heart, brain, lungs, reproductive organs, and nose. They may cause frenzied visions, physical violence, and even death.

Legal drugs can also be abused, **15-11**. Legal drugs include over-the-counter drugs and prescription medications. These drugs should be used only according to package directions or as directed by your doctor. Also, never use someone else's prescription drugs.

Legal drugs also include substances contained in other products not sold for their drug effects. *Caffeine* is one such substance. Caffeine is a stimulant found in coffee, tea, and some soft drinks. These products are marketed as beverages, not as drugs. Consuming large amounts of these products, however, can have negative effects, such as headaches, nervousness, and stomach disorders. Using excessive amounts of these products constitutes drug abuse.

Other products not sold as drugs, but often abused, include spray paint, glue, cleaning supplies, permanent markers, and nail polish remover. These products contain substances known as *inhalants*. People who abuse these

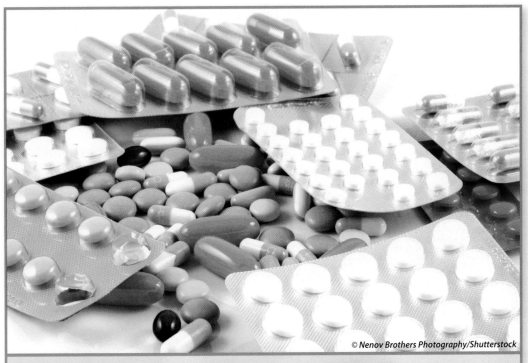

© Nenov Brothers Photography/Shutterstock

15-11 Legal drugs, such as coffee, cold medicines, prescription drugs, and diet aids, can be harmful if abused.

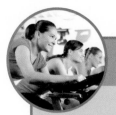

Health Connections

Avoid Risky Behaviors

Have you ever noticed that highly involved people with many interests rarely take risks with their health? They are literally too busy to waste time on tobacco, alcohol, and drugs. You can develop a high standard for your own behavior to avoid risking your health in these ways. Keep busy. For instance, if you love music, take lessons and join a school band. Volunteer for a local community organization that helps others in need.

Sometimes, it is your friends who want you to risk your health by trying to make the behaviors look like fun. You always have a choice. Remember the following options if you are in a situation that feels wrong:

- Practice saying *no* and mean it.
- Provide other safe activities.
- Leave the situation; if needed, call an adult or trusted friend to pick you up.

products intentionally inhale them for their intoxicating effects. This is known as *sniffing*. Abusing inhalants causes damage to the nervous system, kidneys, and blood. Sniffing has also been known to cause severe brain damage and death.

There are many other legal and illegal drugs that can be harmful. A good way to deal with drugs is to use products only in the ways they are intended.

Health Risk Resources

Many sources of help exist for people who want to stop smoking or who have problems with alcohol or other drugs. Many clinics offer programs to help people stop smoking. Every state and many cities and communities have agencies devoted to the treatment of alcohol and drug problems. Churches and hospitals offer programs to help. School nurses, counselors, teachers, or family members may be able to refer you to professional help.

Alcoholics Anonymous (AA) is a well-known and effective self-help organization. Members support each other in their effort to quit drinking. When they are tempted to drink, they call other members who help them fight the urge.

Al-Anon and Alateen are organizations to help people cope with family members who are alcoholics. Regular meetings are held to give family members support with their problems.

Look online or in the yellow pages of the telephone book under "Drug Abuse and Addiction" for sources of help for drug problems. You will find agencies and support groups for drug users and the families of drug users.

Reading Review

1. Give two excuses teens give for smoking and a response to each excuse.
2. True or false. Alcohol speeds up a person's reactions to pain and danger.
3. List four lasting effects alcohol can have on health.
4. Using a drug for a purpose other than one for which it was intended is called _____. *(2 words)*
5. List five sources of help for problems with tobacco, alcohol, or drugs.

First Aid

Objectives

After studying this section, you will be able to
- **identify** types of common injuries and illnesses.
- **follow** recommended treatments for minor injuries and common illnesses.

Key Terms		
calamine lotion	R.I.C.E.	abdominal thrust
sprains	poison	immunizations
strains		

The first aid procedures discussed in the following section are simple and basic. They will help you deal with everyday types of injuries and illnesses.

Treating Common Injuries

Hardly anyone gets through life without a few minor injuries. Such injuries may include scrapes and cuts, falls, minor burns, reactions to poisonings or poisonous plants, choking, or dental injuries. You can treat many minor injuries at home, **15-12**. Some injuries require treatment from medical professionals. Others, still, require emergency medical help.

Scrapes and Cuts

Mild scrapes and cuts happen during everyday activities. Keeping these wounds clean and preventing infection are your main goals for scrapes and cuts. Severe wounds require medical treatment. These include deep cuts, wounds that continue bleeding after applying continuous pressure, and animal bites. For severe wounds, seek emergency medical help by phoning 911 or other emergency number in

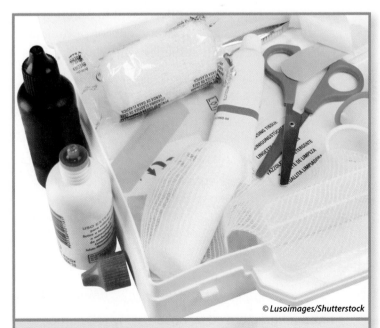

© Lusoimages/Shutterstock

15-12 Having basic first aid supplies organized in a first aid kit can help you deal with injuries calmly and efficiently.

your area. Certain wounds may require stitches or a tetanus shot from a medical professional.

Use the following procedure to treat minor scrapes and cuts:

1. **Stop bleeding.** Apply pressure to the cut or scrape with a clean cloth or sterile gauze until the bleeding stops, usually about 20 minutes. Minor cuts and scrapes often stop bleeding on their own.

2. **Clean the scrape or cut.** Use *clear* water to rinse all dirt or debris from the scrape or cut. It is not necessary to use soap or antiseptic cleaners directly in the wound because they can irritate the skin. You can, however, clean the area around the scrape or cut with soap, water, and a clean cloth.

3. **Cover the scrape or cut.** Use a clean, dry bandage to cover the scrape or cut to keep it clean and free of harmful bacteria. Change the bandage every day or sooner if it becomes wet or dirty.

4. **Observe for signs of infection.** Signs of infection in a scrape or cut may include redness, drainage, or increasing pain or swelling. If you notice any of these signs, call your doctor. If symptoms are severe, call 911 or seek help at your local emergency room.

Insect bites and stings require similar treatment. Wash the area with soap and water and apply cold, wet compresses to help reduce the itching and swelling. **Calamine lotion**, a zinc oxide mixture with a small amount of ferric (iron) oxide, can help reduce itching, too. If the insect has a stinger, be sure to pull it out and wash the area with soap and water. Some people may have allergic reactions that are severe and happen quickly. In such cases, call 911 or other emergency medical number for help.

Falls

Running, walking, or tripping can all cause falls under the right circumstances. These events often result in minor scrapes and cuts, bruises, or bumps. Thoroughly cleaning scrapes and cuts or putting an ice pack on bruises and bumps may be the only treatment required. When falls result in serious injuries, seek emergency medical help immediately.

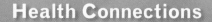

Health Connections

Severe Allergic Reactions

Some people experience severe allergic reactions from a variety of substances. Such substances may include the venom from insect bites and stings, reactions to certain foods, mold, dust, or tree and plant pollens. Call 911 or another emergency medical number if you notice any of the following signs of severe allergic reaction:
- breathing difficulty
- swelling of the lips, mouth, or throat
- hives (characterized by raised, itchy red bumps on the skin)
- nausea and vomiting
- fainting, dizziness, or confusion

Sprains, Strains, and Broken Bones

Sprains and strains are common injuries for teens and young children. **Sprains** are injuries that result from tearing ligaments and tendons, usually at a joint such as a knee, elbow, or ankle. **Strains** are injuries that result from overstretching muscles. Symptoms of sprains and strains often include swelling, bruising, joint or muscle pain, and difficulty moving the injured area. A simple treatment you can do at home is **R.I.C.E.**, which includes *rest, ice, compression,* and *elevation,* **15-13**.

Serious falls may result in broken bones or fractures. Symptoms of a broken bone may be a *snapping* sound during the injury, inability to move a body part or put weight on it, or swelling and bruising. If the injury is to the head, neck, or back, or a broken bone that breaks through the skin, call 911 or other emergency number. Do not move the person with the injury while you wait for medical help to arrive.

If bleeding occurs as the result of a fall, apply pressure with a clean cloth and attempt to stop the bleeding. Loosen clothing around the injured person's neck for easier breathing. Make the person comfortable and do not provide anything to eat or drink. If the fall appears to have caused serious injuries, call 911 or other emergency medical number for help.

The R.I.C.E. Treatment

- **Rest.** Rest the injured body part until the injury is less painful.
- **Ice.** Use an ice pack or cold compress and apply it to the injured body part. Be sure to wrap the ice pack or compress in a towel to avoid direct contact with the skin. Apply the ice for 20 minutes four or more times per day.
- **Compression.** Wear an elastic compression bandage or wrap on the injured area for a minimum of two days.
- **Elevate.** Raise the injured body part above the level of your heart to reduce swelling. For instance, if you have an elbow injury, elevate your arm on a pillow (either sitting or lying down) so the level of your elbow is above your heart.

15-13 Following the steps of the R.I.C.E. method at home can help you treat minor sprains and strains.

Burns

Burns can happen in a number of ways. Bumping a hot pot on a cooktop and burns from hot liquids are common. You can treat mild burns easily at home using the following guidelines:

- Remove clothing from around the burn injury. If any clothing is stuck to the burn, *do not* remove it. Seek medical help.
- Run *cool* water on the burn for several minutes or until the pain decreases.
- *Do not* apply butter, ointments, or other types of remedies. These items can cause infection.
- *Do not* break any blisters that form to help avoid infection.

Serious burns require immediate medical treatment. Such burns may involve large parts of the body (especially the face, hands, and feet), or may come from fire, chemicals, or electricity. Call 911 or other emergency number for immediate assistance.

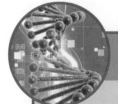

Science Connections

Types of Burns

First-degree burns are the mildest type of burns. Redness, pain, and minor swelling may be visible. This type of burn does not produce blisters because it affects only the top layer of skin. *Second-degree burns* are more serious because they affect several skin layers beneath the top layer. Second-degree burns often result in blisters, severe pain, and redness. *Third-degree burns* are the most severe because they affect all skin layers, underlying tissues, and possibly the nerves. Burn areas may be charred, leathery, or waxy in appearance. Burn area may be numb because of nerve damage. Treatment of a burn depends on the burn type, area affected, and the cause of the burn.

Poisonings

A **poison** can be any substance that harms the human body. Poisons come from many sources. They may include carbon monoxide (a toxic fume), prescription medications, or illegal drugs. Chemicals from household products, indoor and outdoor plants, and metals such as lead and mercury are also poisonous substances. Symptoms of poisoning may include

- drowsiness or unconsciousness
- breathing difficulties
- behavior changes
- mental confusion
- burns or redness around the mouth from drinking poisons
- vomiting

If you suspect poisoning, call 911 or your local poison control center. Follow any treatment directions the poison control center staff gives to you while you wait for help. If carbon monoxide poisoning is a suspect (from a malfunctioning furnace, for instance), get to fresh air immediately.

Reactions to Poisonous Plants

Most people react to plants such as poison ivy and poison oak, **15-14**. Contact with these plants commonly causes redness and itching. There may be blisters and a burning sensation. At times, a headache or high fever may also occur. Do the following to treat a reaction to a poisonous plant:

- Remove clothing that has come in contact with the poisonous plant. Wash the clothing in hot water with a heavy-duty detergent. This will break up the plant oil in the clothes and wash it away.
- Wash affected skin areas with soap and water. Apply a soothing lotion such as calamine lotion or take an oatmeal bath to help relieve itching. The symptoms usually disappear within 48 hours after contact.

Severe reactions to poisonous plants will cover large parts of the body and continue to get worse. At times, the skin may look infected. People who have severe reactions need medical attention.

Electric Shock

In the event of an electric shock, do not touch the injured person or the source of electric current. Turn off the current by unplugging the appliance or turning off the circuit. You may need to separate the injured person from the source of electricity.

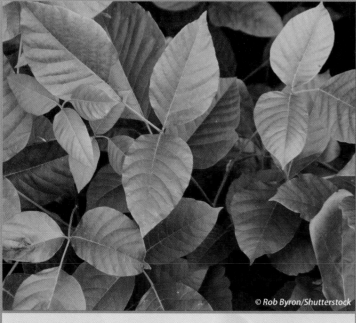

© Rob Byron/Shutterstock

15-14 People commonly contract poison ivy by touching the leaves of the plant, or by coming in contact with something else that has touched it, such as clothing or a pet.

Be careful to protect yourself from the current. For instance, wear shoes with rubber soles or other material that does not conduct electricity. Use a wooden pole or board or some other nonconducting material to do this. Immediately call 911 or other emergency number for medical help.

Choking

Choking occurs when a piece of food or other object gets stuck in a person's throat. The food or object can block the air passage and prevent the victim from speaking or breathing. The lack of air causes the victim's face to turn blue and he or she will collapse. Without removal of the food or object from the air passage, the individual could die within minutes.

If a person is coughing and gagging but can still talk and breathe, observe but do not attempt to dislodge the object. With continued coughing, the person will likely dislodge the food or object on his or her own. If the person cannot breathe or speak, a trained person can use the **abdominal thrust** (or *Heimlich Maneuver*) procedure. Using this procedure can dislodge a piece of food or other item that is stuck in a choking victim's throat. Call 911 or other emergency number if the object cannot be dislodged.

Before attempting to perform the abdominal thrust or CPR, take a first-aid certified training course through your local Red Cross or American Heart Association.

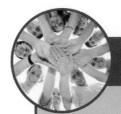

Community Connections

CPR Training

A victim of electric shock may need *CPR*. *Cardiopulmonary resuscitation (CPR)* is a combination of chest compression and rescue breathing that can save lives in an emergency, but you absolutely need to know how to perform it properly. It can only be used on a person who has stopped breathing and who is without a heartbeat. Your school, local Red Cross, or local American Heart Association may offer classes on this technique. Check with these resources in your community if you are interested in learning more about the CPR procedure.

Dental Injuries

Injuries to teeth can happen in a number of ways and are common with teens. Auto accidents, falls, work activities, and sports activities such as soccer, football, baseball, and hockey can all be sources of dental injuries. Such injuries might include a tooth that is knocked out, a loose tooth that is not completely out, or a broken tooth. If you or someone you know experiences a dental injury to a permanent tooth, do the following:
- Pick up the tooth or piece of tooth by the crown, not the root area. If a tooth cannot be put back in its socket, put the tooth in a clean container with *whole milk*, not water.
- Rinse the mouth with warm water.
- Apply a cold compress to the injured tooth area.
- Bite down on a clean gauze pad in the injured area to help stop bleeding.
- Seek emergency dental assistance.

To prevent dental injuries, wear proper protective equipment. For instance, be sure to wear the mouth guards required for sports activities.

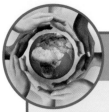

Global Connections

Travel Immunizations

There are some countries for which the Center for Disease Control (CDC) recommends special immunizations. Many are Third World countries with health risks, such as malaria, typhus, dengue fever, or avian flu. Check the *Destinations* page on their website at wwwnc.cdc.gov/travel to see their recommendations by country.

Most vaccines take time to become effective in your body, so make a doctor's appointment at least four to six weeks before your trip. Some vaccines must be given in a series over a period of days or sometimes weeks. If it is less than four weeks before you leave, you should still see your doctor. You can benefit from shots, medications, and information about protecting yourself from illness. The more informed you are about the diseases in your destinations, the more preventable they are.

Treating Common Illnesses

Most people experience a cold or influenza occasionally along with diarrhea, fevers, headaches, and nausea and vomiting. Knowing how to ease the discomfort of these problems without seeing a doctor is important information. If the illness does not clear up in a reasonable amount of time, see a doctor. Table **15-15** explains how to treat these common illnesses. Although common illnesses generally transmit easily from one person to another, it is possible to limit how often you get sick. Using proper hand-washing techniques and washing your hands often can help prevent illness.

Many contagious diseases that are harmful to the human population can be limited or prevented through immunizations. **Immunizations** are treatments that help people's bodies develop antibodies to resist certain diseases, such as polio, tetanus, or measles, mumps, and rubella.

Many doctors agree that giving children immunizations starting at birth can provide the most protection from disease. Some parents disagree, however. They feel that immunizations (or vaccinations) can lead to other diseases. Parents who choose not to immunize their children should understand, however, that if a child contracts one of these diseases, it could cause serious illness or death.

Schools usually require parents to submit immunization records for their children before admission. The American Academy of Pediatrics website provides a recommended list of childhood immunizations from birth through 18 years of age.

Reading Review

1. Describe the procedure for treating minor scrapes and cuts.
2. How do you treat minor sprains and strains?
3. What are two things you should *not* do when treating minor burns?
4. Name three symptoms of poisoning.
5. Treatments that help people's bodies develop antibodies to resist certain diseases are called _____.

Treating Common Illnesses	
Illness and Symptoms	**Recommended Treatment**
Common cold (symptoms may include runny nose, sneezing, sore throat, coughing, and headaches)	For adults, take aspirin, aspirin substitutes, or over-the-counter medications. For children and teens, use aspirin substitutes to avoid triggering Reye's syndrome (an often fatal brain disease in childhood). Such drugs will not cure the cold, but will relieve symptoms. Stay away from other people during the first few days of a cold and wash your hands often. Drink plenty of liquids and get plenty of rest. A vaporizer may help clear nasal passages.
Diarrhea (watery stools)	Drink plenty of clear fluids to avoid dehydration. Do not drink milk. Try to eat, but avoid greasy or fatty foods. See a doctor if diarrhea continues more than 48 hours.
Fever (temperature above 98.6°F)	Wear minimal clothing and coverings and try to avoid shivering. Drink cool fluids. Take fever-reducing drugs. A lukewarm bath may help. See a doctor if the fever is high, occurs with other symptoms, or lasts more than three days.
Influenza (symptoms may include fever, aches, and a tired feeling, as well as all symptoms of a cold)	Follow the directions for treating a cold. Get plenty of rest. If a fever spikes over 100°F, consult a medical professional. Children and older adults, or those with chronic health conditions should see a doctor for treatment. Get a yearly flu shot.
Headache	Headache may be a sign of illness, stress, or anxiety. Try applying an ice pack to the painful area. Ask someone to rub your neck and shoulders to help relieve tension headaches. A short period of rest in a dimly lit room may help relieve the pain. Take an over-the-counter pain reliever if necessary. Children and teens should avoid aspirin. Learning to reduce stress or deal with it can help prevent future headaches related to stress and anxiety.
Nausea and vomiting	Avoid food and increase liquid intake. This is especially important for young children because frequent vomiting can cause dehydration. Over-the-counter medications can make the patient more comfortable. Call a doctor if the condition continues.
Allergies (symptoms may include sneezing and coughing, itchy and watery eyes, rash or hives, difficulty breathing)	Avoid allergens if possible. Use over-the-counter allergy medications according to directions. See a doctor for severe allergies.
Asthma (symptoms may include difficulty breathing, wheezing, coughing, or chest tightness)	Avoid substances that trigger asthma flare-ups. Follow the asthma plan and take controller medications as prescribed by a doctor. Keep medications with you at all times.

15-15 This table offers suggestions for treating common illnesses.

Chapter Summary

Section 15-1. Looking your best begins with following basic practices for good health. Cleaning and caring for your body properly will keep you looking good. Bathing or showering daily will keep your body looking and smelling fresh. Shampooing your hair and keeping it neatly styled will add to your total appearance. Keeping your fingernails and toenails clean and neatly trimmed will make your hands and feet look nice. Brushing and flossing your teeth regularly will help them stay clean and strong. Eating healthful foods, being physically active, and getting plenty of sleep can also help you look and feel your best.

Sometimes change can lead to stress. Anxiety, fear, conflict, and worry can be signs of stress. There are also many physical signs indicating stress. Learn ways to avoid stress if possible. Also, learn healthy ways to handle stress when it does occur.

Section 15-2. Tobacco, alcohol, and other drugs present risks to your health. Teens give many reasons for using these substances, even though they may be aware of the harm they can cause. People who want to help with substance abuse problems can turn to a number of resources. Getting help, or avoiding these risks altogether, is an important step to a more healthful lifestyle.

Section 15-3. Common injuries include scrapes and cuts, falls, burns, poisonings, electric shock, choking, and dental injuries. Knowing how to treat minor injuries can help prevent further injuries and infections. Common illnesses can easily transmit from person to person. Following thorough hand-washing procedures can help limit the transmittal of illness.

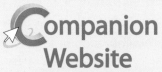

Companion Website

www.g-wlearning.com

Check your understanding of the main concepts for Chapter 15 at the website.

Critical Thinking

1. **Determine.** What can you do to make time for physical activity when you have a busy schedule?
2. **Assess.** What can be done to keep children and young adults from abusing drugs, tobacco, and alcohol?
3. **Analyze.** Why do you think some people avoid having immunizations or having their children immunized? What are some of the advantages and disadvantages of immunizations?

Common Core

College and Career Readiness

4. **Listening.** Interview the school nurse or someone from the local health department on skin cancer and how it can be prevented.

Prepare a list of questions prior to the interview.

5. **Speaking.** Survey 10 people who do not smoke. Ask them how they feel when forced to be around smokers. Summarize your findings in an article for your school website or newsletter.

6. **Writing.** Write a pamphlet about basic first aid procedures. Obtain permission to display the pamphlet in a prominent place in your school.

7. **Listening.** Plan for your school to have a *Health Fair*. Invite local physicians, nurses, dentists, dietitians, or others who would be willing to come and set up a booth. Ideas could include blood pressure checking, cholesterol screening, anti-cancer information, eating disorder information, and dental care stations. Visit your local health department or center and obtain free informational brochures on a variety of topics to pass out at the fair.

Technology

8. **Electronic Presentation.** Prepare an electronic presentation about ways you would advise other teens to say *no* to tobacco, alcohol, and other drugs. As part of your presentation, include research concerning the laws in your state that relate to smoking, drinking, and drug abuse. Share your presentations in class.

Journal Writing

9. Keep a *health habit* journal for one week. In your journal, list all the foods you eat each day. List all the physical activities you do and how many minutes you spend doing them. Record how much sleep you get each night. At the end of the week, evaluate the journal for strong and weak points in your personal health habits. Then create a plan to address any changes you might want to make in your daily health habits.

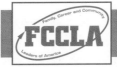

FCCLA

10. *Student Body* is a national FCCLA program that focuses on teaching others how to eat right, be fit, and make healthy choices. Select one or more health related issues teens deal with and create an awareness campaign promoting positive health habits. Use the *FCCLA Planning Process* to develop strategies for your campaign. See your adviser for information as needed.

Chapter 16
Nutrition and You

Reading Prep

College and Career Readiness

Before you read this chapter, go the end of the chapter and read the *Chapter Summary*. The summary highlights the main points of the chapter. How does this activity help you prepare to understand the content?

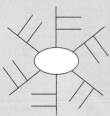

Concept Organizer

Use a diagram like the one shown to identify the six classes of nutrients. List a function and a source for each nutrient.

Companion Website

Print out the concept organizer for Chapter 16 at the website.

Companion Website
www.g-wlearning.com

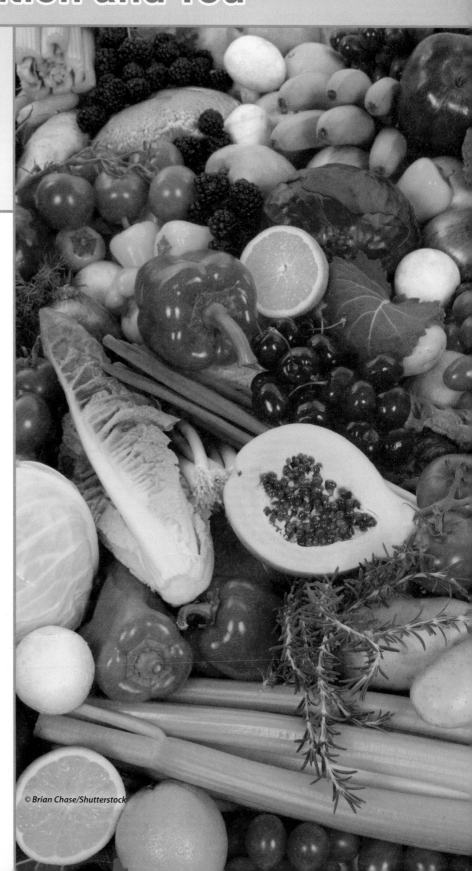

© Brian Chase/Shutterstock

Understanding Nutrients

Objectives

After studying this section, you will be able to
*   **justify** the importance of good nutrition.
*   **list** the essential nutrients and describe their functions and sources.
*   **understand** how needed amounts of nutrients are determined.

Key Terms		
diet	protein	vitamins
nutrition	carbohydrates	fortify
nutrients	deficiency	minerals
malnutrition	fats	

Although you have had years of experience eating food, do you really know enough to make wise food choices? This chapter helps you understand why eating healthful foods is important. It also discusses and provides information about substances in foods your body needs for good health.

Eating for Good Health

When you look in the mirror, what do you see? Do you have a clear complexion, bright eyes, and good posture? Do you have strong white teeth and healthy nails? Is your body the right weight for your body build? These characteristics are signs of good health, **16-1**.

Good health requires a healthful eating pattern, or diet. A **diet** is all the foods you regularly eat and drink. A healthful diet is necessary for good nutrition. **Nutrition** is the study of how your body processes and uses the foods you eat and drink. Good nutrition results when you provide your body with healthful foods that supply needed nutrients. **Nutrients** are the substances in food that are used by your body to grow and function properly.

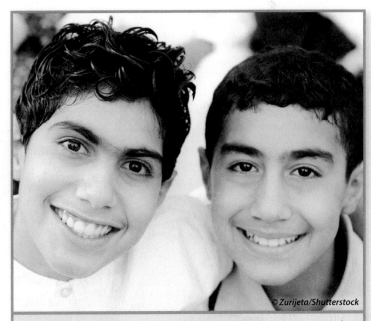
© Zurijeta/Shutterstock

16-1 Bright eyes, shiny hair, a clear complexion, and strong teeth are all signs of good health.

Someone who looks in the mirror and does not see the characteristics described earlier may be suffering from malnutrition. **Malnutrition** results when a person's diet lacks needed nutrients over a period of time. It could be caused by not eating the right amount or selection of foods.

Malnutrition can cause irritability, overweight, underweight, tooth decay, and skin problems. A tired feeling and a lack of resistance to disease are other problems related to poor nutrition. Feeling good about yourself is difficult if you have health problems. By taking care of yourself, you may be able to avoid many of these problems. If you eat foods that are good for you and get plenty of rest and exercise, you are promoting good health. When you are in good health, it is easier to look, act, and feel your best, **16-2**.

What you eat now not only affects how you look and feel today, but also affects your future health. Your body and mind are growing at a rapid rate. Eating the right foods helps you develop to the fullest possible extent. Good health in adulthood benefits all aspects of your life.

Nutrients

You may have heard the expression "You are what you eat." This means eating a combination of foods that supply few or no nutrients could lead to poor health. Likewise, eating a combination of foods that are rich in nutrients promotes good health.

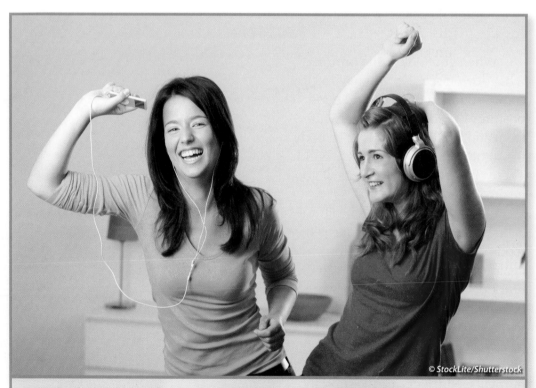

© StockLite/Shutterstock

16-2 Exercise and eating right can help keep you healthy and allow you to do the activities you enjoy.

Selecting a healthful combination of foods requires a basic understanding of nutrients. Six types of nutrients found in foods act to promote growth and development, provide energy, and regulate body functions. These six essential nutrients are proteins, carbohydrates, fats, vitamins, minerals, and water. No single food supplies all the nutrients required to nourish the body. Eating a variety of foods is necessary to obtain all the nutrients your body needs.

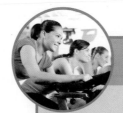

Health Connections

Conditional Amino Acids

Sometimes amino acids that can be made by the body under normal conditions, can no longer be made by the body. These amino acids must then be obtained in the diet. This type of amino acid is called *conditionally indispensable*. Conditions that could cause insufficient production of these amino acids may occur in infants that are born too early. Illness or stress can bring about this change as well.

Protein

Your skin, hair, nails, muscles, blood, and all other body tissues contain protein. **Protein** is needed for growth, maintenance, and repair of tissues. Protein is also needed to control body processes, such as blood circulation, breathing, and digestion. Protein can also be used to supply energy when necessary.

Proteins are made of *amino acids*. Amino acids can be thought of as blocks that your body uses to build the type of protein it needs. The body can make some amino acids. Others, called *indispensable amino acids* (also called *essential amino acids*), cannot be made by the body. They must be obtained through foods.

Meat, fish, poultry, cheese, eggs, milk, processed soy products, beans and peas, nuts, and seeds are all food sources of protein. Protein foods fall into two main groups—complete and incomplete proteins. The protein from animal food sources is called *complete protein*. Complete proteins supply all the indispensable amino acids your body needs. The protein from plant food sources is called *incomplete protein*. Incomplete proteins supply only some of the indispensable amino acids. To meet the body's needs, different incomplete proteins can be combined to provide all the needed amino acids. For instance, red beans and rice are two incomplete proteins that together provide all the needed amino acids. Incomplete proteins that can be combined to supply indispensable amino acids are called *complementary proteins*.

People who do not eat enough protein-rich foods may grow more slowly. They may also develop infections more easily and recover from illnesses at a slower rate. You can see why eating protein foods each day is important.

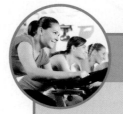

Health Connections

Complementary Proteins

It was once believed that complementary proteins had to be eaten at the same meal to provide all the needed amino acids for the body. Current studies have shown that is not the case. Complementary proteins will be effective when eaten within a day or so of each other.

Carbohydrates

Carbohydrates are the body's main source of energy. When insufficient carbohydrates are eaten to meet your body's energy needs, the body may use protein to meet those needs. Carbohydrates play an important role by sparing proteins for the job of building and repairing tissues.

The two main types of carbohydrates are simple carbohydrates and complex carbohydrates. Simple carbohydrates are called *sugars* and can be used by your body as a quick source of energy. Some sugars occur naturally in foods such as fruit and milk. Other sugars, such as table sugar, are produced from plants and are added to foods. Complex carbohydrates found in foods include *starches* and *fiber*. Starches take longer for your body to use as an energy source than sugars. Potatoes, yams, lentils, and dried beans and peas are good sources of starch. Grains such as wheat, rice, and corn are also rich sources of starches. *Whole grains* that have had little or no processing can also be a rich source of fiber as well as other nutrients, **16-3**. Fiber supplies your body with little or no energy, but provides other benefits. Fiber aids in digestion by helping push foods through the body at the proper speed. Fiber is also found in fruits and vegetables.

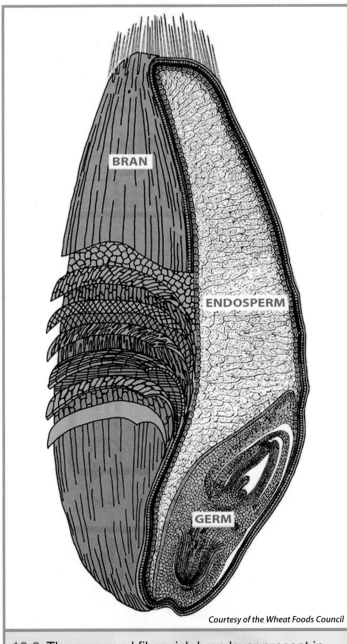

BRAN

ENDOSPERM

GERM

Courtesy of the Wheat Foods Council

16-3 The germ and fiber-rich bran layer present in whole grains are often removed during processing.

The amount of carbohydrates needed each day depends on a person's age, gender, body size, and level of activity. Select carbohydrate sources such as fruits, vegetables, dairy, and whole grains that are also rich in other nutrients, and limit foods containing added sugars such as candy and soft drinks. Excess calories from carbohydrates or other foods can result in weight gain. Your body stores starch and sugar you do not need for energy as fat. If you do not eat enough carbohydrates, you may feel tired. In the United States, an individual rarely suffers from a **deficiency**, or shortage of carbohydrates in his or her diet. He or she is more likely to be consuming too much carbohydrate in the form of added sugars and refined grains, and not enough whole grains.

Fats

Fats are concentrated sources of energy found in both animal and plant foods. They supply more than twice as much energy than is supplied by the same amount of protein or carbohydrate. Fats from animal sources are solid at room temperature and are called *saturated fats*. Fats from plant sources are *unsaturated fats* and are liquid at room temperature. These fats are referred to as *oils*, **16-4**. Oils are important to include in your eating pattern because they provide essential nutrients that your body cannot produce. Oils are needed to keep your body functioning properly. Saturated fats are not necessary for a healthful diet.

Excess calories from protein, carbohydrates, and fat are stored as body fat. Your body fat insulates and protects vital organs such as your heart, liver, and kidneys. It also forms a layer just under your skin that protects your body from cold temperatures. This fat can also be used for future energy needs when food is not available.

Saturated fats are found in foods such as butter, meats, and cheeses. Trans fats are oils that have been processed to create a solid fat. Trans fats are found in shortening, some margarines, and many snack and dessert foods. Diets high in saturated and trans fats are associated with higher risk for certain chronic diseases. Reducing these types of fats in the diet and replacing them with oils may help to lower risk for these diseases. Excess calories from fats as well as carbohydrates and protein may cause weight gain. Excess weight can also result in chronic health problems.

Many experts agree that the types of fat in the diet have more impact on health risk than the total fat in the diet. A more healthful diet replaces saturated and trans fats with oils. You can limit your intake of saturated fat by choosing low-fat dairy products and lean meats (meats containing very little fat). Avoiding too many fried foods is another way you can limit the amount of saturated and trans fats you eat.

Many high-fat foods are also high in cholesterol. *Cholesterol* is a fatlike substance found in every human cell and is part of many hormones. It is not essential to your diet because your body also produces cholesterol. In the diet, cholesterol is found only in animal food sources. Plant foods such as olive oil contain no cholesterol. Health authorities link too much cholesterol in the diet with heart disease. They recommend you limit dietary cholesterol to reduce your risk of health problems.

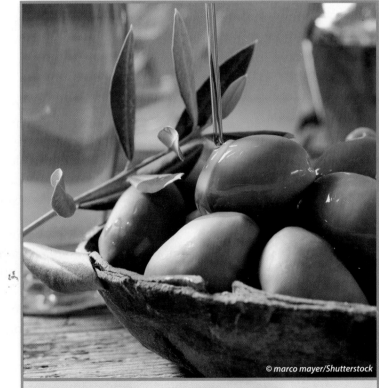

© marco mayer/Shutterstock

16-4 Oil extracted from the fruit of the olive tree is a source of essential nutrients.

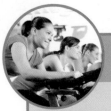

Vitamins

Vitamins are substances needed by the body for growth and maintenance. Vitamins help regulate the chemical processes in your body. They provide no energy, but are necessary for your body to store and use energy for growth and development. Although required in very small amounts, vitamins are essential to life and health. For this reason, the government requires companies to **fortify** some foods by adding certain vitamins or other nutrients. Eating foods that are naturally rich in vitamins does not guarantee your body is receiving them. Many vitamins are damaged by heat and light. To preserve vitamins, limit exposure to light and heat during food storage and preparation.

Vitamins are either fat-soluble or water-soluble. *Fat-soluble* vitamins are carried through your body by fats. You do not need to eat food sources of fat-soluble vitamins every day because they can be stored by your body. In fact, getting more than the required amounts of these vitamins could make you sick.

Water-soluble vitamins dissolve in water, which allows any unused amounts to be expelled with body wastes. Water-soluble vitamins cannot be stored in your body, so you need to eat foods that supply these vitamins every day.

Understanding the role vitamins play in your body and their foods sources will help you choose healthful foods, **16-5**.

Minerals

Minerals are another type of nutrient needed for a healthy body. Much like vitamins, they provide no energy and the body requires them in small amounts. Unlike vitamins, minerals are not damaged by heat or light. Minerals also differ from vitamins in their chemical makeup and structure.

Minerals help regulate many of your body's activities. They help muscles contract and nerves transmit signals to and from the brain. They also help maintain the body's water balance and strengthen bones and teeth.

Minerals are considered either *major minerals* or *trace minerals*, **16-6**. The body needs major minerals in larger quantities than trace minerals. The two types of minerals also differ in the amounts present in the body. Trace minerals are found in much smaller amounts in the body than major minerals. For instance, an average-size male body contains about two and one-half pounds of calcium (a major mineral) and only one-tenth ounce of iron (a trace mineral).

Water

Water is the single most important substance you take into your body. You can get along for days, even weeks, without food. You can only survive a few days without water.

Vitamins and Their Functions

Vitamin	Function
Fat-Soluble Vitamins	
Vitamin A	Aids normal vision, helps body fight infections, needed for normal growth and development Sources: beef liver, sweet potato, broccoli, cantaloupe, spinach, peaches
Vitamin D	Needed for proper development of bones and teeth, controls cell growth Sources: produced by the body when exposed to sunlight, cod liver oil, fortified milk
Vitamin E	Protects cells from possible damage due to exposure to oxygen Sources: vegetable oils, whole-grain breads and cereals, eggs, organ meats, leafy green vegetables
Vitamin K	Helps blood clot Sources: green leafy vegetables, cauliflower, liver, egg yolk
Water-Soluble Vitamins	
Thiamin (vitamin B_1)	Needed for energy production; aids proper heart, nerve, and muscle function Source: whole-grain products, pork, legumes
Riboflavin (vitamin B_2)	Needed for growth and red blood cell production; aids energy production Sources: eggs, green leafy vegetables, lean meats, milk, legumes, nuts
Niacin (vitamin B_3)	Aids digestion, contributes to healthy skin and nerve function, aids energy production Sources: meat, fish, poultry, whole-grain products
Pantothenic acid	Aids growth and development, helps body break down and use food Sources: broccoli, avocado, mushrooms, potatoes, oatmeal, sunflower seeds
Biotin	Aids growth and development, helps body break down and use food Sources: cauliflower, liver, cheese, peanuts
B_6	Needed for production of proteins and red blood cells, aids energy production, promotes healthy nervous system Sources: fortified cereals, bananas, potatoes, liver, garbanzo beans
Folate	Promotes healthy cell growth, critical for healthy development of fetus Sources: dark-green, leafy vegetables, orange juice, liver, sunflower seeds, legumes, fortified cereals
B_{12}	Helps body break down and use food, aids development of red blood cells and healthy nerve function Sources: beef, milk products, shellfish
Vitamin C	Protects cells from possible damage due to exposure to oxygen, aids skin and bone health, helps body use iron, aids healing Sources: oranges, strawberries, broccoli, raw spinach, banana, cauliflower

Lists of food sources are not all inclusive.

16-5 Eating a varied diet will help you obtain all the vitamins your body needs.

Minerals and Their Functions

Mineral	Function
Major Minerals	
Sodium	Helps with nerve and muscle function, maintains fluid balance in the body Sources: table salt, processed foods
Magnesium	Helps with energy production and transport, needed for protein production, aids nerve and muscle function Sources: dark green, leafy vegetables; bananas; avocados; almonds; legumes; whole grains
Phosphorus	Needed for tooth and bone formation, needed for energy storage and protein production, aids body's use and storage of carbohydrate and fat Sources: meats, milk products
Sulfur	Helps maintain acid-base balance in body, aids in removing drugs from the body Sources: all foods containing protein
Chloride	Maintains fluid balance in the body, needed for proper digestion Sources: table salt, tomatoes, lettuce, celery, olives
Potassium	Needed for growth, helps regulate acid-base balance in body, aids in production of proteins, needed for normal heart function Sources: meat, poultry, salmon, cod, soy products, broccoli, sweet potatoes, cantaloupe, bananas, milk, nuts
Calcium	Supports structure of bones and teeth, needed for muscle movement and proper nerve function, helps move blood throughout body, aids in release of hormones and enzymes Sources: dairy foods, broccoli, Chinese cabbage, canned sardines and salmon, fortified foods
Trace Minerals	
Fluoride	Supports the structure of bones and teeth Source: drinking water
Chromium	Involved in body's use and storage of carbohydrate, protein, and fat Sources: meat, whole-grain products
Manganese	Serves as key part of enzymes involved in preventing tissue damage Sources: fresh pineapple, oatmeal, brown rice, tea, coffee
Iron	Helps carry oxygen throughout the body, part of many proteins in the body Sources: Dried beans, dried fruits, lean red meat, dark meat poultry, salmon, whole grains
Copper	Helps red blood cell formation; needed for healthy bones, nerves, blood vessels, and immune system Sources: oysters, shellfish, whole grains, beans, nuts, potatoes
Zinc	Needed for immune system to work properly, aids cell growth and healing, required for senses of taste and smell Sources: meats, dark meat poultry, nuts, whole grains, legumes
Selenium	Helps prevent cell damage Sources: vegetables, fish, meat, grains, eggs
Molybdenum	Required for production of some important enzymes in the body Sources: Peas, beans, some breakfast cereals, liver
Iodine	Helps convert food into energy, required for normal thyroid function Sources: iodized table salt, seafood, dairy products

Lists of food sources are not all inclusive.

16-6 Minerals are found in both plant- and animal-based foods.

About two-thirds of your body is made up of water. Water carries nutrients into cells and carries wastes out of the body. The food you eat cannot be digested and used by the body without an adequate supply of water. Water also helps regulate the internal temperature of your body.

Your body needs about three and one-half quarts of water daily. The water you drink should provide about 75 percent of your daily water needs, or roughly 10½ cups. You get much of the water you need from the liquids you drink and the rest is supplied by the foods you eat, **16-7**.

Nutrient Amounts

You now know the nutrients your body needs for good health, but how much of each nutrient do you need? Nutrient needs differ based on age, sex, body build, and level of activity. Health also affects nutrient needs. People who are sick or injured have special requirements. In the United States, a set of dietary standards called *Dietary Reference Intakes (DRIs)* recommend how much of each nutrient is needed in the diet. The DRIs are used to help nutritionists evaluate the diets of healthy people. These standards are based on broad research. There are four types of DRIs— Estimated Average Requirement (EAR), Recommended Dietary Allowance (RDA), Adequate Intake (AI), and Tolerable Upper Intake Level (UL). These standards are used by health professionals to develop nutrition guidance for healthy Americans as well as those at increased risk of chronic disease.

Water Content of Some Common Foods

Food	Percent Water*
Iceberg lettuce	96
Zucchini squash	95
Tomatoes	94
Watermelon	93
Cantaloupe	91
Green beans	90
Corn	90
Broccoli	89
Strawberries	89
Yogurt	89
Grapefruit	88
Carrots	88
Milk	87
Eggs, hard-cooked	74
Bananas	76
Ice cream	63
Pizza	48
Bread, whole wheat	36

*percent of the total weight of the food product made up by water.

16-7 Some of your body's water needs are supplied by foods.

Reading Review

1. When does malnutrition result?
2. List the six essential nutrients.
3. Explain the difference between complete and incomplete proteins.
4. Why do health experts recommend you limit dietary cholesterol?
5. What factors affect nutrient needs?

Choosing Foods

Objectives

After studying this section, you will be able to
- **understand** the reasons people eat.
- **apply** guidelines to make healthful food choices.

Key Terms		
Dietary Guidelines for Americans	nutrient dense	MyPlate

You eat food to obtain needed nutrients, but have you ever thought about why you are eating at a particular moment or a specific food? Do you choose the best foods to provide the nutrients your body needs? Learning which foods supply needed nutrients will help you make healthful food choices for your body.

Why You Eat

Hunger prompts people to eat. It communicates your body's need for food. Your body needs food to supply energy so you can carry out your daily activities. It also needs food to provide nutrients for growth and repair of tissues. You may think you eat food simply to survive, but eating fulfills more than just physical needs.

People are not always hungry when they eat. People often eat to meet social needs. People eat at parties, sporting events, family gatherings, and other activities enjoyed with friends and family members. Food adds to these occasions because people take pleasure in sharing food, **16-8**.

Food helps satisfy emotional needs for many people. When people are happy, they eat to celebrate. Other people eat when they are depressed. They feel comforted by food. Nervousness, loneliness, and boredom are just a few of the other emotions some people try to relieve with food.

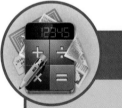

Math Connections

Food Advertising

Roughly $15 billion is spent on advertising U.S. food or candy products every year. Much of these dollars are spent for television advertising directed at children and teens. Some Saturday morning, spend one hour watching a children's TV channel. Keep track of the number of commercials aired during that time. Note how many were for food. List the type of food being advertised—candy bar, cereal, vegetable, milk, fast-food, and so on. Calculate what percent of the total commercials were for food. Next, calculate what percent of the food commercials were for healthful foods such as fruits, vegetables, or dairy products.

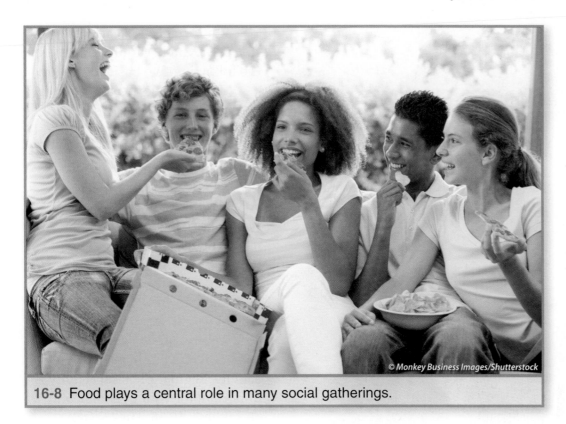

16-8 Food plays a central role in many social gatherings.

Recognizing why you are eating can help you make food choices that benefit your health.

Making Wise Food Choices

A number of factors probably affect your decision about the foods you eat. Often, your food choices are influenced by one or more of the following factors:
- family
- friends
- cultural heritage
- advertising

These factors may or may not be healthful influences. If another family member prepares meals at home, you may not have a choice about what foods you eat, **16-9**. When you are in a restaurant or the school cafeteria, you make your own food choices. As you get older, you are free to make more and more food choices. Learning to choose nutritious foods now will benefit you for a lifetime.

Dietary Guidelines for Americans

The *Dietary Guidelines for Americans* is published by the United States Departments of Agriculture and Health and Human Services. Revised every five years, it serves as basis for many nutrition programs and sources of information in the United States.

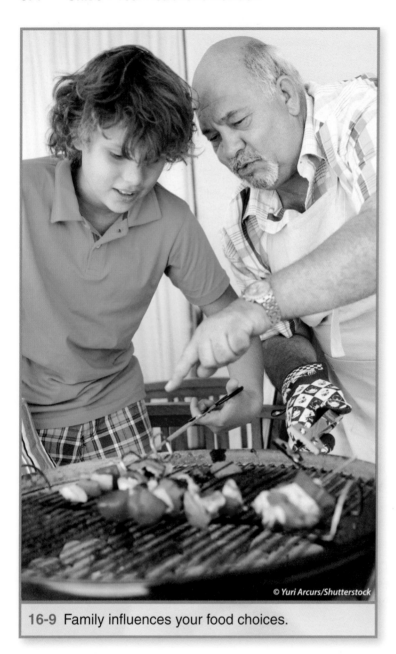

© Yuri Arcurs/Shutterstock

16-9 Family influences your food choices.

The *2010 Dietary Guidelines for Americans* can be summarized in the following two basic messages:

- Maintain calorie balance over time to achieve and sustain a healthy weight.
- Focus on consuming nutrient-dense foods and beverages.

Maintain calorie balance over time to achieve and sustain a healthy weight. At all stages of your life, maintaining a healthy weight positively affects your health and ability to enjoy life. Healthy weight results when the right types of foods are eaten in amounts that balance with your level of physical activity. Regular physical activity is important for your overall health and fitness, **16-10**. The *Dietary Guidelines* recommend you adopt the levels of activity suggested for your age group in the *2008 Physical Activity Guidelines for Americans*.

Focus on consuming nutrient-dense foods and beverages. Foods and beverages that are **nutrient dense** provide vitamins, minerals, and other substances that may have positive health effects with relatively few calories. When a food has added sugars and solid fats, many calories are also added. The added calories act to dilute the food's nutrient density. For instance, to make applesauce, sugar is added to apples as they cook. The nutrients provided by the apples are now diluted by the calories from the added sugar.

MyPlate

The United States Department of Agriculture (USDA) created a tool to help people apply the messages from the *Dietary Guidelines* to their daily life. This tool is the **MyPlate** food guidance system. The MyPlate symbol communicates a simple message about what a healthy plate should look like at mealtime. MyPlate divides foods into five main food groups—fruits, grains, vegetables, protein foods, and dairy. A healthy diet will include foods from each of these groups as well as oils. Oils are not represented on the MyPlate symbol because they are not a food group, but they do provide nutrients your body needs.

For help creating a healthy plate, go to the website ChooseMyPlate.gov. You can create a personalized food plan by entering your age, sex, height, weight, and level of physical activity, **16-11**. The website provides other tools to help you track your food intake and activity, as well as plan a menu. You can also find many tips and resources to help you maintain a healthy weight and make nutrient-dense choices from each food group.

Grains

The grains group includes foods made from wheat, rice, oats, barley, cornmeal, and other grains. For instance, foods in this group include breads, cereals, rice, and pasta. MyPlate divides the grains group into subgroups—whole grains and refined grains. Brown rice, whole-grain breads, popcorn, whole-grain pasta, and oatmeal are examples of whole-grain products. *Refined grains* have been processed in a way that removes the bran and germ. Unfortunately, the many good nutrients the bran and germ provide are removed with them. Examples of refined grains include white rice, white bread, and refined cornmeal. Refined grains that include *enriched* on the label have had some vitamins and minerals added back.

Foods in this group provide a rich supply of carbohydrates. The amount you need from the grains group each day depends on your age, sex, and level of physical activity. Foods in this group are measured in ounce-equivalents. One slice of bread, one cup of ready-to-eat cereal, or one-half cup of cooked rice or pasta counts as one ounce-equivalent.

You should make at least half of your grains whole grains every day. Whole grains are an excellent source of many vitamins and minerals. Choosing whole-grain foods may also reduce your risk for chronic diseases and help with weight management. Whole grains can also be a good source of needed fiber. Limit items high in solid fats and added sugars, such as cakes and cookies. Also, limit your use of spreads and toppings that are high in fat and sugar, such as butter and jam.

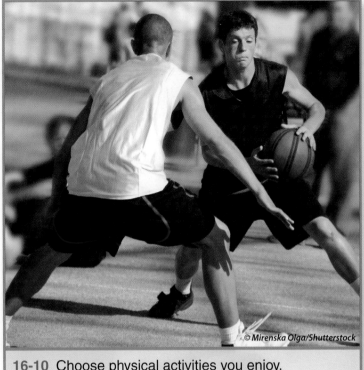

© Mirenska Olga/Shutterstock

16-10 Choose physical activities you enjoy.

Social Studies Connections

White Bread—A Class Issue?

Before advances in the milling process, breads were dark and heavy. During this time, coarsely ground flours made from such things as barley, buckwheat, rice, corn, and even chestnuts were used to make breads. Poorer classes of people ate dark, heavy breads made from these flours. It is believed that the upper class of ancient Rome is responsible for the notion that eating white bread was a sign of status and wealth. They preferred to impress their guests with white breads made with lighter, high quality wheat flour.

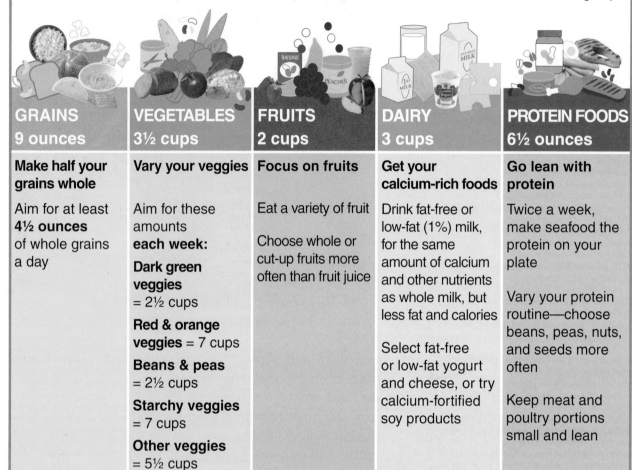

My Daily Food Plan

Based on the information you provided, this is your daily recommended amount from each food group.

GRAINS 9 ounces	VEGETABLES 3½ cups	FRUITS 2 cups	DAIRY 3 cups	PROTEIN FOODS 6½ ounces
Make half your grains whole	**Vary your veggies**	**Focus on fruits**	**Get your calcium-rich foods**	**Go lean with protein**
Aim for at least **4½ ounces** of whole grains a day	Aim for these amounts **each week:** Dark green veggies = 2½ cups Red & orange veggies = 7 cups Beans & peas = 2½ cups Starchy veggies = 7 cups Other veggies = 5½ cups	Eat a variety of fruit Choose whole or cut-up fruits more often than fruit juice	Drink fat-free or low-fat (1%) milk, for the same amount of calcium and other nutrients as whole milk, but less fat and calories Select fat-free or low-fat yogurt and cheese, or try calcium-fortified soy products	Twice a week, make seafood the protein on your plate Vary your protein routine—choose beans, peas, nuts, and seeds more often Keep meat and poultry portions small and lean

Find your balance between food and physical activity

Be physically active for at least **60 minutes** each day.

Know your limits on fats, sugars, and sodium

Your allowance for oils is **8 teaspoons** a day.

Limit calories from solid fats and added sugars to **360 calories** a day.

Reduce sodium intake to less than **2300 mg** a day.

Your results are based on a 2600 calorie pattern   Name: _____

This calorie level is only an estimate of your needs. Monitor your body weight to see if you need to adjust your calorie intake.

16-11 This personalized MyPlate food plan is for a 15-year-old male who is physically active 30–60 minutes daily.

Vegetables

The vegetable group includes all types of fresh, frozen, canned, and dried vegetables as well as vegetable juices. These foods provide you with a variety of nutrients including vitamins, minerals, and fiber.

MyPlate divides vegetables into five subgroups and recommends a certain amount from each group every week based on your individual needs. The subgroups are based on nutrient content and include the following:

- *dark green vegetables* such as broccoli, spinach, and kale
- *red and orange vegetables* such as carrots, red peppers, sweet potatoes, and tomatoes
- *beans and peas* such as black-eyed peas, pinto beans, lentils, and soy beans (Beans and peas also appear in the protein foods group because they are rich in protein as well)
- *starchy vegetables* such as potatoes, corn, and green peas
- *other vegetables* such as avocado, celery, cauliflower, and mushrooms

Fruits

The fruit group includes fresh, frozen, canned, and dried fruit, and fruit juices. Fruits are rich sources of vitamins and fiber. Deep yellow or orange fruits, such as apricots and peaches, are rich in vitamin A. The fruits rich in vitamin C include citrus fruits, strawberries, and cantaloupe.

Choose whole fruit more often than fruit juice. Whole fruit contains fiber and is more nutrient dense than juice, **16-12**. Look for canned fruits packed in juice rather than syrup. Read labels to be sure that you are drinking 100 percent juice rather than a *juice drink*. Juice drinks often contain added sugars.

Dairy

Foods in the dairy group are good sources of calcium. Milk and many foods made from milk are included in this group. Milk products, which contain little or no calcium, such as cream cheese and butter, are not in this group. Calcium-fortified soymilk is also in the dairy group. In addition to calcium, foods in this group supply protein, potassium, and vitamin D.

Most teens should consume three cup-equivalents per day from this group. One cup of yogurt, one and one-half ounces of natural cheese, or two ounces of processed cheese count as one cup-equivalent.

MyPlate recommends choosing fat-free or low-fat milk products most often. The fat found in dairy products is saturated fat, which should be limited in a healthy diet. Choose skim milk, low-fat or fat-free yogurt, and reduced-fat cheeses. These products are lower in fat and calories than their whole-milk counterparts.

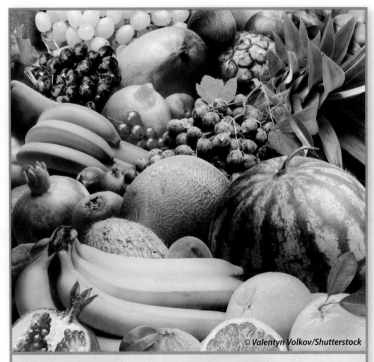

© Valentyn Volkov/Shutterstock

16-12 Fresh fruits are rich, low-fat sources of fiber, vitamins, and minerals.

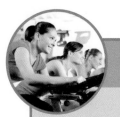

Health Connections

Keep Your Protein Lean

Avoid adding fats to your lean protein during preparation. The USDA suggests the following:

- Grill, broil, roast, poach, or boil your meat or fish instead of frying.
- Drain off fat that appears during cooking.
- Skip or limit breading on meat, poultry, or fish.
- Prepare beans and peas without added fat.
- Choose and prepare foods without high-fat sauces or gravies.

Protein Foods Group

In addition to protein, foods in the protein foods group supply vitamins and minerals. Some foods in this group, such as seafood and nuts, are sources of unsaturated fats that may provide health benefits.

The amount of food you need daily from this group depends on your age, sex, and level of activity. Protein foods are measured in ounce-equivalents. For instance, one-fourth cup of cooked dried beans, one egg, or one tablespoon of peanut butter can be counted as one ounce-equivalent from the protein foods group. An average hamburger or half of a chicken breast weighs three ounces or more. Some restaurants may serve portions twice that size. It is important to know the amount of food you are eating and eat only your recommended daily amount.

Choose lean meats and poultry without skin to limit saturated fat. Choose eggs less often because they are high in cholesterol. Dry beans and peas are good low-fat, high-fiber choices. Try to eat eight ounces of seafood weekly, **16-13**. Smaller amounts of seafood are recommended for children and women who are pregnant.

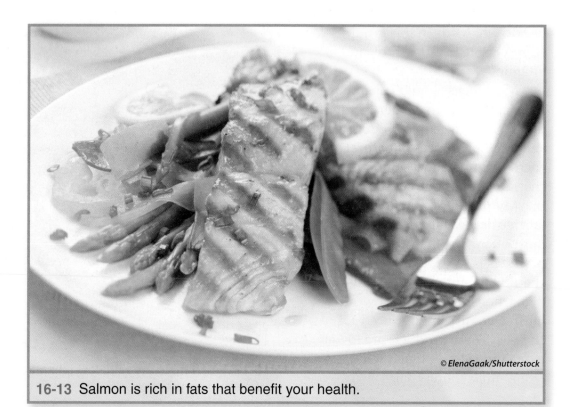

© ElenaGaak/Shutterstock

16-13 Salmon is rich in fats that benefit your health.

Oils

Oils are fats that are liquid at room temperature. Some oils are needed in the diet to provide essential nutrients. They are high in calories and can easily contribute to an imbalance between calories consumed and daily activity level.

Your personalized food plan recommends an allowance for oils. Olive oil, canola oil, and corn oil are common to many people's diets. Foods such as nuts, avocados, olives, and some fish are naturally high in oils. Salad dressing, soft margarine, and mayonnaise are also rich in oils.

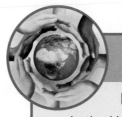

Global Connections

International Dietary Guidelines

In the U.S., Americans follow the *Dietary Guidelines for Americans* and MyPlate. Other countries follow different guidelines that are customized to their diets. For instance, Canada has a Food Guidance System, the United Kingdom has the eatwell plate, and Latvia and France both have food pyramids. Although there are slight differences between guidelines, almost all food guidance systems emphasize the five main groups: grains, vegetables, fruits, dairy, and protein.

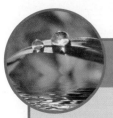

Go Green

Organic Food

You may have heard the phrase "organic food" as a growing *green* term that is often promoted in many grocery stores. *Organic* food means the food has been grown or raised through natural means, without added chemicals, genetic modification, or exposure to radiation. Organic food has both health and environmental benefits. The lack of chemicals used on organic foods ensures that food is more natural and healthy for people to eat. No chemicals also mean fewer pollutants are emitted into the ozone during the cultivation stage. The United States Department of Agriculture has regulations for organic food. You can tell if a food is organic by checking the label printed on the side.

Reading Review

1. List four factors that can influence food choices.
2. What are the two basic messages of the *2010 Dietary Guidelines for Americans*?
3. What are the five main food groups of the MyPlate food guidance system?
4. What does it mean when *enriched* is included on the label of refined grain products?
5. Why should you choose whole fruit more often than fruit juice?

Your Healthy Balance

Objectives

After studying this section, you will be able to

- **compare and contrast** weight and body composition as measures of health and fitness.
- **understand** factors that affect your weight.
- **implement** healthy eating and physical activity behaviors to manage weight.
- **summarize** the effects of common eating disorders on the body.

Key Terms		
body composition	dieting	anorexia nervosa
calories	fad diets	bulimia nervosa
energy balance	fasting	binge-eating disorder
basal metabolism	eating disorder	

Maintaining a healthy weight throughout life is very important for your health and fitness. You must understand what affects your weight to make managing it easier. Adopting some simple guidelines for eating and physical fitness can help you achieve your weight management goals.

What Is Healthy?

It is not always simple to determine what healthy weight is. Your weight is not always the best gauge of your health. The amount of body fat you carry has greater impact on your health than your total weight. For this reason, body composition is a better measure of health and fitness than weight. **Body composition** describes the proportion of body fat to lean mass in your body. Lean mass includes muscle, bone, and water **16-14**. Excess body fat is associated with higher risk for chronic diseases.

Measuring your body composition can be difficult without help from professionals. A formula called *body mass index (BMI)* is used to estimate body fatness. An adult

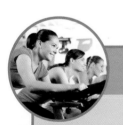

Health Connections

Find Your BMI

Find the *BMI Percentile Calculator for Child and Teen* on the Centers for Disease Control (CDC) website. Have your parent enter your information to find your BMI-for-age percentile. Ask your parent to help you identify ways you can improve your eating habits. Speak with a health professional if you have concerns about your results.

calculates his or her BMI using his or her height and weight. For a teen, determining your healthy weight is more challenging because your body is still growing and developing. For this reason, teens' BMIs are compared to others of the same age and gender. A teen with a high BMI for his or her age and sex may or may not have excess body fat. For instance, some highly trained athletes have high BMIs seeming to indicate they are overweight, but the extra weight is due to muscle mass not fat. In fact, these athletes have healthy body compositions. On the other hand, someone with a normal BMI can have a low amount of muscle mass and high body fat due to lack of physical activity. You may be wondering what weight is right for you. The best person to make that decision is your doctor. Your doctor can also tell you if you are healthy at your current weight.

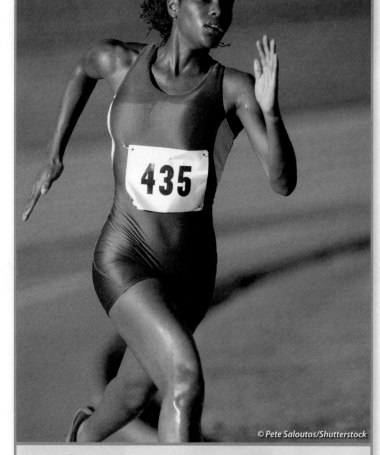

© Pete Saloutos/Shutterstock

16-14 A runner's body has a greater proportion of lean mass.

Factors Affecting Your Weight

Once you understand the factors that affect your weight, you are better able to manage it and live a healthier life. You may have wondered why you are overweight, underweight, or healthy weight. Your actual body weight is influenced by two main factors—heredity and energy balance.

Heredity

Your physical body structure refers to the size and shape of your bones. You inherited your body structure from your parents and other ancestors. You may be tall and thin or short and stocky. You may have wide hips or narrow shoulders. Your bones may be large or small. The structure of your body helps determine what you weigh.

Heredity also influences where and how efficiently your body stores fat. For instance, your body may tend to store fat around your stomach area, but your friend's body stores fat in her thighs. If your body is inefficient at storing fat, you may be prone to underweight. If your body is very efficient at storing fat, it may be more difficult for you to avoid weight gain.

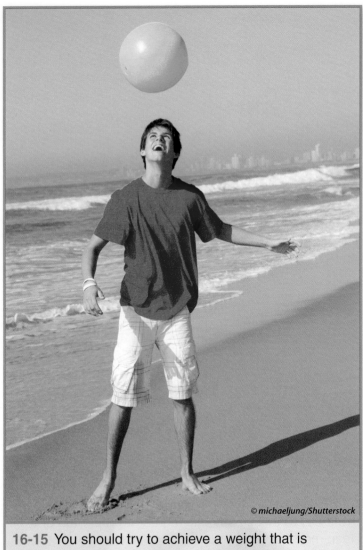

16-15 You should try to achieve a weight that is healthy for your body structure.

© michaeljung/Shutterstock

Your inherited traits make your body unique, **16-15**. You cannot change your body structure, but you can change your body composition. Having a large body structure does not mean you have to be overweight. Likewise, having a small body structure does not guarantee you will be slim. You have to work to maintain the weight that best suits your body structure.

Energy Balance

When you eat, you take energy into your body. Your body uses this energy to fuel physical activity, to digest food, and to support the basic functions needed to live. Energy is commonly measured in calories. **Calories** are units of energy or body fuel provided by carbohydrates, fats, and proteins in food. **Energy balance** results when calories taken in (from food) equal calories used (for physical activity, digestion, and basic functions). To maintain your weight, you must be in energy balance.

When you take in more calories than you use, weight gain will result. When you take in fewer calories than you use, weight loss will result. The energy used to support the basic functions that keep you alive is called **basal metabolism**. This energy supplies fuel for your lungs to breathe, your heart to beat, and so on. The energy used for basal metabolism represents about 60 percent of the total energy used by your body daily, **16-16**. About 10 percent of your daily energy use is needed for your body to digest and use the foods you eat. Physical activity uses the balance of your daily energy. The amount of energy needed for physical activity depends on how active you are and your body size. A soccer player uses more energy for physical activity than a sedentary person. A larger person uses more calories than a smaller person to perform the same activity because it takes more energy to move the bigger weight.

Weight Management

One of the key concepts from the *2010 Dietary Guidelines* is "Maintain calorie balance over time to achieve and sustain a healthy weight."

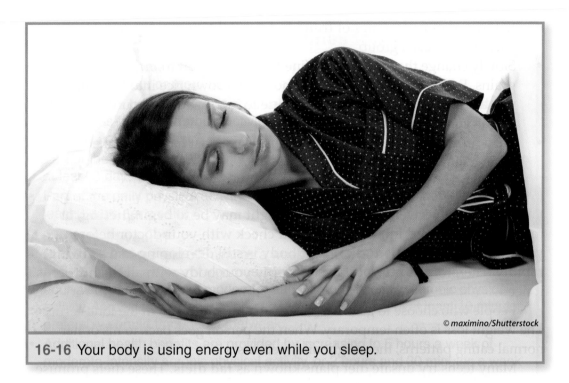

© maximino/Shutterstock

16-16 Your body is using energy even while you sleep.

Achieving and maintaining a healthy weight is known as *weight management*. Your goals for weight management must be realistic and attainable. Attempting to change your body into the ideal images you see in the media can be harmful to both your physical and mental health. Perhaps a good first weight management goal is to improve your health. Weight management requires you adopt healthy eating and physical activity behaviors.

Healthy Eating

Your doctor can help you identify your healthy weight. You are most likely to achieve and maintain healthy weight by changing your eating behaviors. Replace old, unhealthy eating habits with new, healthy habits you can keep for a lifetime, **16-17**. The following tips will move you toward a healthy weight:

- Eat fewer and smaller portions of foods that contain solid fats and added sugars such as sports drinks, sugary cereals, candy, and snack and dessert foods.
- Drink water or fat-free milk instead of soft drinks, juice drinks, and other sugary beverages.

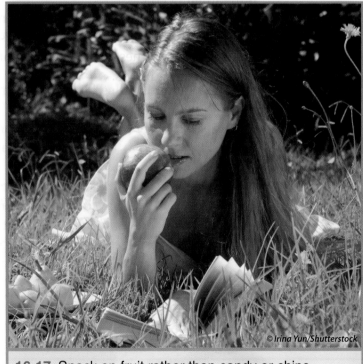

© Irina Yun/Shutterstock

16-17 Snack on fruit rather than candy or chips.

Reaching and maintaining a healthy weight benefits your self-esteem and increases your confidence. You will have more energy and view life more positively, **16-19**.

Maintaining a healthy weight reduces many health risks. Individuals who are underweight may have more problems recovering from illness or surgery. Women who are underweight may have more difficult pregnancies. Lack of energy and inability to stay warm are problems associated with being underweight.

Overweight and obesity are linked to many chronic diseases such as diabetes, cancer, and heart disease. Obesity can also cause problems during pregnancy and surgery. Many social and emotional problems can result from problems with overweight and obesity as well.

Diets that are lacking in nutrients and physical inactivity can cause health problems for individuals of any weight status.

Eating Disorders

Society's emphasis on being thin may be just one factor contributing to the incidence of eating disorders, **16-20**. An eating disorder is an illness that results in abnormal eating patterns which can be life threatening. Eating disorders range from self-starvation to binge-eating. Recovery from these illnesses requires help and support from knowledgeable professionals who study these types of disorders.

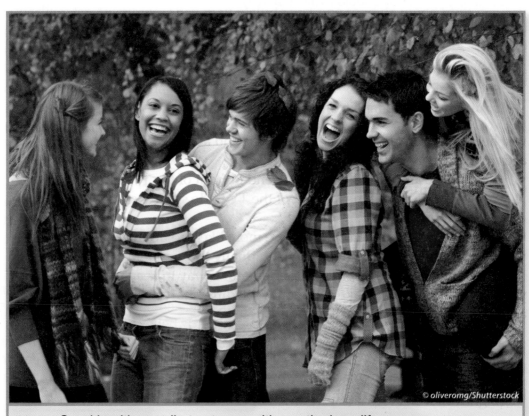

© oliveromg/Shutterstock

16-19 Good health contributes to a positive outlook on life.

Anorexia Nervosa

Anorexia nervosa is an eating disorder that causes people to starve themselves. People with anorexia have a distorted image of their bodies. They can be severely underweight and still see themselves as fat. Anorexia nervosa affects both the body and mind.

Anorexia is most commonly seen in young women, but the number of young men diagnosed is growing. Females are likely to lose weight by not eating. Males are more likely to use excessive exercise to lose weight. Anorexia may begin with a strict weight-loss diet. The victim begins skipping meals and disliking all foods. Excessive exercise is a symptom that usually follows the cutback in food. Many people with anorexia take diet pills to curb the appetite and large doses of laxatives. This constant abuse to the body is harmful.

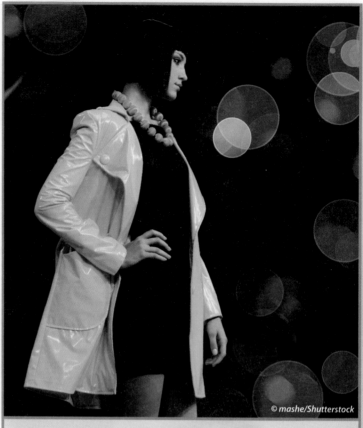

© mashe/Shutterstock

16-20 In recent years, some fashion shows have required that models be within a healthy weight range.

In addition to weight loss, females stop menstruating due to low body fat. The low body fat causes both males and females with anorexia to feel cold. Their bodies attempt to keep warm by growing a covering of fine hair to hold in heat. Insufficient nutrients result in hair loss and skin problems. If the starvation continues, normal growth stops and the body begins to use muscle tissue for energy. Heart muscle is lost, which can result in abnormal function or even death. As the illness progresses, individuals withdraw and suffer from deep depression.

Counseling and a lengthy period of recovery are usually necessary to cure this illness.

Bulimia Nervosa

Another type of eating disorder is bulimia nervosa. Individuals with bulimia nervosa suffer uncontrollable urges to eat large amounts of food followed by behavior to avoid weight gain. Due to intense fear of weight gain and disgust with their behavior, they rid their bodies of the food with forced vomiting. People with bulimia may also take laxatives or diuretics. Excessive exercise is also common. As with anorexia nervosa, people with this disorder have an intense desire to be thin. They know their eating patterns are not normal and often eat in secret.

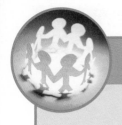

Life Connections

Helping Someone with an Eating Disorder

It may be difficult to decide when and how to help a friend who you suspect has an eating disorder. Body image and eating habits can be a sensitive subject. If you are considering confronting someone who you suspect has an eating disorder, follow these tips:

- Become knowledgeable about your friend's eating habits and the disorder. The more information you have, the easier it will be to understand what your friend is experiencing.
- Be honest. Let your friend know you are concerned for his or her well-being and you want to help.
- Be supportive. Remember to talk about the many positive qualities your friend possesses, beyond physical traits.
- Alert an adult. Your friend may need professional help dealing with the disorder. Getting someone else involved is a good step toward recovery.

There are many resources and hotlines available to help someone with an eating disorder. For more information, visit www.nationaleatingdisorders.org.

Reading and Writing Activity

Read a book that focuses on eating disorders. Write a two-page summary and share your findings with the class.

Bulimia nervosa may cause the body to become unable to digest food. Frequent vomiting results in acids from the stomach damaging the esophagus and teeth. Mineral and fluid balance is upset, which can cause serious health concerns. Eventually, people with bulimia may suffer from malnutrition. Like anorexia nervosa, both medical help and counseling are necessary to help the patient overcome bulimia nervosa.

Binge-Eating Disorder

As with bulimia, people with binge-eating disorder repeatedly eat great amounts of food and feel powerless to stop. People who suffer from this illness are often overweight because behaviors to eliminate the food do not occur. Embarrassed by their behavior, they attempt to stop the eating pattern, but cannot.

Binge-eating disorder can lead to health issues from excess weight. In addition, people with this disorder are likely suffering from emotional problems. Some problems may be the result of chemical imbalances in the body. It is important to seek professional help to avoid long-term health problems.

Reading Review

1. What does body composition describe?
2. What two main factors influence your actual body weight?
3. Why are fad diets rarely successful?
4. List three tips that will help you decrease your sedentary time and adopt healthful physical activity behaviors.
5. What is an eating disorder?

Healthy Eating Across the Life Cycle

Objectives

After studying this section, you will be able to
- **explain** nutrient needs at each life-cycle stage.
- **recognize** special dietary needs for athletes and vegetarians.
- **identify** health conditions that may require modified eating patterns.

Key Terms

vegetarianism	food intolerance	diabetes
food allergy		

Healthy eating is important at every stage of the life cycle. Each stage from pregnancy to older adulthood has unique nutrient needs. As humans age, their needs change and so should their eating patterns.

Pregnant Women and Infants

Pregnancy places great demands on the mother's body. Energy and nutrient needs increase to support the growing fetus. The mother's nutrient needs also increase during pregnancy. Energy needs increase during pregnancy, but to a lesser extent than the need for vitamins and minerals, **16-21**.

Nutrition Before Pregnancy

The mother's health is important at the very moment pregnancy begins. For this reason, it is critical

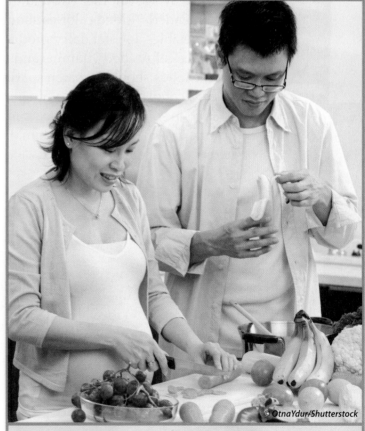

© OtnaYdur/Shutterstock

16-21 Pregnant women should make nutrient-dense food choices to meet increased nutrient needs.

for women to practice healthy eating habits before they get pregnant. A woman with a healthy weight before pregnancy is more likely to give birth to a healthy baby. Women who are either under- or overweight when they become pregnant are more likely to have problems during their pregnancies. There is also a greater risk of babies being born early. These babies have greater rates of illness or death.

Certain vitamins require close attention early in the pregnancy. Inadequate folate supplies very early in the pregnancy can result in serious birth defects. To address this concern, health experts recommend all women of childbearing age consume folate supplements or foods fortified with folate. Vitamin A can cause birth defects when present in the mother's body in unusually high amounts. Vitamin A from food sources alone cannot reach these dangerous levels. The problem occurs when drugs that contain vitamin A are taken.

Nutrition During Pregnancy

Most women with healthy eating patterns are able to meet their nutrient needs during pregnancy. Many doctors prescribe supplements to ensure that the mother is getting all the needed vitamins and minerals. In addition to folate, women often have trouble meeting their increased needs for iron with food alone.

Unlike vitamins, the need for energy does not increase until later in the pregnancy. About 14 weeks into the pregnancy, the mother should increase her food intake by 340 calories. Around the 27th week, an additional 110 calories is recommended. Added calories should come from healthful foods such as fruits, vegetables, low-fat dairy products, and whole grains. These are also good sources of needed vitamins and minerals.

Some foods should be eaten sparingly or not at all during pregnancy. For instance, alcohol should not be consumed at all. Pregnant women should limit foods high in solid fats and added sugars that supply few nutrients and can contribute to unhealthy weight gain. Fish that are likely to contain high levels of mercury should not be eaten.

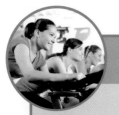

Health Connections

Fish to Limit or Avoid

The Environmental Protection Agency (EPA) and Food and Drug Administration (FDA) recommend the following guidelines for women who are pregnant or may become pregnant and young children:

- Avoid eating shark, swordfish, king mackerel, or tilefish.
- Consume no more than six ounces per week of albacore (white) tuna.
- Check with local authorities about the safety of fish caught in local waters.

Nutrition for Infants

Once the baby is born, his or her nutrient needs must also be met. The first six months is a period of rapid growth. Frequent small feedings are necessary because the infant's stomach is small, but the need for nourishment is great. The best food for an infant is breast milk, **16-22**. Breast milk changes as the infant's needs change. In addition to nutrients, it helps protect the baby from infections and may reduce future risk for overweight or obesity.

Sometimes breastfeeding cannot or should not be practiced. The only other option doctors recommend is iron-fortified infant formulas. There are different types of these formulas to address various health conditions. Doctors should help parents choose the best formula for their baby. Cow's milk is *not* an option and should not be offered until the baby is one year old. Solid foods should not be added to the infant's diet until four to six months of age. Only one food should be added to the baby's diet at a time. This makes it easier to identify foods that may cause problems for the baby.

Babies should not be forced to eat. If a baby rejects a food, it should be offered again a few days later.

Children and Teens

Children and teens continue to grow and develop, but not as rapidly as during infancy. During this time, nutrient needs must be met and healthful eating patterns established.

Nutrition for Children

Around one year of age, children begin to be able to feed themselves.

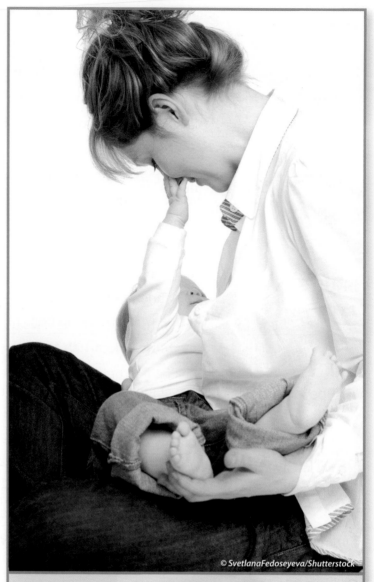

© SvetlanaFedoseyeva/Shutterstock

16-22 Breast-feeding promotes bonding as well as nourishes.

Soft-textured foods from each food group should be offered. Foods should be cut into bite-sized pieces to avoid choking. Meals should include about one tablespoon of each food for each year of age, but the child should not be forced to finish. The child's appetite should determine how much food is eaten. The MyPlate food guidance system can be used for meal planning for children two years and older, **16-23**.

Young children have small stomachs, which prevent them from eating large meals. Snacks are important for ensuring they receive sufficient nutrients. It is important that snack foods are healthful and supply more than just added sugars and fats.

As children get older, their need for nutrients continues to increase due to their increasing size. Children should continue to be offered healthy foods from each food group to meet their increased energy needs. Healthy eating habits should be established to prevent health problems in the future.

My Daily Food Plan

Based on the information you provided, this is your daily recommended amount from each food group.

GRAINS 3 ounces	**Make half your grains whole** Aim for at least **1½ ounces** of whole grains a day
VEGETABLES 1 cup	**Vary your veggies** Aim for these amounts **each week**: **Dark green veggies** = ½ cup **Red & orange veggies** = 2½ cup **Beans & peas** = ½ cup **Starchy veggies** = 2 cups **Other veggies** = 1½ cups
FRUITS 1 cup	**Focus on fruits** Eat a variety of fruit Choose whole or cut-up fruits more often than fruit juice
DAIRY 2 cups	**Get your calcium-rich foods** Drink fat-free or low-fat (1%) milk, for the same amount of calcium and other nutrients as whole milk, but less fat and calories Select fat-free or low-fat yogurt and cheese, or try calcium-fortified soy products
PROTEIN FOODS 2 ounces	**Go lean with protein** Twice a week, make seafood the protein on your plate Vary your protein routine–choose more fish, beans, peas, nuts, and seeds Keep meat and poultry portions small and lean

Find your balance between food and physical activity	**Know your limits on fats, sugars, and sodium**
Children 2 to 5 years old should play actively every day.	Your allowance for oils is **3 teaspoons a day**. Limit extras–solid fats and sugars–to **140 calories** a day. Reduce sodium intake to less than **2300 mg** a day.

Your results are based on a 1000 calorie pattern. Name: _____

This calorie level is only an estimate of your needs. Monitor your body weight to see if you need to adjust your calorie intake.

16-23 This food plan is appropriate for a two-year-old.   *USDA*

Rather than sugary drinks, water or low-fat dairy products should be offered. (Whole-fat milk and milk products are recommended until two years of age.) In addition to healthy eating, children should be encouraged to be physically active for 60 minutes each day. Less time should be spent doing sedentary activities such as watching TV and playing video games. Poor eating habits and lack of physical activity can cause weight problems in children.

Nutrition for Teens

During your teen years, the nutritional needs of your body are extremely high. This is because your body is growing and developing. It is important that sufficient nutrients are available for teens to reach their growth potential. Of course, the body's need for energy and protein are high due to the growth taking place. In addition, iron, calcium, and vitamins A and D require close attention during this time. These nutrients are critical for the bone formation and muscle growth that is taking place. Optimal bone formation during the teen years is important for bone health in older adulthood. All these nutrient needs can be met with healthful food choices. Unfortunately, teens may not always make wise choices. Busy schedules, peer pressure, and increased freedom can all contribute to poor eating habits during this time.

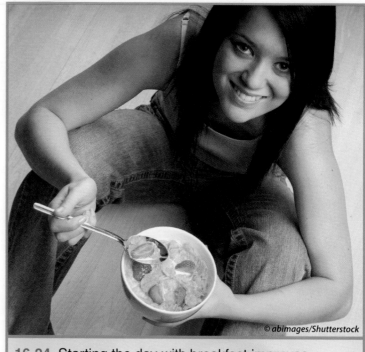

© abimages/Shutterstock

16-24 Starting the day with breakfast improves problem-solving ability and creativity.

Teens who start the day with a good breakfast are better able to concentrate in school, **16-24**. Frequent meals at fast-food restaurants can contribute more fat, sodium, and added sugar than is healthy. These foods should be eaten less often and balanced with foods that are nutrient dense. As with other life-cycle stages, regular physical activity is important to good health and weight management for teens.

Adults

As people age, their energy needs begin to decrease. Continuing to eat as you did when you were a teen can result in unhealthy weight gain. Overweight and obesity increase the risk for many chronic diseases. Maintaining a healthy weight throughout your life is easier than trying to lose weight in adulthood.

Unlike energy needs, the needs for some nutrients increase with age. The body may not absorb nutrients as readily or use them as efficiently as it once did. At this stage, people are more likely to be on prescribed drugs. These drugs sometimes have unintended side effects. Drugs may alter sense of taste or interfere with nutrient absorption. Vitamin D, calcium, zinc, iron, and many B vitamins are nutrients that require attention during this life-cycle stage. For this reason, adults should continue to make nutrient-dense food choices, **16-25**. Some doctors may recommend vitamin and mineral supplements. Adults also benefit from consuming foods rich in fiber and regular exercise to avoid constipation.

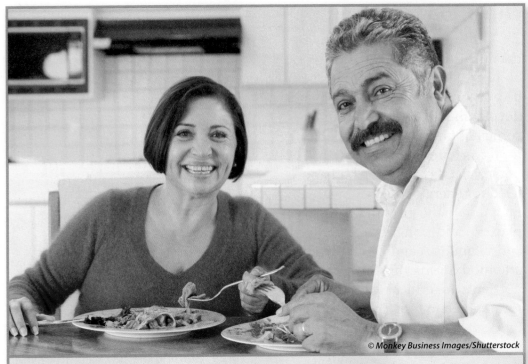

© Monkey Business Images/Shutterstock

16-25 Nutrient-dense food choices become even more important as energy needs decrease with age.

Older adults often have additional factors impacting their nutrition. Declining health may prevent older adults from being physically active. It could hinder their ability to purchase and prepare food. Tooth loss may cause problems with chewing food. Often, older adults experience reduced sense of taste and foods all taste bland. They may feel isolated and lonely and lose interest in food.

Older adults may benefit from assistance shopping for and preparing food. Many community resources are available to help this age group. Older adults should include daily physical activity to the extent they are able. Short walks or exercises while sitting can help with muscle tone and blood flow.

Special Dietary Needs

Various lifestyle choices and health conditions occur during the life cycle. People may choose to become a triathlete or follow a vegetarian diet. Perhaps a child has a food allergy. These choices and conditions can create additional nutritional concerns.

Competitive Athletes

Competitive athletes often engage in more prolonged and strenuous physical activity than nonathletes. This demanding training requires attention to fluid intake, adequate consumption of nutrients, and weight management. These needs can usually be met without major changes to an already healthy diet. The MyPlate food guidance system can serve as the basis for an athlete's eating pattern. Depending on the specific event, the athlete may require amounts of most nutrients greater than those of a nonathlete of the same gender and size, **16-26**. Nutrient-dense food choices are even more important due to the added physical demands. To meet the added energy needs, athletes should consume healthful snacks between meals.

Maintaining his or her body's fluid levels is important to an athlete's health and performance level. To avoid dehydration, athletes need to drink fluids before, during, and after training and events. Cool water meets fluid needs for events lasting less than one hour. For longer events, fluid choices may be needed that deliver calories or minerals.

Weight management is important to athletic performance. Some events such as gymnastics or wrestling place much emphasis on weight. The intense focus on body weight can cause some athletes to use unhealthy weight-loss or -gain strategies. In fact, these practices may result in decreased performance. Weight management concerns should be discussed with a health professional.

Vegetarianism

Vegetarianism is an eating pattern that excludes some or all animal products. There are different types of vegetarian diets, **16-27**. There are also many reasons people practice vegetarianism including

- religion
- health concerns
- environmental
- compassion for animals
- food scarcity

A healthful vegetarian diet requires careful planning to ensure that needed nutrients and amounts

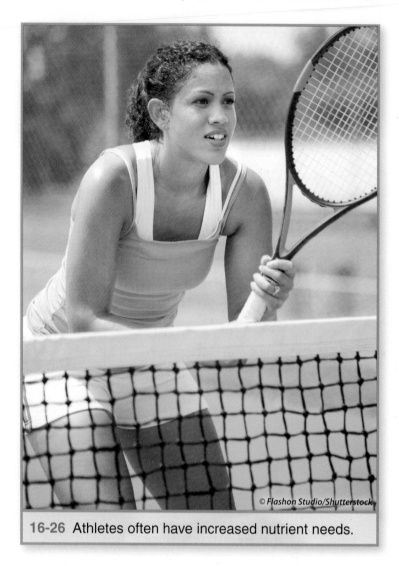

© Flashon Studio/Shutterstock

16-26 Athletes often have increased nutrient needs.

Types of Vegetarians

Lacto-ovo vegetarians
- eat milk products, eggs, and plant foods
- do not eat meat, fish, or poultry

Lacto-vegetarians
- eat milk products and plant foods
- do not eat meat, fish, poultry, or eggs

Ovo-vegetarians
- eat plant food and eggs
- do not eat milk products, meat, poultry, or fish

Pescetarians
- eat plant foods and fish
- do not eat meat or poultry

Vegans
- eat plant foods only
- also called strict vegetarians

16-27 Vegetarian diets can vary greatly.

Nutrition Facts

Serving Size 2 bars (42g)
Servings Per Container 6

Amount Per Serving	2 bars		1 bar	
Calories	190		90	
Calories from Fat	60		30	
		%DV*		%DV*
Total Fat	7g	**10%**	3.5g	**5%**
Saturated Fat	1g	**4%**	0.5g	**2%**
Trans Fat	0g		0g	
Cholesterol	0mg	**0%**	0mg	**0%**
Sodium	180mg	**7%**	90mg	**4%**
Total Carbohydrate	28g	**9%**	14g	**5%**
Dietary Fiber	2g	**8%**	1g	**4%**
Sugars	11g		16g	
Protein	5g		2g	
Iron		4%		2%

Not a significant source of vitamin A, vitamin C and calcium.

*Percent Daily Values (DV) are based on a 2,000 calorie diet. Your daily values may be higher or lower depending on your calorie needs:

	Calories	2,000	2,500
Total Fat	Less Than	65g	80g
Sat Fat	Less Than	20g	25g
Cholesterol	Less Than	300mg	300mg
Sodium	Less Than	2,400mg	2,400mg
Total Carbohydrates		300g	375g
Dietary Fiber		25g	30g

Ingredients: Whole Grain Oats, Sugar, Canola Oil, Peanut Butter (peanuts, salt), Yellow Corn Flour, Brown Sugar Syrup, Soy Flour, Salt, Soy Lecithin, Baking Soda.

CONTAINS PEANUT, SOY; MAY CONTAIN ALMOND AND PECAN INGREDIENTS.

16-28 Food labels must clearly state ingredients that are the cause of most food allergies.

Health Connections

DASH Diet

The goal of Dietary Approaches to Stop Hypertension (DASH) is to reduce sodium in your diet while increasing other nutrients that help reduce or avoid high blood pressure. Eating foods high in nutrients such as potassium, calcium, and magnesium can help lower blood pressure. The DASH diet is a healthy way of eating for individuals of all ages and may reduce risk for other diseases as well. Search the Internet to find the DASH Eating Plan issued by the Department of Health and Human Services (HHS).

are eaten. Failure to do so can result in health problems. When properly designed, vegetarian diets provide less saturated fat and cholesterol and more vitamins and minerals than meat-based diets. This results in lower risk for overweight, some cancers, and heart disease.

Food Intolerances and Allergies

It is not unusual to hear someone claiming to have a food allergy. A **food allergy** occurs when a food protein you have eaten triggers a response by your body's immune system. Milk, eggs, tree nuts, peanuts, soy, wheat, fish, and shellfish are the most common causes of this type of reaction. The body's reaction to food allergies can be serious and sometimes fatal. Fortunately, more often people have food intolerances. **Food intolerance** is a reaction to a food that is unpleasant, but not the result of an immune response.

Both food allergies and intolerances can be avoided by removing the offending food from the diet. This requires careful planning when meals are being prepared at home. Food labels must be read to identify ingredients that might trigger a reaction, **16-28**. Recipes may need to be modified. When eating away from home, even more care must be taken when communicating with your server. More and more restaurants are providing food allergy training for their employees and information on menus.

Health Conditions

A number of common health conditions such as diabetes and high blood pressure require modified eating patterns.

Diabetes is a disease that limits or prevents the body's ability to properly use energy from food. People with diabetes must plan healthy meals in controlled amounts and eat them at about the same time every day. Often their doctor will prescribe medicine to help control their diabetes as well. Exercise also plays an important role in managing this disease. Maintaining a healthy weight and regular physical activity can reduce the risk for developing some types of diabetes.

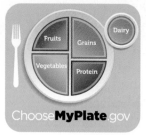

MyPlate Tip

Salt and Sodium

Think fresh. Most of the sodium Americans eat is found in processed foods. Eat highly processed foods less often and in smaller portions—especially cheesy foods such as pizza; cured meats such as bacon, sausage, hot dogs, and deli/luncheon meats; and ready-to-eat foods like canned chili, ravioli, and soups. Fresh foods are generally lower in sodium.

Source: MyPlate 10 tips Nutrition Education Series

Blood pressure rises and falls naturally due to certain activities and states. For instance, your blood pressure rises during exercise and returns to normal when you finish exercising. Persistent high blood pressure that does not return to a normal level can weaken blood vessels over time. There are many risk factors for high blood pressure. Risk factors you can control include lack of physical activity, obesity, and too much sodium in the diet. Reducing the amount of table salt you use and limiting processed foods will help you decrease your sodium intake. In addition, increasing the amounts of fruits and vegetables in your diet will supply your body with more potassium. Potassium-rich diets have also been proven to help keep blood pressure at healthy levels. A diet that combines sodium reduction with increased potassium-rich foods is more effective at reducing blood pressure than only reducing sodium intake. It is important that you obtain the potassium from foods *not* supplements.

Reading Review

1. Which foods should be eaten sparingly or not at all during pregnancy?
2. Which is the best food for an infant?
3. During the teen years, why are nutritional needs of the body extremely high?
4. List five reasons people practice vegetarianism.
5. Distinguish between a food intolerance and a food allergy.

Chapter Summary

Section 16-1. Good nutrition results when you provide your body with healthful foods that supply needed nutrients. The essential nutrients are proteins, carbohydrates, fats, vitamins, minerals, and water. Eating a variety of foods is necessary to obtain all the nutrients your body needs. Nutrient needs differ based on age, sex, body build, and level of activity. Health also affects nutrient needs.

Section 16-2. People eat for a variety of reasons. Food choices are influenced by factors such as family, friends, cultural heritage, and advertising. The *Dietary Guidelines for Americans* and the MyPlate food guidance system can help you to make wise food choices. MyPlate divides foods into five main food groups—grains, vegetables, fruits, protein foods, and dairy.

Section 16-3. Maintaining a healthy weight is important for health and fitness. Body composition is a better measure of health and fitness than weight. Heredity and energy balance influence your actual body weight. Maintaining a healthy, fit body benefits both your mental and physical health. The incidence of eating disorders, such as anorexia nervosa, bulimia nervosa, and binge-eating disorder may be related to society's emphasis on being thin. These illnesses result in abnormal eating patterns that can be life threatening.

Section 16-4. Healthy eating is important at each stage of the life cycle. Nutrient needs vary at each life cycle stage from pregnancy to older adulthood. In addition, athletes and vegetarians have special dietary needs. People with food intolerances and allergies, as well as people with certain health conditions, may require modified eating patterns.

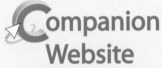

Companion Website

www.g-wlearning.com

Check your understanding of the main concepts for Chapter 16 at the website.

Critical Thinking

1. **Analyze.** Make a list of all the foods you eat for one day. Then analyze the factors that affected each of your food choices. What factors seem to affect your choices most?
2. **Compare.** Find a magazine or newspaper article that describes a diet. Compare the foods in the diet with the foods suggested in the MyPlate food guidance system.
3. **Determine.** What can you do to educate young adults on the dangers of dieting improperly?

Common Core

College and Career Readiness

4. **Listening.** Invite a dietitian to talk to your class about the functions of food in the body.

5. **Speaking.** Divide the class into small groups. Have each group write a TV commercial about a different nutrient to *sell* to the public. Use creative ways to make the nutrient appealing. Present the commercials in class.

6. **Reading.** Research current articles about eating disorders, such as anorexia nervosa, bulimia nervosa, and binge-eating disorder. Find out about what can lead to these disorders, the long-term health problems that can result, and how people who suffer from these disorders can get help.

7. **Writing.** Imagine you are the editor of a popular teen blog. Write an article promoting healthy eating and physical activity. (You may want to submit your article to the school website or newsletter.)

Technology

8. **Electronic presentation.** Many communities have organizations that promote healthy eating. Prepare an electronic presentation about healthy eating. Ask a dietitian to review the presentation for accuracy. Then make any adjustments and present it at a community event.

Journal Writing

9. Keep a food and physical activity log for one week. At the end of the week, write about your food choices and physical activity by answering the following questions: What influenced your food choices? How well did your food choices reflect the recommendations of the *Dietary Guidelines* and the MyPlate food guidance system? Was your physical activity adequate? Were you in energy balance? What adjustments would you make now and in the future?

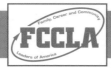

FCCLA

10. Develop a *Focus on Children STAR Event* that teaches children about nutritious eating and includes the major nutrient categories and key vitamins and minerals. Host a family night or visit an elementary classroom that teaches others how to prepare and/or select healthy and easy snacks. Use the *FCCLA Planning Process* to create your project strategies. See your adviser for information as needed.

Chapter 17
Meal Considerations

Sections

Reading Prep

College and Career Readiness

On separate sticky notes, write five reasons why the information in this chapter is important to you. Think about how this information could help you at school, work, or home. As you read the chapter, place the sticky notes on the pages that relate to each reason.

Concept Organizer

Factors for Meal Appeal	Examples

Use a T-chart diagram to list factors that contribute to an appealing meal. Give a specific example for each factor.

Companion Website
Print out the concept organizer for Chapter 17 at the website.

Companion Website
www.g-wlearning.com

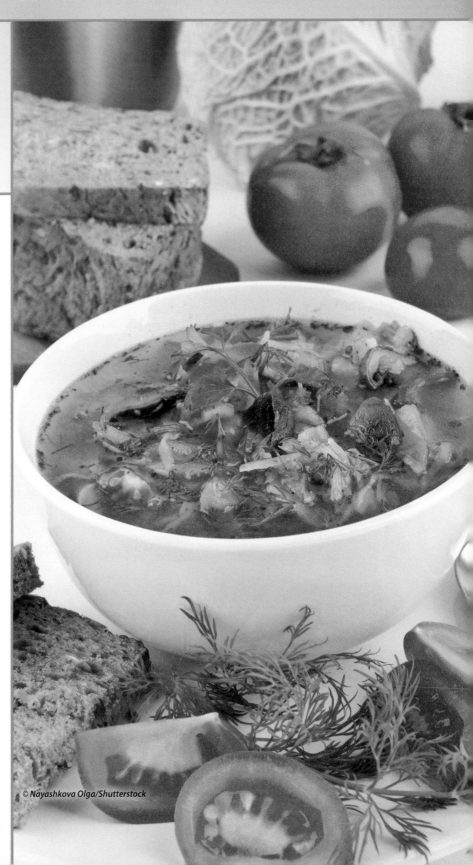

© Nayashkova Olga/Shutterstock

Section 17-1

Cultural Food Influences

Objectives

After studying this section, you will be able to
- **relate** how geography, tradition, and religion can influence food customs.
- **list** foods that are typical of different regions of the United States.

Key Terms		
geography	soul food	potluck
traditions	creole foods	

Would it seem strange to you to have rice with every meal? What about beef? The way you react to these ideas depends on your food customs. To the Japanese, eating rice with meals is common. Indians who are Hindu would not consider eating beef.

Food customs vary from culture to culture. *Culture* includes the way people live, how they act (their customs), and what they believe. It is passed from one generation to the next. It also tends to be shared by people from a certain region or country.

Influences on Food Customs

You may wonder why people in the same culture eat similar foods. Why are foods that are common in one culture rarely eaten in another culture? Many factors within a culture affect food customs. These include geography, religion, and traditions.

Geography

People in most cultures make dishes from foods that can be found nearby. These foods vary in different cultures because of the region's geography. Geography includes the location and climate of a land. It also includes the type of soil and water sources. The lay of the land—whether it is flat, hilly, or mountainous—is another part of geography.

The geography influences the types of foods that are easily found or grown in an area. For instance, fish are plentiful in areas near oceans or lakes. Citrus fruits thrive in lands with a long warm season. Rice grows well in marshy regions, **17-1**.

Foods that are readily available play a central role in a culture's food customs. For instance, many native Japanese dishes contain rice and fish because Japan is surrounded by oceans and has much marshy land.

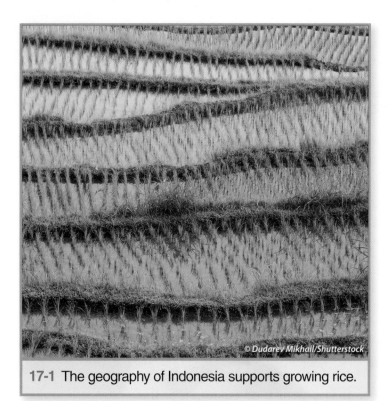

17-1 The geography of Indonesia supports growing rice.

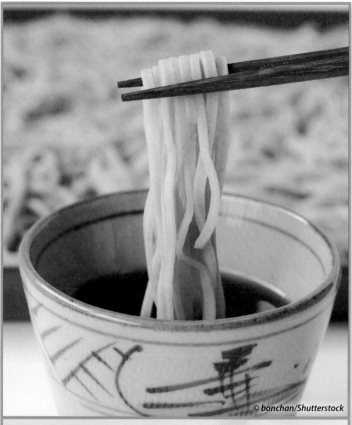

17-2 A Japanese New Year's tradition suggests good luck will come to those who can swallow a soba noodle without chewing or breaking it.

Scandinavian countries have a long cold season and many mountains. They cannot grow much produce, but they can raise livestock on their land. They are also close to oceans. Since growing and harvesting seasons are short, much food is preserved. Therefore, cheeses, dried fruits, and smoked meats and fishes are common in this culture.

Religion

Religion also influences the foods of cultures. For instance, unleavened (or flat, thin) bread is a part of the Jewish Passover meal. It is a symbol of their ancestors being forced to leave Egypt quickly.

Christian religions also give meanings to foods. Bread and wine taken during communion symbolize Christ's body and blood. Easter eggs symbolize rebirth. In Germany, pretzels are a symbol of prayer. A rich Russian cheesecake with the letters *XB* on it celebrates Easter. The letters stand for "Christ has risen" in Greek.

Some religions restrict the eating of certain foods. People of the Hindu religion eat no beef because they consider cows sacred. In the Islam faith, eating any kind of pork is forbidden.

Tradition

A culture's traditions also affect the foods eaten. **Traditions** are customs that are passed from generation to generation. Many traditions center on holidays. Holiday traditions often call for special foods. For instance, the Chinese celebrate their new year with a ten-course dinner, **17-2**.

Other traditions are based on folklore. These traditions become a part of food customs. According to Swedish folklore, eating "dream herring" or "dream porridge" on

Midsummer Eve is a way to find out about the future. In China, black teas are called *red teas* because bad luck is associated with the color black.

Traditions related to art also affect food customs. In Japan, food is an art form. For their spring festival, the Japanese arrange foods to depict the mountains, rivers, trees, and flowers of springtime in Japan.

Food Customs of the United States

The United States is a country with many cultures. People have come from many different lands to live here. They brought their cultures' recipes and ingredients for their favorite foods with them. For this reason, the United States is rich with a variety of food customs.

Each group of newcomers to the United States kept strong ties with their old culture. They used old recipes and adapted local foods. Gradually, food styles from different cultures blended to create new cooking styles.

Early Influences

The English, Spanish, and French were some of the first settlers in North America. They brought their own food customs from their homelands. They also learned about American foods from the Native Americans. Some foods introduced by Native Americans include corn, pumpkins, squash, peppers, cranberries, and peanuts, **17-3**. Native Americans also taught colonists to hunt and fish. Colonists used local foods in recipes from their homelands.

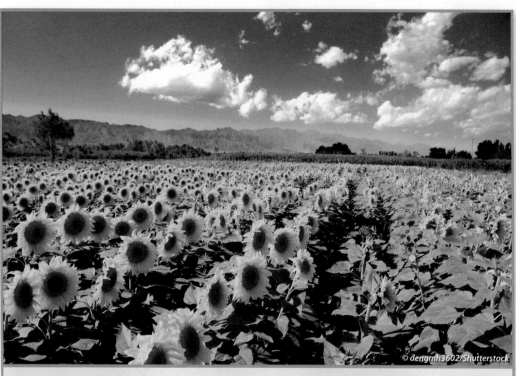

© dengmh3602/Shutterstock

17-3 Native Americans introduced sunflower seeds into the diets of early settlers.

As the colonies grew, slaves worked on farms and plantations. From the 1700s to the mid-1800s, Africans were taken from their homelands and forced to be slaves. Most slaves worked on farms and plantations in the South. Africans brought their own style of cooking, making spicy, stewlike dishes. They also brought okra, a native African vegetable, to America.

Around the 1800s, people from other cultures *immigrated* (moved from their former country to a new one) to the United States. Immigrants came from Germany, Ireland, Italy, and Slavic countries. Many European Jews immigrated at this time as well. Asians also came to the United States and settled along the West Coast. Each culture brought more new food customs to the United States.

Regional Differences

When people first came to the United States, they tended to settle with others from their culture. The native cultures of these people influenced food customs in that region. As a result, different regions of the United States are noted for distinct cooking styles.

Transportation and communication links have improved greatly since the 1800s. For this reason, foods from different regions can be found throughout the United States. You can find regional produce, such as California avocados and New England cranberries, in grocery stores across the country. You may be able to sample regional foods at local restaurants.

Northeast and Middle Atlantic States

These states are close to the Atlantic Ocean. Their climate is fairly cool. Although winters are long and harsh, berries, apples, beans, corn, and squash can be grown there during warm seasons. Maple trees flourish and are used to make maple syrup, **17-4**.

The northeast states are known as New England. These states were settled by English Pilgrims. The Pilgrims learned much about food from the Native Americans. They developed many American dishes with English ties. These include baked beans, pumpkin pie, cranberry sauce, and clam chowder. New England is also known for seafood and wild game. These include lobster, crab, turkey, duck, and pheasant.

The middle Atlantic states were home to Dutch, German, Swedish, and English settlers. Many Jewish

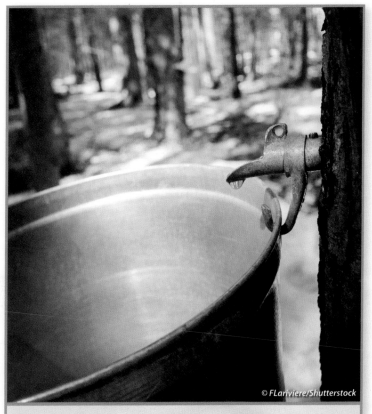
© FLariviere/Shutterstock

17-4 Sap collected from maple trees is boiled down until it becomes syrup.

Europeans settled in this area, especially New York. Because so many cultures settled in this region, the foods are diverse. Specialties of this area include doughnuts, waffles, chicken and dumplings, bagels, lox, sausages, hot dogs, and pretzels. This region also has many seafood dishes.

South

The southern states are bordered by the Atlantic Ocean on the east and the Gulf of Mexico on the south. They have long, warm growing seasons that allow many crops to be grown. Corn, rice, sugarcane, sweet potatoes, peaches, and peanuts grow well in this climate, **17-5**. Pork and chicken are raised for meat. Catfish, bass, trout, and turtle are also used in foods. Citrus fruits are grown in Florida.

Settlers in the South were mainly from the British Isles, Spain, Africa, and France. Influences from these cultures can be seen in Southern cooking. Barbecued pork ribs, fried chicken, smoked ham, and biscuits are Southern foods. Sweet potato pie and pecan pie are popular desserts.

Two unique cooking styles were founded in the South. One is **soul food**, which is based on the food customs of African Americans. Catfish, fried chitterlings (hog intestines), and hush puppies (cornmeal dough made into small balls and fried) are some soul foods. Many stewlike dishes are made with vegetables such as squash, black-eyed peas, okra, and greens.

Creole is another cooking style found mainly in New Orleans. **Creole foods** have roots in the French, Spanish, African, and Native American cultures. Many creole dishes contain mixtures of rice, tomatoes, okra, seafood, poultry, hot sausage, and meat. Many dishes are very hot and spicy. Gumbo (a stewlike dish) and jambalaya (a spicy casserole) are two popular creole dishes.

West and Southwest

Much of the land in the West and Southwest is rocky or sandy. Raising large crops is difficult. Cattle farms are common in these regions. Sheep are raised in the West. Some fruits and vegetables are grown. Potatoes are a major crop in Idaho, Montana, and Wyoming.

Southwestern cooking has been influenced by Mexicans, Spaniards, and Native Americans. Hot peppers are used in much Southwestern cooking. Barbecued beef, chili, tamales, and nachos are popular Southwestern dishes.

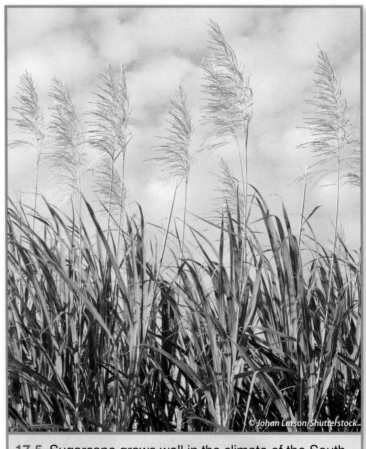

©Johan Larson/Shutterstock

17-5 Sugarcane grows well in the climate of the South.

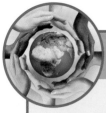

Global Connections

Influence of the Aztecs

The first people to live in Mexico were the Aztec Indians. Their culture was very advanced in art and learning for its time. In the 1500s, Spanish explorers came to Mexico. They gained control of Mexico and had a strong influence on Mexican culture. Most Mexicans have a mixed Aztec and Spanish heritage.

Aztec foods included chocolate, vanilla, corn, peppers, avocados, beans, sweet potatoes, pineapples, and papayas. The Aztecs would boil much of their food to make stewlike dishes. Other food was steamed or broiled. Spaniards brought oil, cinnamon, peaches, rice, wheat, chicken, and cattle to Mexico. They introduced frying to the Aztecs. These foods and cooking methods have been combined in Mexican cuisine.

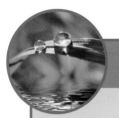

Go Green

Local Foods

Eating locally grown foods is a growing *green* trend and has many benefits. Local foods are fresher because they do not have to travel hundreds of miles to get to their destination. Because foods are already in the community, the amount of chemicals used to ensure a long shelf life are less than those used with shipped foods. Packing materials and carbon dioxide emissions involved with shipping are also reduced. Instead, foods are offered to consumers at their peak ripeness. Buying locally also aids local farmers within the area, which overall benefits the community and the environment.

Western foods also have Spanish and Native American influence. Barbecued beef and lamb are popular in this region. Thick stews made with meat, vegetables, and potatoes are also common in this area.

Midwest

The Midwest has rich soil and flat land that is good for farming. Although winters are cold, the growing season is warm. This region is nicknamed the nation's "breadbasket" because so much corn, grain, and soybeans are grown there. In fact, these crops supply many other parts of the nation and world. Many fruits and vegetables are grown. Farms also raise cattle, dairy cows, pigs, and chickens.

Many different ethnic groups settled in the Midwest. These include Scandinavian, Swiss, German, French, Polish, Irish, and Greek immigrants. These groups contributed cheeses, sausages, lasagna, pot roast, apple pie, and many other foods to the midwestern diet.

The farming culture of the Midwest is known for serving large dinners with much simple, but tasty food. After a hard day's work, farmworkers would sit down to tables laden with food. Beef, pork, chicken, mashed potatoes, vegetables, breads, pies, and cakes would all be served. Midwesterners are also known for having potluck dinners. At a **potluck**, families would eat together and each family would bring one or two dishes for everyone to enjoy.

West Coast States

The Pacific Ocean supplies much seafood to states along the West Coast. Southern California has warm weather throughout the year. Many fruits and vegetables grow well there. Fruits include oranges, avocados, grapes, papayas, nuts, and dates. Vegetables include lettuce, tomatoes, and Chinese cabbage. Northern California, Oregon, and Washington have cooler, but mild weather. Crops include apples, peaches, apricots, and berries.

California attracted many settlers from other parts of the United States. Many came to seek their fortunes by finding gold. Many Mexicans and Asians also settled in California. Dishes often include seafood and fresh produce. Tuna, salmon, lobster, crab, and shrimp are used in many recipes.

Settlers in Oregon and Washington came mainly from other parts of the United States. Seafood such as crab, clams, and salmon is favored. Beef and pork are also popular.

The west coast states are known for their sourdough bread. Sourdough bread is made from a special starter that gives the bread a fermented, sour flavor. Sourdough bread was a staple food for gold prospectors. This is because the starter could be kept and used over long trips. Sourdough bread is still served in many homes and restaurants along the West Coast.

Alaska

Alaska is surrounded by ocean on three sides. Part of the state is in the Arctic region. This land has long, cold winters that make natural food supplies scarce. The southern part of Alaska has a milder climate. Some fruits, vegetables, grain, and dairy cows can be found on farms in this region. Wild caribou, reindeer, rabbit, and bear can also be used for food.

Many Alaskans are native to the land. Others came from other parts of the United States during the gold rush. These people contributed foods from their regions to Alaskan food customs. Other Alaskan foods include caribou sausage, reindeer steak, king crab, salmon, and trout, **17-6**. Huckleberry pie and cranberry ketchup are other favorites.

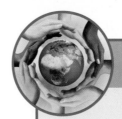

Global Connections

Foods of China

The People's Republic of China (called China) is located in Asia. China is a large country with eastern coastlines and many mountains in the west. Much like the United States, northern parts of China are quite cold, but southern parts have long warm seasons. Because the western part is so mountainous and dry, few people live there. Most of China's people live in the eastern part. This region has good land for growing crops.

Many crops are grown in the eastern part of China. These include rice, wheat, and corn. Vegetables include Chinese celery and pea pods, turnips, radishes, water chestnuts, mushrooms, and eggplants. Some fruits including oranges, pears, grapes, and kumquats are grown. Ducks, chickens, and pigs are the main animals raised for food. Historically, China raised very little dairy cattle. As a result, milk, cheese, and other dairy products were rare in China. In the past 40 years, China has made great strides to increase dairy production.

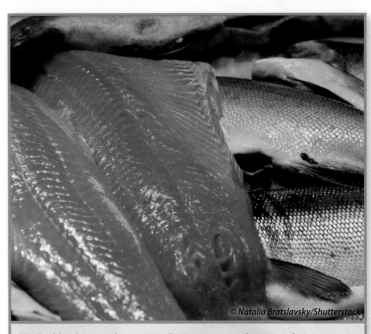

© Natalia Bratslavsky/Shutterstock

17-6 Alaskan salmon are important to the state's economy.

Hawaii

Hawaii is made up of several islands in the South Pacific. It has a mild climate and long growing season. Tropical fruits such as pineapples, mangoes, coconuts, and papayas grow well there. Vegetables, such as snow peas, water chestnuts, Chinese cabbage, and squash, also grow well in Hawaii's warm climate.

Hawaii's first settlers were Polynesians. Later, Americans of European background, Chinese workers, and Japanese settlers came to the islands. The Polynesians brought coconuts and breadfruit. Europeans brought chicken, pork, and sugarcane. The Chinese contributed rice and various Chinese vegetables. The Japanese brought many rice and fish dishes. They also introduced a thick, slightly sweet food marinade called *teriyaki*.

Popular Hawaiian foods include roast pig, mahimahi (a tropical fish) and other seafood, and coconut bread. Poi, a smooth paste made from the taro plant, is served with many Hawaiian meals.

Reading Review

1. List three factors within a culture that affect food customs.
2. Name six foods introduced to the first settlers in North America by Native Americans.
3. Name two unique cooking styles founded in the South.
4. What are potluck dinners?
5. What is poi?

Planning Meals

Objectives

After studying this section, you will be able to
- **implement** healthful meal planning.
- **recognize** the factors that make a meal appealing.
- **identify** strategies for eating healthful meals away from home.

Key Term
garnishes

Planning healthful meals—both at home and away from home—can be easy when you are armed with the necessary tools. If you can recognize nutrient-dense food choices and know the amounts from each food group you need daily, you can plan a healthful meal. With a little thought, that healthful meal can be appealing as well.

Healthful Meals

Your eating pattern describes all the foods you regularly eat and drink. It may or may not be a healthful eating pattern. There are a number of resources available to help you plan a healthful one. ChooseMyPlate.gov is one of these resources. The first step is to determine the amounts from each food group to meet your daily needs. You can do this by entering your height, weight, gender, and level of activity to create a personalized food plan.

Once you know the food amounts you need, you can plan your meals for the day. ChooseMyPlate.gov has a *Food Planner* tool to help you plan healthful meals. As you build your menu for the day, the planner shows your progress toward meeting your daily amounts for each food group, **17-7**.

You can also plan healthful meals without the use of the website. You can arrange the food amounts from your personalized food plan over the number of meals you usually eat in a day. For instance, suppose you choose to eat three meals and a snack each day. If your food plan recommends two cups of fruit daily, you may choose to eat some fruit at each meal.
- *Breakfast:* one-half cup of orange juice
- *Lunch:* snack container of applesauce
- *Dinner:* small bunch (16) of grapes
- *Evening snack:* one plum

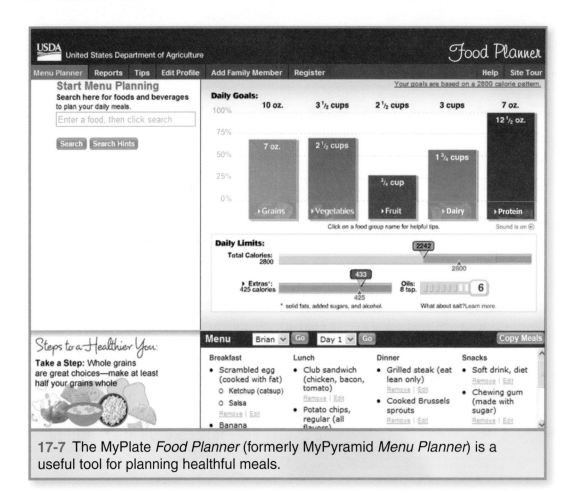

17-7 The MyPlate *Food Planner* (formerly MyPyramid *Menu Planner*) is a useful tool for planning healthful meals.

You can arrange the food amounts over your meals as you prefer. The following suggestions will help you provide your body with a steady supply of nutrients throughout the day.

Breakfast

Make time to eat breakfast every day. You may have heard that breakfast is the most important meal of the day. In fact, teens that routinely eat breakfast are more likely to

- maintain a healthy body weight
- be more creative
- perform well in school
- be physically active

Breakfast should give your body at least one-fourth of the nutrients it needs for the day. Foods should be nutrient dense. Including at least one serving each of whole grains, low-fat dairy, fruit or vegetable, and protein will supply your body with a steady stream of energy and nutrients for hours.

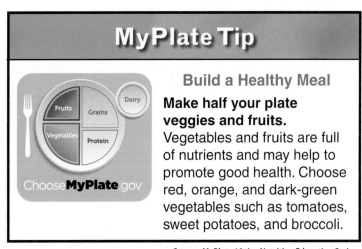

MyPlate Tip

Build a Healthy Meal

Make half your plate veggies and fruits.
Vegetables and fruits are full of nutrients and may help to promote good health. Choose red, orange, and dark-green vegetables such as tomatoes, sweet potatoes, and broccoli.

Source: MyPlate 10 tips Nutrition Education Series

You may be skipping breakfast so you can sleep a little longer. Actually, you may find that eating breakfast will help you more than the extra sleep. Studies show that students who eat breakfast stay more alert in class. They are also better able to concentrate on their work.

Perhaps you do not eat breakfast because you dislike traditional breakfast foods. If foods such as toast and eggs do not appeal to you, choose other foods you enjoy more. Nutritious foods are nutritious no matter what time of day they are eaten. For instance, an orange and a ham and cheese sandwich on whole-grain bread can serve as a healthy breakfast, **17-8**.

Lunch

Your body needs nutrients to keep it going in the middle of the day. Lunch is especially important if you have a full schedule. Your body needs a supply of energy to keep up a fast pace. Do not allow your busy schedule to keep you from eating lunch.

Lunch should provide you with about one-third of the day's nutrients. Choosing a variety of foods in the middle of the day will help supply you with the nutrients you need. Many school cafeterias serve hot lunches. You can also make nutritious food choices when packing your lunch. Many nutritious foods are tasty and easy to pack.

Dinner

In the evening, you need to replace some of the nutrients your body has used during the day. Like lunch, dinner should provide you with about one-third of your daily nutrient requirements. Again, choosing a variety of foods is the best way to get all the nutrients you need.

Mix and Match Your Breakfast			
Grains	*Fruits and Vegetables*	*Protein Foods*	*Dairy (fat free or low fat)*
Brown rice	Banana	Walnuts	Milk
Whole-grain bagel	Orange	Egg or egg whites	Yogurt
Whole-wheat tortilla	Applesauce	Peanut butter	Cheese (cheddar,
Oatmeal	Raisins	Turkey bacon	mozzarella, Swiss,
Whole-grain muffin	Strawberries	Pinto beans	Parmesan)
Whole-grain corn bread	Cantaloupe	Lean ham or turkey	Fortified soymilk
Low-fat granola	Pineapple chunks	Sunflower seeds	Cottage cheese
Whole-wheat toast	Orange juice	Turkey sausage	Ricotta cheese
Whole-wheat pancakes	Blueberries	Canned tuna	
Whole-wheat waffles	Grapefruit		
Whole-grain pizza crust	Tomato salsa		
Whole-grain, ready-to-eat cereals	Tomato juice		
	Vegetables (for pizza toppings or in scrambled eggs)		

17-8 Select amounts from each group to meet your nutrient needs and food preferences.

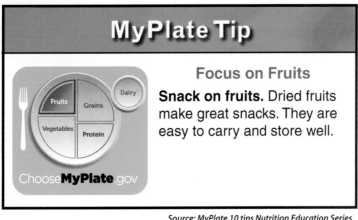

MyPlate Tip

Focus on Fruits

Snack on fruits. Dried fruits make great snacks. They are easy to carry and store well.

Source: MyPlate 10 tips Nutrition Education Series

Snacks

Snacks are foods that are eaten at times other than mealtimes. Snacks are part of your daily food intake. They should help you meet any energy and nutrient needs not met by the foods you eat at meals. If you eat regular meals, you need to limit your snacking. On the other hand, if your schedule forces you to miss meals, you need to snack more.

When snacking, avoid processed snack foods such as candy and chips. These snacks tend to be high in sugar, fat, and salt. Instead, select nutritious snacks such as fresh fruits and vegetables, nuts, cereals, and popcorn. Food choices for snacks should also be nutrient dense.

Meals with Appeal

Planning appealing meals requires giving some thought to how foods look and taste together. Coming up with ideas for appealing meals may be difficult for you as a beginning cook. Cookbooks offer many different types of recipe and menu suggestions. Magazines, newspapers, TV, and the Internet might also give you ideas for planning tempting meals. As you look for menu ideas, remember to keep your plans simple at first. Trying to prepare big, complicated menus may lead to frustration.

Meals with appeal are attractive, interesting, and varied. Choosing foods with different colors, flavors, textures, shapes, sizes, and temperatures helps create interest. You and your family are more likely to enjoy meals with appeal.

Color

Plan meals that include a variety of colors. Picture a meal consisting of baked chicken with cream sauce, white rice, cauliflower, white bread, and vanilla pudding. A meal such as this would look boring because all the foods are white or cream colored. Sweet potatoes could be substituted for the rice. A golden-brown roll could be served in place of the bread. Green beans could be served instead of cauliflower and chocolate pudding instead of vanilla. These simple changes would add color and interest to this meal.

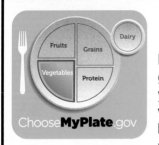

MyPlate Tip

Add More Vegetables to Your Day

Make your garden salad glow with color. Brighten your salad by using colorful vegetables such as black beans, sliced red bell peppers, shredded radishes, chopped red cabbage, or watercress. Your salad will not only look good, but also taste good.

Source: MyPlate 10 tips Nutrition Education Series

Foods that decorate a dish or plate are called **garnishes**. They are used to add color and zest to meals. Parsley, lemon slices, or a sprig of rosemary are examples of garnishes.

Flavor

Think about how the flavors of your foods will blend when planning a meal. Certain foods taste good together. Turkey and dressing, spaghetti and meat sauce, and baked chicken with mashed potatoes are natural combinations. Take advantage of these well-liked combinations to make your meals appealing and save you planning time.

Including contrasting flavors in the same meal provides interest. For instance, sweet and sour chicken is a successful dish because it features the contrast of sweet and sour flavors. Varying the flavors of your foods in this way will add interest to your meals.

Texture

Texture refers to the feel of food in your mouth when you are eating it. Foods are often described as crisp, soft, tender, crunchy, chewy, or creamy. A general rule is to include at least three different textures in each meal. A meal of tender poached fish, chewy wild rice, and crisp lettuce salad would provide a nice variety of textures.

Shape and Size

Choose foods with different shapes and sizes. Meatballs, Brussels sprouts, and cherry tomatoes are too similar in shape and size to be served at the same meal. To make a more attractive meal, you might serve the meatballs with broccoli spears and slices of tomato. This would add a variety of shapes and sizes.

Temperature

Your meals should include both hot and cold foods. For instance, you might serve a cold salad with a hot entree to give your meal a variety of temperatures. Remember to serve hot foods piping hot and cold foods icy cold, **17-9**.

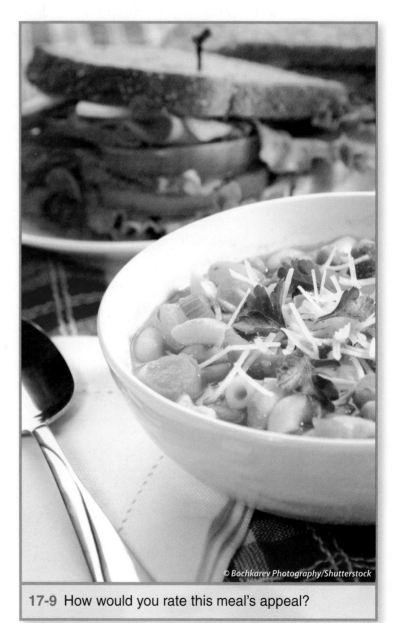

© Bochkarev Photography/Shutterstock

17-9 How would you rate this meal's appeal?

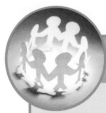

Life Connections

Meals Away from Home

Many families eat meals away from home on occasion. This is due partly to busy lifestyles. Setting aside time to prepare meals is often hard for working parents or teens with full schedules. Many families also think eating out is fun. It may be a treat to eat at a special restaurant.

Making healthful food choices when eating out is becoming easier. Many more restaurants are offering healthful menu choices. Making substitutions can help you choose a healthful meal.
- Order fat-free or low-fat milk or water instead of a carbonated beverage.
- Choose broiled chicken over fried, breaded chicken sandwiches.
- Order a hamburger rather than a cheeseburger.
- Substitute fruit or steamed vegetables for French fries.
- Do not add extra salt to your food.
- Select pizza with vegetables instead of extra meat and cheese.

Research Activity

More restaurants are being required to provide nutrition information for their menus. Check several restaurant websites for menus and nutrition information to help you make healthful choices.

Reading Review

1. When using ChooseMyPlate.gov to create a personalized food plan, what information do you need to enter?
2. What do studies show about students who eat breakfast?
3. When snacking, what foods should you avoid and why?
4. How do you create meals with appeal that are attractive, interesting, and varied?
5. Give two examples of how you can make substitutions to help you choose a healthful meal at a restaurant.

Section 17-3

Using Recipes

Objectives

After studying this section, you will be able to
- **identify** the parts of a recipe.
- **explain** how to measure dry ingredients, liquid ingredients, and shortening.
- **use** a conversion factor to change recipe yield.
- **define** common cooking terms used in recipes.
- **recognize** a healthful recipe.

Key Terms		
recipe	yield	recipe conversion
ingredients	preheat	

Cooking involves a language, set of skills, and tools that are unique. Before you begin to prepare your meal, you should be familiar with these basics of cooking. Arming yourself with this knowledge improves your chances of success in the kitchen.

Understanding Recipes

Recipes are often used when preparing meals. A **recipe** is a set of instructions used to prepare a food product. Before you begin to cook, you need to understand how to read and use recipes.

All recipes include the ingredients needed and how to assemble them. **Ingredients** are food items needed to make a certain food product. The list states the amount of each ingredient that is needed to prepare the recipe properly. The directions explain how the ingredients are combined to produce the desired dish. Oven temperature and length of cooking time are given for baked and cooked products. Recipes also include a **yield** that states the number of servings the recipe produces. All recipes include this information, but may organize it in different ways. Three common recipe formats are standard, action, and narrative, **17-10.**

Using simple recipes is a good idea when you are first learning to cook. Give yourself a chance to develop some basic cooking skills before trying more involved recipes.

Recipe Formats

Standard Format — Souper Rice

Yield: 6 servings

1½ c. white rice
1 can (10½ oz.) condensed cream of mushroom soup
1½ c. water

1. Coat a 2-quart casserole with cooking spray or butter.
2. Combine rice, soup, and water in the casserole and stir until blended.
3. Cover and bake rice in 350°F oven for 30 to 45 minutes or until liquid is absorbed and rice is tender and fluffy.

Action Format — Souper Rice

Yield: 6 servings

Coat a 2-quart casserole with cooking spray or butter.
Combine 1½ c. white rice, 1 10½-oz. can condensed cream of mushroom soup, and 1½ c. water in casserole and stir until blended.
Bake covered casserole in 350°F oven for 30 to 45 minutes or until liquid is absorbed and rice is tender and fluffy.

Narrative Format — Souper Rice

Yield: 6 servings

Coat a 2-quart casserole with cooking spray or butter. **Combine** 1½ c. white rice, 1 10½-oz. can condensed cream of mushroom soup, and 1½ c. water in casserole and stir until blended. **Cover and bake** rice in 350°F oven for 30 to 45 minutes or until liquid is absorbed and rice is tender and fluffy.

17-10 The standard recipe format is most common.

Tips for Using Recipes

Most recipes are tested before they are featured in cookbooks. Recipes that have been tested are more likely to produce consistent, high-quality dishes. Despite testing, a recipe may not always produce the end result you desire. This can make you feel frustrated. A failed food product means wasted time, energy, and money. Before you start cooking, follow these tips to improve your chances for a successful dish.

- Read the recipe carefully before you begin cooking. As you read, check for understanding of the terms and procedures in the recipe, **17-11**.
- Verify that you have all the ingredients listed.
- Locate the equipment you will need.
- Confirm you have enough time to prepare the food product.
- Note the yield—you may need more or less food than the recipe makes. If this is the case, you may need to adjust the recipe to produce the desired yield.
- Gather all the ingredients and utensils you need. You will find working easier if you have everything you need within reach.

Your recipe may tell you to preheat the oven. **Preheat** means to turn on the oven before beginning to cook. This allows the oven to heat to the correct temperature before you place food in it. Be sure you set the oven to the temperature stated in the recipe.

As you begin to prepare a recipe, follow all directions exactly. Carefully measure the amount of each ingredient. Mix the ingredients in the order given using the techniques stated.

Bake or cook foods as indicated on the recipe. You should use correct pan sizes and follow stated times and temperatures. Each of these factors affects the outcome of a food product.

Measuring Ingredients

Using the correct amount of each ingredient is crucial to the success of a recipe. Even small changes in the amounts of some ingredients may affect the outcome of a dish.

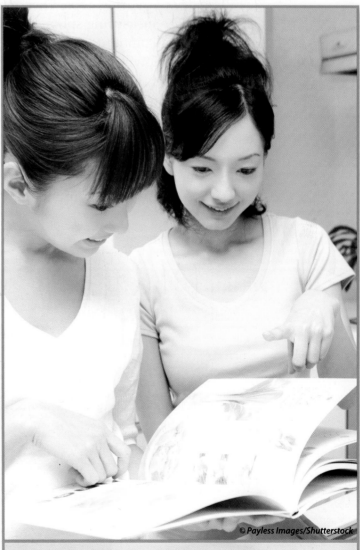

© Payless Images/Shutterstock

17-11 Read through a recipe before you begin to prepare it.

Experienced cooks may combine a "pinch" of one ingredient and a "sprinkle" of another when cooking. Beginning cooks, on the other hand, need to measure ingredients carefully. Accurate measuring helps ensure a desired final product.

Abbreviations

Amounts of ingredients are often given as abbreviations. Learning these abbreviations enables you to read recipes quickly and measure accurately, **17-12**.

How to Measure

To measure ingredients correctly, you must use standard measuring tools and proper methods. Liquid and dry measuring cups and measuring spoons are marked for measuring exact amounts.

Measuring Dry Ingredients

Use dry measuring cups when measuring dry ingredients such as sugar and flour. Use measuring spoons when measuring baking powder, salt, spices, or small amounts of any dry ingredient. Fill the measuring cup or spoon to overflowing. Then level it off with a narrow spatula or the straight edge of a knife.

Most dry ingredients should not be packed down when they are measured. Packing causes you to have more than your recipe tells you to use. Brown sugar is measured differently. It is always packed lightly into measuring tools. As with other dry ingredients, the measuring cup or spoon is first overfilled and then leveled. Brown sugar should hold the shape of the measuring tool when you turn it out.

Measuring Liquid Ingredients

Liquid ingredients such as water, milk, oil, syrup, and juices should be measured in liquid measuring cups. Liquid measuring cups are made from clear material that you can easily see through. Small amounts of liquid ingredients can be measured in measuring spoons.

Liquid measuring cups should be placed on a flat, level surface before you pour in the liquid. Carefully fill the measuring cup to the line indicating the amount you need. For an accurate measure, you should check the amount of liquid at eye level. Bend down to check the measurement while the cup is on the flat surface, **17-13**. (Holding the

Abbreviations Used in Recipes	
Abbreviation	*Unit of Measure*
tsp. or t.	teaspoon
Tbsp. or T.	tablespoon
c. or C.	cup
pt.	pint
qt.	quart
gal.	gallon
oz.	ounce
lb. or #	pound

17-12 Measurements are often abbreviated in recipes.

cup up to your eye does not give an accurate measure.) You will see that the liquid curves upward slightly along the sides of the measuring cup. Be sure to use the lowest part of the curve for your measurement.

Measuring Shortenings

Use dry measuring cups to measure solid shortening. Use measuring spoons when measuring less than ¼ cup. Shortening is easier to measure at room temperature. Firmly press the shortening into the measuring tool as you overfill it. Be sure no air spaces are left in the measuring tool. Next, level it with a narrow spatula or straight-edged knife. Remove the shortening from the cup with a rubber scraper. This technique is also used when measuring foods such as peanut butter and mayonnaise.

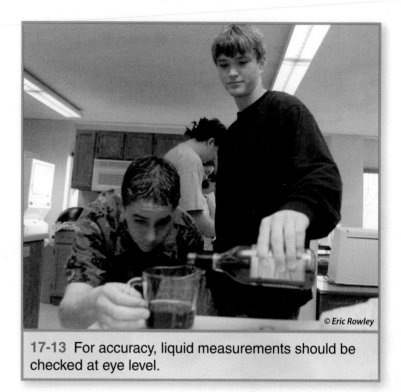
© Eric Rowley

17-13 For accuracy, liquid measurements should be checked at eye level.

Butter and margarine often come in quarter-pound sticks. The wrappers on the sticks are marked with lines. These lines divide each stick into eight tablespoons. Use these lines as guides and cut through the wrapper to measure the amount of butter or margarine needed.

Changing Recipe Yield

Sometimes you need more servings than a recipe yields. At other times, you may need fewer servings. Changing a recipe's yield up or down is called **recipe conversion**. When you perform a recipe conversion, you need to increase or decrease the amount of each ingredient. You determine the new ingredient amounts by applying a conversion factor. You calculate the conversion factor using the following simple math:

Desired yield ÷ Current yield = Conversion factor

For instance, suppose you have a recipe that yields 12 servings, but you only need 6 servings. Your desired yield is 6 and your current yield is 12. You would calculate your conversion factor as follows:

6 (desired yield) ÷ 12 (current yield) = ½ (conversion factor)

The next step is to apply your conversion factor to each ingredient amount.

Conversion factor x Original ingredient amount = New ingredient amount

If your recipe calls for three cups of flour, you would calculate the new amount as follows:

½ (conversion factor) x 3 cups flour = 1½ cups flour

To perform recipe conversions properly, you need to learn measurement equivalents. (An *equivalent* is something that is equal to something else.) For instance, three teaspoons are the equivalent of one tablespoon. If you are cutting a recipe in half that calls for one tablespoon of sugar, you would first convert the tablespoon to teaspoons because there is not a measuring spoon for half tablespoon. To calculate, divide three teaspoons in half to get one and one-half teaspoons sugar, **17-14**.

Be sure to perform your recipe conversions before you start cooking to avoid mistakes.

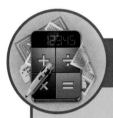

Math Connections

Converting a Recipe

Suppose you are baking chocolate chip cookies for your scout troop. The recipe ingredients listed below make 36 cookies, but you need 72 cookies. Calculate the conversion factor and then use it to adjust each ingredient amount.

Chocolate Chip Cookies

1 c. butter	1 tsp. vanilla extract
½ c. sugar	2¼ c. flour
½ c. brown sugar, packed	1 tsp. baking soda
	½ tsp. salt
2 eggs	2 c. chocolate chips

(*Answer:* conversion factor = 2; ingredient amounts 2 c. butter, 1 c. sugar, 1 c. brown sugar, 4 eggs, 2 tsp. vanilla extract, 4½ c. flour, 2 tsp. baking soda, 1 tsp. salt, 4 c. chocolate chips)

Measurement Equivalents

3 teaspoons = 1 tablespoon

2 tablespoons = ⅛ cup

4 tablespoons = ¼ cup

5 1/3 tablespoons = ⅓ cup

8 tablespoons = ½ cup

10 2/3 tablespoons = ⅔ cup

12 tablespoons = ¾ cup

16 tablespoons = 1 cup

2 cups = 1 pint

4 cups = 1 quart

17-14 Knowing measurement equivalents makes changing a recipe's yield easier.

Food Preparation Terms

If you are a beginning cook, you may not know what some of the terms in recipes mean. For instance, do you know how to *dredge* a food? What does *marinate* mean? Do *mix* and *blend* mean the same thing? What is the difference between *stir* and *beat*? Understanding common cooking terms will help you follow recipes exactly, **17-15**.

Choosing Healthful Recipes

As you are selecting recipes to prepare, keep in mind that you are also making a choice about your health. By choosing a healthful recipe, you are taking a step toward good health.

To identify a healthful recipe, you must look at two factors—the ingredients and the cooking method. If the ingredients are nutrient dense and the cooking method does not require large amounts of fat, the recipe is likely to be good for you.

Healthful ingredient options can be found in every food group, **17-16**. Look for recipes that use oils rather than solid fats when possible. Find recipes that include nutrient-dense ingredients or try making your own more healthful substitutions.

Food Preparation Terms

- **Baste.** Periodically moistening food with a liquid as it cooks. The liquid used may be pan drippings or a cooking sauce. Basting can be performed with a brush, baster, or spoon. Meats, such as roasts and spareribs, are basted to keep them moist.
- **Bread.** A procedure that coats food in flour, then liquid—usually milk or beaten egg—and then crumbs. Crumbs are usually made from crackers, bread, or cereal. Foods, such as chicken and fish, are breaded to give them a delicate crust.
- **Brush.** To lightly coat foods with a liquid before, during, or after cooking using a food preparation brush. The liquid may be melted butter or some type of sauce. Brushing is done to foods, such as turkey and grilled items, to keep them moist during cooking.
- **Dredge.** Coating a food with a dry ingredient—usually flour or sugar— by "dragging" it through the ingredient until it is coated. Excess coating is removed by gently shaking food. This is the first step in the breading procedure. Some cookies and candies are dredged in sugar. Chicken or beef cuts may be dredged in flour.
- **Marinate.** To soak food in a seasoned liquid for a period of time. Tougher cuts of meats are often marinated to add flavor and make them more tender.
- **Mash.** To crush a food until it has a smooth texture. Potatoes are commonly mashed to be served as a side dish.
- **Pare.** To remove the skin or thin outer covering of a food using a knife or peeler. Apples and potatoes are often pared to keep their skins from interfering with the texture of foods.
- **Peel.** To remove the skin or outer covering of a food. Peel and pare are often used to mean the same thing, but peeling is usually done by hand.

Food Cutting Terms

- **Chop.** To cut food into small, uneven pieces that are not uniform in shape. Cut the food into small pieces if the recipe calls for a finely chopped ingredient. Cut the food into bigger pieces if the recipe calls for a coarsely chopped ingredient. Vegetables are often chopped when being added to salads and casseroles.
- **Core.** To remove the center, inedible area of a fruit. Apples, pears, peaches, and pineapple may be cored before serving.
- **Cube.** To cut food into uniform box shapes about one-half to one inch in size. Meats and potatoes are often cubed for adding to soups and stews.
- **Dice.** Cut food into small, even cubes, about ¼ inch in size. Vegetables may be diced before cooking.
- **Grate.** To cut food into very fine pieces by rubbing it across a rough surface. Cheese is often grated before it is sprinkled on foods.
- **Julienne.** To cut food into a size and shape similar to a matchstick. Julienne vegetables are often used in salads.
- **Mince.** To cut or chop food into very tiny pieces using a knife or scissors. Parsley and onions are often minced. Mincing helps spread their flavors through a food without overpowering the food with large pieces.
- **Shred.** To cut, grate, or pull apart food to form long thin strips. Cabbage is shredded to make coleslaw.
- **Slice.** Use a knife to cut foods into flat pieces of even widths. Your recipe should tell you how thick the slices need to be. Vegetables are often sliced before cooking. Bread and meat loaf are sliced after cooking.

(Continued)

17-15 Understanding these terms will help you prepare recipes correctly.

Food Preparation Terms *(Continued)*

Mixing Terms

- **Beat.** To mix ingredients with a fast up and over motion bringing the contents to the top of the bowl and then down again. Beating is done with a spoon, rotary beater, or electric mixer. Eggs are beaten when making scrambled eggs.
- **Blend.** To stir ingredients so they are completely combined, but not beaten. Liquid ingredients are blended with dry ingredients when making muffins.
- **Combine.** To mix two or more ingredients together. Several dry ingredients may be combined before mixing with liquid ingredients.
- **Cream.** Beating fat and sugar to add air and create a soft, smooth mixture.
- **Cut in.** To combine fat with a dry ingredient using knives or a pastry blender. Fat should be roughly pea-size pieces when finished. Solid shortening needs to be cut into a flour mixture when making biscuits and pastry.
- **Fold.** To gently mix a light, airy ingredient with a heavier ingredient using a scraper in a circular motion. Mixing is done gently and slowly to maintain airy quality.
- **Stir.** Using a spoon, scraper, or whisk in a circular motion to mix ingredients. Be sure to stir around the outside of the bowl or pan as well as in the center.
- **Toss.** To mix ingredients by flipping them lightly with a spoon and a fork, one in each hand. Push the spoon down one side of the bowl and the fork down the other. Bring the utensils up through the center. Continue tossing until the ingredients are thoroughly mixed. Salads are often mixed in this way.
- **Whip.** Use the same up and over motion used in beating, but much faster using a wire whisk, rotary beater, or electric mixer. The mixture expands due to the added air. Whipping cream is whipped to change the liquid cream to foam.

Cooking Methods

Dry Heat

- **Baking.** Food, often covered, is surrounded by hot air in an oven. Used to cook foods with added sauce or other moisture such as lasagna.
- **Broiling.** Food is placed under a direct flame or heat source. Food is placed on a rack to allow fat to drip away and is turned so both sides are exposed to the heat source.
- **Deep frying.** Food is fully immersed in hot fat. Item may be coated in breading or batter before frying.
- **Grilling.** Food is placed above a heat source on a grate. Fat drips off and is lost.
- **Panbroiling.** Food is placed in a preheated skillet with no lid and with no fat added. This method is used on foods such as meats that contain fat. Food is turned so both sides are exposed to the heat source.
- **Roasting.** Similar to baking, food is surrounded by hot air in an oven using a shallow pan. Food is left uncovered.
- **Sautéing.** Food is placed in a preheated pan with a small amount of hot fat over high heat to cook quickly. Food is turned so both sides are exposed to the heat source.

Moist Heat

- **Boiling.** Food is placed in liquid that is heated to the highest temperature possible. Boiling liquid has rapidly forming, large bubbles.
- **Poaching.** Food is placed in liquid that is heated just to the temperature where it barely moves and small bubbles form only occasionally. This method is used on delicate foods such as eggs and fish.
- **Simmering.** Food is placed in liquid that is heated to slightly below boiling temperature. The liquid moves steadily and bubbles form constantly.
- **Steaming.** Food is placed on a rack and surrounded by vapor created from boiling liquid.

Combination

- **Braising.** Food is first browned on all sides in a small amount of fat and then simmered in a flavored liquid for a long period. Food is usually covered during simmering.

A healthful cooking method should add little or no additional fat to a recipe. Grilling, broiling, roasting, baking, poaching, and steaming require no addition of fat. Sautéing and panbroiling can be performed using very small amounts of oil rather than butter or shortening. Some nutrients are destroyed by high temperatures. Healthful cooking methods use either high temperatures for shorter periods or lower temperatures for longer periods. Braising cooks food in liquid using a lower temperature for a longer period. Nutrients that leach into the cooking liquid are preserved because the cooking liquid is served as a sauce with the dish.

Even small steps in the right direction are good. Perhaps the recipe you choose has some less healthful ingredients, but is more healthful than your old recipe. For instance, choosing a banana bread recipe that calls for a large amount of sugar, but uses half whole-wheat flour is a positive step. Once you adapt to the taste of the new recipe, you could consider ways to reduce the amount of sugar.

Identifying Healthful Ingredients

In the grains group, look for
- *whole grain* or *whole wheat* in the name, such as whole-wheat pasta or whole-grain cornmeal
- less processed grains such as rolled oats rather than instant oatmeal or brown rice rather than white rice

In the vegetable group, look for
- vegetables that are in season or frozen vegetables
- canned vegetables labeled *low sodium*
- vegetables that are high in potassium such as sweet potatoes, white potatoes, white beans, tomato products, beet greens, soybeans, lima beans, spinach, lentils, and kidney beans more often

In the fruit group, look for
- fruits that are in season
- fruits that are canned or frozen without added sugar
- fruits that are high in potassium such as bananas, prunes and prune juice, dried peaches and apricots, and orange juice more often

In the dairy group, look for
- low-fat or fat-free milk products or soymilk
- cheeses that are naturally lower in fat such as Parmesan or feta

In the protein foods group, look for
- cuts of meat that include *round* or *loin* in the name and are leaner
- ground beef, turkey, or chicken that is labeled as 90% (or greater) lean
- skinless poultry cuts
- seafood such as salmon, trout, or herring
- beans, peas, or soy products such as pinto beans, split peas, or tofu as a replacement for meat or poultry
- nuts or seeds as a replacement for meat or poultry

17-16 Use these tips to help you identify healthful ingredients.

Reading Review

1. List three common recipe formats.
2. Why should you note the yield on a recipe?
3. Why is using the correct amount of each ingredient crucial to the success of a recipe?
4. Why is it necessary to understand common cooking terms?
5. What two factors help you to identify a healthful recipe?

Healthy Recipes

Granola Baked Apples

Yield: 4 servings

4 cooking apples
(Rome Beauty
or Granny
Smith)

¾ c. low-fat granola
2 Tbsp. brown sugar
⅛ tsp. cinnamon

1. Wash and core apples.
2. Scoop out center of apples to leave ½-inch shell. Chop ½ cup apple from the center and reserve. Cut a strip of peel ½-inch wide around the top of the apple.
3. In a medium bowl, mix granola, reserved ½ cup chopped apple, brown sugar, and cinnamon.
4. Fill scooped out apples with granola mixture and place in a shallow baking dish. Add ¼ inch of water to baking dish.
5. Cover apples and bake in 350°F oven for 45 minutes or until tender.

© Marcie Fowler - Shining Hope Images/Shutterstock

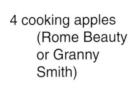

Healthy Recipes

Roasted Sweet Potato Fries

Yield: 6 servings

¼ c. extra virgin
olive oil
1 clove garlic,
chopped
½ tsp. fresh rosemary,
chopped

⅛ tsp. paprika
⅛ tsp. onion powder
¼ tsp. black pepper
¼ tsp. salt
2 sweet potatoes

1. Preheat oven to 450°F and line cookie sheet with parchment paper.
2. Place oil in bowl and mix in garlic, rosemary, and seasonings.
3. Wash and peel sweet potatoes.
4. Cut sweet potatoes into fries approximately ⅜-inch x ⅜-inch x 3-inches
5. Place sweet potatoes in oil mixture and toss to coat.
6. Spread sweet potato fries on parchment paper and place in oven.
7. Turn fries after 15 minutes and cook another 10 to 15 minutes until brown and crispy.

© Robyn Mackenzie/Shutterstock

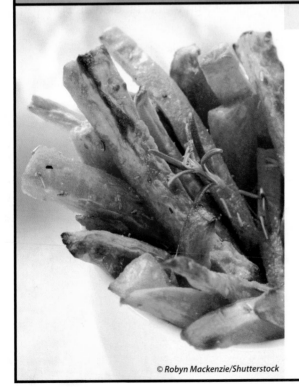

Healthy Recipes

Black Beans and Rice

Yield: 8 servings

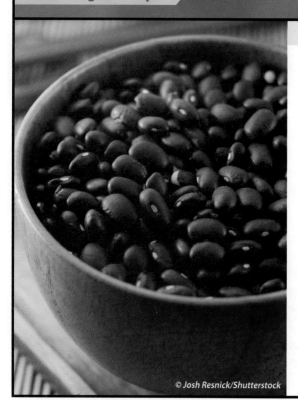

© Josh Resnick/Shutterstock

1½ tsp. canola oil
1 small onion,
   chopped
4 cloves garlic, minced
½ c. brown rice
¼ c. white rice
1½ c. chicken stock
1 tsp. ground cumin
¼ tsp. cayenne pepper

¼ tsp. salt
1 jalapeño pepper,
   pickled
1 c. tomatoes,
   small dice
3½ c. canned black
   beans, drained
1 Tbsp. lime juice

1. Place oil in pot and heat over medium heat. Sauté garlic and onion for 5 minutes. Add brown and white rice and sauté for another 2 minutes.
2. Add chicken stock and spices to pot and bring to a boil. Reduce heat and cover to simmer for 20 minutes.
3. Add pepper, tomatoes, and black beans to pot and simmer for another 10 minutes stirring occasionally.
4. Mix in lime juice and serve.

Healthy Recipes

Sautéed Spinach

Yield: 6 servings

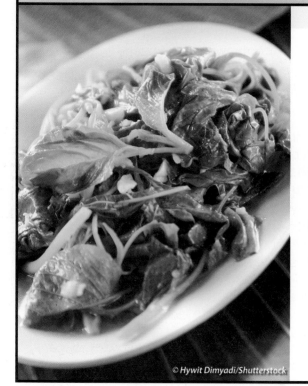

© Hywit Dimyadi/Shutterstock

1½ lb. baby spinach leaves
2 Tbsp. olive oil
6 cloves garlic, sliced
¼ tsp. lemon juice
salt and pepper to taste

1. Rinse spinach well and pat dry.
2. Heat oil in a large pot over medium heat. Add garlic and sauté for about 1 minute—do not let garlic brown.
3. Add spinach, salt, and pepper to pot and stir about 1 to 2 minutes until wilted.
4. Place spinach in serving bowl and drizzle with lemon juice.

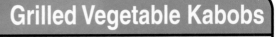

Healthy Recipes

Grilled Vegetable Kabobs

Yield: 6 servings

1 zucchini
1 each red, yellow, and green bell peppers
12 oz. button mushrooms
1 red onion
1 pint cherry tomatoes
2 Tbsp. canola oil
Salt and pepper to taste

1. Preheat grill to medium.
2. Wash and trim vegetables. Cut zucchini, peppers, and onion into 1½ inch chunks.
3. Thread vegetables onto skewers, alternating for color. (If using wood skewers, soak in water for 30 minutes prior to using.)
4. Brush oil on skewered vegetables. Salt and pepper to taste.
5. Use tongs to place vegetable kabobs on a preheated grill.
6. Cook kabobs for about 10 minutes. Turn kabobs with tongs halfway through cooking time.

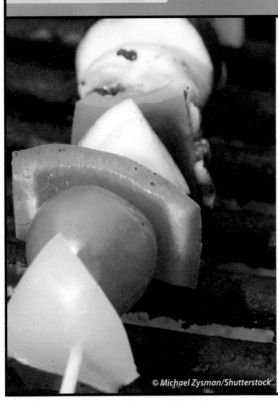

© Michael Zysman/Shutterstock

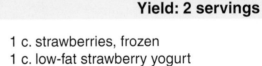

Healthy Recipes

Strawberry Yogurt Shake

Yield: 2 servings

1 c. strawberries, frozen
1 c. low-fat strawberry yogurt
1 c. low-fat or fat-free milk
1 tsp. vanilla

1. Combine strawberries, yogurt, milk, and vanilla in a blender.
2. Blend on high speed for 20 seconds or until mixture is smooth.

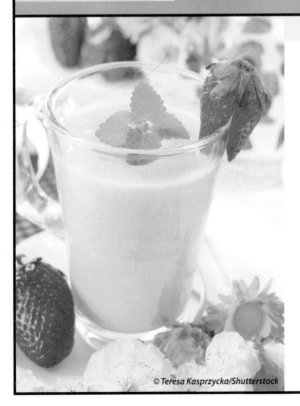

© Teresa Kasprzycka/Shutterstock

Healthy Recipes

Grilled Peach Salad

Yield: 6 servings

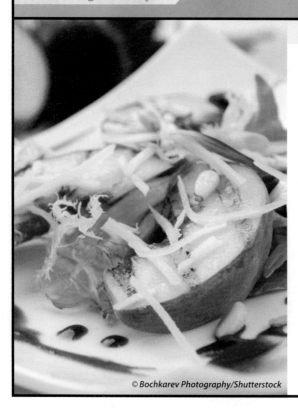

1½ Tbsp. vegetable oil
4 firm, ripe peaches
1 oz. Parmesan cheese, large shred
3 Tbsp. pine nuts, toasted
4 oz. baby lettuce
¼ c. balsamic vinaigrette

1. Preheat a grill to medium heat.
2. Halve and pit unpeeled peaches. Cut each half into 3 wedges and lightly brush with oil.
3. Place pine nuts on a sheet pan in a 300°F oven for 10 minutes until lightly browned. Shake pan after about 5 minutes to ensure even browning.
4. Place wedges on grill. Cook for about 2 minutes on each side.
5. Arrange 4 wedges on a bed of lettuce. Sprinkle with cheese and pine nuts. Drizzle with vinaigrette.

© Bochkarev Photography/Shutterstock

Healthy Recipes

Marinated Cherry Tomatoes

Yield: 6 servings

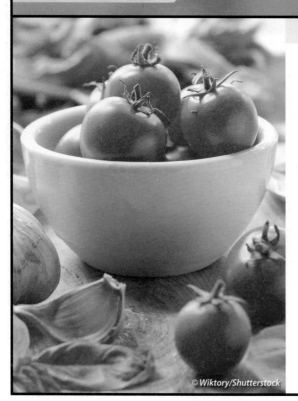

½ tsp. salt
¼ c. lemon juice
¾ c. oil
1 clove garlic, crushed
½ tsp. basil
½ tsp. thyme
1 Tbsp. parsley, chopped
2 pints cherry tomatoes

1. Mix all ingredients except tomatoes in a bowl.
2. Wash cherry tomatoes and remove stems.
3. Add tomatoes to dressing and chill 2 hours or overnight.

© Wiktory/Shutterstock

Healthy Recipes

Hearty Corn Bread

Yield: 8 servings

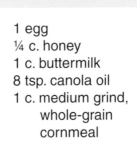

1 egg
¼ c. honey
1 c. buttermilk
8 tsp. canola oil
1 c. medium grind,
   whole-grain
   cornmeal

1 c. all-purpose flour
2 tsp. baking powder
½ tsp. baking soda
½ tsp. salt

1. Prepare 8-inch baking dish with cooking spray.
2. Beat egg in a medium-size mixing bowl. Add honey, buttermilk, and oil to egg and mix well.
3. Place cornmeal, flour, baking powder, baking soda, and salt in a separate bowl and stir to combine ingredients.
4. Add dry ingredients into liquids and stir until ingredients are thoroughly incorporated.
5. Pour corn bread batter into baking dish and bake at 410°F for 20 minutes.

© David P. Smith/Shutterstock

Healthy Recipes

Chicken Stir Fry

Yield: 4 servings

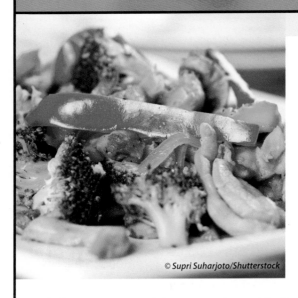

1 lb. boneless, skinless
   chicken breasts,
   slightly frozen
1 red pepper
¼ tsp. ginger, ground
2 Tbsp. soy sauce
1 Tbsp. cornstarch

⅔ c. cold water
2 Tbsp. sesame or
   vegetable oil
1 12-oz. bag broccoli
   florets, frozen
3 c. brown rice,
   cooked

1. Slice chicken breast into thin slices.
2. Using a different knife and cutting board, wash red pepper then remove stem and seeds. Slice into thin strips.
3. Combine ginger, soy sauce, cornstarch, and water in a small bowl.
4. Preheat a wok or large skillet over medium high heat.

© Supri Suharjoto/Shutterstock

5. Carefully add 1 Tbsp. plus 2 tsp. of oil to wok or skillet. Add chicken and cook until chicken is lightly browned, stirring constantly. Remove chicken from wok and hold in warm oven.
6. Add remaining 1 tsp. oil to wok. Add red pepper and broccoli stirring constantly for 2 to 3 minutes.
7. Add chicken back into wok with vegetables.
8. Add mixture from step 3 to chicken and vegetables. Bring to a boil and cook until mixture thickens slightly.
9. Serve over hot rice.

Healthy Recipes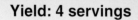

Marinated Chicken Breasts

Yield: 4 servings

¼ c. cider vinegar
¾ tsp. dried thyme
¾ tsp. dried oregano
¾ tsp. dried rosemary
3 Tbsp. whole-grain mustard
2 cloves garlic, crushed
½ c. canola oil
4 chicken breasts, boned and skinned

1. Mix the vinegar, herbs, mustard, garlic, and oil in a resealable bag. Add chicken to bag, seal, and shake to coat with marinade. Refrigerate until ready to cook.
2. Preheat grill to medium-high. Remove chicken from marinade. Allow excess marinade to drip off before placing on grill. Turn chicken once grill marks form and continue cooking until chicken reaches 165°F.

© Elena Elisseeva/Shutterstock

Healthy Recipes

Breakfast Oatmeal

Yield: 2 servings

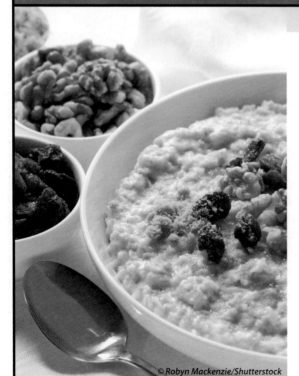

¾ c. oatmeal, old fashioned
⅛ tsp. cinnamon, ground
½ c. raisins
1 c. nonfat milk
½ c. water
⅓ c. walnuts, chopped
2 tsp. brown sugar

1. Place oatmeal, cinnamon, raisins, milk, and water in a microwave-safe dish. (Use a dish that is large enough to accommodate oatmeal as it doubles in volume.)
2. Microwave on high for 3½ minutes. Stir oatmeal mixture and microwave for another minute or until it reaches desired consistency.
3. Divide nuts and sugar between two cereal bowls. Pour half of oatmeal mixture in each bowl and mix.

© Robyn Mackenzie/Shutterstock

Chapter Summary

Section 17-1. Food customs are influenced by culture. They are also influenced by geography, religion, and tradition. The United States was settled by people from many different lands. Therefore, the food customs of the United States have been influenced by many cultures. As immigrants from different countries settled in various parts of the United States, distinct regional cuisines evolved. Certain foods are characteristic of the northeastern, southern, western, midwestern, and west coast states, as well as Alaska and Hawaii.

Section 17-2. You can plan healthful meals at home and away from home. Using resources such as ChooseMyPlate.gov can help. Plan meals that are nutritious and appealing. Your eating pattern may or may not include breakfast, lunch, dinner, and snacks. In either case, choose a variety of foods to meet your nutritional needs throughout the day. Choose foods with a variety of colors, flavors, textures, shapes, sizes, and temperatures. These factors can make a meal more appetizing. You can also develop strategies for eating healthful meals away from home.

Section 17-3. Understanding the meaning of recipe information and knowing how to use it are basic skills for kitchen success. Measuring ingredients accurately is important to the success of a food product. Become familiar with recipe abbreviations to be sure you are measuring the right amounts. Use the correct techniques for measuring each type of ingredient and understand measurement equivalents so you can increase or decrease the recipe yield. Learning the exact meanings of food preparation terms will help you be sure you are using the correct techniques when preparing foods. Choose healthful recipes by checking the ingredients and cooking method.

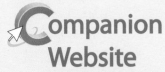

Companion Website

www.g-wlearning.com

Check your understanding of the main concepts for Chapter 17 at the website.

Critical Thinking

1. **Determine.** Should school lunch programs offer a wide variety of foods for people of different cultures and religious backgrounds? Why?
2. **Analyze.** Have you or anyone you know ever made a measuring mistake while cooking? What was the mistake? How did it affect the food product?
3. **Predict.** If you could develop a new kind of breakfast cereal, what would the ingredients be? What would you call it?

Common Core

College and Career Readiness

4. **Listening.** Interview someone from another country or another region of the United States. Ask about typical foods and food customs in that country or region. Share your findings in class.

5. **Math.** Copy a recipe from a cookbook, online source, magazine, or newspaper. Draw two columns down the page to the left of the ingredient list. In the first column, list the amount of each ingredient you would need to double the recipe. In the second column, list the amount of each ingredient you would need to halve the recipe.

6. **Reading.** Obtain a take-out menu from a fast-food restaurant. Analyze the menu options. What would you order from that menu? Where would your selections fit in the MyPlate plan?

Technology

7. **Electronic presentation.** Prepare an electronic presentation to show how to use the MyPlate plan as a resource in planning healthful meals.

Journal Writing

8. Imagine you are a world-famous chef and could work in any restaurant in the world. Write about where you would work and what kinds of meals you would prepare.

FCCLA

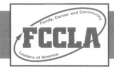

9. Explore the backgrounds of the different cultural and ethnic groups at your school. Create an *FCCLA Families First* project that educates others on your school and community's diversity through cultural food practices—complete with ethnic holidays and recipes. See your adviser for information as needed.

10. Cooking for one or two people can often be challenging. Collect a number of your favorite recipes, alter them to serve two people, and develop a *Cooking for Two* cookbook. Include a cost analysis of cost-per-serving and nutrition with each recipe for an *FCCLA Community Service* project. Use the cookbooks for a fund-raiser and donate the proceeds to an organization that feeds hungry people. See your adviser for information as needed.

Chapter 18
Buying and Storing Foods

Sections

College and Career Readiness

Reading Prep
Describe how this chapter relates to another class. Make a list of the similarities and differences.

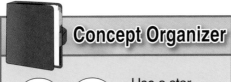

Concept Organizer

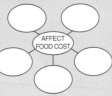

AFFECT FOOD COST

Use a star diagram like the one shown to list five factors that affect food costs.

Companion Website
Print out the concept organizer for Chapter 18 at the website.

Companion Website
www.g-wlearning.com

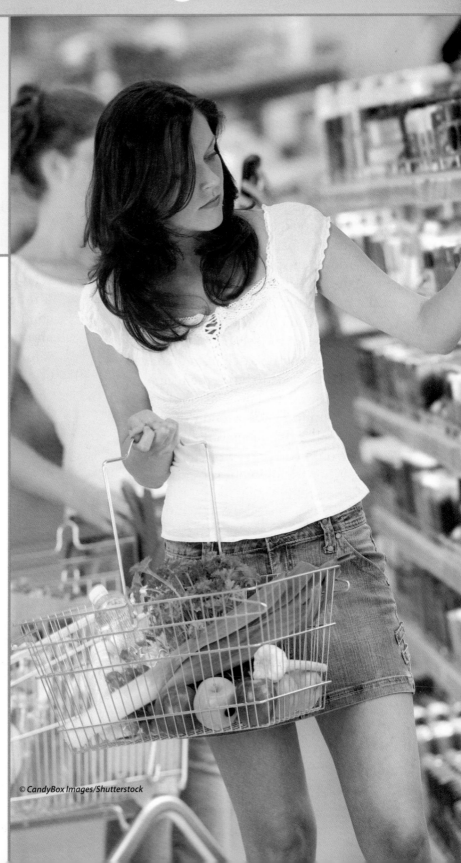

© CandyBox Images/Shutterstock

Shopping for Food

Objectives

After studying this section, you will be able to

- **compare** types of food stores.
- **recognize** the benefits of using a shopping list.
- **explain** the various factors that affect food costs.
- **calculate** a unit price.

Key Terms

produce in season	generic products	unit price

Shopping for food takes thought and planning. Understanding how your choices impact your food costs will help you spend your money wisely.

Know Where to Shop

Deciding the best place to shop takes some homework. Each type of food store offers different products and services. You can choose the type of store that best meets your needs.

Supermarkets sell a wide variety of products. Aside from food, supermarkets sell household items such as cleaning supplies and paper goods. Some supermarkets also provide pharmacies, banking services, and floral arranging, **18-1**.

Supermarkets offer a full range of fresh, frozen, and canned food products. Some supermarkets have special departments such as delicatessens and bakeries. They carry most canned and frozen products in a number of brands and sizes. The large selection makes it easier to find the exact items you want.

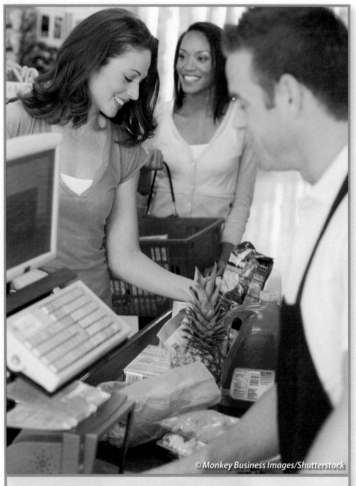

© Monkey Business Images/Shutterstock

18-1 Supermarkets often provide cashier checkout as well as an option for self checkout.

Discount or *warehouse supermarkets* sell grocery items at lower prices. These stores often provide less variety and fewer services than regular supermarkets in order to keep their prices low. Items are often sold in large sizes or bulk units. Some of these stores may charge a membership fee and shoppers may have to bag their own groceries. Despite these disadvantages, the cost savings can be worthwhile for shoppers that buy large quantities.

Convenience stores carry a more limited selection of food and household items than supermarkets. Convenience stores are generally open for longer hours and are well located. Despite the higher prices charged at these stores, some shoppers might feel the convenience is worth the price.

Specialty stores focus on one type of food item. Bakeries and butcher shops are specialty stores. The prices at these stores are often higher. Many shoppers think the freshness and high quality of the items is worth the cost.

Farmers' markets and *roadside stands* sell fruits and vegetables just picked from the fields, **18-2**. Farmers are able to sell their fresh fruits and vegetables, also called **produce**, at a lower price because they are selling directly to consumers rather than through another party. As a result, consumers are able to buy fresh produce for less.

Make a Shopping List

Being a wise shopper involves planning. Planning begins with writing a grocery list before you go to the store. Your list should include items needed to prepare the meals and snacks for the week's menu. Planning ahead also helps make effective use of leftovers. Have your weekly menus

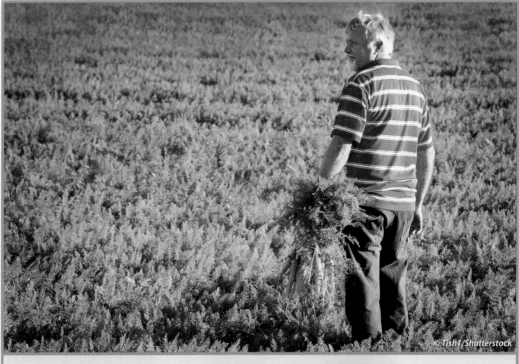

©Tish1/Shutterstock

18-2 Farmer's markets and roadside stands sell products that are in season.

and any needed recipes on hand when you write your shopping list. Check to be sure you do not already have the ingredients in your storage areas.

Your list should also include basic items such as milk and eggs that need to be restocked. Have a special place in your kitchen for your grocery list. Jot down staple items as you run out to ensure you buy more the next time you shop.

A list saves you time and money when shopping. You avoid wasting time trying to remember what to buy. Organizing your list according to the layout of the store can save you time as well. In addition, a list provides guidance so you are less likely to spend money on unneeded items, **18-3**.

Buying items you do not need is often the result of impulse buying. Impulse buying is making an unplanned purchase of an item that suddenly appeals to you. This type of buying causes you to spend more money than planned.

Control Food Costs

Smart shoppers know not only where to buy what they need, but also the right price to pay. To control your food costs, you must understand the factors that affect it and how to compare pricing.

Factors That Affect Food Costs

Consider the following factors when planning your meals. Use this knowledge to build menus based on foods that provide the best value. This strategy helps control food costs.

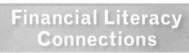

The Influence of In-Store Advertising

Companies often use in-store advertising to encourage impulse buying. Strategies such as displays are used to draw interest. Displays feature pairings of foods such as soup and crackers to encourage shoppers to buy two items rather than just one.

Store managers know that once shoppers notice display items, they are more likely to buy them. To ensure displays are seen, they are placed in key locations. For instance, candy is placed at checkout to tempt shoppers waiting in line.

Samples and demonstrations are other techniques used to encourage impulse buying. Customers are more likely to buy foods after tasting a sample or seeing it demonstrated.

Inviting aromas from the bakery and deli are used to encourage hungry shoppers to buy.

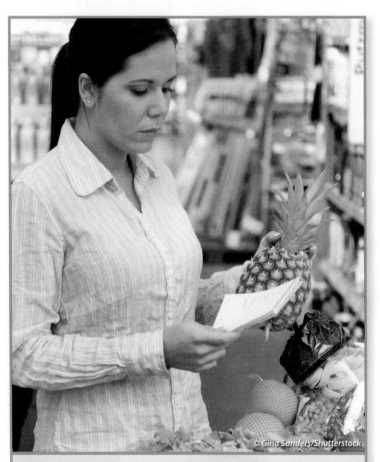

© Gina Sanders/Shutterstock

18-3 A shopping list helps you avoid unnecessary purchases.

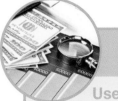

Financial Literacy Connections

Use Ads and Coupons to Save

Check newspaper advertisements and store sales fliers as you make your grocery list. Look for foods in your weekly menus that are on sale. Consider changing your menu to include sale items. Read ads carefully to ensure featured items are on sale. Not all foods listed in ads are sale items.

Avoid buying items just because they are on sale. Buy only products you need. Unused sale items are not bargains. Stock up on sale items you use often.

Find coupons in newspapers, leaflets, magazines, and on Internet coupon websites. Check the expiration date and use the coupons before they expire. Avoid buying products you will not use just because you have coupons.

Go Green

Shop with Less Packaging in Mind

Packaging not only drives up cost of a product, but also impacts the environment. Food packaging makes up about two thirds of total packaging waste. Try buying foods with less packaging. When possible,
- buy foods in bulk
- purchase food and drink packaged in glass jars or metal cans more often—and recycle
- prepare foods from scratch rather than highly packaged prepared foods

Amount of Processing

Products that are fully or partially prepared cost more because you are paying for the preparation. For instance, convenience products such as shredded cheese or ready-made pastry cost more than shredding your own cheese or making your own pastry dough.

Supply

When a supply of food is great, the price for that food is less. Foods are usually most plentiful and at peak flavor at their time of harvest when they are **in season**. When a fruit is in season, the supply is greater and the price is lower. For instance, apples and oranges are least expensive in the fall and winter when these fruits are in season. The best time to buy peaches is late summer when they are in season—the prices are low and flavor is at its peak.

Weather conditions in growing areas affect the supply of a food product. When parts of Florida experience unusually cold temperatures, citrus crops are lost. The reduced supply of oranges pushes the price of orange juice up.

Freshness

Freshly sliced deli meats and cheeses cost more than those in the refrigerator case. Likewise, you pay more for fresh rolls from the bakery than for those in the bread aisle. Fresh foods are fresh for only a short time. If the food does not sell during that time, it is often wasted. This contributes to the higher cost for freshness.

Packaging

A food's packaging sometimes costs more than the food itself. Items that are individually wrapped or in single-serving packages often have high prices. On the other hand, foods sold in bulk can save you money.

Transportation

Where you live also impacts the price you pay for food. For instance, pineapples cost less in Hawaii than in other places because they grow in Hawaii. There is little added cost to transport the pineapples. As you see fuel prices rise, the higher cost of transporting foods drives food prices up as well.

Comparing Prices

The store is selected, the shopping list is written, and you know the foods you need to buy. How do you decide which can of tomatoes or container of orange juice to buy? Comparing prices of the various sizes, brands, and forms of a food product helps you make the most cost effective choice, **18-4**.

Size

Purchasing the larger product size is often the best buy, but not always. Sometimes the larger size may be more economical, but the smaller size may better suit your needs. For instance, if you are unable to use the entire product before it spoils, the waste may erase any cost savings. In this case, buying the larger size may not be to your advantage. Large size products also require more storage space.

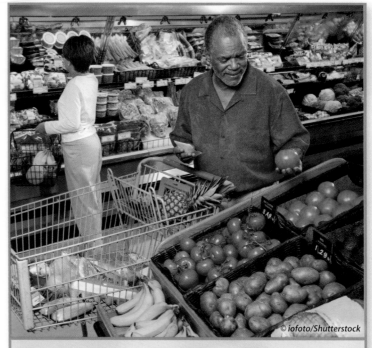

© iofoto/Shutterstock

18-4 Fresh tomatoes in season may cost less than canned tomatoes.

Brand

Consider product brands when making your food choice. Prices for the same food product can vary greatly based on the brand. Food companies use *national brands* to sell their products throughout the country. Food companies spend much money advertising their national brands to drive consumer recognition. Advertising costs are passed along to consumers in the form of higher prices.

Each major store chain sells food products using its *store* or *house brand*. Store brands usually cost less than national brands because there is little or no advertising cost.

Many stores also sell **generic products** that have no brand names. Generic products usually cost less than both national and store brands due to reduced packaging costs and varying quality. Labeling and packaging for generic products is simple. These products may vary in grade, color, size, and texture.

Form

Many products are available in more than one form. For instance, you can buy fresh orange juice in the refrigerator case. You can also buy canned or frozen, concentrated juice. The costs of the different forms can vary greatly.

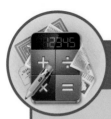

Math Connections

Calculating Unit Price

Suppose you are shopping for cereal. The store offers the following sizes and prices of your favorite cereal:

9-oz. box for $2.50
14-oz. box for $2.84
18-oz. box for $2.98

Calculate the ounce unit price for each box of cereal. Compare the unit prices and select the box size with the lowest unit price. (Round your answers up to the second decimal place.)

(*Answer:* $2.50 ÷ 9 = $0.28/oz., $2.84 ÷ 14 = $0.21/oz., $2.98 ÷ 18 = $0.17/oz.; The 18 ounce box has the lowest unit price.)

Use Unit Pricing

To choose the best size, brand, or form of product for the cost, compare unit prices. The **unit price** is the cost for each measure of a product. The unit price may be given in cents per ounce (gram), pound (kilogram), quart (liter), or dozen. Many grocery stores print this information on the shelves under each food item, but you can calculate unit prices easily yourself. Use the following formula to calculate unit price:

Cost of product ÷ Quantity = Unit price

Suppose you want to learn the price per cup for a quart of milk. The unit in this example is cup. A quart contains four cups. If the price for a quart of milk is $1.92, you calculate the price per cup as follows:

$1.92/quart ÷ 4 cups/quart = $0.48 per cup unit price

Use unit pricing to help you compare the costs of your purchase options and make the best choice to control your food costs.

Reading Review

1. List five types of stores where you can shop for foods.
2. What is impulse buying?
3. List five factors that affect food costs.
4. When buying food, what are three factors you should compare to make the most cost effective choice?
5. What is unit pricing?

Reading Food Labels

Objectives

After studying this section, you will be able to

- **use** label information to make wise food choices.
- **recognize** information that is required by law on food labels.

Key Terms

food additive	universal product	open dating
Daily Values	code (UPC)	
organic foods		

Do you read food labels when you shop? They can give you valuable information to help you make wise food purchases.

Required Label Information

According to federal laws, certain information must appear on the labels of food products. The *name and form of the food* must be on the label. This information can help you understand what type of food you are buying. For instance, if you need sliced pineapple, the statement of form can help you avoid buying the crushed type, **18-5.**

The *weight of the contents*, including any liquid used in processing and packing the product, is required to appear. The *name and address of the manufacturer*, *packer*, or *distributor* must also be shown on the label.

On canned and packaged foods, the *ingredients* must be listed on the label. The ingredient present in the largest amount by weight is listed first. The ingredient present in the second largest amount is listed second, and so on. Manufacturers are required to clearly state the presence of ingredients that contain protein from any of the eight major *allergens*—milk, egg, fish, crustacean shellfish, tree nuts, peanuts, wheat, or soybeans.

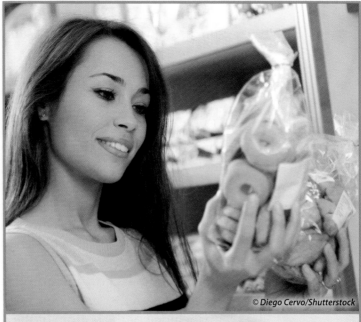

© Diego Cervo/Shutterstock

18-5 Read labels to ensure you are buying the product that best meets your needs.

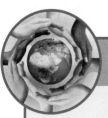

Global Connections

Country-of-Origin Labeling (COOL)

Federal law requires food stores to provide the consumer with information about the country from which foods originate. Only certain foods require this country-of-origin labeling including

- muscle cuts of beef (including veal), lamb, pork, chicken, and goat
- ground beef (including veal), lamb, pork, chicken, and goat
- fish and shellfish (wild and farm raised)
- fresh and frozen fruits and vegetables
- peanuts, pecans, and macadamia nuts
- ginseng

Next time you are in the supermarket, look for the COOL to find out where your favorite fruit originated.

Allergens are substances that cause an allergic response in people.

The list of ingredients must also include food additives. A **food additive** is any substance added to a food to improve the final product. Food additives include ingredients such as salt and sugar that you use every day. Other additives, such as guar gum or tocopherol, may not be as familiar to you.

Additives are used in foods for one or more of the following purposes:

- *To maintain or improve nutritional value.* Some foods, such as breads and cereals, are enriched with added vitamins and minerals to make them more nutritious.
- *To maintain freshness.* Foods last longer on the shelf or in the refrigerator because of these additives.
- *To make foods more appealing and attractive.* Some additives make foods more appetizing and colorful.
- *To help in processing or preparation.* Some additives affect the texture and performance of food products.

Foods must also include certain nutrition information on the label. The following information is found in the Nutrition Facts panel on most foods:

- *Serving size.* This represents a portion size that a typical person would eat. It is given in both household and metric measures. Serving sizes for similar food products are the same. This way you can easily compare products with one another.
- *Servings per container.* This tells you how many portions the package contains.
- *Calories.* Both the calories per serving and the calories from fat in each serving are listed.
- *Nutrients amounts.* Amounts per serving are given for certain nutrients. Some of these nutrients, such as total fat, saturated fat, trans fat, cholesterol, and sodium, should be limited in the diet. Other nutrients listed—dietary fiber, vitamins A and C, calcium, and iron—are often lacking in diets and should be increased. The remaining nutrients listed on the panel include total carbohydrate, sugars, and protein. The amount given for sugars includes both naturally occurring sugar and added sugar.
- *Percent Daily Values.* **Daily Values** are references used on food labels to show consumers how food products fit into an overall diet. Daily Value recommendations for key nutrients for both 2,000 and 2,500-calorie diets are included at the bottom of the Nutrition Facts panel. The *Percent Daily Values* are listed to the right of each nutrient amount the product contains. The Percent Daily Values are based on a 2,000-calorie diet.

Make a habit of reading and comparing nutrition labels as you shop for food. Information provided on food labels is especially important for individuals with nutrition-related health conditions. This information enables you to make nutritious food choices, **18-6**.

Other Labeling

You may see other information on food labels that is of interest to you. This information is not required by law, but the government often sets requirements that must be met before it can be placed on the label.

Claims

Claims often appear on product labels. Words such as *light, low cholesterol*, and *fat free* are just a few of the many claims you might see. Manufacturers use these words to appeal to consumers who are interested in healthy eating. These terms can be confusing if you do not understand what they mean. To avoid claims that are confusing or misleading, the government wrote definitions for each, **18-7**.

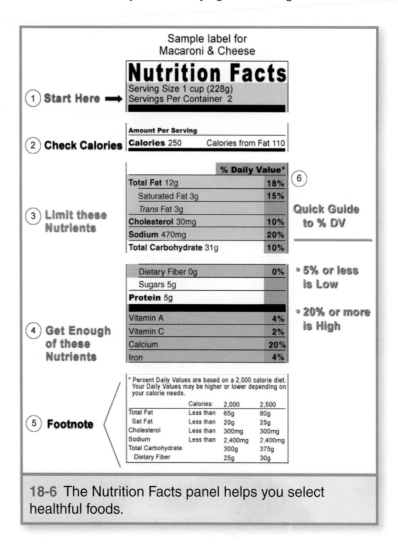

18-6 The Nutrition Facts panel helps you select healthful foods.

Organic Labeling

Some people are interested in buying and eating organic foods. Foods must meet certain requirements before being labeled *organic*. **Organic foods** are raised without the use of pesticides, fertilizers, and drugs that are commonly used for crops and livestock. Organic farmers might use manure or compost to enhance the soil. Animals must be fed organic feed and have access to the outdoors. Look for the United States Department of Agriculture (USDA) seal when shopping for organic foods, **18-8**.

Universal Product Code

Another feature found on food labels is the **universal product code (UPC)**. This is the group of bars and numbers that appears on product packaging.

The UPC is used by stores and producers to track their products. In the supermarket, cashiers pass the codes over a scanner. The scanner reads the bars on each item and automatically enters the price and product information into the computer. The UPC is also useful for gathering details about how goods are selling.

What Do Label Claims Mean?

Cholesterol free: less than 2 milligrams of cholesterol and 2 grams or less of saturated fat per serving

Fat free: less than 0.5 grams of fat per serving

Fresh: food is raw, has never been frozen or heated, and contains no preservatives

High fiber: 5 grams or more fiber per serving (Foods making high-fiber claims must also meet the definition for low fat, or the level of total fat must appear next to the high-fiber claim.)

Light/Lite: a nutritionally altered food product containing one-third fewer calories or half the fat of the "regular" version of the food. This term can also be used to indicate that the sodium of a low-calorie, low-fat food has been reduced by 50 percent. In addition, labels may state that foods are light (lite) in color or texture.

*Low calorie: 40 calories or less per serving, 120 calories or less for meals or main dishes

*Low cholesterol: 20 milligrams or less of cholesterol and 2 grams or less of saturated fat per serving

*Low fat: 3 grams or less of fat per serving

*Low sodium: 140 milligrams or less sodium per serving

Reduced calories: at least 25 percent fewer calories per serving than the "full-calorie" version of the food

Sodium free: less than 5 milligrams of sodium per serving

Sugar free: less than 0.5 grams of sugar per serving

*Foods with a serving size of 30 grams or less or 2 tablespoons or less must meet the specified requirement for portions of 50 grams of the food.

18-7 A food must meet established criteria before a claim can be made on the label.

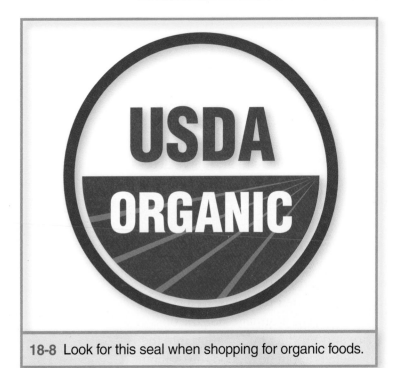

18-8 Look for this seal when shopping for organic foods.

Many food companies are beginning to use quick reference (QR) codes on their products labels. When scanned using a smartphone, this graphic takes the shopper to a website providing added interaction with the product. For instance, some seafood producers are using this code on their labels. Scanning the QR code on their product takes the shopper to a website where he or she can learn where and when the fish was caught.

Open Dating

Open dating is a method used to help store employees and consumers know when a food product is fresh.

Dates are stamped or imprinted on perishable and semiperishable food products, such as dairy and bakery products. The employees use these dates to know when products should be removed from the shelves and no longer offered for sale. Consumers use the dates to tell them which products to use first. Open dating is not required by law.

Several different types of open dating are used. Understanding the different types will help you make the freshest food choices.

The *freshness date* tells when a product should be used to assure peak quality. This type of date is often found on baked goods.

The *pack date* tells when a food was packaged. You can use it to decide which products were packaged most recently. Pack dates are often found on canned foods.

The *sell* or *pull date* indicates the last day a product should be sold. A cushion is built into this type of date so you have time to use products after you buy them. Yogurt, ice cream, and cold cuts are often labeled with pull dates, **18-9**.

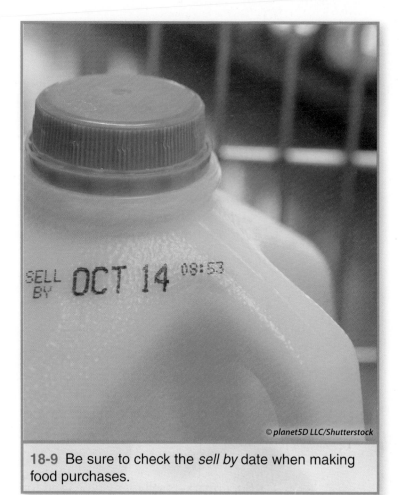

© planet5D LLC/Shutterstock

18-9 Be sure to check the *sell by* date when making food purchases.

The *expiration date* is the date when a food product is no longer flavorful, useful, or safe. Yeast has an expiration date after which it no longer helps dough rise.

You can use these dates to help you manage your food at home and ensure proper *food rotation*. This requires placing the foods with the newest dates behind foods with the oldest dates. This encourages you to use older foods first.

Reading Review

1. True or false. Ingredients are listed in alphabetical order on the food label.
2. List four reasons food additives are used in foods.
3. True or false. The amount given for sugars on the Nutrition Facts panel represents only sugars added to the food.
4. How can you be sure the food you are purchasing is organic?
5. Why is food rotation important?

Fruits and Vegetables

Objectives

After studying this section, you will be able to
- **apply** knowledge of types and forms of fruits and vegetables to selection process.
- **explain** how to store fruits and vegetables to maintain their quality.

Key Terms	
legumes	cruciferous vegetables

Eating fruits and vegetables adds flavor and variety to your diet. Most fruits and vegetables have no fat, so they are more nutrient dense.

Fruits and vegetables taste best when they are carefully chosen and stored. By knowing your options, you can get the most flavor and nutrition for your money.

Buying Fruits and Vegetables

Supermarkets sell many types and forms of fruits and vegetables. In addition to a wide variety of produce, they also stock frozen, canned, and dried fruits and vegetables. With so many options, choosing what to buy can be hard. Understanding how these products differ can help you make wise consumer choices.

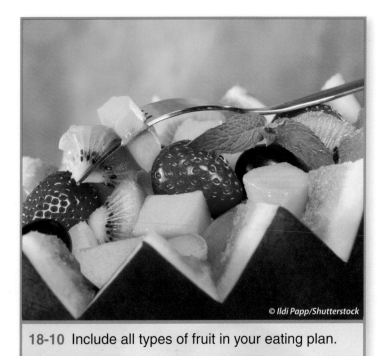

18-10 Include all types of fruit in your eating plan.

© Ildi Papp/Shutterstock

Types of Fruits

Fruits add flavor and nutrition to meals. Most fruits are naturally sweet. Many are good sources of vitamins A and C. Most fruits also supply some B vitamins, minerals, and fiber.

Fruits are grouped according to how they grow. The types of fruits include berries, drupes, pomes, melons, citrus fruits, and tropical fruits, **18-10**. Some examples of each of these types follow:
- *Berries*—grapes, blackberries, strawberries, raspberries, and blueberries
- *Drupes*—fruits that contain a pit, or stone, at their center such as cherries, apricots, peaches, and plums

- *Pomes*—apples and pears
- *Melons*—watermelon, cantaloupe, and honeydew
- *Citrus fruit*—oranges, grapefruits, lemons, limes, and tangerines
- *Tropical fruits*—avocados, bananas, pineapples, and dates

Types of Vegetables

Vegetables provide a number of important nutrients without adding many calories to the diet. Vegetables can be good sources of fiber, many minerals, and vitamins A, B, and C.

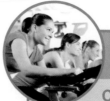

Health Connections

Cancer and Cruciferous Vegetables

Some studies have shown a possible connection between cruciferous vegetables in the diet and decreased risk for certain types of cancer. The reasons are still unclear, but these vegetables may guard against colorectal cancer. Vegetables in this family include broccoli, cabbage, cauliflower, turnips, kale, mustard greens, and collards. The American Cancer Society suggests that eating many types of vegetables—including cruciferous—decreases your risk for cancer.

Vegetables can be classified in a number of ways. They may be grouped by how they grow. For instance, some vegetables grow underground and others may be the stems, leaves, fruits, flowers, or seeds of plants. **Legumes** are the edible seeds of plants. Legumes include vegetables such as pinto beans, lentils, soybeans, and peanuts. This type of vegetable is often a good source of protein.

Vegetables can also be classified by their flavor. They may be mild or strong in flavor. **Cruciferous vegetables** are strong-flavored vegetables that include Brussels sprouts, cauliflower, turnips, onions, broccoli, and cabbage. These vegetables are high in sulfur, which contributes to the strong flavor. The flavors of these vegetables tend to be stronger after cooking. For this reason, some people prefer to eat these vegetables raw. You can use special techniques when cooking these vegetables to make the flavors milder.

MyPlate organizes vegetables into five groups—dark green, red and orange, beans and peas, starchy, and other vegetables.

Forms of Fruits and Vegetables

You can purchase both fruits and vegetables in a variety of forms including fresh, frozen, canned, and dried. Each form has benefits and drawbacks. Select the form that best meets the needs of your dish and budget. For instance, if you are preparing a fruit platter, fresh fruit might be the best choice. Frozen vegetables, however, would be more convenient and work just as well as fresh vegetables when making a soup.

With careful shopping, you can save money without giving up quality of fruits and vegetables. If you prefer fresh, buy items that are in season. You may even find these items to be less costly than canned or frozen items. If you want a fruit or vegetable that is not in season, frozen or canned may be a better buy. Canned items are usually less expensive than frozen.

You can save money on frozen, canned, and dried items by choosing generic or store brands. These often cost less than name brands even though they are similar in quality.

Fresh

Many fresh fruits and vegetables are available only at certain times of the year. In-season fruits and vegetables are at peak flavor, abundant, and cost less, **18-11**. For instance, strawberries are harvested April through July. The supply is greatest during these months, so they cost less. Although strawberries may be available in other months, they ship from other states or countries. In order to ship, perishable fruits are picked before they are fully ripened. Flavor suffers when produce is picked before ripening. The shipping also adds to the cost of the product.

Many people prefer the flavors and textures of fresh produce to canned, frozen, or dried products. Fresh produce cannot be stored as long as other forms. When buying fresh products, quality factors vary for different foods.

Peak Seasons for Fresh Fruits and Vegetables (shaded areas)

	Jan	Feb	Mar	Apr	May	June	July	Aug	Sept	Oct	Nov	Dec
Apples	▓	▓	▓	▓					▓	▓	▓	▓
Bananas	▓	▓	▓	▓	▓	▓	▓	▓	▓	▓	▓	▓
Blueberries					▓	▓	▓	▓				
Broccoli	▓	▓	▓	▓	▓	▓				▓	▓	▓
Cabbage	▓	▓	▓	▓	▓	▓	▓	▓	▓	▓	▓	▓
Cantaloupes					▓	▓	▓	▓	▓			
Cherries					▓	▓	▓					
Corn					▓	▓	▓	▓	▓			
Cucumbers					▓	▓	▓	▓				
Grapes						▓	▓	▓	▓	▓	▓	▓
Green beans					▓	▓	▓	▓	▓	▓		
Lemons	▓	▓	▓	▓	▓	▓	▓	▓				
Lettuce	▓	▓	▓	▓	▓	▓	▓	▓	▓	▓	▓	▓
Limes	▓	▓	▓	▓	▓	▓	▓	▓	▓	▓	▓	▓
Onions	▓	▓	▓	▓	▓	▓	▓	▓	▓	▓	▓	▓
Oranges	▓	▓	▓	▓	▓						▓	▓
Peaches						▓	▓	▓	▓			
Pears	▓	▓	▓					▓	▓	▓	▓	▓
Peas			▓	▓	▓							
Peppers, bell							▓	▓	▓	▓		
Pineapples			▓	▓	▓	▓	▓					
Plums						▓	▓	▓	▓			
Potatoes, sweet									▓	▓	▓	▓
Strawberries				▓	▓	▓	▓					
Tomatoes					▓	▓	▓	▓	▓	▓		

18-11 Peak seasons may vary in different parts of the country.

For instance, if you buy bananas that are not fully ripe, they will ripen at home. If you buy strawberries that are not fully ripe, they will decline in quality instead of ripening. You need to learn which quality factors are important for each type of fresh food. In addition, produce may lose quality and nutrients during storage. To get your money's worth, buy only as much as you can eat within a few days.

Frozen

Buying frozen fruits and vegetables has benefits. For instance, fruits and vegetables are often harvested and frozen at their peak flavor and nutrition. The freezing process prevents (or greatly slows) the loss of both flavor and nutrients. In fact, frozen produce may have greater nutrient content than its fresh counterpart that has spent days or weeks in shipping and storage before being eaten. When thawed or cooked, these products taste much like fresh. On the other hand, freezing affects the texture and appearance of most produce, which can be a drawback for some uses.

Life Connections

Tips for Choosing Produce

When buying produce, you want to select the best quality possible. You must learn to identify good produce without tasting (most stores frown on this practice!). Use the following tips to help you select the best produce:

- Select mature, ripe fruits and vegetables. These are usually medium in size. Immature produce is often small. Unusually large produce may be overripe.
- Check the firmness of the product. Oranges, apples, carrots, and cucumbers should be firm to the touch. Peaches, nectarines, tomatoes, and pears should be a little less firm. Never press too hard on produce; it bruises easily.
- High-quality citrus fruit, such as oranges and grapefruit, is heavy for its size. The heavier the fruit, the juicier it will be.
- Look for bright colors in fruits and vegetables. Skins should not be bruised (having dark, soft spots) or faded.
- Do not buy produce with bruises, cracks, wilting, shriveling, yellowing, or soft spots. These are signs of old, overripe, low-quality produce. This produce has declined flavor and nutrient value.

Food Science Activity

Practice selecting fresh produce. Choose one type of fruit and obtain this fruit in its underripe, ripe, and overripe forms. State your hypothesis on how the fruit will differ at each stage. Compare the differences by recording how each fruit looks, feels, tastes, and smells at each stage.

Unlike fresh produce, you can buy most frozen fruits and vegetables year-round. They will keep in your freezer for months. This makes them more convenient to use than fresh produce. If you have sufficient freezer space, you can stock up when items are on sale and save money. When buying frozen fruits and vegetables, make sure the items are completely frozen. Items that are partially thawed do not last as long and may not taste as good. Select packages that are clean and free of rips or holes.

Canned

Canned fruits and vegetables are convenient because they are available year-round. In addition, less money is spent on storage. Canned goods can be stored at room temperature on a shelf. A drawback is the canning process can change the flavors of fruits and vegetables. Textures are also changed.

Fruits and vegetables are canned whole, sliced, or in pieces. Most vegetables are packed in water. Look for canned vegetables that are labeled *low salt* if you are trying to reduce sodium in your diet. Fruits are packed either in their own juices or in syrup. Syrup adds unneeded sugar and calories to fruits. Some fruits and vegetables may be packed in sauces, such as creamed corn or cherry pie filling.

When buying canned items, choose cans that are free of dents, bulges, or leaks. Foods in these cans have a high risk of causing food poisoning.

Dried

Dried fruits and vegetables last several months without refrigeration or freezing. They are lighter than other forms of fruits and vegetables because the water in them is removed. Their small size and weight makes them handy for traveling and camping. The flavors and textures of dried items differ from fresh, even if they are *rehydrated* (have the water added back to them). Some people enjoy the unique flavor and texture of dried foods.

Dried fruits are more common than dried vegetables, **18-12**. Fruits that are often available in dried form include raisins, prunes, figs, apricots, apples, bananas, pineapples, and peaches. Some dried fruits, such as raisins and apricots, are fairly soft and pliable. Others, such as bananas, are designed to be crisp like chips. Dried fruits are popular as snack foods. They may also be added to cakes, cereals, and other foods.

Legumes are the vegetables most often dried. Other dried vegetables are used in dried soup mixes or food packages designed for hiking and camping. Dried vegetables have a hard, brittle texture. They are usually rehydrated and cooked before eating.

Storing Fruits and Vegetables

Careful buying assures that you get high-quality fruits and vegetables. If you do not store them properly, fruits and vegetables may lose quality before you use them. Produce is highly perishable and spoils quickly. Careful storage is needed to keep fresh produce from spoiling too quickly. Proper storage also helps frozen, canned, and dried items last longer.

Storing Fresh Produce

Time, light, heat, and moisture destroy vitamins in fruits and vegetables. Proper storage helps preserve the nutrients, flavors, and freshness.

Wash all fruits except berries, cherries, and citrus fruits before you store them in the refrigerator. Use berries as soon as possible because they are very perishable, **18-13**.

Bananas ripen at room temperature. If ripe bananas are not to be used soon,

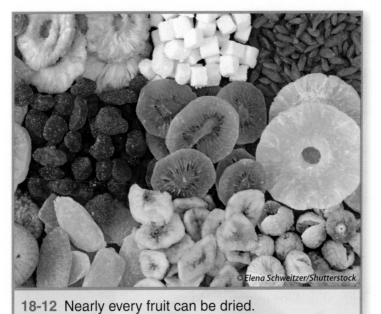
© Elena Schweitzer/Shutterstock

18-12 Nearly every fruit can be dried.

they can be stored in the refrigerator. The peels turn dark brown, but the texture and flavor of the fruit is still good.

Fresh onions, potatoes, and sweet potatoes should be stored in a cool, dry place. They do not need to be refrigerated, although they can be.

Wash celery, lettuce, and other salad greens before storing. They will be crisp when you are ready to use them. Trim away any wilted or damaged parts and refrigerate vegetables in separate containers.

You do not need to wash other vegetables before storing them. Water sometimes causes brown spots to appear and hastens spoiling. Vegetables must be washed before using them. Even if they look clean, they may have pesticides and other chemicals on them.

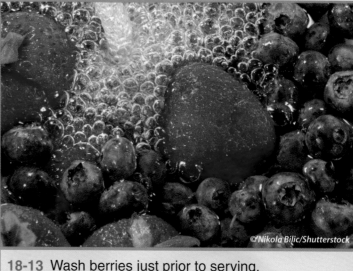

©Nikola Bilic/Shutterstock

18-13 Wash berries just prior to serving.

Storing Other Fruits and Vegetables

Frozen fruits and vegetables should be stored in the coldest part of the freezer. Storage space in the freezer door may not be cold enough. Fruits are often thawed before serving. Vegetables retain their quality better if they are cooked from the frozen state. Once thawed or cooked, items should not be refrozen. Store uneaten portions in the refrigerator. Thawed items do not last as long as frozen, so use them as soon as possible.

Canned goods should be stored in a cool, dry place. Do not store them over a stove, under the sink, in the garage, or in a damp basement. Be sure to rotate older cans forward and place newer purchases at the back to avoid waste and spoilage. You can eat commercially canned fruits and vegetables with or without cooking them. Cover and store unused portions in the refrigerator.

Dried items can be stored in a cool, dry place even if the packages have been opened. Dried foods are packaged in sealed bags or boxes. Resealing these packages after opening extends their shelf life. Some dried fruits are sold loose. Make sure you place such fruit in tightly sealed bags or jars before storing. Exposure to moisture during storage causes dried foods to spoil. If you rehydrate fruits or vegetables, eat them right away or store in the refrigerator.

Reading Review

1. List the six types of fruit and give an example of each.
2. True or false. Legumes are often a good source of protein.
3. In-season fruits and vegetables are at peak flavor, abundant, and cost _____.
4. Time, light, heat, and moisture destroy _____ in fruits and vegetables.
5. Describe how to store canned goods.

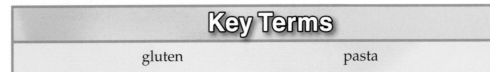

Section 18-4

Grain Products

Objectives

After studying this section, you will be able to
- **summarize** options for selecting and buying grain products.
- **identify** appropriate storage for various grain products.

Key Terms	
gluten	pasta

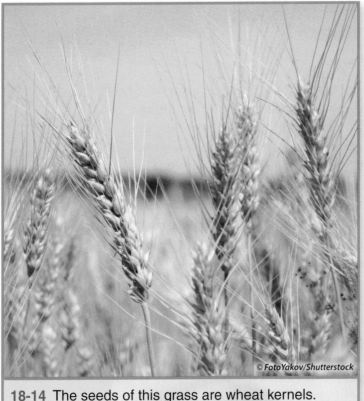

18-14 The seeds of this grass are wheat kernels.

© FotoYakov/Shutterstock

Grains play a major role in the diets of people around the world. Understanding what is available helps you choose the products that best fit your needs and budget. Proper storage helps you get the most flavor and quality from the grain products you buy.

Types of Grain Products

Grains are the seeds from various types of grasses, **18-14**. There are many types of grains including
- wheat
- corn
- rye
- barley
- oats
- rice
- quinoa

These grains are sometimes prepared and served as a single food such as oatmeal. Often, the grains are processed to varying degrees and used as ingredients. For instance, corn is ground into cornmeal or cooked and rolled into flakes for breakfast cereal.

Whole-grain products still contain most of the beneficial parts of the grain due to little or no processing. This makes whole grains a more nutrient-rich choice. To be sure you are buying whole-grain products, read the label.

Choose breads, tortillas, pastas, flours, and crackers labeled *whole grain*. Look for ingredients that contain the word *whole* at the beginning of the ingredient list on the label.

Nearly any grain can be ground into flour and used to make a variety of grain products such as pastas, cereals, and breads. Some grains, such as rice, can be prepared and served on their own.

Flours

Flour is made by grinding grain into powder. Any grain can be used to make flour, but wheat flour is the most common in the United States. Flour is used most often to make baked products such as bread. It is also used as a thickener in sauces, soups, and gravies.

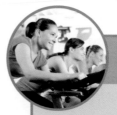

Health Connections

Gluten in Foods

Some people are unable to eat foods that contain gluten. These individuals have a disease, which causes an immune response when they eat gluten. As a result, they experience stomach pain and diarrhea. In addition, this causes damage to the intestines.

Grains such as barley, wheat, and rye contain gluten. Foods made from these grains also include gluten and must be avoided. Some grains that are gluten free include buckwheat, corn, quinoa, and rice. Sometimes these grains are contaminated with gluten during processing, which must be noted on the label.

More and more gluten-free food products are appearing on supermarket shelves, such as pastas made from quinoa flour.

Different flours give different flavors and textures when used in cooking. They may work well for some uses, but poorly for others. A flour's gluten level influences how it is used. **Gluten** is a protein found in many grains that provides structure for baked goods. Some food products, such as yeast breads, benefit from the use of flours with higher levels of gluten. On the other hand, flour with lower gluten content is preferred for cakes, **18-15**.

Types of Flours and Their Uses

Type of Flour	Uses
All-purpose	General baking and cooking
Buckwheat	Pancake mix, Asian noodles
Cake	Cakes and other baked products with delicate textures
Instant or quick mixing	Thickener for gravies and sauces
Rice	Asian noodles, low protein breads
Rye	Rye breads
Self-rising	Bread products, such as biscuits
Semolina	Pastas
Whole wheat	Whole-wheat baked goods

18-15 Choose the flour that best meets your need.

Pasta

Macaroni, spaghetti, and noodles are made by rolling out and shaping flour dough. These products are called **pasta**. Pastas are most often made from wheat flour, but common types of Asian noodles are made from buckwheat or rice.

Many shapes and varieties of pasta are available. Pasta shaped like shells, bows, or corkscrews adds interest to meals.

Other ingredients can be added to change the flavor and appearance of pasta. Noodles have whole eggs or egg yolks added. Vegetables such as spinach or tomatoes can be added to pasta. Seasonings such as basil or cinnamon may also be added.

Pasta is sold in dried, fresh, and frozen forms. Dried pasta is most commonly used for cooking. It is inexpensive and easy to store.

Breakfast Cereals

Breakfast cereals may be made from grains such as wheat, oats, corn, and rice. Cereals are sold in both ready-to-eat and cooked forms. Cereals can differ greatly in nutrient content and price.

Ready-to-eat cereals may be eaten straight from the box or with milk. Some types have dried fruits or nuts added.

Cooked cereals are prepared by cooking the cereal in liquid. Oatmeal and farina are two types of cooked cereals. Regular, quick-cooking, and instant types are available. Regular cereals (also called *old-fashioned*) must be cooked for several minutes. Quick-cooking cereals are ready in only a few minutes. Instant cereals can be prepared by simply adding hot water to them. Cooked cereals may have fruit or other flavorings added to them.

Many ready-to-eat and instant cereals can be high in sugar and fat. Read labels carefully to avoid too much added sugar or fat.

Breads

Many types of breads including white, whole wheat, rye, oatmeal, pumpernickel, and raisin are available to consumers, **18-16**. Bread products are sold in different forms such as rolls, tortillas, pita breads, muffins, bagels, and buns as well.

Mass-produced breads are prepackaged and sold on supermarket shelves. These breads are fairly inexpensive because they are produced in large quantities. Freshly baked breads are sold in bakeries and bakery sections of stores. They can

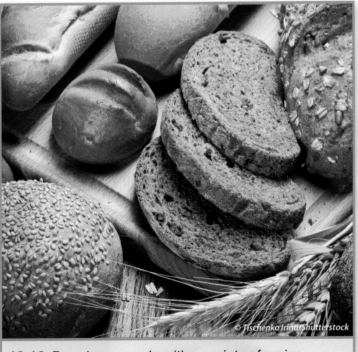

© Tischenko Irina/Shutterstock

18-16 Breads are made with a variety of grains.

be more costly than mass-produced items. Many people, however, prefer the flavor and texture of freshly baked breads.

Some convenience bread products can be baked at home. Brown-and-serve products are partially baked. You can brown them quickly in your oven before serving. Refrigerated doughs are ready to be arranged on a tray and baked at home. Frozen doughs must be thawed and baked. You may need to allow the dough time to rise before baking. These products vary in price. They can be more costly than making baked goods from scratch, but may be less expensive than prebaked items.

Rice

Rice is often served as a side dish. White rice has the outer hull and other portions of the grain removed. As with many other refined grains, white rice is enriched. Brown rice is whole grain because only its outer hull is removed. It has a nutty flavor and is chewier than white rice.

A variety of rice products are available, **18-17**. You may buy long grain or short grain rice. When cooked, the long grains do not cling to each other as easily as short grains. Instant rice has been precooked so it cooks rapidly. It takes only a few minutes to prepare, but costs more than regular rice. Wild rice is a whole grain with a nutty flavor. It is often added to other rice due to its high cost.

Many rice mixes with seasoning packets are sold. These are tasty and convenient, but might cost more than plain rice and be high in salt. Frozen packages of rice may be boiled in the pouch and served. These pouches are fast and easy to prepare. They are more expensive than uncooked rice.

Finding the Best Buys

When buying grain products, avoid packages that are damaged or ripped. Make sure bags or boxes are tightly sealed. Dampness, insects, and dirt can harm the quality of grain products.

The freshness of baked goods affects their price. Older products are often sold at reduced prices. These items may only have a few days before they reach their freshness date. You may be able to use the product quickly or freeze it until you are ready to use it. Warming stale bread in an oven can also make it softer.

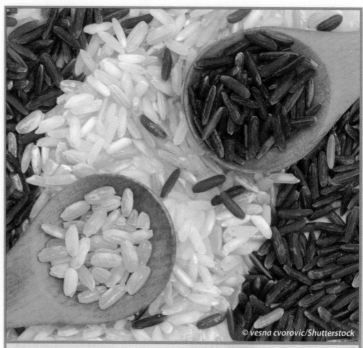

© vesna cvorovic/Shutterstock

18-17 These are just a few of the many types of rice available.

Storing Grain Products

Most grain products can be stored in a cool, dry place for several months. Store them in tightly closed containers to keep out moisture and insects, **18-18**. Store grains separate from foods with strong odors such as onions. This prevents the grain product from absorbing the flavor of the onion.

Properly stored breakfast cereals will keep for two or three months. Refined rice and pasta products stored in tightly closed containers keep for about one year. Whole-grain products do not last as long on the shelf because they contain a small amount of oil. Keep whole-wheat flour in the refrigerator or freezer. When stored at room temperature, both brown and wild rice will keep for up to six months. They will last longer when stored in the refrigerator or freezer.

Most breads can be stored for about a week in a cool, dry place. After this time, breads may become stale or moldy. Bread can be stored for several months in the freezer. You can thaw slices as you need them. As with all grain products, bread must be stored in tightly sealed packaging. Excess moisture can harm the quality of bread whether it is at room temperature or frozen.

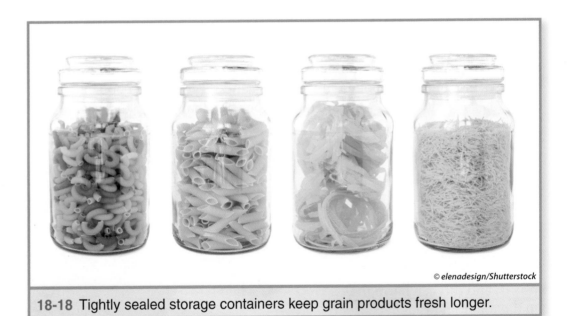

© *elenadesign/Shutterstock*

18-18 Tightly sealed storage containers keep grain products fresh longer.

Reading Review

1. Grains are the _____ from various types of grasses.
2. True or false. Gluten provides sweetness to baked goods.
3. List two whole-grain rice products.
4. Why do whole-grain products benefit from refrigerator or freezer storage?

Dairy Products

Objectives

After studying this section, you will be able to
- **compare** and contrast a variety of dairy products.
- **list** points to consider when buying and storing dairy products.

Key Terms

pasteurization
ultra high temperature
  (UHT) milk

evaporated milk
sweetened condensed
  milk

stabilizers

The smooth, creamy flavor of milk makes dairy products popular foods. A variety of dairy products are produced from milk, which contribute a rich flavor either as ingredients or single foods.

Types of Dairy Products

Many different types of dairy products are available to consumers. These include milk, cheese, frozen milk products, yogurt, cream, and butter, **18-19**.

All dairy products sold in the United States must be pasteurized. Pasteurization is a process in which products are heated to destroy much of the harmful bacteria they contain. This process prevents illness that may be caused by some bacteria. It also helps milk stay fresh longer.

Milk and milk products are often fortified. Because there are not many food sources of vitamin D, it is added to most milk products. Vitamin D improves the body's ability to use the

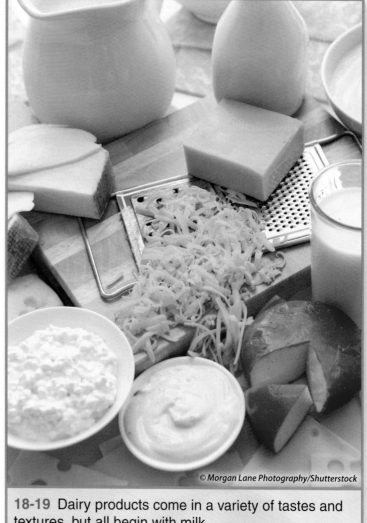

© Morgan Lane Photography/Shutterstock

18-19 Dairy products come in a variety of tastes and textures, but all begin with milk.

MyPlate Tip

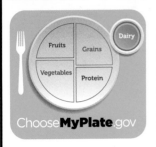

ChooseMyPlate.gov

Got Your Dairy Today?

Can't drink milk? If you are lactose intolerant, try lactose-free milk, drink smaller amounts of milk at a time, or try soymilk (soy beverage). Check the Nutrition Facts panel to be sure your soymilk has about 300 mg of calcium. Calcium in some leafy greens is well absorbed, but eating several cups each day to meet calcium needs may be unrealistic.

Source: MyPlate 10 tips Nutrition Education Series

Levels of Fat in Milk

Product	Percent Fat
Whole milk	Minimum 3.25
Reduced fat milk	Maximum 2.1
Low-fat or light milk	Maximum 1.2
Fat-free or skim milk	Maximum 0.2

18-20 The government establishes minimum standards for milk sold in the United States.

calcium in milk. Because vitamin A is supplied by the fat portion of milk, vitamin A is often added to milk products from which fat has been removed.

Milk

Milk is sold in many different forms including fresh fluid, UHT, dried, and canned.

Fresh Fluid Milk

Fresh fluid milk is liquid in form. It is commonly used for drinking and cooking. Types of fluid milk vary in fat content, **18-20**. The fat in milk is called *butterfat*. The butterfat gives milk a rich taste. Milk with high butterfat content also has more calories.

Other fluid milk products include flavored milks. Chocolate milk is the most common flavored milk. Buttermilk has a special type of bacteria added. The bacteria cause the milk to become somewhat sour and thick. Buttermilk is mainly used in baking.

UHT Milk

Ultra high temperature (UHT) milk is sterilized by heating to a very high temperature for a few seconds. All bacteria normally found in milk are killed in this process. The milk is then put in sterilized, airtight cartons. Most fluid milk lasts about a week when it is refrigerated. UHT milk can last about three months without refrigeration. Once the carton is opened, the milk must be refrigerated.

Dry Milk

Water is removed from fluid milk leaving a powder or dry milk. It may be whole fat, with all its fat content, or nonfat. Dry milk keeps without refrigeration for many months. Once water is added, the milk is similar to fresh fluid milk and must be refrigerated.

Some people do not like the flavor of dry milk and do not drink it for this reason. Instead, people often use it for cooking. Others may mix dry milk and fresh fluid milk for drinking. Dry milk is usually less expensive than fresh fluid milk.

Canned Milk

Canned milk is processed and canned so it can be kept without refrigeration for a long time. Once the can is open, canned milk products must be refrigerated.

Evaporated milk is a form of canned milk. It is made from whole milk from which 60 percent of the water has been removed. When it is mixed with an equal amount of water, evaporated milk can be used like fresh whole milk.

Sweetened condensed milk is also made from whole milk that has about 60 percent of its water removed. Sugar is then added and it is cooked to a syrupy consistency. Sweetened condensed milk is fairly expensive and high in calories compared to other forms of milk. It is mainly used in cooking and baking. Sweetened condensed milk is too sweet to be substituted for evaporated milk in recipes.

Cheese

Cheese is made from milk by thickening the milk protein. The solid portion of the thickened milk (called *curds*) is separated from the liquid (called *whey*), **18-21**. From this solid portion, hundreds of different cheeses can be produced. Cheeses may be classified as natural or processed.

Natural Cheeses

Natural cheeses may be unripened or ripened. Unripened cheeses include cottage cheese and cream cheese. These cheeses are prepared to be shipped to stores as soon as the whey is removed from them. They have soft textures and mild flavors. They must be refrigerated and used within a fairly short period of time.

Ripened cheeses are stored at a certain temperature to develop flavor and texture. Certain amounts of special bacteria, mold, yeast, or enzymes are used during ripening. These cheeses are more firm and flavorful than unripened cheeses. They vary in texture from smooth and fairly soft to hard and crumbly. Ripened cheeses can be kept much longer than unripened cheeses. Swiss, Cheddar, Colby, and Parmesan are examples of ripened cheeses.

Processed Cheeses

Processed cheeses, such as American cheese, are made by blending natural cheeses through a heating process. They may have moisture and other ingredients added during the process. After cheese is processed, it does not ripen anymore. This type of cheese melts easily and has a mild flavor.

Processed cheeses are sold as slices, blocks, and spreads. They may have spices or flavorings added to them. These cheeses are especially popular for sauces and casseroles.

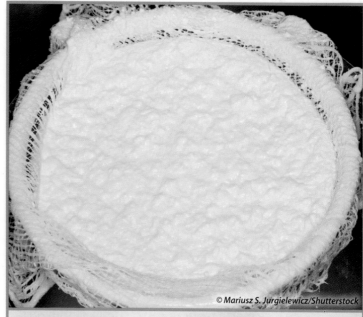

© Mariusz S. Jurgielewicz/Shutterstock

18-21 Cheese curds are easy to identify in cottage cheese.

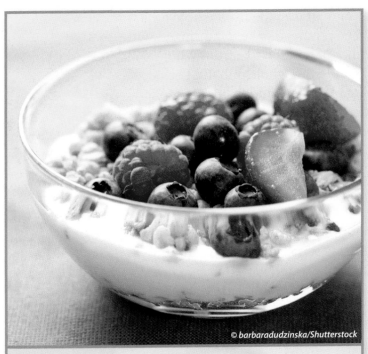

© barbaradudzinska/Shutterstock

18-22 Add granola and fresh fruit to plain yogurt for breakfast.

MyPlate Tip

Got Your Dairy Today?

Choose sweet dairy foods with care. Flavored milks, fruit yogurts, frozen yogurts, and puddings can contain a lot of added sugars. These added sugars are empty calories. You need the nutrients in dairy foods—not these empty calories.

Source: MyPlate 10 tips Nutrition Education Series

Imitation cheese is made with vegetable oil instead of butterfat. Its texture differs from that of real cheese. Imitation cheese may not have the same qualities as other cheese when it is cooked or melted.

Yogurt

Yogurt is made from whole- or low-fat milk. A special type of bacterium is added to the milk. This mixture is held at a temperature that encourages the bacteria to grow. This causes it to become thick and creamy. The finished product has a somewhat sour taste. Yogurt must be refrigerated, but it stays fresh longer than milk.

Yogurt may have fruit or other flavorings added to it, **18-22**. Plain or flavored yogurt may be used in cooking and baking. Plain yogurt can be used as a substitute for sour cream on baked potatoes. It can also be used instead of mayonnaise as a base for creamy salad dressings. Plain yogurt is lower in calories than these other items.

Frozen Milk Products

Frozen desserts containing milk products include ice cream, sherbet, frozen yogurt, and frozen custard. Some frozen dairy products contain reduced amounts of fat. Their labels might read *reduced fat, light, low fat,* or *fat free*. These products also vary in the amount of sugar they contain.

They come in a variety of flavors. The ingredients affect how rich products taste and how high in calories they are.

Ice cream is made from milk, sugar, cream, flavorings, and stabilizers. **Stabilizers** are additives that maintain an ice cream's smooth, creamy texture. Sherbet has about twice the sugar of ice cream, but less fat. Frozen yogurt is made from yogurt, sugar, stabilizers, and flavorings. It is lower in fat than ice cream. Frozen custard is ice cream with egg yolks added. It is richer and higher in fat than ice cream.

Cream

Cream products contain mainly the fat portion of milk. They vary in the amount of butterfat they contain. Heavy whipping cream contains the most fat. It is used in baking and cooking and can be whipped to put on desserts. Light cream has less fat. It is often used in coffee or in cooking. Half-and-half is half cream and half milk. Many people use it instead of light cream in coffee and cooking because it is lower in calories.

Sour cream is made by adding special bacteria to light cream. The bacteria give the cream a thick texture and sour taste. Sour cream is used in baked goods, casseroles, dips, and sauces. It is popular as a topping for baked potatoes and fruits.

Imitation cream products are not made from real cream. They may contain vegetable fats and gums, soy protein, and other substances to make them taste and feel like cream products. Nondairy creamers, whipped toppings, and imitation sour cream are examples of these products.

Butter

Butter is made by churning, or continually mixing, cream. It is usually salted to add flavor and help it stay fresh longer. Sweet butter is made without salt. It is more perishable than salted butter. It is also a little more expensive.

Butter is mainly sold in one-pound packages that are solid or wrapped in individual quarters, **18-23**. Solid packages are often less expensive than quartered packages. Whipped butter, which has air added into it, is sold in tubs. It is a little softer and easier to spread than solid butter. It is also more expensive. Margarine is not a dairy product, but it is often used as a substitute for butter. Margarine is made from vegetable oil rather than butterfat. It has the same amount of fat as butter and usually costs less.

Buying and Storing Dairy Products

Dairy products require care when buying and storing. Once you buy the product, proper storage will keep it fresh and wholesome for as long as possible.

Considering Cost

The government has set standards for content of many dairy products. If two products differ in price, it is probably due to packaging or other factors. For instance, milk may be sold in gallons, half gallons, quarts, and pints. Milk sold by

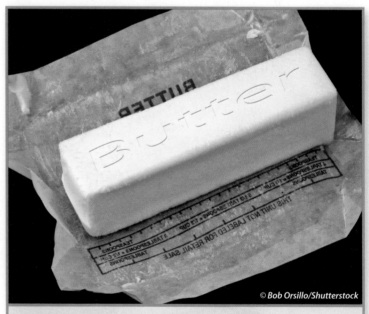

© Bob Orsillo/Shutterstock

18-23 Wrappers for quarter-pound sticks of butter are often marked for ease of measuring.

the half gallon is often more expensive per ounce than milk sold by the gallon. There are also different brands of milk. A well-known name brand may cost more, but the milk may taste the same as other brands.

Most dairy products are fairly similar in taste and other qualities due to the government standards. As a result, you can save money by looking for the least expensive product without giving up quality. On the other hand, the least expensive product may not always be the best buy. For instance, if you cannot use a gallon of milk before it spoils, the waste may erase any savings. Even though it costs more per ounce, a half gallon may be a better buy for you.

Items such as cheese and frozen milk products do vary in quality and flavor. There are minimum standards for these products, but some products use more expensive ingredients to improve the quality. For instance, extra fat and expensive nuts or chocolate can be added to ice cream. This makes it richer, but more expensive. Cheese may be aged for a longer time to give it a smoother, more mellow flavor, and a higher price.

When shopping, you must decide whether the extra cost is worthwhile. When combining cheese with other ingredients, you can save money by using a less costly cheese, **18-24**.

Most dairy products are fairly perishable. Be sure to check freshness dates before you buy. Unless you are using a product quickly, get the latest date possible.

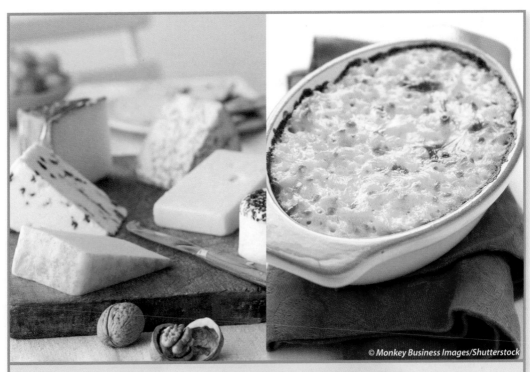

© Monkey Business Images/Shutterstock

18-24 If you are serving cheese and crackers, you might choose a higher quality cheese than you would for use in a casserole.

Storage

Proper storage of dairy products is important because they are perishable. Keep them in the coldest part of the refrigerator. When you are using the product, take just what you need. Return the rest to the refrigerator right away. Milk products tend to pick up flavors and odors from other foods. Keep milk containers tightly closed to avoid picking up flavors.

Dried and canned milk products should be stored in a cool, dry place. Keep packages tightly closed. Once water is added to dry milk, store it in the refrigerator. Canned milk products should be stored in the refrigerator after opening.

Ripened cheeses can last for a long time if properly stored. Wrap tightly so they do not get moldy or dry out. Wrapping also prevents the spread of odors and flavors to or from the cheese. Cheese should be refrigerated.

Keep frozen milk products in the coldest part of the freezer. Also, keep them tightly closed to prevent other flavors and moisture from affecting them. If these foods are not completely frozen, it can harm their textures.

Butter and margarine keep longer than milk, but they should be refrigerated. These products keep even longer if they are frozen. Be sure to tightly close the packages before freezing.

Reading Review

1. Give two reasons for pasteurizing milk.
2. True or false. UHT milk has had the water removed from it.
3. List two types of unripened cheese.
4. What is added to milk to make yogurt?
5. True or false. Milk products tend to pick up flavors from other foods.

Protein Foods

Objectives

After studying this section, you will be able to

- **recognize** factors to consider when buying meat, poultry, fish, and eggs.
- **explain** how to properly store meat, poultry, fish, and eggs.

Key Terms	
marbling	freezer burn

Protein foods are expensive compared to other foods such as produce and grain products. In addition, there are more factors to be considered when buying and storing these foods.

Buying Protein Foods

Understanding protein foods requires a little more effort than other foods. The same type of protein may come in different forms. These forms can vary in flavor and tenderness. Some forms may be appropriate for certain dishes or cooking methods and not for others. For instance, you may know you want beef, but you may not be sure what cut, **18-25**. An arm

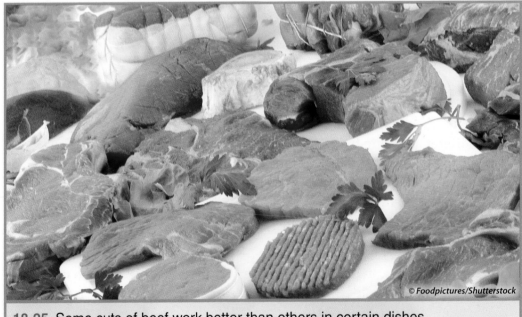

© Foodpictures/Shutterstock

18-25 Some cuts of beef work better than others in certain dishes.

pot roast is inexpensive, low in fat, and not very tender. A rib steak, on the other hand, is expensive, higher in fat, and very tender. If your plan was to cook out on the grill, the pot roast would be a poor choice.

In the United States, meat, poultry, fish, and eggs are the foods people choose most often for protein. Some basic information about these types of foods will help you make better purchases.

Meat

Meat includes cuts from beef, veal, pork, and lamb. *Beef* comes from mature cattle. *Veal* is from very young cattle—usually less than five months old. *Pork* is meat from hogs. *Lamb* is the meat from very young sheep.

Beef is red in color with creamy white fat. Beef cuts tend to vary more in terms of tenderness than other types of meat.

Veal has a delicate flavor and is light pink in color. Because veal comes from young animals, the meat is very tender. Veal does not have as much fat as beef.

High-quality pork is grayish-pink in color. Pork usually comes from young animals, so most cuts are fairly tender. Some cuts are higher in fat than others. Bacon, which comes from the belly, is very high in fat.

Lamb is pinkish-red in color and has very white fat. It has a mild flavor. Most lamb cuts are very tender because they come from young animals.

Choosing Cuts of Meat

Different cuts of meat vary in tenderness and flavor. The amount of fat in a meat and the toughness of the muscle affect how tender it is.

Fat makes meat more juicy and tender. It also adds flavor. The soft, white- or cream-colored part of meat is the fat. You can often see fat surrounding the muscle part of meat. There is also fat mixed in with the muscle. This fat is called **marbling**. The more marbling meat has, the more tender and flavorful it is.

The location of the muscle on the animal affects the flavor and tenderness of the cut of meat. This is especially true with beef, **18-26**. Muscles that are used more tend to be tougher and have less fat. For instance, the shoulder muscle is an active muscle needed during standing and moving. Meat from this area of an animal tends to be less tender. Muscles that are less active are more tender and have more marbling. For instance, muscles in the rib section are less active and known for their tenderness. Identifying the part of the animal different cuts are from will give you a good idea of their tenderness.

Just because meat is naturally tender does not always make it the best choice. Meat with less fat is lower in calories and cholesterol. There are cooking methods that can make less tender cuts of meat more juicy and flavorful. These cuts also tend to be less expensive than more tender cuts.

Quality Grading

Quality grading can help you select meats. Beef, veal, and lamb cuts in retail stores are often graded. Pork is considered so tender that it is not usually graded for retail sale.

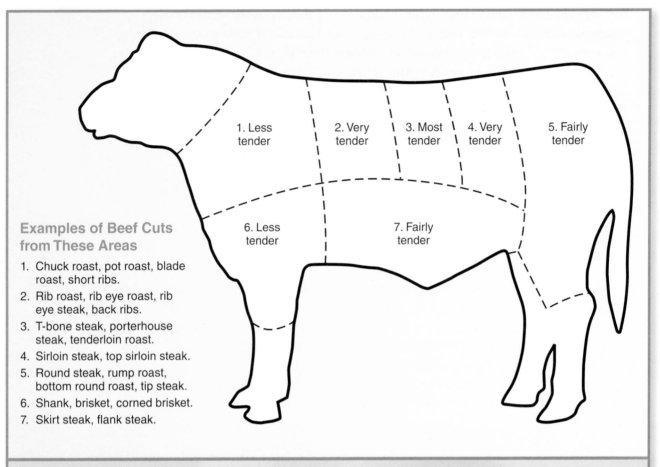

Examples of Beef Cuts from These Areas

1. Less tender
2. Very tender
3. Most tender
4. Very tender
5. Fairly tender
6. Less tender
7. Fairly tender

1. Chuck roast, pot roast, blade roast, short ribs.
2. Rib roast, rib eye roast, rib eye steak, back ribs.
3. T-bone steak, porterhouse steak, tenderloin roast.
4. Sirloin steak, top sirloin steak.
5. Round steak, rump roast, bottom round roast, tip steak.
6. Shank, brisket, corned brisket.
7. Skirt steak, flank steak.

18-26 Cuts of meat vary in tenderness and flavor depending on the part of the animal from which they originate.

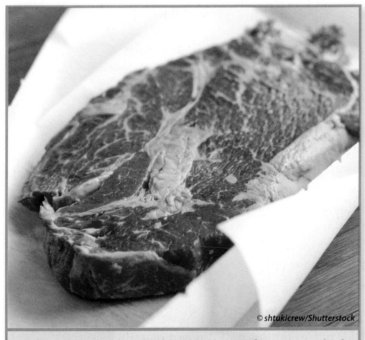

© shtukicrew/Shutterstock

18-27 The marbling in this prime cut of meat results in a tender, flavorful steak.

The quality grades you find most often on meats are prime, choice, select, and standard. *Prime* meats are very tender because they have a lot of marbling, **18-27**. They are mainly sold to restaurants and cannot be found in supermarkets. You may read on a menu that a restaurant serves prime cuts of meat. Prime meats are the most expensive of the grades.

Choice meats have a good amount of marbling, but not as much as prime. They are the highest quality found in most supermarkets and meat markets. Choice meats are less expensive than prime, but more expensive than other grades.

Select meats have less marbling than choice meats. They are less tender and flavorful. Select grade meats may be healthier choices if you are trying to limit fat and cholesterol. Select meats are less expensive than choice meats.

Standard meats have little marbling. They are less tender and flavorful than select meats. Standard meats are not often sold in grocery stores, but when available, they are less expensive. With the right cooking methods, standard meats can be made more tender. They can be inexpensive, but tasty meat choices.

Poultry

Poultry includes chicken, turkey, duck, and goose. Most poultry is very tender. Chicken and turkey are fairly low in fat. Duck and goose are fairly high in fat. Removing the skin greatly reduces the fat content of poultry.

Chicken and turkey contain both white and dark meat. White meat is found in the breast area. Dark meat includes the legs and thighs. White meat is lower in fat than dark meat. White meat can be a little dry if not cooked properly. Duck and goose contain only dark meat. Dark meat tends to be more tender and higher in fat than white meat.

The age of a bird affects the tenderness of the meat. Younger birds are the most tender. They are good for most types of cooking. Older birds are less tender and usually less expensive. Older birds might be used in soups, stews, and casseroles.

When buying poultry, look for plump, meaty breasts, thighs, and legs. The skin should be a clean, light color rather than dull and yellow. The skin should also be free from bruises and blemishes. If you buy frozen poultry, make sure it is frozen solid. Do not buy packages with rips or tears.

Fish

Fish is gaining popularity as a main dish in the United States. This is partly because people have become more health-conscious. Fish is lower in fat and calories than most other protein sources. It is a great source of many nutrients. Fish is also becoming more popular because shipping and packing have improved greatly. Fresh or fresh-frozen fish is available daily almost everywhere in the United States.

There are many types of fish. Some, such as swordfish, flounder, and cod, are lean fish. These fish are light, flaky, and very low in fat. Their flesh is white when cooked. Fish that contain more fat include catfish, salmon, and tuna. They have firmer textures and slightly

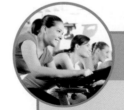

Health Connections

Eat Fatty Fish

The fats found in fish are considered oils and are more healthful than the solid fat present in meat, poultry, and eggs. Some of the oils found in fish are linked with decreased risk for heart disease. Fatty fish such as salmon, trout, and herring are richest in these beneficial nutrients. The *Dietary Guidelines* recommend increasing the amount and variety of fish you consume as part of a healthy eating pattern.

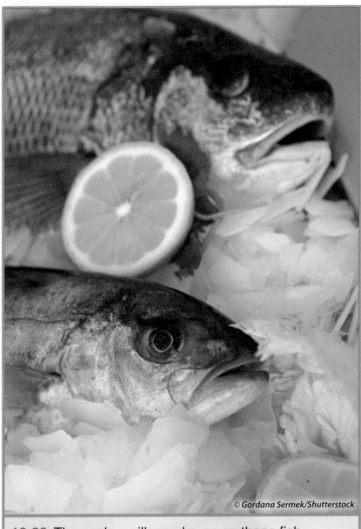

© Gordana Sermek/Shutterstock

18-28 The scales, gills, and eyes on these fish indicate freshness.

stronger flavors. The flesh from fatty fish may be pink, yellowish, or gray in color.

Many types of fish are more plentiful at certain times of the year. Like produce, fish is higher quality and less expensive during this time. Some fish may be unavailable or only sold in frozen form at other times of the year. It is much more expensive at these times.

When buying fresh fish, look for firm flesh that is not slimy. Whole fish should have tight scales, red gills, and bright, bulging eyes, **18-28**. The fish should not have a strong or foul odor. Frozen fish should be frozen solid.

Shellfish

Shellfish are types of seafood that have hard outer coverings or shells. They include lobster, shrimp, crab, oysters, scallops, and clams. Their flesh is more firm and rich tasting than the flesh of most fish.

Lobster and crab are sold live or cooked and frozen. Fresh lobster and crab must be cooked from their live state. Canned lobster and crabmeat is also available. Shrimp are sold fresh, fresh frozen, cooked and frozen, or canned. Oysters and clams are sold live in the shell and fresh, frozen, or canned without the shell. Scallops are sold without the shell fresh or frozen.

When buying fresh shellfish, look for bright, clear colors. Shellfish should not be dull or slimy. They should have no strong odor. Live shellfish should be quick to respond when touched. Frozen shellfish should be frozen solid.

Eggs

Eggs are thought to be one of the most perfect protein foods available. In addition to being a good source of protein, eggs are high in many vitamins and iron. Egg yolks are also high in cholesterol. For individuals who are trying to reduce cholesterol in their diet, they should limit their intake of egg yolks.

Fresh eggs are most often sold in cartons by the dozen. Eggs are available in different sizes—small, medium, large, extra large, and jumbo. Most recipes call for medium or large eggs. These are the sizes most popular with consumers.

When buying eggs, open the carton and check the eggs carefully. The eggs should be smooth and clean. They should also be free from cracks.

Egg substitutes supply the flavor of eggs without the cholesterol. They contain real egg whites with added vegetable oils and other ingredients to replace the egg yolk. Egg substitutes are sold frozen in cartons.

Making the Most of Your Protein Food Buys

Care when selecting and buying protein foods is important because they are expensive. The lowest price may not always save you the most money. You need to select the right food for the dish to turn out correctly.

Be sure you choose protein foods that fit your needs. If you want to save money, plan recipes that make the most of inexpensive meats, **18-29**. These recipes employ cooking methods that work well with less tender cuts of meat. (You will read more about this later in the chapter.) If you choose the wrong cut of meat for a recipe and cooking method, the result may be inedible. The resulting waste could cost you more than buying the cut that costs a little more.

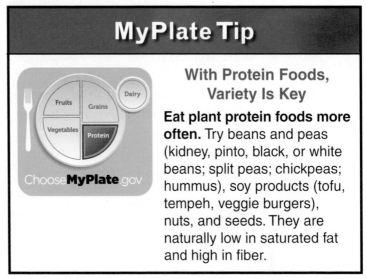

MyPlate Tip

With Protein Foods, Variety Is Key

Eat plant protein foods more often. Try beans and peas (kidney, pinto, black, or white beans; split peas; chickpeas; hummus), soy products (tofu, tempeh, veggie burgers), nuts, and seeds. They are naturally low in saturated fat and high in fiber.

Source: MyPlate 10 tips Nutrition Education Series

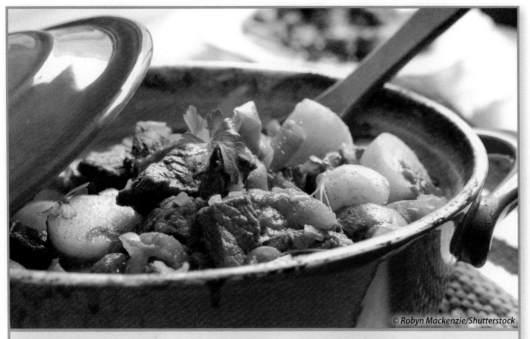

© Robyn Mackenzie/Shutterstock

18-29 Long, slow cooking with moist heat makes less expensive cuts of meat very appealing.

Other than eggs, most protein foods are sold by the pound. Be sure to compare the price per pound, not the total price. This will give you a better idea of which items cost more.

The price per pound alone may not give you a true picture of the cost of protein foods. You also need to consider waste. Bones, fat, and other portions of protein foods are not always edible. Protein foods in this form are usually less expensive per pound, but may not be a better value. For instance, when you buy a whole chicken, you are paying for the bones and skin that are not eaten. When you buy boneless, skinless chicken breast, there is no waste. It may cost more per pound, but may not be more expensive when you consider the cost of waste with the whole chicken.

Many protein foods are placed on special from time to time. Turkey is usually less expensive during November and December. Different types of fish are less expensive at certain times throughout the year. Ground beef and other meats for grilling are often on special during summer months. Taking advantage of these specials can save you money on high-quality protein foods.

Storing Protein Foods

Proper storage of protein foods is important. Most protein foods are even more perishable than fresh produce. Improper storage can lead to loss of flavor and nutrients. More importantly, it can cause illness. Because protein foods are expensive, it is worth your effort to store them properly.

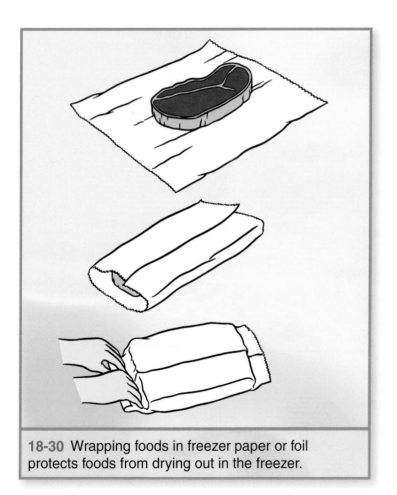

18-30 Wrapping foods in freezer paper or foil protects foods from drying out in the freezer.

Meat and Poultry

Meat and poultry should be stored in the coldest part of the refrigerator. They should be wrapped well so they do not dry out or drip on other foods.

Most meat can be stored three to four days in the refrigerator. Ground beef and poultry should be stored only one or two days.

If you do not plan to use your purchases soon, they should be frozen. Meat and poultry purchased frozen can be left in its original packaging. Meat and poultry purchased fresh should be rewrapped before freezing, **18-30**. Remove the store wrappings and rewrap in a freezer bag, freezer paper, or heavy aluminum foil. You may want to separate a large package of meat or poultry into smaller portions before rewrapping. Be sure to wrap tightly so air cannot reach the meat or poultry. Exposure to air causes food to become freezer burned. **Freezer burn** is a white or gray-colored spot where food has dried out. Parts of food with freezer burn are dry and tasteless.

Frozen items should not be thawed and refrozen. If an item still has ice crystals on it, then it can be refrozen. If an item becomes completely thawed, use it right away. Meat and poultry can be refrozen after cooking.

Fish

Fresh fish is more perishable than poultry. Fish should be wrapped tightly in waxed paper or foil. It should be stored in the coldest part of the refrigerator and eaten within one or two days.

Fish can be stored for a longer time if it is frozen. Like meat and poultry, it should be wrapped well before freezing. Fish bought frozen can be left in its original package.

Fish should not be refrozen once it is thawed. Some fish sold in stores is shipped frozen, then thawed for display. Be sure to check the labels carefully—this fish should not be refrozen.

Eggs

Eggs are not as perishable as meat, fish, and poultry. Eggs are at their highest quality if used within a week of purchase. When properly stored, eggs are safe to use for up to five weeks.

Eggs should be stored in the refrigerator in their original carton, **18-31**. Eggs may pick up flavors and odors from other foods. Storing eggs in their carton prolongs their freshness and reduces absorption of strong odors from other foods.

Whole eggs out of the shell, egg yolks, and egg whites can be frozen for longer storage. A little salt or sugar must be added to egg yolks or whole eggs before freezing. The egg should be poured into a freezer container and tightly sealed before freezing.

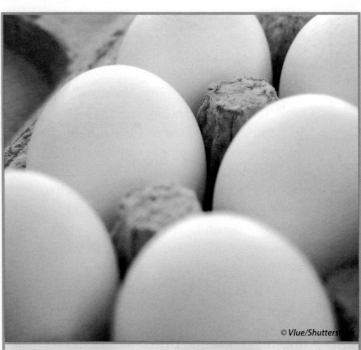

© Vlue/Shutterstock

18-31 Store eggs in the refrigerator in their original carton.

Reading Review

1. True or false. The flavor and tenderness of cuts of beef vary.
2. How is light meat from poultry different from dark meat?
3. List four factors to look for when selecting fresh whole fish.
4. True or false. The protein food with the lowest price per pound is always the best value.
5. Why is it important to tightly wrap protein foods before freezing?

Chapter Summary

Section 18-1. When shopping for food, you can follow some guidelines to help you get your money's worth. Choose the type of store that meets your needs. Make a shopping list to help you remember everything you need. Be aware of factors that affect food costs. These include amount of processing, supply, freshness, packaging, and transportation. When comparing food prices, consider size, brand, and form. Unit pricing can help you make these comparisons easily.

Section 18-2. Reading food labels helps you make food choices that best meet your needs. Certain information is required by law and must appear on the label. Other information, such as *high fiber* and *organic*, must meet requirements set by the government before they can appear on the label. The universal product code found on food labels helps stores and producers track their products. Open dating on food labels allows store employees and consumers to identify freshness of products.

Section 18-3. Fruits and vegetables add variety, flavor, and nutrients to your meals. Fruits and vegetables are sold fresh, frozen, canned, and dried. You should choose the type and quality that gives you the best buy and suits your planned use.

Fresh fruits and vegetables need to be stored carefully to preserve nutrients, flavors, and freshness. Frozen fruits and vegetables should be stored in the coldest part of the freezer. Canned and dried products should be kept in a cool, dry place.

Section 18-4. Grains are seeds from various types of grasses. Grain products can be prepared and served as a single food or used as an ingredient. Grains are ground into flour to make pasta, breakfast cereal, and breads. Grain products should be stored in a cool, dry place in tightly closed containers.

Section 18-5. A variety of dairy products are made from milk including fresh fluid, ultra high temperature, dry, and canned milk. Natural and processed cheeses, frozen milk products, yogurt, cream, and butter are also made from milk. These products vary in level of fat content and added ingredients. Choose the items that best meet your needs.

When buying dairy products, compare different brands and package sizes to get the best buys. These products are perishable and must be stored carefully to maintain their freshness.

Section 18-6. Protein foods are expensive compared to other foods such as produce and grain products. Use the cut and grade to help you select meat. Age affects the tenderness of poultry. The time of year can affect the cost of fish. Buy eggs that are clean and free from cracks. Select protein foods based on the needs of your dish and your budget. Compare the price per pound to help you make the best buy. Remember to consider waste when comparing cost.

Meat, poultry, and fish should be wrapped securely and stored in the refrigerator. Meat should be used within three to four days. Poultry and fish should be used within one or two days. For longer storage, these foods can be frozen.

Eggs should be stored in the refrigerator in their original carton and use within five weeks of purchase.

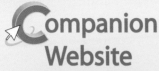

Companion Website
www.g-wlearning.com

Check your understanding of the main concepts for Chapter 18 at the website.

Critical Thinking

1. **Create.** Imagine you are a manager of a supermarket. Describe a new strategy you would use to encourage customers to buy a product on impulse.
2. **Analyze.** List the individual foods that make up your favorite meal. Next to each food, note whether the food is processed and, if so, the type of processing.
3. **Design.** Select a food product and design an improved nutrition information label. Identify where on the packaging the label would appear.

Common Core

College and Career Readiness

4. **Math.** Calculate and compare the unit price for fresh, frozen, and canned forms of your favorite fruit or vegetable.

5. **Speaking.** Prepare and give an informative speech on how to select a quality plant-based protein of your choosing.
6. **Math.** Create a bar graph comparing the unit prices for organic, brand name, and store brand milk products.
7. **Writing.** Research how fish are farm raised and write a brief summary.

Technology

8. **Identify uses.** Research to learn ways quick reference (QR) codes are being employed in the food industry. Consider ways you would like to see a QR code used on food labeling.

Journal Writing

9. Select and prepare a grain you have never before eaten. Write a journal entry describing why you selected this grain, if you liked it, and if you will be adding this grain to your diet.

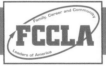 ## FCCLA

10. Create a new cereal product for a *Food Innovations STAR Event*. Develop a cereal prototype along with packaging ideas for long-term storage. Conduct focus groups to taste-test your product. Develop a marketing strategy for promoting your product. Design a display that illustrates the product-development process and your packaging ideas. See your adviser for information as needed.

Unit 6
Preparing Meals and Dining Out

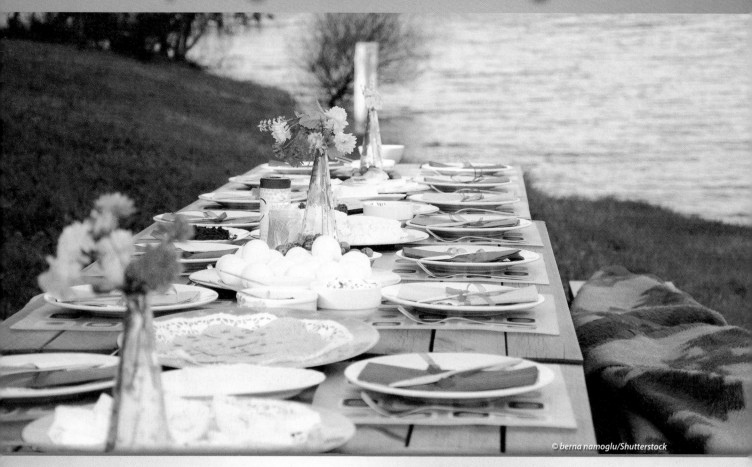

© berna namoglu/Shutterstock

Unit Essential Question

What role does the selection and preparation of food have in the lives of people worldwide?

Exploring Career Pathways

Hospitality and Foodservice Careers

Are you a person with strong organizational skills and the ability to multitask? Do you enjoy working with people? Perhaps a career in hospitality or foodservice is for you. Here are some careers in this pathway in which many people succeed.

Concierge

Whether working in a hotel, apartment complex, or office building, the main responsibility of a concierge (kahn-see-EHRZH) is to help people meet their personal needs. Perhaps when on vacation, you had a concierge give you a dining recommendation or make sightseeing arrangements. These workers need to know how to provide good customer service. A high school diploma is a basic requirement for a concierge. Many people hired for this position work with a mentor for several months to a year. Vital personal characteristics include integrity, carefulness about details, flexibility, and an ability to cooperate well with others.

Chef

Chefs have great passion for cooking and using their creativity with food. Along with cooking ability, chefs are responsible for guiding cooks and other kitchen staff. They develop recipes, plan menus, prepare food cost estimates, and make sure the facility runs efficiently. Ensuring workers and the facility comply with all sanitation and safety regulations is an important responsibility. Chefs need some postsecondary training. Many earn associate's or bachelor's degrees in culinary arts. Good chefs are skillful communicators, strong leaders, and know how to motivate others. Most states require health certificates showing that foodservice workers are free from communicable disease.

Meeting, Convention, and Event Planner

Meeting, convention, and event planners ensure that events run smoothly, and without flaw. Their many responsibilities include searching for event sites, such as hotels or convention centers. They also coordinate services such as catering, photography, displays, transportation, and security. Planners meet with clients to establish needs for the event, plan budgets, and monitor all aspects of the event. The work is fast-paced with demanding deadlines. Most employers require planners to have a bachelor's degree in areas such as marketing, public relations, or hospitality management. Excellent verbal and written skills, along with computer and financial skills are necessary for people who work in this field. Achieving the Certified Meeting Professional credential is a benefit for career advancement.

Is this career path for you? Pursue one or both of the following activities to determine if you are suitable for a career in hospitality or foodservice.

- Try your hand at event planning by helping plan a school event. Record your experiences in a photo journal. Evaluate the process. Did you enjoy and excel at these work activities?
- Take the O*NET *Interest Profiler* self-assessment on the Internet to see if you have the interest it takes for a career in hospitality or foodservice. Write a summary of what you learned about yourself from this self-assessment.

Chapter 19
Getting Ready to Cook

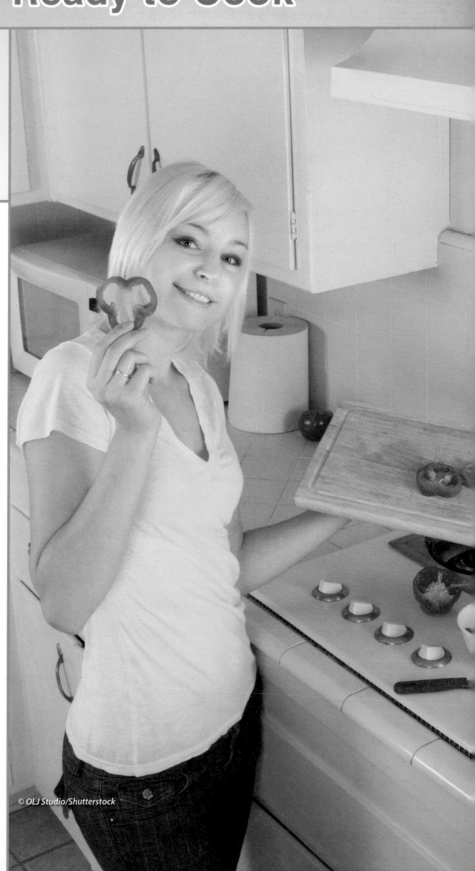

Sections

Reading Prep

College and Career Readiness

Find an article online that relates to the topic covered in this chapter. Print the article and read it before reading the chapter. As you read the chapter, highlight sections of the news article that relate to the text.

Concept Organizer

Food Contaminant	Examples

Use a T-chart to identify the different types of food contaminants and give an example of each.

Companion Website

Print out the concept organizer for Chapter 19 at the website.

Companion Website
www.g-wlearning.com

© OLJ Studio/Shutterstock

Sanitation and Food Safety

Objectives

After studying this section, you will be able to
- **understand** what causes foodborne illness.
- **apply** sanitation practices to promote a safe kitchen.
- **explain** safe food handling techniques.

Key Terms

contaminants	cross-contamination	temperature danger
bacteria	sanitation	zone
foodborne illness		

Before beginning to cook, it is important to have a basic understanding of how to prepare and serve safe food. A responsible cook prepares food that is flavorful as well as wholesome.

Foodborne Illness

People eat food because they like the way it tastes. People also eat food to nourish their bodies. Sometimes neither of these is possible because harmful substances, called **contaminants**, have been introduced to the food. Contaminants can be physical, chemical, or biological. The following are examples of each type of contaminant:
- *Physical*—hair, pieces of glass, or bits of packaging
- *Chemical*—cleaning products or toxic metals such as mercury in fish
- *Biological*—a variety of small, living organisms including *bacteria*, viruses, fungi, or parasites

Bacteria are one-celled organisms that live in soil, water, and the bodies of plants and animals. In fact, bacteria can be found nearly everywhere, **19-1**.

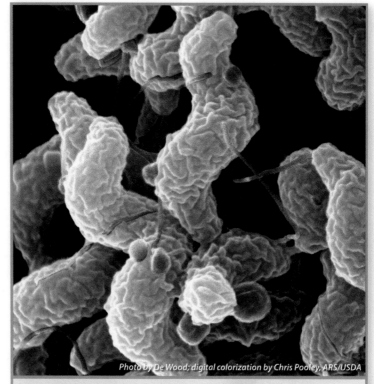

Photo by De Wood; digital colorization by Chris Pooley, ARS/USDA

19-1 This type of bacterium is often found in contaminated water, raw milk, and raw or undercooked meat, poultry, or shellfish.

Occasionally food is contaminated during processing, but most often it is contaminated during preparation.

Contaminants either cause food to spoil or be unsafe. Some types of bacteria can cause food to go bad even when refrigerated. These foods are generally no longer appealing, but they do not usually cause you to be sick.

Foods are contaminated most often with harmful bacteria. Many people become sick each year from eating contaminated food. Sickness caused from eating contaminated food is called foodborne illness. Different types of foodborne illnesses are caused by different types of bacteria, viruses, parasites, and fungi. Symptoms of these illnesses vary, but they often include vomiting, diarrhea, severe headaches, stomach cramps, and fever. These symptoms can occur as quickly as 30 minutes after eating the contaminated food or may take weeks to appear. Some types of foodborne illness can be fatal. The good news is that most foodborne illness can be avoided with proper sanitation and safe food handling.

Sanitation

When bacteria are transferred to food by people, insects, rodents, pets, unclean utensils, or other unsanitary objects, it is called cross-contamination. The bacteria can then be transferred to the people who eat the food.

Proper sanitation helps prevent cross-contamination. Sanitation is the process of making conditions clean and healthy. Sanitation is especially important in food preparation. Keeping utensils and work areas clean can help prevent food from becoming contaminated.

Personal cleanliness also plays an important part in kitchen sanitation. Always wash your hands with soap and warm water before handling any food. Be sure to clean under your fingernails. If your hair is long, tie it back to keep it from falling into the food. Make sure your clothes are clean, 19-2.

Safe Food Handling

Foods are often contaminated with harmful bacteria through improper storage or handling. Handling and storing food properly is important to help prevent contamination. Your responsibility for safe food handling begins when you are shopping for food and ends after the food is eaten. Everything that happens to the food between those two points has the potential to threaten the safety of the food.

Time and Temperature

Time and temperature are key factors for safe food handling. Bacteria multiply rapidly at temperatures between 40°F and 140°F, called the temperature danger zone. As food remains longer in this range, the number of bacteria increases and so does the risk for foodborne illness. For this reason, food should not sit at room temperature for more than a total of two hours.

Practice Sanitation in the Kitchen

Handwashing

Wash hands

- for 20 seconds or more with warm, soapy water and wear gloves to handle food if you have a cut or infection.
- after using the bathroom.
- any time you touch something else such as your hair, nose, refrigerator handle, telephone, oven knob, your pet, or faucet handle.
- before beginning to prepare a different food.
- when you are done preparing food.

Food Contact Surfaces and Utensils

Wash

- counters, knives, dishes, and cutting boards with hot, soapy water before and after each food you prepare.
- produce before preparing, including the rinds of melons and banana skins.
- can lids before opening cans.
- can openers after each use.
- thermometers between each use.
- tasting spoon each time you sample your food; or get a clean one.

Cutting Boards

- Use a clean cutting board for food preparation.
- When possible, designate one cutting board for preparing produce and a different board for cutting raw meat, poultry, and fish.
- Sanitize cutting boards with a mixture of 1 tablespoon of unscented, liquid chlorine bleach in 1 gallon of water.
- Replace cutting boards that have deep, hard to clean cracks or grooves.

General

- Sponges and dishcloths harbor bacteria and should be changed or sanitized daily.
- After cleaning, sanitize countertops and handles for appliances using the mixture for cutting boards or undiluted white distilled vinegar. (When using vinegar, allow to sit for 10 minutes to be effective.)
- After cleaning, sanitize sinks and faucet handles.
- Keep books, purses, backpacks, and shopping bags off food contact surfaces.
- Direct sneezes and coughs away from food.

19-2 Follow these sanitation guidelines to prepare wholesome food.

To limit time food spends in the danger zone, keep hot foods hot and cold foods cold. Serve hot foods as soon as they are prepared and refrigerate leftovers promptly. If you cannot serve hot foods immediately, maintain a temperature of 140°F or higher. Likewise, if you will not be serving a cold food right away, keep it in the refrigerator.

Life Connections

Using a Food Thermometer

The best way to check that food is at a safe temperature is with a food thermometer. There are different types of food thermometers—oven-safe, digital, disposable, and dial instant-read thermometers. The dial instant-read thermometer is easy to use, inexpensive, and can be purchased at most food stores. Certain guidelines must be followed when using a thermometer.

- The thermometer should be placed in the thickest part of the food. Make sure it is not touching bone, fat, or gristle. For combination dishes, such as casseroles, place thermometer in the center. Dishes containing eggs or ground meat or poultry should be checked in several places.
- To obtain an accurate reading with this type of thermometer, the stem must be submerged at least two inches into the food.
- The thermometer must be cleaned with hot, soapy water before and after each use to avoid cross-contamination.
- Calibrate the thermometer on a regular basis.

Calibration Activity

- To calibrate a dial instant-read thermometer:
  1. Fill a container with crushed ice and add cold water.
  2. Use the clip on the dial thermometer sheath to hold the thermometer upright in ice water for one minute.
  3. If the dial reads 32°F, the thermometer is calibrated. If it does not, use the wrench on the thermometer sheath to adjust the nut located under the dial face until it reads 32°F.

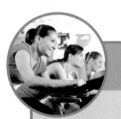

Health Connections

Refrigerator Temperature

Check your refrigerator temperature periodically to ensure it is cold enough to keep your food safe. Temperature controls that are built into the refrigerator are not always accurate or effective. Use an appliance thermometer to check that your refrigerator is cooling to 40°F or below. You can check the freezer as well to confirm it is at or below 0°F.

Shopping Carefully

Being a careful shopper can help you avoid buying food that may already be spoiled. Bacteria can get into damaged food packages. When buying food, make sure bags and boxes are intact. Do not buy dented cans or jars that are not securely sealed. Avoid buying frozen foods that have thawed in the display case. Buy eggs with clean, uncracked shells.

Be aware of open dating on packages when you shop. Do not buy items if the pull date or expiration date has passed. Keep raw meat, poultry, fish, and eggs apart from other foods in your shopping cart and refrigerator.

Put refrigerated and frozen foods in your shopping cart last. Avoid buying these products if you will not be going straight home from the store. When you get home, put away these foods quickly. The time food spends in the shopping cart and in your car, is time spent in the danger zone and should be limited. On days when the temperature outside is over 90°F, consider bringing a cooler to transport your perishable foods or refrigerate foods within one hour.

Storing Foods Properly

Foods can be stored for only a limited amount of time. To keep foods safe, use them within the recommended time, **19-3**.

Wrap foods properly for storage. Use moisture-proof, vapor-proof paper to wrap foods for freezer storage. For the refrigerator, use covered containers to keep harmful bacteria out of foods. Do not store raw meat, poultry, and fish over ready-to-eat foods. The juices from the raw foods could drip into the ready-to-eat foods and contaminate them. Be sure to thaw frozen foods in the refrigerator—not at room temperature.

Cold Storage Chart

Product	Refrigerator (40°F, 4°C)	Freezer (0°F, -18°C)
Eggs		
Fresh in shell	3 weeks	Do not freeze
Hard cooked	1 week	Do not freeze well
Salads		
Egg, chicken, ham, tuna, and macaroni salads	3 to 5 days	Do not freeze well
Hot Dogs		
Opened package	1 week	1 to 2 months
Unopened package	2 weeks	1 to 2 months
Luncheon Meat		
Opened package or deli meat	3 to 5 days	1 to 2 months
Unopened package	2 weeks	1 to 2 months
Bacon and Sausage		
Bacon	7 days	1 month
Sausage, raw (chicken, turkey, pork, beef)	1 to 2 days	1 to 2 months
Hamburger and Other Ground Meats		
Hamburger, ground beef, turkey, veal, pork, lamb, and mixtures	1 to 2 days	3 to 4 months
Fresh Beef, Veal, Lamb, and Pork		
Steaks	3 to 5 days	6 to 12 months
Chops	3 to 5 days	4 to 6 months
Roasts	3 to 5 days	4 to 12 months
Fresh Poultry		
Chicken or turkey, whole	1 to 2 days	1 year
Chicken or turkey, pieces	1 to 2 days	9 months
Soups and Stews		
Vegetable or meat added	3 to 4 days	2 to 3 months
Leftovers		
Cooked meat or poultry	3 to 4 days	2 to 6 months
Chicken nuggets or patties	3 to 4 days	1 to 3 months
Pizza	3 to 4 days	1 to 2 months

19-3 The USDA provides guidelines for length of time foods can be stored in the refrigerator or freezer.

Source: USDA Kitchen Companion: Your Safe Food Handbook

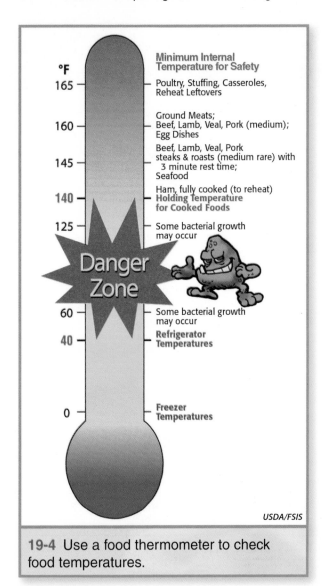

°F

165 — Poultry, Stuffing, Casseroles, Reheat Leftovers

Minimum Internal Temperature for Safety

160 — Ground Meats; Beef, Lamb, Veal, Pork (medium); Egg Dishes

145 — Beef, Lamb, Veal, Pork steaks & roasts (medium rare) with 3 minute rest time; Seafood

140 — Ham, fully cooked (to reheat) **Holding Temperature for Cooked Foods**

125 — Some bacterial growth may occur

Danger Zone

60 — Some bacterial growth may occur

40 — Refrigerator Temperatures

0 — Freezer Temperatures

USDA/FSIS

19-4 Use a food thermometer to check food temperatures.

Cooking Foods Safely

Time and temperature are not only important when purchasing and storing foods. These factors are key to cooking and reheating foods safely as well. Food must be cooked to a temperature that is high enough to kill the harmful bacteria that may be present in the food. You cannot know that food is cooked to a safe temperature simply by looking at it. Using a thermometer is the best way to ensure food reaches a safe temperature. Different foods must be cooked to different temperatures to be safe, **19-4**. Once a food reaches a safe temperature, it must either be served or held at 140°F or above.

Packing Food Safely

Keeping food for school lunches at safe temperatures can be a problem. You must take steps to protect food even when you do not have access to hot or cold storage.

Use a thermos to keep foods at safe temperatures. Before adding hot food to a thermos, rinse the inside with boiling water. Rinse the thermos with ice water if you are using it to carry cold food.

Pack something cold in a lunch bag if you are unable to refrigerate your lunch. A well-chilled canned drink or a frozen gel pack helps keep your lunch cool.

Make sandwiches ahead of time and freeze them so they stay cool until lunchtime. Avoid freezing lettuce, tomatoes, and sandwich fillings containing mayonnaise as these items do not freeze well.

You might even want to make a week's worth of sandwiches and freeze them all. This will save time as you pack lunches throughout the week. Wrap each sandwich separately in aluminum foil or a tightly closed plastic bag.

Cooking and eating should be healthy, enjoyable activities, so use care in the kitchen. Follow safety and sanitation guidelines when you prepare food.

Reading Review

1. List the three types of food contaminants.
2. True or false. Food is contaminated most often during processing.
3. Why is proper sanitation in the kitchen important?
4. Why are time and temperature important to food safety?
5. True or false. Raw meat, poultry, fish, and eggs should be stored apart from other foods in your shopping cart.

Kitchen Utensils and Appliances

Objectives

After studying this section, you will be able to
- **identify** basic kitchen utensils and their uses.
- **understand** how cookware and bakeware differ.
- **recognize** the purposes of common kitchen appliances.

Key Terms		
kitchen utensil	double boiler	convection oven
cookware	skillets	microwaves
bakeware	appliance	superheating

Kitchen equipment allows you to store and prepare foods more easily and with greater success. Using the right tool for each food preparation task can also save time. As with any tool, knowing how to use it safely is important.

Kitchen Utensils

A **kitchen utensil** is a handheld, hand-powered tool used to prepare food. To be a well-informed cook, you need to learn how to use each utensil correctly and safely.

Be sure to care for utensils properly. Clean them after every use to prevent cross-contamination. You can wash most utensils in warm, soapy water. Read any care instructions included on the utensil's packaging.

You can perform most common food preparation tasks with a basic set of inexpensive tools. As you gain cooking experience, you may wish to learn about some of the more specialized utensils that are available. Basic tools can be grouped according to the types of tasks they perform, **19-5**.

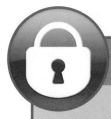

Safety Connections

Edge of Safety

Follow these guidelines to prevent injuries:
- Do not place cutting utensils in a sink of sudsy water.
- Wash sharp knives individually. Soaking knives may cause wood handles to loosen.
- Run a paper towel along the back of the blade to dry knives.
- Cut food away from yourself.
- Keep blades sharp.
- Use a cutting board for chopping and slicing.
- Store knives apart from other utensils.
- Remove lids and carefully place in bottom of can before disposing—do not leave lid attached to can.
- Sweep broken glass onto paper or cardboard to throw away. Use a damp paper towel to wipe up slivers.
- Keep fingers away from blender, food processor, and food waste disposer blades.

Kitchen Utensils

Measuring Utensils	Cutting Utensils *(Continued)*

Measuring Utensils

- *Dry measuring cups*: measure dry ingredients such as flour and sugar. Cup is overfilled and a flat edge is used to scrape off excess. They commonly come in sets of four, including ¼-cup (50 mL), ⅓-cup (85 mL), ½-cup (125 mL), and 1-cup (250 mL) sizes.

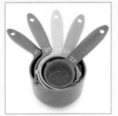
© WhitePlaid/Shutterstock

- *Liquid measuring cups:* measure liquid ingredients such as milk and oil. They are available in 1-cup (250 mL), 2-cup (500 mL), and 4-cup (1 L) sizes.

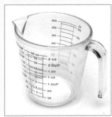
© M. Unal Ozmen/Shutterstock

- *Measuring spoons*: measure small amounts of liquid and dry ingredients. Measuring spoons usually come in sets of four, including ¼-teaspoon (1 mL), ½-teaspoon (2 mL), 1-teaspoon (5 mL), and 1-tablespoon (15 mL) sizes.

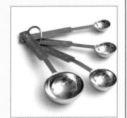
© Freddy Eliasson/Shutterstock

Cutting Utensils

- *Paring knife*: used for small cutting jobs, such as trimming and peeling vegetables and fruits.

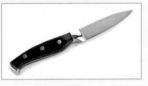
© Darryl Brooks/Shutterstock

- *Chef's knife*: used to chop, dice, and mince fruits and vegetables.

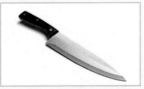
© Picsfive/Shutterstock

Cutting Utensils *(Continued)*

- *Serrated knife*: used for slicing bread and tender vegetables such as tomatoes.

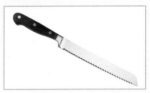
© Matt Valentine/Shutterstock

- *Cutting board*: protects both the countertop and the knife's edge when cutting foods.

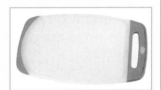
© sevenke/Shutterstock

- *Peeler*: trims away skin on foods such as carrots, potatoes, and apples.

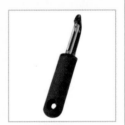
© shutswis/Shutterstock

- *Kitchen shears*: used for snipping herbs, such as parsley. Can also be used for cutting soft foods, such as pizza, meats, dough, and dried fruits.

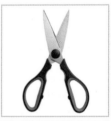
© Lev Kropotov/Shutterstock

- *Can opener:* cuts lids away from canned foods.

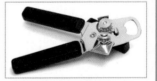
© terekhov igor/Shutterstock

- *Grater*: shreds and shaves foods such as cheese, cabbage, and potatoes.

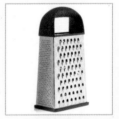
© Jaroslav74/Shutterstock

(Continued)

19-5 Use the kitchen utensil best suited to the job.

Kitchen Utensils *(Continued)*

Mixing Utensils

- *Mixing bowl*: holds ingredients as they are being combined. Bowls may be glass, metal, or plastic. Often sold in sets including bowls of various sizes.

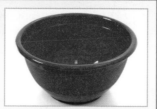
© Artistic Endeavor/Shutterstock

- *Kitchen spoons*: used to mix, baste, and stir foods during preparation. Choose a spoon with a wood or plastic handle to avoid burning your hand when stirring hot foods.

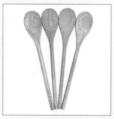
© Jeff Lueders/Shutterstock

- *Silicone spatula*: used to fold ingredients in, and for cleaning the sides of mixing bowls.

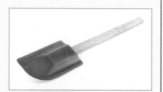
© Marc F Gutierrez/Shutterstock

- *Pastry blender*: cuts shortening into pieces and blends them with flour.

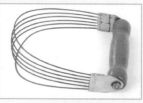
© Scott Sanders/Shutterstock

- *Sifter*: adds air and removes lumps from dry ingredients.

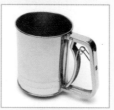
© M. Unal Ozmen/Shutterstock

- *Rotary beater*: hand-powered blades used to beat, blend, and whip foods.

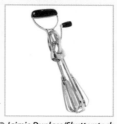
© Jaimie Duplass/Shutterstock

Cooking Utensils

- *Kitchen fork*: holds meat and poultry for slicing.

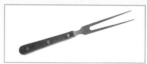
© Ganko/Shutterstock

- *Offset spatula or turner*: lifts and flips foods such as hamburgers, pancakes, and eggs during cooking.

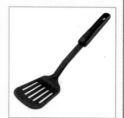
© Coprid/Shutterstock

- *Tongs*: used to turn or move foods without piercing.

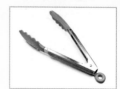
© ribeiroantonio/Shutterstock

- *Ladle*: used to serve punches, soups, and stews.

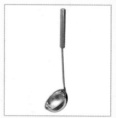
© Dudaeva/Shutterstock

Other Kitchen Utensils

- *Slotted spoon*: used to remove foods from cooking liquids.

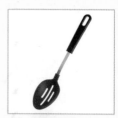
© EuToch/Shutterstock

- *Colander*: holds food while allowing liquid from cooking or rinsing to drain off. Often used for draining cooked pasta and noodles.

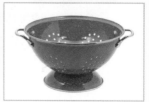
© Shawn Hempel/Shutterstock

(Continued)

Kitchen Utensils (Continued)

Other Kitchen Utensils (Continued)

- *Strainers*: used to separate solids from liquids. Used for foods that are too fine to drain in a colander. Can also be used to sift small amounts of dry ingredients.

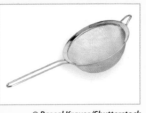

© Pascal Krause/Shutterstock

- *Rolling pin*: flattens dough into a thin, even layer. Used when making pastry, cookies, and other dough products.

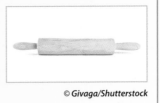

© Givaga/Shutterstock

- *Timer*: measure cooking and baking time to prevent overcooking.

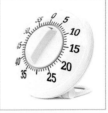

© saiko3p/Shutterstock

- *Thermometer*: measures the temperature of foods. Different types are used for meats, candies, and hot fat.

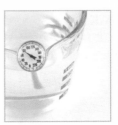

© Carlos Yudica/Shutterstock

Cookware and Bakeware

Special kitchen tools are needed to hold food as it is being cooked or baked. The term **cookware** refers to pots and pans used on top of the range. **Bakeware** refers to items used to cook food in an oven. Items used in a microwave oven are often called *microwave cookware*.

Saucepans are used for many types of cooking chores. It is helpful to have saucepans in a few different sizes with tight-fitting lids.

A **double boiler** is a small pan that fits inside a larger pan. This tool is used for cooking delicate foods. The food is placed in the small pan and water is placed in the larger pan. The food is cooked by the heat of the steam from the water in the larger pan. This type of heat is gentler than the direct heat of the range.

Skillets, or *frying pans*, are used for panfrying, panbroiling, and braising foods. They are often made out of heavier materials than saucepans, **19-6**.

A number of bakeware pieces are used for baking cakes. *Square pans* and *round pans* are used to bake layer cakes. Square pans are also used for baking coffee cakes and bar cookies. *Tube pans* are used to bake angel food, sponge, and chiffon cakes. *Jelly roll pans* are used for making sheet cakes.

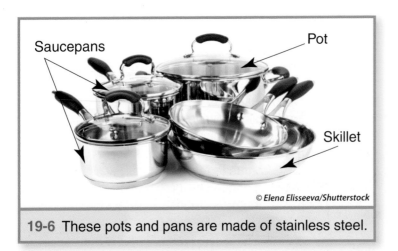

Saucepans

Pot

Skillet

© Elena Elisseeva/Shutterstock

19-6 These pots and pans are made of stainless steel.

They are also used for making jelly rolls and bar cookies. *Muffin pans* are used to bake cupcakes as well as muffins.

Other bakeware pieces include *cookie sheets*, *pizza pans*, *loaf pans*, and *pie pans*. The names of these items explain their uses, 19-7.

A *cooling rack* is a wire rack that allows air to circulate around baked goods. This causes them to cool faster and more evenly. A *covered cake server* is used to store cakes and keep them fresh and moist.

Materials

A number of different materials are used to make cookware and bakeware. Metals such as copper, aluminum, and stainless steel are popular for cookware items. Cast iron is used to make some skillets. Plastics are often used to make microwave cookware. Glass, as well as aluminum and stainless steel, is frequently used to make bakeware.

These various materials may also be found in other uses, although less commonly. For instance, some plastics can be used in a conventional oven. Some glass can be used on top of the range. Some metals can be used in a microwave oven.

Not all materials are suited for every use. Always read cookware and bakeware labels before using a new item. This information tells you the types of uses for which each piece is suited.

Small Appliances

A kitchen **appliance** is a piece of equipment run by gas or electricity that is used to store, process, or cook food. Small kitchen appliances, including items such

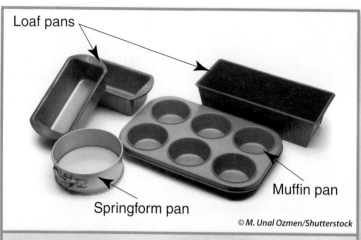

Loaf pans

Springform pan

Muffin pan

© M. Unal Ozmen/Shutterstock

19-7 These bakeware items are used for foods cooked in an oven.

Safety Connections

Materials for Microwaving

The USDA Food Safety and Inspection Service recommends the following when using microwave ovens.

Safe to use:
- Any utensil labeled for microwave use.
- Heatproof glass (such as Pyrex).
- Glass-ceramic (such as Corning Ware).
- Oven cooking bags.
- Baskets (straw and wood) lined with napkins for quick warm-ups of rolls or bread.
- Most paper plates, towels, napkins, and bags. For optimal safety, use white, unprinted materials.
- Wax paper, parchment paper, and heavy plastic wrap. Do not allow plastic wrap to touch food; vent it to allow a steam escape.
- Heat-susceptor packaging.

Not safe to use:
- Cold storage containers such as margarine tubs, and cottage cheese and yogurt cartons. These materials are not approved for cooking and chemicals can migrate into food.
- Brown paper bags and newspapers.
- Metal pans.
- Foam-insulated cups, bowls, plates, or trays.
- China with metallic paint or trim.
- Chinese take-out containers with metal handles.
- Metal twist ties on package wrapping.
- Food completely wrapped in aluminum foil.
- Food cooked in any container or packaging that has warped or melted during heating.

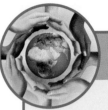

Global Connections

Mongolian Hot Pot

The Mongolian Hot Pot is also called the *Chinese Hot Pot*, *Chinese Fondue Pot*, or simply *Fire Pot*. Used by nomadic tribes of China in ancient times, this appliance is still used in Asian kitchens today. A large pot is filled with hot broth and placed in the middle of the table. The pot has a heat source to maintain the temperature. Platters of raw, thinly sliced meats, seafood, and vegetables are also served. Guests use long-handled forks to spear the pieces of food and place in the hot broth to cook. A variety of dipping sauces are often served so guests can flavor their meal to their own tastes.

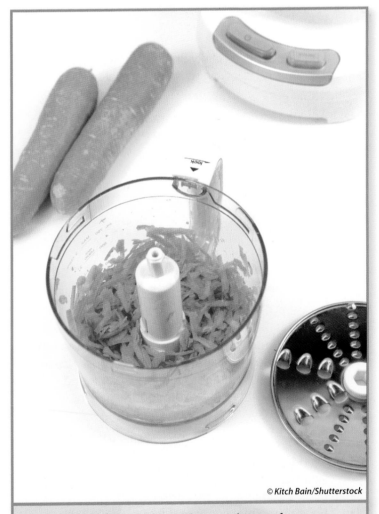

© Kitch Bain/Shutterstock

19-8 Food processors can be used to perform many food preparation jobs.

as mixers, toasters, and blenders, are called *portable appliances*. Portable means you can move them from one place to another with ease.

Small kitchen appliances make preparing food much easier. Many appliances can be used for several jobs. For instance, a food processor can be used to chop nuts, slice vegetables, and mix dough, **19-8**.

Some small appliances help save energy and cut down on fuel costs. For instance, it costs less to prepare toast in a toaster than in an oven.

Some small appliances may not save energy, but are easy to use. Electric can openers use more energy than hand-operated can openers, but the electric models are faster and require less effort to use. Unplugging small appliances when not in use saves energy. It is also an extra precaution against small kitchen fires.

Using appliances correctly helps them last longer and work better. Proper use also reduces the risk for accidents and safety problems. Appliances come with instruction booklets that describe how to operate and care for them properly. Some appliances should be wiped with a damp cloth or sponge after every use. The instructions tell you what pieces can and cannot be washed or placed in the dishwasher. Reading and following this information will keep your appliances in good working order.

Toasters

Toasters brown bread and bread products, such as waffles, bagels, and English muffins. Most toasters can hold two or four slices of bread at a time. You can adjust the toaster setting to the level of darkness you prefer. The bread automatically pops up when it is done. Do not stick a knife or fork into the toaster to dislodge stuck food—utensils made of metal can conduct electricity. Instead, unplug the toaster and use a wooden utensil to remove the food.

Toaster ovens can be used for baking and broiling foods as well as toasting. They use less energy than full-size ovens and can be a good choice when preparing small food items.

Electric Skillets

An electric skillet can perform many food preparation tasks. It can be used to stew meat and fry chicken. It can also be used for making soups and baking casseroles.

Electric skillets are convenient to use. They have *thermostats* that maintain the temperature at the desired setting. Most have coated cooking surfaces to keep foods from sticking. Many can be immersed in water for easy cleanup.

Blenders

Blenders are helpful when making milk shakes, dips, dressings, soups, and many other blended foods. Most blenders have a number of speeds to perform a range of blending tasks. They can shred, puree, and liquefy foods quickly, **19-9**.

Many blenders have measurements marked on the side of the blender container. This makes measuring ingredients easy. Blender containers may be made of glass or plastic and should have tight-fitting lids.

Electric Mixers

Electric mixers are handy kitchen appliances. They can be used for mixing doughs and batters. They can be used to beat eggs and whip cream. They can also be used for a number of other stirring, blending, and mixing jobs.

Electric mixers may be standard mixers or hand mixers. *Standard mixers* are larger, heavier appliances. They are attached to a stand that sits on the countertop. The stand holds a bowl. The bowl or the beaters turn when the mixer is running. This type of mixer may have attachments that allow it to knead dough, make juice, or do other tasks.

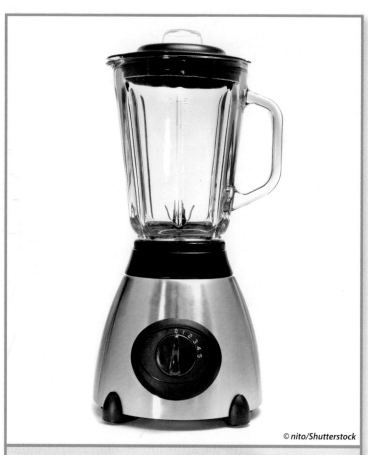

© nito/Shutterstock

19-9 Blenders have different speed settings for different tasks.

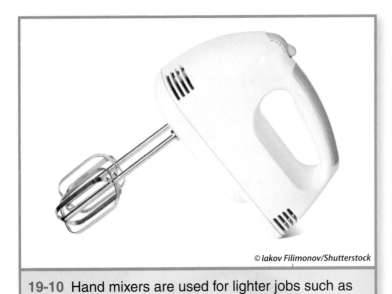

© Iakov Filimonov/Shutterstock

19-10 Hand mixers are used for lighter jobs such as mixing cake batter.

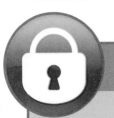

Safety Connections

Kitchen Fire Safety

Keep a fire extinguisher in the kitchen and know how to use it. Choose a multipurpose extinguisher that can be used on all types of fires.

To prevent burns and fires,

- turn pan handles toward the center of the range
- use potholders to handle hot utensils
- lift lids on pots and pans so that steam is directed away from you
- do not reach over open flames, hot range units, or steaming pans
- strike match before turning on gas to light a gas stove or oven
- never leave food on the range unattended
- ensure food is free from water droplets or ice crystals before putting in hot oil

A *hand mixer* is held in one hand while it is being used. This type of mixer is not as sturdy as a standard mixer, but is useful for many lightweight mixing jobs, **19-10**.

Large Appliances

Large kitchen appliances include ranges, microwave and convection ovens, and refrigerators. These are the main cooking and food storage appliances in the kitchen. Automatic dishwashers, food waste disposers, and trash compactors are also major appliances.

Most major appliances are sold in a number of styles. They are available with a variety of features. Appliances are also sold in a range of sizes. These options allow people to buy appliances that best meet their needs.

As with small appliances, you need to use and care for large appliances properly. This ensures your safety and keeps the appliances working right. The booklets that come with appliances are the best sources of use and care information.

Ranges

Kitchen ranges usually include one or more ovens, a cooktop with burners, and a broiler. Ranges can be freestanding or built-in to the cabinetry. Ranges are usually positioned under a hood that vents fumes and odors away from the kitchen. Ranges can either be gas or electric powered. The oven in a range can either be standard or convection.

Standard versus Convection Ovens

A standard, or conventional, oven is an insulated box with heated air. The hot air surrounds the food to cook it. A **convection oven** is a conventional oven with the addition of a fan that circulates the hot air, **19-11**. This forced air cooks food more quickly than the still air in a conventional oven. Convection cooking also saves energy because oven temperatures can be lowered.

Microwave Ovens

One of the most convenient kitchen appliances is the microwave oven. Microwave cooking is done with high-frequency waves called **microwaves**. Microwaves enter food and cause tiny particles in the food to vibrate. This movement causes friction that, in turn, creates heat to cook the food. This cooking action takes place in as little as one-fourth the time of conventional cooking.

In addition to saving time, microwave ovens save energy. The cooking time is shorter, which reduces the total energy needed to cook the food. In addition, since the oven does not heat up, the kitchen stays cooler.

Microwave ovens stay cool because the energy is absorbed only by the food. On the other hand, microwave ovens can heat liquids beyond their boiling points with no bubbles being produced. This is called **superheating**. Superheating is one reason microwaves account for more hospital visits due to scald burn injuries than any other kitchen appliance. Cookware may become hot from the heat of the food, so pot holders should be used to remove food from the microwave oven.

Microwave cooking helps preserve nutrients in some foods. Vegetables retain more vitamins and minerals when cooked in a microwave oven due to shorter cooking times. Microwave cooking uses less water, which means fewer nutrients are dissolved and lost in the cooking water.

Proper use of the microwave oven can make the difference between a successful food product and a failure. You should become aware of basic guidelines before working with a microwave oven. Each microwave oven model is a little different. Be sure to read the manufacturer's use and care booklet for special instructions about your model.

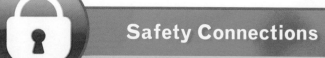

Safety Connections

Cooking Fires

When a cooking fire occurs,
- it is best to leave and close the door behind you to contain the fire
- call 911 or other local emergency number after you leave
- be sure others are notified and you have a clear path to exit before trying to fight the fire

If oil catches fire on your stove,
1. wearing an oven mitt, carefully slide a lid on top of the pan
2. turn off the burner
3. carefully slide pan off heat source
4. keep pan covered until cool to avoid fire restarting

If oil overflows the pan and is on fire, get everyone out of the house and call the fire department.

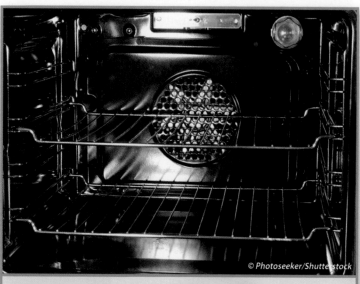

© Photoseeker/Shutterstock

19-11 The fan located at the back of the oven cavity circulates the hot air in convection ovens.

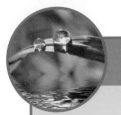

Refrigerator

Refrigerators are an important appliance in the kitchen because they keep foods cold. The cold temperature slows the growth of bacteria and preserves the safety of the food. Refrigerators usually have a freezer compartment to hold frozen foods. Options such as icemakers and water dispensers are available as well.

For a refrigerator to function well, it must be maintained. Refrigerators work by pulling heat out of the refrigerator compartment. This heat is expelled into the space around the appliance. If there is not sufficient space around the refrigerator, it causes extra strain on the appliance. The refrigerator coils need to be cleaned periodically. The door seal should also be washed with warm, soapy water a couple times per year.

Dishwasher

Automatic dishwashers are common in many kitchens today. They can be built-in or portable and come in different sizes. To avoid wasting water and electricity, only run dishwashers that are full. Wipe down the outside of your dishwasher as needed with warm, soapy water. Be sure to clear any clogged holes in the sprayer arms to ensure proper function. Dishwashers may not be recommended for cleaning some dishes and glassware—be sure to read the labels before purchasing.

Reading Review

1. Give examples of two ingredients that would be measured in dry measuring cups.
2. True or false. A chef's knife is the best choice for slicing bread.
3. List three jobs a food processor can perform.
4. True or false. A convection oven cooks foods more quickly than a conventional oven.
5. A microwave oven can heat liquid beyond its _____ point with no bubbles being produced.

Section 19-3

Getting Organized

Objectives

After studying this section, you will be able to
- **recognize** a work triangle in a kitchen layout.
- **explain** how to organize equipment and supplies in the kitchen to improve workflow.
- **use** a work plan to prepare a meal.

Key Terms		
work triangle	work plan	multitasking

Organization is key to being an efficient and effective cook. This is true whether you are cooking alone, with family at home, or with classmates in the school foods lab.

Kitchen Layout

Good kitchen layout enhances workflow during food preparation. Food preparation centers around three points in the kitchen—refrigerator, sink, and range. A well-designed kitchen includes a **work triangle** that allows for easy movement between these three points, **19-12**. A work triangle saves time and energy during food preparation. Cabinets and counters are located in and around the work triangle to provide storage and work space.

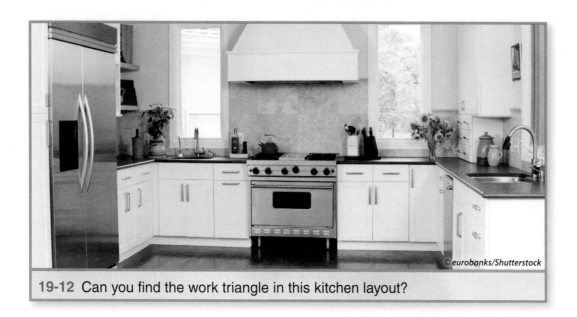

© eurobanks/Shutterstock

19-12 Can you find the work triangle in this kitchen layout?

Organize Equipment and Supplies

The size of a kitchen is not as important as how well the space is used. You may not be able to change a kitchen's layout, but you can control how effectively you use the existing space.

Equipment and supplies should be stored close to the work area in which they are used. For instance, pots and pans should be stored near the range. Food storage containers should be stored near the refrigerator. This eliminates extra steps and saves time and energy during food preparation.

Items you often use together should be stored in the same location. For instance, flour, sugar, salt, and baking soda are ingredients commonly used in baked products. Storing these items in the same location improves workflow during baking.

Equipment and supplies you use most often should be stored within easy reach. Items you use less often can be stored in less handy locations. You might store cooking spoons at the front of a drawer. A lemon juicer, on the other hand, could be stored at the back of a drawer. Store everyday dinnerware on an easy-to-reach shelf. Store a seldom-used serving platter on a high shelf or at the back of a low cabinet.

You can find many special racks and storage units designed to hold kitchen equipment and supplies. Spice racks, flatware trays, and wrap and bag holders are just a few examples. These items are not necessary, but make organizing your kitchen easier, **19-13**.

You can make your own racks and containers for storing kitchen equipment and supplies. For instance, you could hang pans and utensils from hooks on a piece of pegboard mounted on the wall.

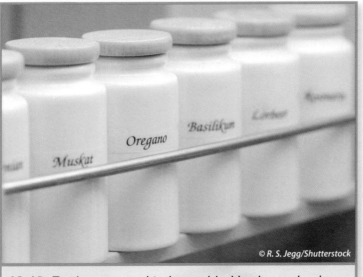

© R. S. Jegg/Shutterstock

19-13 Racks are used to keep dried herbs and spices organized.

Create a Work Plan

When preparing a meal, your goal is to have all the dishes ready at the desired serving time. You want hot foods to be hot and cold foods to be cold. To accomplish this goal, you need to organize your food preparation tasks. This takes careful planning and good management.

Before you begin working, create a work plan. A work plan is a list of meal preparation tasks, who is assigned to each task, the time each task should be performed, and the equipment and ingredients needed. Work plans are especially helpful in a foods lab when a number of people are working on the same meal. Work plans are also useful when cooking at home. It is best to create your work plan two or three days in advance of the meal preparation.

To create a work plan, you must start with a menu. The menu may be determined by your parents, your teacher, or you and your lab partners. Gather recipes for each dish on the menu. Read recipes to ensure you understand the techniques required for preparation. Estimate how much time it takes to prepare each recipe so you know when to start preparing each dish. On the work plan, note the time preparation for each dish. Plan to prepare foods that require the longest cooking time at the beginning of the meal preparation period. Be sure to include any preparation that

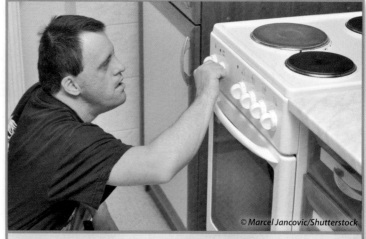

© Marcel Jancovic/Shutterstock

19-14 Be sure to include tasks such as preheating the oven in your work plan.

must be done in advance in your work plan. For instance, you may need to place frozen meat in the refrigerator to thaw the day before you are cooking. Include such tasks as preheating the oven or chopping vegetables in the work plan, **19-14**.

The menu is also used to make a list of all the tasks that need to be done. Next to each task on the work plan, assign an individual who is responsible. Some assignments may involve tasks other than food preparation such as setup and serving. Look for opportunities for multitasking. **Multitasking** means accomplishing more than one task at a time. For instance, the same person who prepared the casserole can make iced tea while the casserole is in the oven. Be sure to include cleanup tasks in the work plan. Maintaining a clean and orderly workstation is important during food preparation. Cleanup duties should be shared by the entire group.

The last step in the work plan is verifying that all the necessary ingredients and equipment are available. Use the recipes to make a list of ingredients and equipment needed. Check that each item is available and that equipment is in working order.

When working as a group in the foods lab, be sure that each person has an opportunity to perform the various tasks. To accomplish this, rotate people through different assignments for future meals. If a person is assigned to host and serve guests for this meal, make sure he or she is involved in food preparation for the next meal.

Reading Review

1. List the three points that create a work triangle in the kitchen.
2. True or false. Items that are often used together should be stored in the same location.
3. True or false. A work plan is only helpful when working in groups in the food lab.
4. How far in advance should you create your work plan?
5. To create a work plan, you must start with a(n) _____.

Chapter Summary

Section 19-1. Contaminants can cause foods to spoil or be unsafe. Foodborne illness results from eating unsafe foods. Proper sanitation and safe food handling can prevent most cross-contamination of foods. Time and temperature are key factors to be controlled for safe food handling.

Section 19-2. Cooks must be able to identify and select the proper kitchen equipment for the job. Kitchen utensils, cookware, and appliances must be cleaned and maintained to prevent cross-contamination. Reading care and user's manuals that come with equipment is necessary for safety in the kitchen.

Section 19-3. Cooking a meal requires organization. A good kitchen layout saves time and energy during food preparation. Equipment and supplies should be stored in the area of the kitchen where they are used most often. Creating and using a work plan to prepare meals is useful at home and in the foods lab.

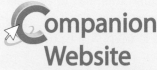

Companion Website
www.g-wlearning.com

Check your understanding of the main concepts for Chapter 19 at the website.

Critical Thinking

1. **Determine.** What can you do to improve food safety in your home?
2. **Plan.** Develop a schedule for cleaning and maintaining various appliances in your home kitchen.
3. **Critique.** Review the organization of equipment and supplies in your kitchen at home. Write suggestions for reorganization to improve the workflow in the kitchen.

Common Core

College and Career Readiness

4. **Speaking.** Find a reported instance of foodborne illness in the news or online. Present a brief summary of the incident including the cause, possible prevention, and results of the outbreak.
5. **Science.** Some scientists are linking foodborne illness to incidence of chronic disease and permanent damage to the body. Research to learn what scientists believe happens in the body to cause these results.
6. **Reading.** Locate and read a user's manual for a kitchen appliance at home or online. Form an opinion on the readability of the manual and share with the class.
7. **Listening.** Interview a chef or caterer to learn how he or she plans for a meal or event.

Technology

8.   **Investigate technologies.** Research new technologies related to food safety. Select one that interests you and share your findings with the class.

Journal Writing

9.   Write a journal entry about a meal you prepared that did not turn out as well as you hoped. Critique your meal planning and preparation noting what you learned from this experience. Include changes you would make to improve the outcome of your next meal preparation. Be sure to include aspects of your planning and preparation that went well.

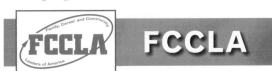 **FCCLA**

10.   Create an *FCCLA Community Service* project that educates older adults on the potential for foodborne illness. Explore various ways people can get foodborne illnesses and create a one-page information sheet that includes visuals and emergency numbers. Partner with a local organization that serves older adults to distribute the information. See your adviser for information as needed.

11.   Use the FCCLA Planning Process to organize a kitchen rummage sale. Collect small appliances (in good working condition) and equipment from peers, teachers, parents, and local organizations. Then host a kitchen equipment and appliance rummage sale as an *FCCLA Community Service* project. Consider donating the money to a local food pantry so they can update their equipment and utensils. See your adviser for information as needed.

12.   Research potential careers in the culinary industry. Consider work environment, skills needed and job outlook as you develop your *Leaders at Work* project. Share your findings in an illustrated report. See your adviser for information as needed.

Chapter 20
Preparing Foods

Sections

College and Career Readiness

Reading Prep

Before reading, skim the chapter and examine how it is organized. Look at the bold or italic words, headings of different colors and sizes, bulleted lists or numbered lists, tables, captions, and boxed features.

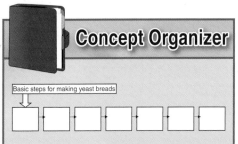

Concept Organizer

Basic steps for making yeast breads

Use a diagram like the one shown to list the basic steps of making yeast breads in correct order.

Companion Website

Print out the concept organizer for Chapter 20 at the website.

Companion Website
www.g-wlearning.com

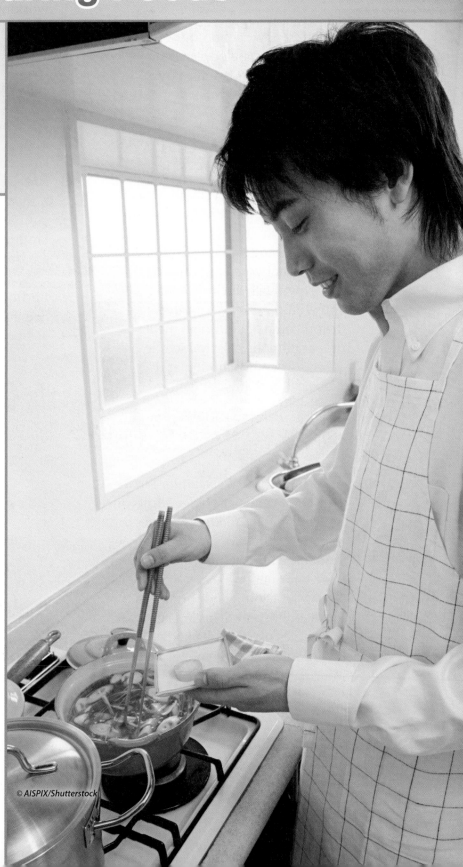

© AISPIX/Shutterstock

Section 20-1

Fruits and Vegetables

Objectives

After studying this section, you will be able to

- **differentiate** between how to prepare raw fruits and vegetables.
- **describe** how to cook different fruits and vegetables.

Key Terms

ascorbic acid	vegetable brush	rehydrated
translucent	stir-frying	

Fruits and vegetables taste good on their own, so they take minimal preparation for eating. They may be raw or cooked, served plain, or mixed with other foods, sauces, or seasonings. With some basic food preparation knowledge, you will be able to make many types of fruit and vegetable dishes.

Preparing Fruits

Many people enjoy simply washing and eating raw fruits. You can also combine a raw fruit with other foods. Fresh fruit served with dip, strawberry shortcake, and gelatin fruit salads are examples. Fruits can be sliced and arranged to garnish meals or desserts. Serve the fruit after preparing it as soon as possible.

Raw Fruits

Always wash fresh fruits under running water before eating or serving to remove pesticides and dirt. Some fruits, such as apples, peaches, and bananas turn brown after slicing. To prevent this problem, dip the cut fruit in lemon, orange, grapefruit, or pineapple juice. The **ascorbic acid** in citrus fruits prevents cut slices from browning.

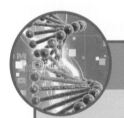

Science Connections

Genetically Modified Crops

The term *genetically modified* simply means that some DNA of a fruit or vegetable crop has been changed to improve its production. It is also called *food biotechnology*. Genetic modification occurs naturally in plants and animals, but scientists have discovered quicker, more precise methods to bring about desired changes. For instance, some vegetables, such as corn and tomatoes, have been modified (or engineered) to produce larger, insect-resistant produce. Growing enough fruits, vegetables, and other crops to feed the world's growing population has made biotechnology a necessary field. Today, crops can grow faster, need less water, and feed more people. Unless labeled organic, the produce in stores today has probably undergone some type of genetic modification during the last 100 years. For instance, carrots and celery look entirely different and taste better today than they did a century earlier. The FDA regulates all foods for consumer safety including those genetically modified.

Most uncooked fruit dishes are easy to prepare and allow the fruits' natural flavors to come through. Examples of basic fruit snack combinations are in **20-1**. Mix or layer the ingredients and then serve.

Raw fruits also come in frozen, canned, and dried varieties. Allow frozen fruits to thaw slightly when you serve them. Fully thawed fruit is mushy compared to fresh fruit. Leaving some ice crystals makes the fruit seem crisper. Canned fruit can be eaten straight from the can. You may want to chill or drain it for some uses. You can eat dried fruits directly from the bag or box. Some side dishes and desserts also list them as ingredients.

When preparing fruit salads with gelatin, let the gelatin become slightly firm before adding fruit. If the gelatin is not firm, the fruit will float to the top. Also, do not add fresh pineapple to gelatin. Fresh pineapple contains a substance that prevents gelatin from becoming firm. This is not a problem with canned pineapple.

Cooking Fruits

Cooking changes the flavors and textures of fruits. You may simmer, stew, bake, broil, or microwave most fruit. Cooked fruits are popular for desserts, breakfast, or side dishes. Some fruits, such as apples and pears, taste good baked on their own, **20-2**. Simply add a little butter, sugar, and spices for flavor. Small pieces of fresh, canned, or dried fruit can be stirred into most cake or muffin batters. They add flavor and moisture.

When simmering or stewing fresh fruits, use a small amount of water to keep the best flavors. Add some sugar to help the fruit hold its shape and add flavor. Keep the amount of sugar to a minimum, though, because too much sugar makes cooked fruit tough. Cook fruit on low heat until tender and translucent. **Translucent** means clear enough to allow light to pass through, but not transparent.

Broiling fresh fruits, such as orange or grapefruit halves, bananas, and pineapple slices make tasty breakfast or snack foods. Sprinkle with a little brown sugar or honey before broiling. Fruits broil within a few minutes, so watch them closely.

Fruit Snack Combinations		
Fruits	**Spreads**	**Toppings**
apples	peanut butter	chopped nuts
pears	marshmallow cream	coconut
bananas	cream cheese	cinnamon sugar
peaches	cheese spreads	raisins
	dessert sauces	shredded carrots
		granola

20-1 You can create a variety of tasty and nutritious fruit snacks by combining different fruits, spreads, and toppings.

You can also cook fruit in the microwave—with little to no water. When cooking several pieces of fruit, the sizes should be similar. This allows more even cooking. If leaving the skin on a fruit, pierce it with a fork several times to allow steam to escape.

When cooking frozen fruits, do not thaw them before cooking. They will keep their shape better if they are still frozen when cooked. Canned fruits can be heated in their juice. Drain canned fruit before using in baked products. Dried fruits are usually soaked in hot water for an hour before simmering. Add dried fruits to baked products, however, without soaking.

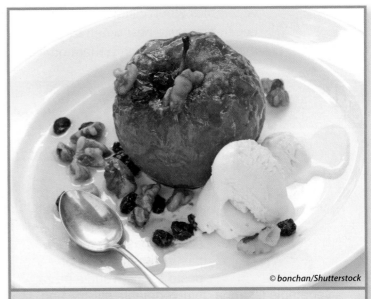
© bonchan/Shutterstock

20-2 This apple baked with cinnamon sugar, nuts, and raisins makes a delicious dessert when paired with ice cream.

Preparing Vegetables

Vegetables' bright colors add to the appeal of a meal or snack. Enjoy raw vegetables as snacks and in salads. Cooked vegetables can be the main course or side dishes, as in casseroles, and used in soups.

Raw Vegetables

Raw vegetables are crisp and refreshing. Celery, lettuce, cucumbers, radishes, peppers, tomatoes, and carrots are vegetables many people prefer to eat raw. People may enjoy other raw vegetables, such as cauliflower, pea pods, broccoli, and mushrooms.

Some salad vegetables, such as carrots and cabbage, may also be shredded. Salads may be served with cold or hot dressings. Most people enjoy savory dips with raw vegetables, **20-3**. Many raw vegetables also taste good with peanut butter, cream cheese, or cheese spreads.

Raw vegetables tend to have more dirt on them than fruits. Wash them carefully in cool running water. You may need to use a **vegetable brush** with stiff bristles to remove some dirt. Do not soak

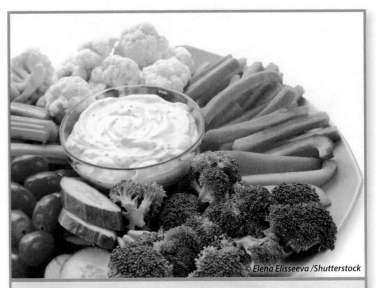
© Elena Elisseeva /Shutterstock

20-3 Cut vegetables into sticks, slices, or wedges and arrange on trays for snacks or appetizers.

vegetables when cleaning or storing them because it causes nutrient loss. Raw vegetables taste best when they are cold. Serve raw vegetables straight from the refrigerator or keep them on ice to preserve freshness and taste.

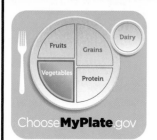

MyPlate Tip

Healthy Eating for Vegetarians

Make simple changes. Many popular main dishes are or can be vegetarian—such as pasta primavera, pasta with marinara or pesto sauce, veggie pizza, vegetable lasagna, tofu-vegetable stir-fry, and bean burritos.

Source: MyPlate 10 tips Nutrition Education Series

Cooking Fresh Vegetables

The cooking process changes the texture of vegetables. They become soft and easier to eat. The flavors and colors of vegetables change through cooking, too. For the most flavor, cook vegetables until they are tender, but slightly crisp. Always cut fresh vegetables into similar sizes so they cook evenly.

Fresh vegetables are most often simmered, steamed, stir-fried, roasted, or microwaved. The way you simmer vegetables depends on the type of vegetable. Cook mild-flavored vegetables, such as corn and green beans, in a small amount of water for a short time. Cover the pan during cooking.

In contrast, make sure stronger-flavored vegetables, such as cauliflower and cabbage, are totally covered by water during simmering. To release the strongest flavors, cook them in an uncovered pan for a short time.

Steam fresh vegetables by placing them in a steaming basket over simmering water in a tightly covered pan. This method works best with tender vegetables, such as broccoli spears and sliced green beans. Vegetables cooked this way retain more nutrients than simmered vegetables.

Stir-frying means to fry quickly over high heat in a lightly oiled pan while stirring continuously. Stir-fried vegetables retain their flavor, texture, color, and nutrients making it a healthful cooking option. An oriental cooking pan called a *wok* is ideal for stir-frying, **20-4**.

Roasted vegetables add wonderful flavors to meals without a lot of fat and calories. Any vegetable can be roasted in an oven or on a grill. Simply mix the cut vegetables with a small amount of olive oil and seasonings, and then bake or grill. The length of roasting time depends on the vegetable's denseness. For instance, potatoes, broccoli, cauliflower, and carrots take longer to cook than garlic, squash, or tomatoes.

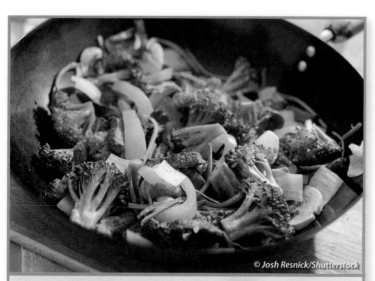

© Josh Resnick/Shutterstock

20-4 A wok is perfect for stir-frying because it is a deeper skillet with high, curved sides to prevent the ingredients from falling out of the pan.

Microwave ovens are also good for cooking fresh vegetables. This method keeps most of the vegetables' natural colors, flavors, and nutrients. Cook vegetables until they are still a little firm in a covered, microwave-safe dish with very little water. Stir a few times during cooking to assure even heating. Let the vegetables stand for a few minutes after the allotted time in the microwave. They will continue to cook during this time.

Cooking potatoes is little different from other vegetables. They are often boiled, mashed, baked, or fried. Different types of potatoes work best for certain cooking methods. Choose a type recommended for the cooking method you will use. Cook potatoes until you can easily push a fork into the center of them. Fried potatoes should be browned on the outside and fluffy on the inside.

Cooking Other Vegetables

Vegetables also come frozen, dried, and canned. Methods for preparing frozen vegetables are similar to preparing fresh ones. Cooking times are usually a little shorter, though. Always cook frozen vegetables in their frozen states without thawing.

Dried vegetables must be **rehydrated**, or restored to their natural state by adding water, before cooking. Soak dried peas and beans in cold water overnight before cooking. Another time-saving option is to boil them in hot water for about an hour. Even when rehydrated, cook dried beans and peas longer than most other vegetables. They turn out best if simmered or baked in liquid until fork tender.

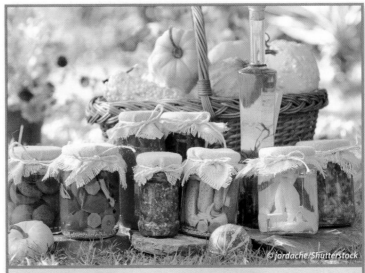

Canned vegetables are already cooked, so they only need a thorough heating. Canned vegetables are not as crisp as fresh or frozen ones, and they become mushy if overcooked. Home-canned vegetables are an exception to these guidelines, however, **20-5**. Boil vegetables canned at home for 10 to 20 minutes before eating to protect against food poisoning.

©jordache/Shutterstock

20-5 Home-canned products can be a tasty treat.

Reading Review

1. How can you prevent fruits such as apples, peaches, and bananas from turning brown when they are cut?
2. How do you help simmered fruit hold its shape?
3. Why should you avoid soaking vegetables when cleaning or storing them?
4. True or false. Strong-flavored vegetables should be cooked in a small amount of water with the pan covered.

Grain Products

Objectives

After studying this section, you will be able to
- **describe** techniques for cooking starchy grain products for optimal quality.
- **explain** basic steps in preparing quick breads and yeast breads.

<table>
<tr><th colspan="3">Key Terms</th></tr>
<tr><td>starch</td><td>carbon dioxide</td><td>dough</td></tr>
<tr><td>gelatinization</td><td>leavening agent</td><td>knead</td></tr>
<tr><td>al dente</td><td>batter</td><td>yeast</td></tr>
</table>

Grain products are a part of nearly every meal, and most are cooked in some way before they are eaten. Cooking directions are on product boxes and in recipes. If you follow the directions, you should get a good finished product. Keeping some tips in mind can help make cooking grain products easier for you.

Cooking Starchy Grains

Starch is the complex carbohydrate portion of grain plants, such as wheat, corn, barley, oats, or rice. In fact, refined grains like flours are mostly starch. The basic concepts of *starch cookery* are the same for cooking almost any grain product. Starch will not dissolve in cold water. Starch granules swell, however, when they are heated with liquid. The grain's starches absorb very hot liquid, making the product soft and thick in a process called **gelatinization**. It is an important aspect of cooking grain products.

The swelling of starch granules in gelatinization during cooking causes grain products to increase greatly in volume. Different products increase by different amounts. Figure **20-6** shows the volume increases of some common grain products. Keep this increased volume in mind when deciding how much of a grain product to prepare.

Volume Increases of Cooked Grain Products	
1 Cup Uncooked	**Cooked Equivalent**
Pasta	2 cups
White rice	3 cups
Oatmeal (old fashioned)	3 cups
Brown rice	4 cups
Farina	5 cups
Hominy grits	6 cups

20-6 Grain products increase in volume during the cooking process.

Temperature is also important when cooking starchy grain products. Starch granules need heat to swell properly, but too much heat causes them to lump together. When cooking, stir gently to prevent lumps. If you stir the product too quickly or too often during cooking, however, the starch granules break down. When this happens, the cooked product may not thicken properly.

Using Thickeners

Refined grain products, such as flours and cornstarch, are used as *thickeners* in cooking. Use them when making gravies, sauces, puddings, pie fillings, or other cooked foods that need to thicken. Extra steps are necessary, however, to prevent lumping when using thickeners. Use any of the following techniques to keep starch granules separated:

- Coat the starch with fat before adding liquid.
- Combine the starch with sugar.
- Mix the starch with a small amount of liquid to form a paste.

Once the granules are separated, you can heat them with liquid to form a smooth, creamy finished product. Most recipes indicate which method is best to prevent lumps for that dish.

Cooking Pasta

Pasta is often served as a side dish or as a main course with meat, vegetables, or a sauce. Spaghetti with meatballs and macaroni with cheese are two examples. You can also use pasta in cold salads, **20-7**.

Because pasta increases in volume when it cooks, you need to boil it in a lot of water. Use about eight cups of water for each eight ounces of pasta to cook. A deep pot prevents water from boiling over when cooking pasta. Make sure the water is boiling rapidly *before* adding the pasta. This keeps pasta from sticking together during cooking. Add the pasta slowly so the water keeps boiling. Adding too much pasta at once lowers the water temperature. Stir gently several times during cooking. You can also add a little olive oil to the water to prevent the pasta from sticking together. Remember, though, that oil prevents sauce from coating the cooked pasta.

Pasta should be cooked al dente. **Al dente** (al den' tay) means there is a slight resistance in the center when the pasta is chewed. Overcooked pasta is mushy. Test the pasta before draining it in a colander. Do not rinse cooked pasta because it washes nutrients away.

Cooking Rice

Rice is popular as a side dish or as part of a meat dish. Sauces and seasonings add flavor and variety. Rice may also be used in cold salads with fruit or vegetables added.

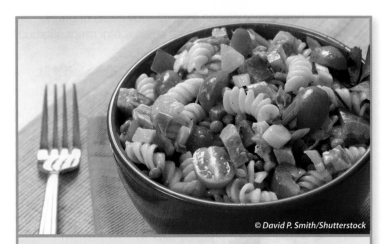

© David P. Smith/Shutterstock

20-7 Toss pasta with vegetables, meats, cheeses, nuts, and dressings for a hearty side dish, lunch, or dinner choice.

Section 20-3

Dairy

Objectives

After studying this section, you will be able to
- **explain** the guidelines for cooking with milk and cheese.
- **give tips** for preparing foods made with dairy products.

Key Terms	
curdle	scalding

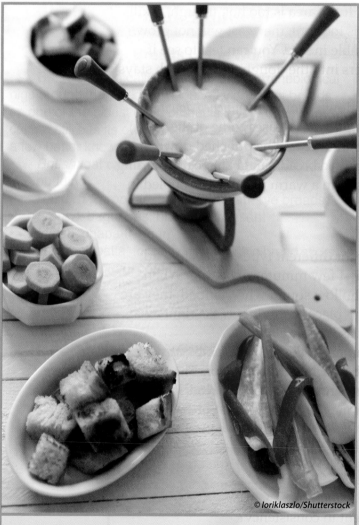

20-11 Cheese fondue is a delicious appetizer or dinner treat that is typical of dairy cooking. If overcooked, it will be rubbery and lose flavor.

© loriklaszlo/Shutterstock

Milk and other dairy products are essential cooking ingredients. They add a creamy, rich flavor to sauces, soups, casseroles, and other foods. You may find many recipes that call for dairy products.

Tips for Cooking with Dairy Products

A few guidelines will help you as you prepare these foods. The milk proteins in dairy products tend to scorch, or burn, when milk gets too hot. The scorching causes a bitter, off taste. To prevent problems, cook dairy products slowly at lower temperatures, **20-11**. Using a double boiler is also helpful.

Cooking with Milk

When milk is not cooked properly, it can **curdle**, or form lumps of milk proteins. Cooking milk at too high a temperature causes curdling. Certain ingredients that are high in acids, enzymes, salts, and other substances can also cause curdling.

These include fruits and vegetables, especially tomatoes, brown sugar, and salt-cured meats. Prevent curdling by using fresh milk and low temperatures. Thickening the milk before adding ingredients also helps.

Some recipes call for scalded milk. **Scalding** means heating to just below the boiling point. To scald milk, heat it slowly at a medium-low temperature until bubbles form around the edge. A thin film will form on the top of the milk. Remove this film because it will not dissolve if stirred into the milk. Although these milk particles from the film are not harmful, they may affect the texture of your finished product.

Cooking with Cheese

When cooking with cheese, the most important thing to remember is that overcooking makes cheese tough. The type of cheese determines the cooking method as well. For instance, cooking cream cheese is much different from cheddar or parmesan. Follow your recipe's instructions closely. A few tips can help you avoid overcooking.

When melting cheese or using it in recipes, grate or cut it into small pieces so it will melt faster. If you sprinkle cheese on a casserole, you may want to put it on the casserole at the end of the cooking cycle. Also, wait until the last few minutes of cooking time to add cheese to sauces and soups.

Cheese melts well in the microwave. Heating cheese at high power settings, however, can cause it to become rubbery. A medium to medium-high power setting melts cheese without it becoming tough.

Preparing Other Dairy Products

Butter, margarine, cream, and yogurt are common cooking and baking ingredients. Butter contains some milk proteins, so it may burn or scorch if cooked too long or at too high a temperature. Be sure to watch butter carefully and use low temperatures when melting it. Using the microwave to melt butter avoids problems with scorching. Margarine does not contain milk proteins, so it is not as likely to scorch. You may use stick margarine like butter for baking, but do not use spread margarine. The higher water content in spreads does not substitute well for butter in baked goods.

Many recipes call for cream to be whipped, **20-12**. Whipping cream adds air so that it becomes thick and fluffy. Whip cream to the thickness called for in the recipe. Cream is at its thickest when *firm peaks* form as you take out the beaters. Do not beat cream beyond this point. The cream will start to separate into solid and liquid forms.

Yogurt is used cold to make dressings, dips, and drinks. Yogurt is sometimes a healthful substitute

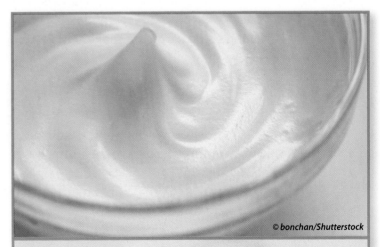

© bonchan/Shutterstock

20-12 For the best results, chill the cream, bowl, and beaters before whipping.

Science Connections

Components of an Experiment with Dairy

Say you need to choose which type of milk to use in a frozen dairy recipe you are making. Your choices are fat free, whole, or light cream. Does the percentage of fat in milk affect the time it takes to freeze? You suspect that cream takes the longest to freeze, but you can easily experiment to learn the answer.

All scientific experiments have the same components: the *question*, *purpose*, your *hypothesis*, *materials* needed, and the *procedure*. The experiment then yields a *result* that either confirms or disproves your original hypothesis. Determine the experiment components of the situation just described.

for sour cream in some recipes. Because yogurt is high in milk proteins, cook it carefully. Use low temperatures and cook just until the yogurt is heated through.

Preparing Desserts

Puddings, custards, ice creams, and other frozen desserts are popular items prepared with dairy products. Puddings and custards are also ingredients in some pies, cakes, and bakery desserts. They are made by cooking milk, flavorings, and a thickener, such as cornstarch. When making puddings and custards, keep in mind the principles of both starch and dairy cookery. Moderate temperatures, gentle stirring, and separating starch granules will help your pudding products turn out smooth and creamy.

Many recipes for ice cream and other frozen desserts are available. You can prepare them using an ice cream maker or the freezer compartment of your refrigerator. The ice cream mixture must be cooked according to directions before it is frozen.

Temperature is an important factor in preparing frozen desserts. To freeze properly, the freezer must be colder than 32°F (0°C). This is not a problem if you use an electric ice cream maker. You must use a mixture of salt and ice to get a nonelectric ice cream maker cold enough though. Be sure to check the manufacturer's directions for the correct proportions of salt and ice.

Stirring is also important when preparing frozen desserts. Stirring prevents large ice crystals from forming in the desserts. Large ice crystals give frozen products a grainy texture, whereas small ice crystals make them smooth and creamy. Electric ice cream makers stir the mixture automatically as it is freezing. Nonelectric ice cream makers have a hand crank to stir the mixture manually.

Reading Review

1. How do you prevent milk from curdling?
2. In the microwave, heating cheese at high power settings can cause it to become _____.
3. True or false. Whip cream until it becomes firm peaks when the beaters are lifted.
4. For frozen desserts to freeze properly, the freezer must be colder than _____.
5. Why is stirring important when preparing frozen dairy desserts?

Proteins

Objectives

After studying this section, you will be able to
- **describe** ways to tenderize meat.
- **select** the appropriate cooking methods for preparing various protein foods.

Preparing protein foods does not have to be difficult. In fact, some of the simplest cooking methods yield very tasty results.

Cooking Protein Foods

When you prepare a protein food, choose a cooking method that best brings out its flavor and tenderness. Dry-heat and moist-heat methods cook most protein foods well. Remember to allow frozen protein foods to defrost in the refrigerator to prevent foodborne illness. Raw eggs are also a health risk.

Cooking Meat

Meats are often seasoned before cooking to make them more flavorful. Depending on the cut of meat, you may choose a dry- or moist-heat cooking method. For instance, dry-heat methods work best on larger, tender cuts of meat, **20-13**. You can broil any meat as long as it is 1-inch thick or less.

Less tender cuts of meat turn out better using moist-heat cooking methods. You can also **tenderize** less tender meats before cooking by pounding them or adding powdered tenderizers. Marinating meats can make them more tender and tasty, as well. Marinades usually contain vinegar and/or citrus juice, oil, and seasonings. Meats usually remain in marinades from two hours to overnight before cooking.

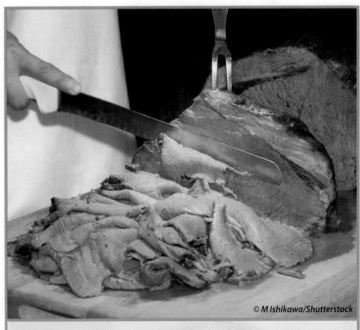

© M Ishikawa/Shutterstock

20-13 Large, tender cuts of beef are roasted and often served at large events at carving stations.

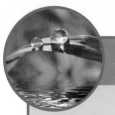

Go Green

One-Pot Cooking

A one-pot meal is exactly what it sounds like—a meal containing a grain, protein, and vegetable made using just one pot. One-pot cooking is both healthful and delicious. It saves the time and energy used for both cooking and the cleanup. Use a Dutch oven, wok, or large skillet on the range. Rice is often a staple that is on hand. Pair it with any vegetables and protein sources you have in the refrigerator and add your favorite spices or sauce. Then enjoy your wonderful, environmentally friendly meal.

You can cook beef and lamb to different levels of doneness depending on your tastes without fear of food poisoning. *Rare meat* is brown on the outside, but pinkish-red and juicy on the inside. *Medium meat* is brown on the outside and pink toward the center. *Well-done meat* has no pink color in it at all.

Cook pork and veal until they are well done to prevent food poisoning. Fresh pork, veal, and cured hams (not precooked) should reach an internal temperature of 160°F (71°C). You can test the internal temperature of any meat with a meat thermometer. Place the thermometer in the thickest part of the muscle without touching bone or fat. To read the internal temperature correctly, leave it in until the temperature indicator stops moving. Be careful not to overcook meat. When you cook it longer than necessary for the level of doneness, meat becomes tough and dry.

Cooking Poultry

Most poultry is young and tender, so dry-heat methods cook poultry the best. Use moist-heat methods for older turkeys and chickens that are less tender.

Use a meat thermometer to judge doneness. Place it in the thickest part of the breast or the center of the thigh not touching the bone, **20-14**. If cooking a whole bird, you can also test for doneness by twisting the drumstick. If it separates easily from the joint, the meat is done. Breast meat is done when you can easily pierce it with a fork and see clear juices.

As with meat, do not overcook poultry. Some types of poultry, such as large turkeys, will still be pink near the bone even when the meat has reached the proper temperature. A chemical reaction causes this pink color. The pink color is harmless, and more cooking will not make it go away.

©Jeff Cleveland/Shutterstock

20-14 Cook poultry to an internal temperature of 165°F (74°C) on a meat thermometer.

Cooking Fish

Whether fatty or lean, all fish is naturally tender. You may use dry- or moist-heat cooking methods. Fish with a higher-fat content, such as salmon, tuna, herring, and trout turn out especially good when grilled. Lean fish, however, such as halibut, cod, and other white fish, tend to fall apart when grilling. In contrast, fatty fish falls apart more easily when poached or steamed.

Fish is done when the flesh is firm and flakes easily with a fork. Fish cooks very quickly, faster than meat or poultry. You must watch it carefully to make sure it is not undercooked or overcooked. Undercooked fish has an unpleasant taste and rubbery texture. It may also cause food poisoning. Overcooked fish becomes tough and dry.

Shellfish are any fish that live inside shells. They include lobster, crab, shrimp, clams, and scallops. You may choose to partially cook live lobster and crab and fresh shrimp in boiling, salted water. Then cooking can be finished with another method. Most shellfish are usually broiled or baked.

MyPlate Tip

With Protein Foods, Variety Is Key

Choose seafood twice a week. Eat seafood in place of meat or poultry twice a week. Select a variety of seafood—include some that are higher in oils and low in mercury, such as salmon, trout, and herring.

Source: MyPlate 10 tips Nutrition Education Series

Cooking Eggs

Never eat raw eggs, including raw-egg drinks and uncooked batter or dough made with eggs. If you only need to use an egg's yolk or the white, do not use the shell to separate them. Using the shell as a separator risks bacteria from the shell's exterior contaminating the egg. Use an egg separator, a kitchen tool that allows the white to slide away as the yolk remains in the cup.

Cooking methods for preparing eggs are different from other protein foods. Eggs cook faster than other protein foods because they have a high liquid content. They become tough and rubbery when overcooked. Frying, poaching, and cooking in the shell are common ways of preparing eggs. Eggs are also used to make meringues, custards, and soufflés.

Frying

Fry eggs by melting a little fat in a skillet and adding the eggs. The skillet should be hot when adding the eggs or the whites will spread too thin. Eggs are done when the whites are firm and not runny. Some people prefer to have the yolks cooked, too. Covering the skillet for most of the cooking time helps eggs cook evenly.

Scrambled eggs and omelets are also fried. Before frying, add liquid and seasonings to the beaten eggs. About one tablespoon of liquid per egg is appropriate. Too much liquid can make the eggs runny. Stir scrambled eggs gently while cooking. For an omelet, allow the eggs to set on the bottom and add other ingredients, such as cheese or ham. Then gently lift and fold the omelet to allow the uncooked egg to reach the bottom of the

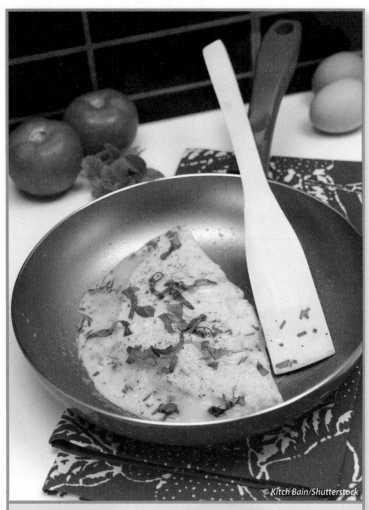

20-15 Get creative with your omelet fillings and serve it for breakfast, lunch, or dinner.

© Kitch Bain/Shutterstock

skillet, **20-15**. Omelets usually take longer to cook thoroughly than scrambled eggs, which may also be cooked in the microwave.

Poaching

Poaching is a fat-free option for cooking eggs. Break the eggs into hot water that has not yet boiled and let simmer for several minutes. You can add a little vinegar in the water to help the eggs keep their shape. Eggs are done when the whites are firm and yolks are semiliquid.

An **egg poacher** is a useful kitchen tool for preventing poached eggs from separating. It contains one to six cups for holding the eggs. Place the poacher over boiling water in a covered pan and the steam then poaches the eggs.

Cooking in the Shell

Eggs may be hard-cooked or soft-cooked in the shell. **Soft-cooked eggs** have a firm white, but the yolk is runny. In **hard-cooked eggs**, the white and yolk are firm because they cook for a longer time.

Cooking eggs in their shells involves cooking them in water. The guideline is to use about one pint (two cups) of water per egg. You can start with either cold or simmering water.

When starting with cold water, cover the eggs with the water in the pan. Bring the water to a boil, cover the pan, and remove it from the heat. For soft-cooked eggs, leave the eggs in the water for one to four minutes. For hard-cooked eggs, leave them in the water for 15 to 17 minutes depending on the size.

When starting with simmering water, add the eggs when the water starts to simmer. Do not let the water boil as the eggs are cooking. Simmer soft-cooked eggs for one to four minutes. Simmer hard-cooked eggs for 13 to 15 minutes.

Cool hard-cooked eggs immediately after cooking. Place them under cold running water to cool. Otherwise, the eggs will continue to cook and become overcooked. A greenish ring will form around the yolk of an overcooked egg in the shell. Although the green ring is not appealing, it is harmless.

Life Connections

Cooking with Convenience Foods

A number of food products are designed to save you time in the kitchen. These products are called *convenience foods* because a portion of the preparation is already done for you. Some convenience foods, such as frozen dinners or canned meat sauce, may require only heating. Others, like a casserole mix, need more ingredients and some additional preparation. All you may need to do is add a cooked protein and liquid, then mix and bake. Preparing convenience foods takes much less time than making dishes from scratch and using fresh ingredients.

Convenience products have some disadvantages though. They often cost more than foods made from scratch. Some may not taste as good as homemade foods. Despite these disadvantages, many cooks are willing to pay more and sacrifice some flavor for the time they save.

Planning Activity

Convenience products are so common that it may seem hard to plan meals without them. When shopping, look at the cost of convenience foods compared to the cost of making the same product at home. Find out how many servings a convenience product yields. Look at the nutrition label. Read the directions to see if you need to add other ingredients. Think about how it will taste. Consider the time savings. Then use this information to help you decide which convenience foods you will use when preparing an evening meal.

Reading Review

1. List three ways to tenderize meat.
2. Which cooking method is best for tender poultry?
3. True or false. Fish cooks faster than poultry.
4. What happens when hard-cooked eggs are not cooled immediately after cooking?

Chapter Summary

Section 20-1. Fruits and vegetables can be eaten raw or cooked. Raw produce is popular for salads and snacks. Cooked fruits are often served as desserts, and cooked vegetables are commonly served as side dishes. Cooked fruits and vegetables may be prepared many ways including simmering, stewing, baking, broiling, or microwaving.

Section 20-2. Grain products contain starch, which greatly affects the cooking processes of the different products. When heated, starch granules absorb water, causing them to soften and expand. Starch granules need to be separated before heating with liquid to avoid lumps. Bread is one of the chief grain products. The two types of breads are yeast and quick breads. Air, steam, or leavening agents cause all breads to rise and become light and porous. Quick breads, such as pancakes, waffles, muffins, and biscuits rise quickly during baking. Yeast breads must have a longer time to rise before baking.

Section 20-3. Following some basic principles helps achieve good results when cooking with dairy products. Cook milk products slowly on low temperatures to avoid scorching and curdling. Avoid overcooking cheese to prevent it from becoming tough and rubbery. Frozen desserts must reach the proper temperature and be mixed well to obtain smooth, high-quality products.

Section 20-4. Dry-heat cooking methods work best when preparing tender protein foods. Moist-heat cooking methods are better for preparing less tender protein foods. Fish is done when the flesh is firm and flakes easily with a fork. Fish cooks very quickly, faster than meat or poultry. You cook eggs by frying, poaching, or cooking them in the shell.

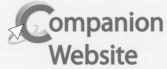

Companion Website
www.g-wlearning.com

Check your understanding of the main concepts for Chapter 20 at the website.

Critical Thinking

1. **Analyze.** Do you think pesticides should be used on fruits and vegetables when they also leak into and contaminate drinking water? Give reasons to support your opinion.
2. **Determine.** Why is the price of processed cereals high when the producer (farmer) receives only a small percentage of the profit?
3. **Cause and effect.** Many people are vegetarians. This means they do not eat any meat products. What are some reasons people choose to be vegetarians?

Common Core

4. **Math.** Visit a grocery store and make a list of the available canned fruits and vegetables. Compare those prices with that of the same fruits and vegetables in fresh and frozen forms. What are the reasons for the differences?

5. **Speaking.** Describe your favorite grain product to the class. Explain why it is your favorite and which nutrients it contains.

6. **Writing.** Find three different recipes for preparing dairy products; one should be a frozen dessert. Copy them and bring to class to compile into a student cookbook—along with the tips for preparing dairy foods to achieve best results.

Technology

7. **Electronic research.** Conduct research on the computer to learn all the ways you can get the recommended amount of milk products each day without adding too much fat to your diet. Write a summary paragraph about your findings.

Journal Writing

8. Write a journal entry planning a healthful, nutritious dinner using recipes from the fruits and vegetables, grains, dairy, and protein groups. Include the recipes and actually make the dinner one evening for your family or friends.

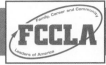 ## FCCLA

9. Create a dairy awareness campaign as part of an *FCCLA Student Body* project. During lunch or after school, demonstrate how to make delicious dairy snacks such as smoothies or yogurt milk shakes. As you prepare the dairy snacks, describe facts about dairy products to educate your peers on the benefits of drinking milk and eating dairy foods.

10. Chili is one food that is high in protein. Host a chili cook-off with high-profile community members serving as the chefs, and feature different chili recipes from beef, to pork to vegetarian. Be sure the chefs display tips for buying high-quality ingredients for their chili. Charge an entry and tasting fee and donate the money to a local food pantry. Submit your project for recognition in the national *FCCLA Community Service* category. See your adviser for information as needed.

Chapter 21
At the Table

Sections

Reading Prep

College and Career Readiness

As you read the chapter, record any questions that come to mind. Indicate where you can find the answer to each question: within the text, by asking your teacher, in another book, on the Internet, or by reflecting on your own experiences. Pursue the answers to your questions.

Concept Organizer

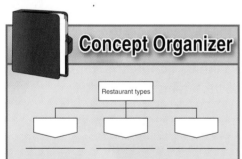

Use a diagram like the one shown to list the three types of restaurants with one example of the type of meal service that may be found in each.

Companion Website

Print out the concept organizer for Chapter 21 at the website.

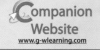

Companion Website
www.g-wlearning.com

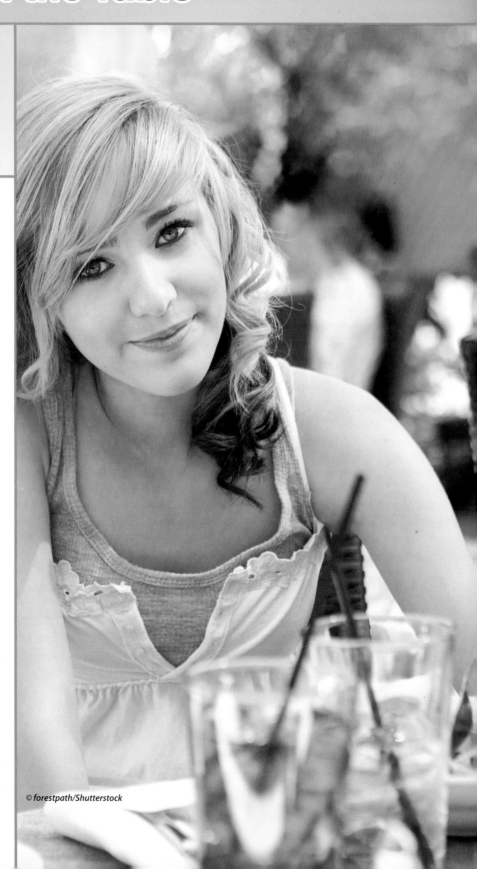

© forestpath/Shutterstock

Eating at Home

Objectives

After studying this section, you will be able to
- **demonstrate** how to set a table according to accepted traditions.
- **identify** different types of meal service.
- **demonstrate** proper mealtime etiquette.

Key Terms		
cover	linens	plate service
dinnerware	family service	RSVP
glassware	buffet service	Regrets only
flatware		

For most people, meals involve more than just eating. Mealtime is also a time for talking with family members or friends. People often celebrate special occasions over meals.

Preparing a meal for family or friends takes time and effort, **21-1**. When you care enough to prepare a good meal, it is worth the extra effort to create a pleasant mood for dining.

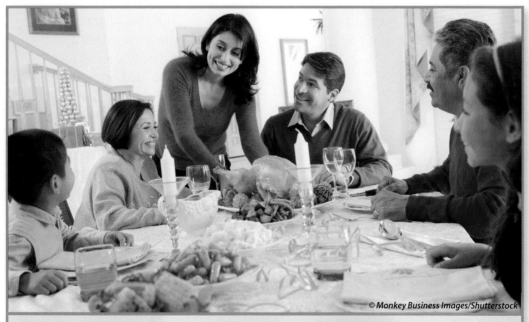

© Monkey Business Images/Shutterstock

21-1 Entertaining is more fun when you know the basics of table setting, meal service, and mealtime etiquette.

Setting the Table

Part of meal preparation is setting an orderly, attractive table for your diners. Tables can be set in more than one way. There are some standard guidelines, however, for setting any table. With practice, setting an orderly table will be easy for you. A pretty table helps put people in the mood for the good food to come. With some creativity, you can add special touches to the table to make even a simple meal seem special.

The Cover

The main part of proper table setting is learning to set a cover. The **cover** is the table space in front of a person's seat. It is also sometimes called a *place setting*.

Dinnerware includes plates, cups, saucers, and bowls. **Glassware** is all types of drinking glasses. **Flatware** includes forks, knives, and spoons. Use only the correct dishes, glassware, and flatware for the foods and drinks you are serving. For instance, bowls and soupspoons are necessary if you serve soup. You may want to set two forks, one for dinner, and one for dessert.

As you begin placing items, be aware of how you handle them. Do not handle areas that will be touched by food. For instance, hold flatware by the handles. Hold glasses near their bases.

To set a cover, place the dinner plate in the center of the cover. The plate should be about one inch from the edge of the table and the other items placed as needed, **21-2**. The following steps can help you set an attractive table:

- Place flatware in the order of use with the first piece to be used set farthest from the plate. For instance, suppose you are using both salad and dinner forks. Because salads are usually served first, the salad fork should be farthest from the plate.
- Place forks to the left of the plate and knives and spoons to the right. The knives are closest to the plate with the blades facing the plate. Turn fork tines and spoons upward. Align the flatware with the lower edge of the plate.
- Place the napkin to the left of the forks or on top of the plate when using a napkin ring.
- Place drinking glasses just above the tip of the knife. If you are having water and another

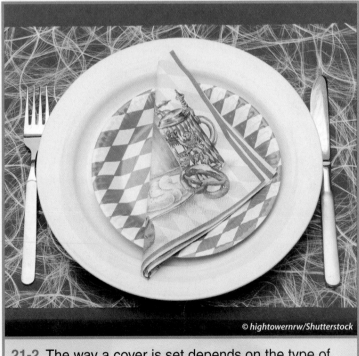

© hightowernrw/Shutterstock

21-2 The way a cover is set depends on the type of meal served.

beverage, the water glass is above the knife with the second glass to its right. Coffee cups, if needed, go to the right of the spoon.

- If you are serving salad, place that plate above the forks and a little to the left. Salad plates or soup bowls can also be on the dinner plates. These pieces are for the first courses and then removed before the main course using the dinner plate.
- You may choose to have a small plate for bread and butter. Bread and butter plates also go above the forks. For a more formal meal, a butter knife rests across the top of the bread and butter plate.

Cover Choices

Think about the type of mood that you want to create for your dinner. Will it be formal and elegant or casual and cozy? The type of meal affects your choices of dinnerware, flatware, glassware, and linens. Fine china, sterling silverware, and crystal glasses are appropriate for very formal meals, **21-3**. Wash formal tableware by hand to prevent damage. Disposable or casual plates, cups, and flatware work well for picnics and barbecues.

The dinnerware, flatware, and glassware you use for most meals, however, falls in between the very formal and very casual. Everyday dinnerware is made of glazed ceramics or durable porcelain. Flatware is made of stainless steel and the glassware is made of glass. Casual tableware is dishwasher safe.

Linens and Centerpieces

If you are celebrating a holiday, you may want to give the table extra attention. **Linens** are the table's place mats, napkins, and tablecloths. Tablecloths and place mats help protect the table from spills. All these items come in a variety of colors, styles, and prices.

A centerpiece adds personality and interest to the table. Centerpieces are good places to express your creativity. Flower arrangements are common centerpieces, but fruits, vegetables, or anything else that complements the occasion is acceptable. The centerpiece should

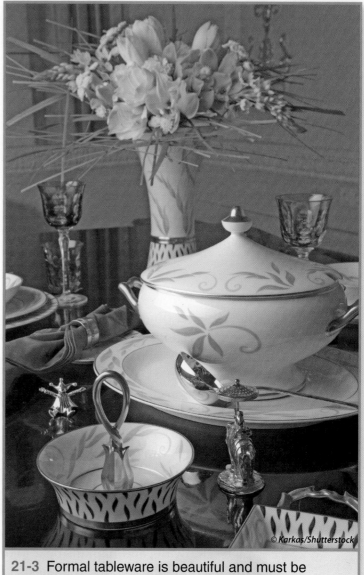
© Karkas/Shutterstock

21-3 Formal tableware is beautiful and must be handled with care.

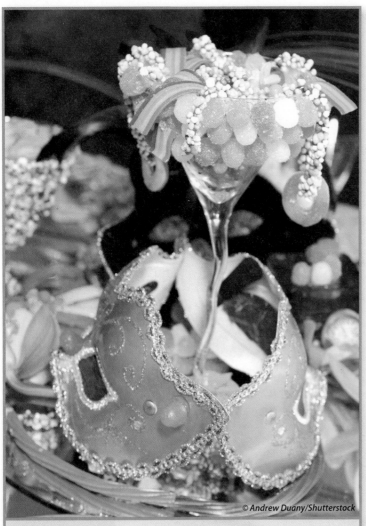

© Andrew Duany/Shutterstock

21-4 This colorful centerpiece could be for a birthday or for a Halloween or Mardi Gras celebration.

fit the type of meal you are serving. You might use a basket of holiday decorations for a holiday dinner. For a Chinese-theme meal, you could use colorful, oriental paper fans. Make sure that the centerpiece does not block people's views across the table.

Work with what you have on hand to decorate the table and save money. Look for items around the house or garden to use in a new way. An old pitcher might make a great vase. You might use real ivy and small flowers from your garden to decorate the center length of a table. You can easily set an attractive table with a little imagination, **21-4**.

Meal Service

There are many ways to serve meals. Three common styles in the United States are family service, buffet service, and plate service. The meal service you will want to use often depends on the number of people and your family's customs.

Family Service

Family service is a quick, easy way to serve food. **Family service** is passing serving dishes around the table for diners to fill their own plates. People begin eating when the serving is complete.

Family service is casual and popular for dinners with family and good friends. Fill the serving dishes in the kitchen and place them on the dinner table with serving utensils. People are free to place as much or as little as they want on their plate. To keep family service working smoothly, pass the serving dishes in the same direction.

Buffet Service

For large dinners and parties, a buffet is a convenient way to serve guests. **Buffet service** allows people to help themselves to foods in serving dishes set on a separate table. Guests move along the buffet table in a line. Place the plates, flatware, and napkins next to the food or set them on the dinner table. After serving themselves, the guests take their seats at the dinner table. When everyone at a table is seated, guests may begin eating.

Depending on the food and table setting, buffets can be elegant or casual. Temperature affects both the flavor and safety of food. Keep hot foods at the proper temperature, **21-5**. Keep cold items, such as salads or ice cream, cool on ice.

Plate Service

Use plate service at home to serve small groups of guests. **Plate service** is filling plates in the kitchen and then serving them to each seated guest. Serve second helpings from the kitchen or from serving dishes at the table.

Plate service saves guests the trouble of passing dishes and serving themselves. Plate service is a more formal serving option because it compares to restaurant dining.

Clearing the Table

People may wish to sit and talk at the table after dinner or during the dessert course. They will feel more comfortable doing so after the table is cleared. Clear the dishes and utensils from the table only when all guests are done eating. Brush any crumbs from the table onto a plate. Store leftover foods in the refrigerator or freezer right away. Wait until guests have left to wash the dishes.

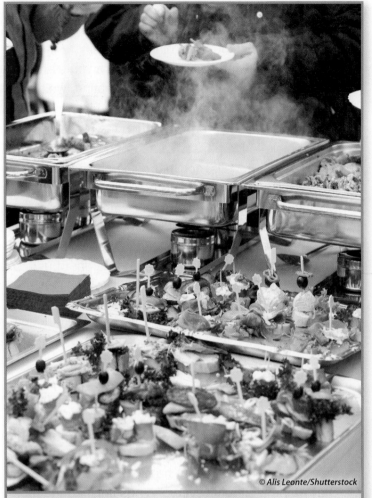

© Alis Leonte/Shutterstock

21-5 To keep hot foods hot, serve immediately or use warming trays.

Mealtime Etiquette

Etiquette is proper behavior in social settings. Learning and practicing etiquette helps you feel more confident when eating with others. A list of good table manners is in **21-6**. Using good manners shows you are thoughtful of others at the table.

Entertaining

You may decide to invite a few friends for dinner. Ask them in advance to be sure they are free that evening. You could invite them on the telephone, through e-mail, or in person. Let your guests know the date and time.

When you invite guests for dinner, try to finish most of the food preparation before your guests arrive. Use recipes you have made before so you will not have to worry about how the food turns out. Then you can relax and concentrate on your guests.

Etiquette for Meals

- Arrive on time if you are a dinner guest.
- Lay your napkin across your lap before you start eating. Never tuck a napkin in your collar.
- Unless the host invites you to begin eating, wait for him or her to start the meal.
- Use good posture throughout the meal and avoid putting your elbows on the table.
- Keep conversation pleasant during the meal. Do not gesture with flatware in your hand.
- Ask to have foods passed rather than reaching across the table or in front of someone.
- Use serving utensils, not your own flatware, to serve yourself from a dish.
- Try a small portion of all foods offered to you. Do not discuss foods you do not like or refuse to eat.
- Some foods, such as bread, chips, small pickles, olives, nuts, and cookies should be eaten with the fingers. Fried chicken may be eaten with the fingers or a fork and knife depending on the setting.
- Eat and drink quietly. Do not slurp, chew with your mouth open, or talk while you are chewing.
- Flatware is placed on the table in the order of use. Use the outermost pieces first. When uncertain about which eating utensil to use, watch the host or hostess. If you drop a utensil, leave it there; the host will offer you another one.
- Cut only a few bites of food at a time and eat those before cutting more.
- If food is too hot, wait for it to cool on its own rather than blowing on it.
- If you have a bone or pit in your mouth, remove it behind a napkin. Never use toothpicks at the table.
- Use a napkin to cover your mouth and turn your head away from the table when sneezing or coughing.
- Place used flatware on a plate or saucer, not on the table.
- Place your knife and fork across the center of your plate when you finish your meal. Before you leave the table, place your napkin beside your plate.
- Stay at the table until everyone has finished the meal. If you must leave the table early, ask the host if you may be excused.

21-6 Good table manners are not just for special occasions.

Your guests look to you to indicate the type of plate service. Sometimes you may need to prompt guests. For instance, you might say, "Chris, would you start passing the corn around the table?"

You might use a combination of styles for holiday meals. A common meal style is to have a carved turkey or ham as the main dish. Guests fill their plate with the meat in a buffet style. You may choose to serve all the food or just the main dish this way. You can also pass side dishes family style.

Parties

Parties are the most common way to entertain larger groups. You can mail, e-mail, or hand deliver written invitations. Be sure to include the date, time, place, and reason for the party. If you want to know how many people will attend, ask for a response. Write **RSVP**, which means *please respond*, on the invitation. RSVP indicates that people should call you to let you know if they will or will not be attending. **Regrets only** written on an invitation means you want only those who *cannot* attend to respond. Include the best way for people to contact you.

Food is the biggest part of most parties. Plan a simple menu to make entertaining easier. If you have a theme, your menu can reflect it. For instance, you might serve little heart-shaped pizzas and red velvet cupcakes for a Valentine's Day party. Many people like to munch on snacks at a party, so you may serve appetizers rather than a full meal. Buffets are popular for serving guests at larger parties. A buffet allows guests easy access to the food and they can eat when they are hungry.

Picnics and Barbecues

Eating outside is a nice change of pace. You might pack ready-to-eat foods for a picnic or cook the food outside for a barbecue.

Finger foods are best for picnics and barbecues. These include sandwiches and raw vegetables with dip. Foods that require the use of flatware, such as salads or baked beans, work well if guests can eat at a picnic table.

When you barbecue, keep the menu simple. Plan to grill one or two items and prepare the other dishes in advance. For instance, you might grill chicken and corn-on-the-cob. You could serve coleslaw, rolls, and fresh fruit with these items.

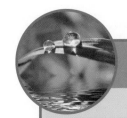

Go Green

Green Picnics

When you think of picnics, do paper plates, napkins, and foam cups come to mind? A better option is reusable plates, cups, and cloth napkins for greener picnics. Although paper products with no plastic on them are biodegradable, they cannot be recycled when exposed to food. Foam is a nonbiodegradable substance, so it remains in landfills indefinitely. The production of foam products also contributes to air pollution. Foam products contain *styrene*, which is a petroleum-based synthetic compound. When styrene is heated, hazardous fumes release into the air and leach from the material. To avoid potential health hazards, remove foods from foam containers before reheating them in the microwave.

Food safety is important when eating outdoors. Thermal ice chests keep drinks and foods that can spoil cold until they are ready to eat. It is simple to add fresh ice as needed. Eat foods from the grill before they have a chance to cool and/or spoil.

Reading Review

1. The table space in front of a person's seat is called a(n) _____.
2. Where is the drinking glass placed when setting a table?
3. The style of meal service in which people serve themselves from serving dishes as they are passed is called _____.
4. What should you do with your flatware at the end of a meal?
5. What information should you include in a party invitation?

Eating Out

Objectives

After studying this section, you will be able to
- **describe** the different types of restaurants.
- **select** nutritious foods from a menu.
- **demonstrate** proper mealtime etiquette in restaurants.

Key Terms		
carryout cafeteria style	maître d'	tip

Eating in restaurants is common in the United States. People spend millions of dollars each year on meals outside the home. Eating out saves people the time and work of shopping, cooking, and cleaning up. It also gives people chances to try new foods in a social setting. Proper restaurant etiquette is important whenever dining out.

Types of Restaurants

The type of food offered, service, price range, and decor differ greatly by restaurant. Three main types of restaurants are fast-food, family, and formal. There are also many types of specialty restaurants, **21-7**.

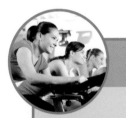

Health Connections

Fast-Food Options

Many items at fast-food places are grilled or fried. Although foods are prepared more quickly using these methods, they are higher in fat and calories. Premade salads are often the only form of vegetables offered. Therefore, you may have trouble getting a well-balanced meal. Occasional fast-food meals are not harmful as long as you eat balanced meals the rest of the day. A steady diet of fast food can lead to nutrition problems. Many fast-food restaurants now offer nutrition information for their menu items at the restaurant or on their website. Before you place an order, check the nutrition information to make choices that are more healthful.

Fast-Food

Fast-food restaurants offer quick service at fairly low prices. At these restaurants, you place your order at a counter or drive-through window. It often takes less than five minutes to get your order. You may eat your food in the restaurant or take it home to eat as **carryout**.

Fast-food meals are inexpensive partly because you serve yourself and the choices are limited. Fewer workers are needed to prepare and serve food, so labor costs are low.

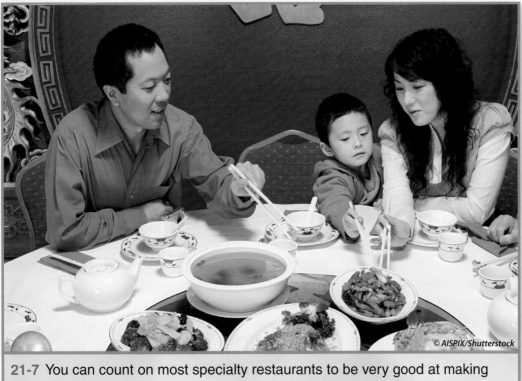

© AISPIX/Shutterstock

21-7 You can count on most specialty restaurants to be very good at making their specialty foods.

Fast-food restaurants often make a small profit on each item they sell. Because they can sell many items quickly, however, the total profit is high.

Family

Family restaurants offer home-style cooking at reasonable prices. Main courses might include fried or baked chicken, roast beef, and spaghetti, **21-8**.

A server takes your order at your table, serves your food, and clears your table at most family restaurants. Some family restaurants are cafeterias. **Cafeteria style** occurs when people choose their foods along a counter and carry it to a table for eating. Cafeterias offer several main dishes, side dishes, and desserts. A busperson may bring you drink refills and clear the table.

Most family restaurants offer a clean, pleasant, and relaxed setting. The ingredients are often fresh and

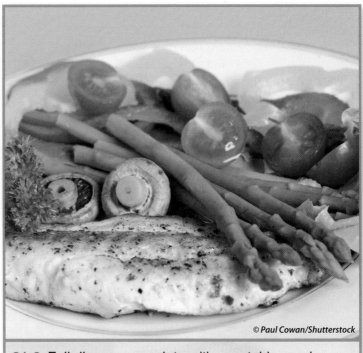

© Paul Cowan/Shutterstock

21-8 Full dinners, complete with vegetables and salad, are on most family restaurant menus.

more healthfully prepared. They can make large amounts of food at one time and keep it warm until ordered. The prices at family restaurants are usually higher than fast-food places, but lower than formal dining restaurants.

Formal

Formal restaurants serve unique and often expensive meals. The servers are very attentive and the décor may be elegant. At these restaurants, a host or hostess, sometimes called a **maître d'** (may tra de') seats you. A server takes your order and serves you. In some formal restaurants, more than one person may wait on you. One person may bring your drinks and another takes your order. A third person may bring your food and clear the table.

A professional chef prepares the high-quality food at formal restaurants. Each meal is prepared individually to order. Many times, a chef creates his or her own recipes to serve. Plate presentation is appealing, too.

Because of the food preparation and special service, meals in formal restaurants can take several hours. Many people enjoy taking their time and relaxing at formal restaurants. For a special treat, you may not mind the extra cost.

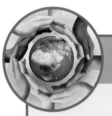

Global Connections

Ethnic Restaurants

Ethnic restaurants are specialty restaurants featuring cuisine of a different culture. Mexican, Greek, and Chinese restaurants are common choices. Ethnic restaurants give you a chance to try foods of different cultures. These foods may be quite different from the foods you eat at home. Some ethnic restaurants give you a taste of different customs, too. For instance, you may try eating with chopsticks at a Chinese restaurant. It is common in Moroccan restaurants to eat at low tables where diners sit on pillows. In some Moroccan restaurants, the country's custom of eating with your fingers and flatbread pieces (instead of utensils) is encouraged.

Specialty Restaurants

Many restaurants specialize in a certain type of food or cuisine. For instance, some specialty restaurants feature pizza with many choices of toppings. They may offer different types of pizza, such as thin crust, deep dish, stuffed, and whole wheat. Other types of specialty restaurants include seafood, barbecue, or steak. Specialty restaurants may be fast-food, family, or formal restaurants.

Making Nutritious Food Choices

Most restaurants offer healthful, nutritious food options. Look for vegetables, fruits, salads, soups, and nonfried items on the menu. You can order water, low-fat milk, or fruit juice instead of a soft drink at a restaurant. Then be sure to choose a variety of foods for your meal. Some restaurants highlight menu items that fit special nutritional needs. For instance, they might mark entrees under 500 calories or designate some as *heart healthy*, meaning lower in fat.

Ordering from the Menu

Your choice of food items appears on a restaurant's menu. Look for some terms that you might find on a menu in **21-9**. Menus are often printed, but they may be written on a large display board. Read the menu carefully and ask your server about preparation methods, ingredients, or any other questions you might have. Many servers will suggest foods you might enjoy if you ask. Servers can also describe specials that are not listed on the menu.

Explain any dietary concerns or restrictions to your server. Special dishes can be prepared to meet your needs. Check to see whether side dishes are priced separately or as part of the main dish. Many menus tell you the sizes of items. Most servers will look at one person to start the ordering. After he or she finishes, the next person to the left orders, and so on. This sequence makes it easier for the server to remember each guest's order.

Restaurant Etiquette

Use the same good table manners that you do at home. Some restaurant situations are a little different, however. These guidelines will help you handle situations that do not apply to home meals.

Common Menu Terms

- **à la carte:** items are priced individually.
- **à la mode:** served with ice cream.
- **au gratin:** covered with melted cheese.
- **au jus:** served in its natural juice, usually referring to meat.
- **du jour:** item of the day, such as soup du jour, which means soup of the day.
- **en brochette:** cooked or served in small pieces on a skewer.
- **entrée:** the main dish of a meal.
- **hors d'oeuvre (appetizer):** a food that is served before the entrée.

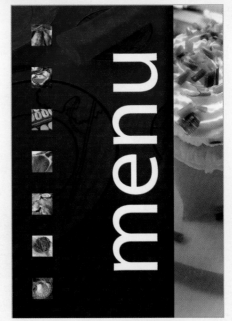

© Jacques PALUT/Shutterstock

21-9 Restaurant meals are more enjoyable if you understand the terms on the menu.

Paying the Bill

Decide in advance how to pay the bill when dining with other people. If you are each paying for your own meal, ask for separate checks. Before placing your order, let the server know if you want separate checks.

Unless someone has said in advance that they will pay for the meal, assume you are paying for your own meal and drinks. Make sure you have enough money for the type of meal you order. Asking to borrow money from a friend at the end of a meal is awkward for both of you.

Some servers give you time to relax before bringing the check. If you have limited time, however, let the server know you are ready for your check. Look over the bill to make sure it is correct. If you notice a mistake, politely let the server know.

In many restaurants, the server brings your check to you and then takes your payment and returns with your change. In other restaurants, you pay the cashier on the way out. If you are unsure who to pay, just ask your server.

Tipping

When someone serves you in a restaurant, you should leave a tip. A **tip** is money for the service you receive. It shows your gratitude. In most cases, 15 to 20 percent of the food total before tax is appropriate. Tipping is not expected in fast-food restaurants.

The amount of your tip is based on the level of service you receive. Therefore, you may leave some servers a higher percent of the bill than others. Reward excellent service with a good tip. A good server is prompt and friendly and will try to honor special requests, **21-10**. He or she will check several times to see if you need anything. Likewise, you may tip less for poor service.

Because servers are often paid less than minimum wage, they depend on tips as a large part of their income. In addition, servers must tip the other people who help them, such as the busperson, from their own tips. You should always leave a reasonable tip unless the service is

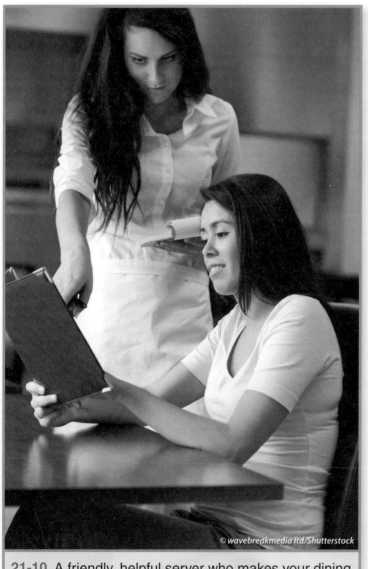

© wavebreakmedia ltd/Shutterstock

21-10 A friendly, helpful server who makes your dining experience enjoyable deserves a good tip.

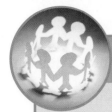

Life Connections

Restaurant Etiquette

Keep the following in mind when eating at a restaurant:
- Put any personal belongings on the floor by your chair, not on the table.
- Talk in a tone of voice for those at your table. Avoid loud laughter.
- If you need something from your server, call him or her in a clear but soft voice as the person goes by your table. If the server is too far away to call, try to catch his or her attention with eye contact or a little hand wave. Never yell loudly for your server.
- If you spill something, let your server know so he or she can clean it up. Apologize briefly and thank the server for cleaning it.
- If someone stops at your table to talk, stop eating until the person leaves. If you want to talk with someone at another table, excuse yourself from your table and make the visit very short.
- If you need to comb your hair or fix makeup, excuse yourself and do so in the restroom, not at the table.
- If your food is unsatisfactory or not as you ordered, let your server know right away. Explain the problem quietly. Good servers will attempt to get you exactly what you ordered.

Writing Activity

Write a paragraph describing a bad experience you either had or witnessed in a restaurant. Now that you know proper etiquette, would you handle the situation differently?

extremely poor. Leave the tip on the table where the server can easily find it. If a check tray is on the table, leave the tip on it. When paying with a debit or credit card, add the tip on the receipt where indicated.

Consider the cost of tax and tip when choosing a restaurant. Be sure you have enough money to cover these costs before ordering a meal.

Reading Review

1. Give an example of a fast-food, family, formal, and specialty restaurant.
2. What items should you look for on a restaurant menu when making healthy, nutritious choices?
3. True or false. The term *à la mode* means served with ice cream.
4. What should you do if your food is not served the way you ordered it?
5. What percent of the food total before tax is an appropriate tip for good service?

Chapter Summary

Section 21-1. Setting a neat, attractive table makes meals at home pleasant. There are several ways to serve meals in an orderly manner: family, buffet, and plate service. When entertaining, set covers with the correct dinnerware, glassware, and flatware in the right positions. Linens and creative centerpieces provide interest to a table as well. Using proper etiquette will help you and your guests feel comfortable.

Section 21-2. Eating out can be a fun change of pace from eating meals at home. Fast-food, family, formal, and specialty restaurants can all offer good nutrition if you select foods carefully. When eating at a restaurant, you need to use the same mealtime etiquette you use at home. Knowing how to order, pay the bill, and leave a tip can make your restaurant experience more enjoyable from start to finish.

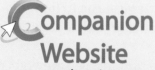
Companion Website
www.g-wlearning.com

Check your understanding of the main concepts for Chapter 21 at the website.

Critical Thinking

1. **Solve.** What would you do if one of your dinner guests had poor table manners? Why?

2. **Choose.** If you could host a dinner party anywhere in the world, where would it be? Why?

3. **Conclude.** Write a questionnaire about eating out. Include questions about where people eat, why they eat where they do, and how often they eat out. Use the questionnaire to survey five people. Compile your responses with those of your classmates. What are your conclusions about your survey and how do they compare to the overall class's survey?

Common Core

College and Career Readiness

4. **Speaking.** As a class, create some role-plays in which you demonstrate examples of poor table etiquette. Then act out the role-play again using proper manners. Perform your role-plays for another class. Hold a discussion on how using good etiquette can help build your confidence.

5. **Writing.** Write a menu for a dinner you would serve to eight guests. Draw a diagram of a cover to show how you would set the table for this meal. Then write a paragraph explaining which style of meal service you would use and why.

6. **Listening.** Watch a movie or TV show featuring a dinner or a party. Describe the type of meal service, how the table was set, the centerpieces, and linens. Was the dinner or party a success? Why or why not?

7. **Math.** Figure the tip for your meal at a specialty restaurant where the service was merely adequate. Your dinner was $10.99, dessert was $4.99, and iced tea was $1.50.

Technology

8. **Online Research.** Conduct research online to find the nutritional values of food items at two fast-food restaurants. Write a one-page report comparing the items at the two places. Which ones do you recommend from a nutritional standpoint?

Journal Writing

9. Write a journal entry about your favorite holiday dinner or party. Describe the meal service, place settings, linens, and centerpieces.

Why is it your favorite holiday dinner or party? If you could change something, what would it be?

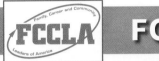

FCCLA

10. Create a *Family Ties* project and set a goal to eat a minimum number of family dinners together. Try a variety of formal and informal meal configurations and poll your family on which they prefer. Pledge to continue this tradition even after your project is completed. Share your project findings with the class. See your adviser for information as needed.

11. Develop an *FCCLA Community Service* project by researching different organizations in your school, community, and online that provide resources and assistance for youth who desire to stay fit and maintain a healthy weight. Create an awareness campaign that promotes healthy lifestyle choices when eating away from home. Use the *FCCLA Planning Process* to develop your strategies. See your adviser for information as needed.

Unit 7
The Clothes You Wear

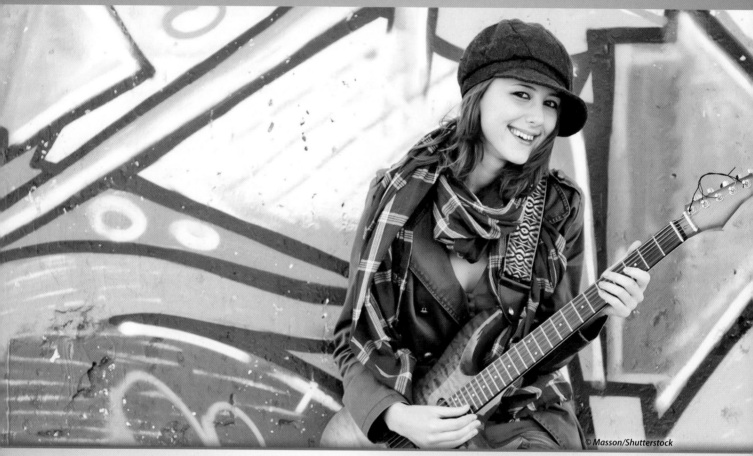

© Masson/Shutterstock

Unit Essential Question

Who benefits from the clothes advertising encourages you to buy?

Exploring Career Pathways

Clothing and Fashion Careers

Do you have a flair for fashion and design? Perhaps you have expert sewing skills or strong interest in selling clothes. The following careers are among those to which many people aspire.

Retail Sales Associate

With ability to engage people in friendly conversation, the main responsibility of retail sales associates is to help customers select and purchase clothing and accessories that meet their needs. Sales associates are required to register sales electronically, take payments (cash, check, or credit), and give correct change and receipts. These workers must count accurately and maintain high ethical standards. No formal training or degree is required for retail sales. Most duties are learned on the job. Those who aspire to move into a management position need education beyond high school.

Tailor, Dressmaker, or Custom Sewer

Tailors, dressmakers, and custom sewers have exceptional sewing abilities. They use a variety of sewing equipment and tools. They often alter, fit, or make custom clothing to their customer's and/or manufacturer's specifications. These workers have good math skills and understand garment design. Knowledge of clothing construction and textiles is essential. Postsecondary training from a technical school or an associate's degree is required for this career. Many receive on-the-job training, too. These people work in boutiques, department stores, dry cleaners, or may have their own businesses. Savvy customer service skills, ability to communicate well, and creativity are other necessary traits.

Fashion Designer

Fashion designers have a strong appreciation for beauty and a good eye for color and design details. They study fashion trends before designing clothing and accessories. Fashion designers excel in art, creating hand-drawn sketches of their designs. Many use computer-aided design (CAD) software for design creation, allowing others to have a virtual view of the designs. Fashion designers may work for apparel manufacturers. Others freelance for various companies. An associate's or bachelor's degree is required for fashion designers. They need an understanding of textiles and fabrics, patternmaking, and sewing skills. Designers must communicate their ideas to others who make the patterns and sew their designs. Many designers start out as sketching assistants to designers with experience.

Is this career path for you? Use the following activities to determine your interest in or ability for a clothing and fashion career.

- Work with an art teacher or fashion designer to develop your drawing skills. Then try sketching some designs. Have the art teacher or designer critique your work. Make refinements as needed.
- Interview a manager of a retail clothing shop. What personal traits and skills does this manager feel are essential for a retail apparel career? How do your traits and skills relate? Write a summary of your findings.

Chapter 22
Clothing Choices

Sections

Reading Prep

College and Career Readiness

As you read the chapter, put sticky notes next to any sections where you have questions. Write your questions on the sticky notes. Discuss the questions with your classmates or teacher.

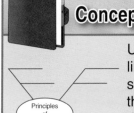

Concept Organizer

Principles of Design

Use a diagram like the one shown to list the principles of design and give two examples of each in fashion design.

Companion Website

Print out the concept organizer for Chapter 22 at the website.

Companion Website
www.g-wlearning.com

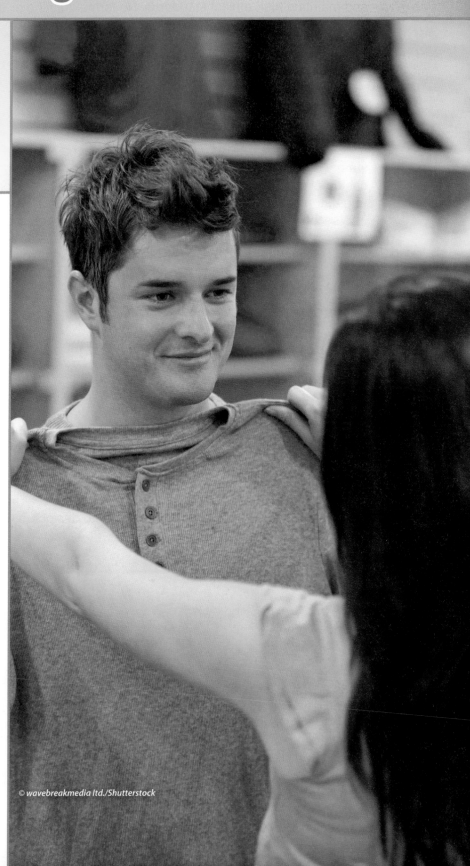

© wavebreakmedia ltd./Shutterstock

Clothing Design

Objectives

After studying this section, you will be able to
- **list** the elements and principles of design.
- **describe** how the elements and principles of design are used in fashion.
- **apply** the elements and principles of design to select the best clothing for you.

Key Terms

elements of design	line	harmony
hue	illusions	balance
value	texture	proportion
warm colors	form	rhythm
cool colors	principles of design	emphasis
neutrals		

A well-designed garment is visually pleasing. Every part looks like it belongs together. Understanding the elements and principles of design makes choosing the best clothing for you much easier. For instance, some colors look better together than others. Certain design elements can make people look shorter, taller, heavier, or thinner.

The Elements of Design

Color, line, texture, and form are the **elements of design**. Fashion designers must consider all the elements of design carefully. When the right colors, lines, textures, and forms are used, the design will usually be a success. Consider the elements of design when you select, buy, or make clothes.

Color

Color is a very exciting part of life. Everyone has a favorite color. In fact, the clothes in your closet often reflect your favorite colors. You can look and feel cheerful, healthy, and full of energy when wearing certain colors, **22-1**.

Colors	Feelings or Moods
Red	Excitement, power, danger, aggression, anger, passion, love, energetic
Orange	Lively, cheerful, friendly, energetic, warmth
Yellow	Cheerful, bright, sympathy, cowardice, wisdom, warmth
Green	Refreshing, restful, peaceful, luck, envy, hope
Blue	Calm, serious, reserved, dignified, serenity
Purple	Dignified, regal, mysterious
Black	Sophisticated, somber, mourning, wisdom
White	Innocence, purity, faith, peace

22-1 Some colors can also affect or express your moods and feelings.

The Language of Color

Hue is the name of a color. Red, yellow, blue, or any other color name are hues. The lightness or darkness of a color is its **value**. Adding white to the color produces a *tint*. For instance, pink is a tint of red. Adding black to the color produces a *shade*. Maroon is a shade of red. Navy is a shade of blue.

Intensity is the brightness or dullness of a color. Bright colors are intense. For instance, kelly green has a high intensity, but mint green is softer and less intense.

The Color Wheel

The *color wheel* shows how colors relate to each other, **22-2**. Red, blue, and yellow are the primary colors. Mixing the primary colors produces the *secondary* colors of green, purple, and orange. Yellow and blue make green; red and blue make purple; red and yellow make orange.

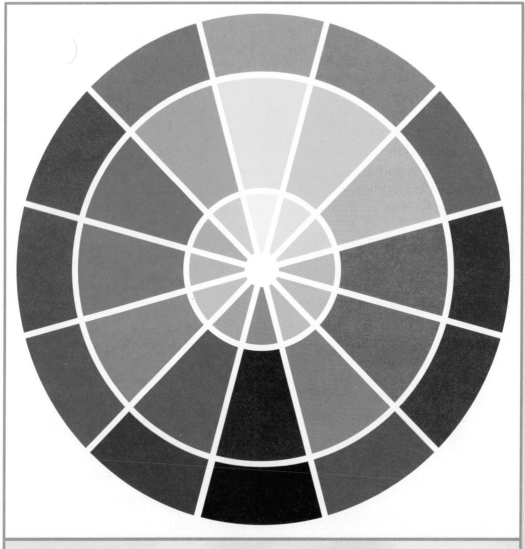

22-2 The inner ring on the color wheel shows the colors' tints, while the outer ring shows the shades.

Combining a primary and a secondary color produces an *intermediate* color. Intermediate colors include red-orange, red-violet, blue-green, blue-violet, yellow-green, and yellow-orange.

Warm and Cool Colors

The color wheel has warm and cool sides. **Warm colors** are red, yellow, orange, and their different variations. They are brilliant, warm like the sun, and suggest activity. Warm colors advance, or appear to move forward.

Cool colors are blue, green, purple, and their variations. Terms to describe them include restful, calm, and relaxing. Cool colors recede, appearing to move away or stay in the background.

In **22-3**, notice how the red sweater (warm color) advances and the blue sweater (cool color) recedes visually. If you want to appear larger, wear warm, lighter colors. These colors draw attention. If you want to appear smaller, wear cool, darker colors because they recede.

Color Schemes

Every outfit you choose has a color scheme. Three common color schemes are monochromatic, analogous, and complementary, **22-4**.

A *monochromatic color scheme* is variations of a single hue on the color wheel. For instance, you would have a monochromatic outfit if you wore blue jeans and a light blue shirt or blouse. People who are shorter can appear taller in one-color outfits.

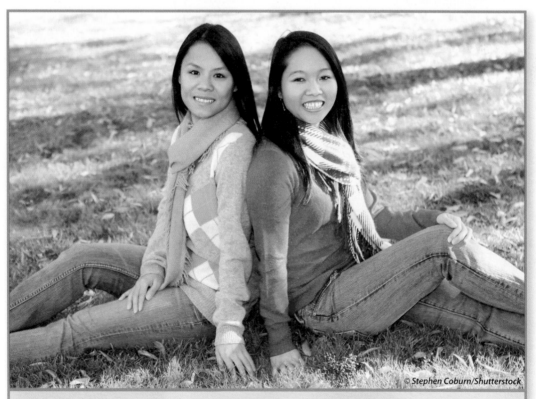

© Stephen Coburn/Shutterstock

22-3 If warm colors advance and cool colors recede, which sweater did you notice first?

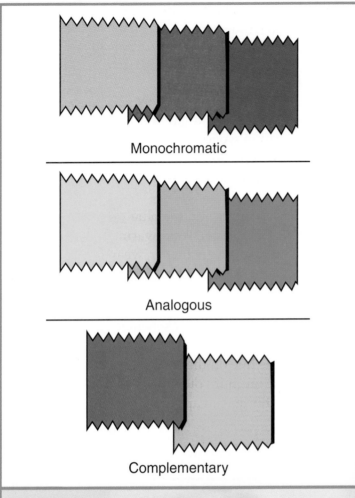

Monochromatic

Analogous

Complementary

22-4 As you select clothes for an outfit, try these familiar color schemes.

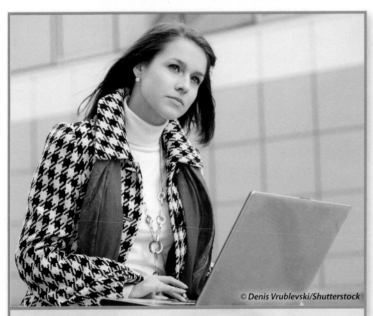

© Denis Vrublevski/Shutterstock

22-5 When paired with neutral black and white, this red scarf looks more vibrant.

An *analogous color scheme* is the colors that are next to each other on the color wheel. Wearing blue pants or a skirt with a green top is an analogous color scheme. The colors are more similar to each other than different.

A *complementary color scheme* is the two colors that are directly across from each other on the color wheel. Complementary colors are contrasting, or opposite, colors. They make each other look brighter and more intense. Red and green are complementary colors. People who are taller often appear shorter when the top and bottom of an outfit are of contrasting colors.

Neutrals

White, gray, ivory, and black are neutral colors. **Neutrals** are not true colors. White is the absence of color. It reflects light and makes objects appear larger than they really are. Black, however, is the combination of all colors. The combination of all colors makes black dense. Black absorbs light and objects appear smaller than they really are. For instance, you appear to be smaller than you are when wearing a black outfit rather than a white one.

Neutral colors are versatile. They work well alone, but also complement any true color. Use a neutral with a small amount of another color to make the other color look brighter, **22-5**.

Line

Line gives direction to a design. In clothing design, lines are structural or decorative. Seams create the structural lines of a garment. Decorative lines are part of the fabric design, visible topstitching, or trims added to the garment. Lines in clothing can be *vertical* (up and

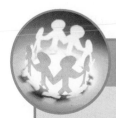

Life Connections

Your Best Colors

Choosing the right colors of clothing is an important decision. They are the ones that bring compliments each time you wear them. The best colors for you are in harmony with your unique coloring. Consider the following when choosing clothes:

- **Your Skin Tone.** The most important consideration in finding your best colors is your skin tone. The five basic skin tones are black, red-brown, yellow-brown, yellow, and white—with many variations. To test how different colors look on you, sit in front of a large mirror in the daylight. Drape different-colored fabrics around your shoulders, covering your other clothing. Study the effects each color has on your skin. Some look good immediately, while others clearly do not. Your favorite color may not go well with your skin tone. You can still wear it, just not around your face. Choose skirts, pants, belts, or shoes in that color.
- **Your Hair Color.** The main hair colors are blonde, red, and brunette (brown and black). Blondes and redheads wear warm shades like oranges, yellows, and rusts well. Taupe, tan, and white also bring out the warm tones in blonde and red hair colors. Redheads look good in shades of green. Most colors flatter brunettes, including reds, oranges, and pinks, plus jewel tones of green and blue.

Research Activity

Find books, websites, and even services that are devoted to *color analysis*. These resources advise people about colors that look best on certain skin tone, hair, and eye color combinations. For easy reference, the color categories are grouped by season. Learn about your season and create a poster showing your best colors.

down), *horizontal* (across), *diagonal* (slanted), or *curved* (rounded), **22-6**.

Lines and Illusions

Lines create **illusions**, or make things appear different from what they are. The direction of lines in a garment can make you seem taller, shorter, thinner, or heavier. When choosing clothes, it is important to know how different lines create various illusions.

Vertical lines carry the eye up and down. They have a slimming effect and make people look taller and slender. Stripes are vertical lines. Any

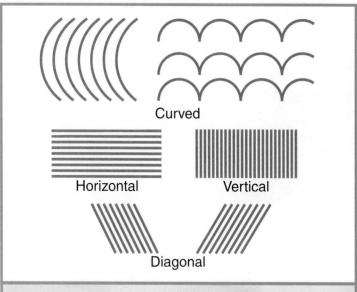

22-6 These lines create very different illusions when used in apparel design.

fabric with a vertical design has the same effect, however. This includes dots, prints, or other designs in a line.

Horizontal lines carry the eye across from side to side. They have a widening effect. Very tall, thin people wear horizontal stripes well. A wide belt creates a horizontal line in an outfit and makes a person look shorter and heavier. The belt halts the upward movement of the eye and cuts the person into two distinct parts.

Diagonal lines are slanted. They add interest to a design. They create the same illusions as vertical and horizontal lines depending on the slant.

Curved lines are rounded as in part of a circle. They give a soft, relaxed look to garments. Fabrics with wavy lines or circles and round collars are examples of curved lines. For instance, a person with a square face looks better in a round neckline than someone with a round face.

Texture

Texture is how a fabric feels and looks. Words describing texture include bulky, fuzzy, dull, furry, nubby, rough, scratchy, shaggy, sheer, shiny, smooth, or soft. The textures of fabrics affect clothing design. Combining textures is desirable in fashion, as long as they are not too different from each other, **22-7**.

Some fabrics are better for certain designs. For instance, sweaters and other comfortable garments are often made with bulky, fuzzy, or shaggy fabrics. These textures rarely show up in formal attire designs. More luxurious fabrics such as silk, satin, or velveteen are more appropriate.

Textures can affect the apparent size of the wearer. For instance, thick, textured leggings make legs appear wider. Sheer, flimsy fabric makes the wearer seem smaller.

Textures also affect colors differently. The color of a shiny, smooth fabric appears lighter and brighter. This texture reflects light and tends to add visual weight or size. For instance, a red satin blouse appears more intense than the same red in a fuzzy sweater. Dull-textured fabrics, such as denim, do not reflect light. They tend to decrease visual weight or size because dull surfaces absorb light.

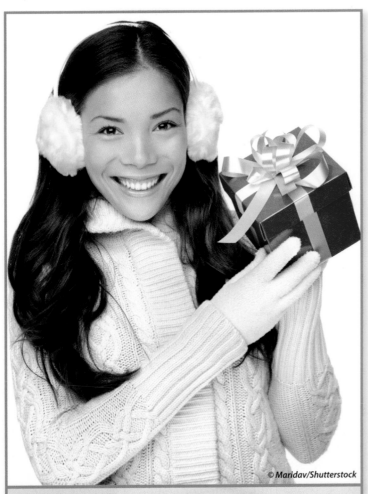

© Maridav/Shutterstock

22-7 Can you find the different textures in this outfit?

Form

Form refers to the shape of an object. It is the overall outline. In clothing design, form is called a *silhouette*. Clothes with a wide, fuller silhouette tend to make a person appear larger and heavier. Examples of these include full skirts or pants with extra-wide legs.

Clothes in a tubular silhouette tend to make a person appear taller and thinner. Examples of these include pencil skirts, straight-leg pants, or a sheath dress without a belt.

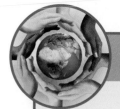

Global Connections

The World of Fashion

Paris, France and Milan, Italy have long been considered the world's centers of high fashion or *haute couture* (oat kootur'). French and Italian designers, such as Dior, Chanel, Gucci, and Prada are still among the best known. Successful high fashion designers, however, are now cropping up across the globe, including the United States. New York and Tokyo, Japan have highly attended international fashion shows. Buenos Aires, Argentina is also emerging as a new center of fashion. The new names in fashion design, such as Kenzo, Betsey Johnson, Vera Wang, and Efrin Africa reflect the global economy.

The bell-shaped silhouette is flattering to most people. A-line skirts and pants with flared legs are examples of the bell form.

The Principles of Design

The **principles of design** are guides for using the elements of design. They are balance, proportion, rhythm, and emphasis. **Harmony** is the goal of good design, which is the result of using the principles of design properly.

Balance

Well-designed garments are balanced. **Balance** is having equal visual weight on both sides. Color, line, form, and/or texture work together to achieve balance. When a garment is well balanced, the eye is drawn to both parts equally.

Proportion

Proportion is how the sizes of parts relate to each other and to the whole. Proportion is sometimes called *scale*. In clothing design, proportion refers to how separate pieces of an outfit look together and how the whole outfit looks on the body.

Proportion is not as pleasing when all areas are exactly equal in size. Garment designs that match the structure and proportion of the human body are best. For instance, dresses usually have smaller bodices than skirts. Fashions that flatter the natural figure are visually pleasing and remain in style.

Proportion also relates to accessories and the scale of fabric prints. For instance, a very large handbag looks out of proportion on a smaller person. Fabrics with small, repeating prints look better on smaller body types than larger ones.

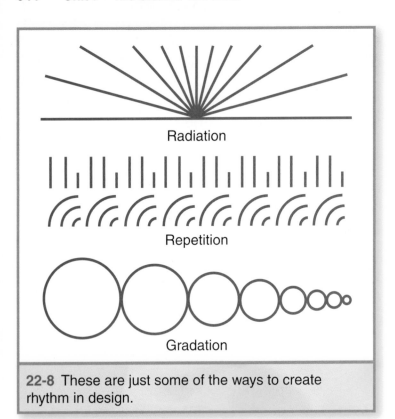

Radiation

Repetition

Gradation

22-8 These are just some of the ways to create rhythm in design.

Rhythm

Rhythm creates a feeling of movement. Your eye easily moves from one part of the design to another. Repetition, gradation, and radiation of colors, lines, shapes, and textures form rhythm, **22-8**. Rhythm is broken when lines, trim, or fabric patterns do not match at the seams.

Emphasis

Emphasis is the center of interest in a design. It is where your eye looks first. To emphasize a waistline, wear a colorful belt. To draw attention away from the waistline, wear a bright scarf at the neckline or a necklace. Bright colors can also be used for emphasis.

To appear taller, place the area of interest higher on the body. The emphasis draws the eye upward instead of downward. If you want to appear shorter, make the area of emphasis at the hip or hemline.

Reading Review

1. List the elements of design.
2. Explain the difference between a *tint* and a *shade*.
3. Which two primary colors are warm?
4. True or false. Fabrics with dull textures tend to decrease visual weight and apparent size because they absorb light.
5. List the principles of design.
6. The goal of design is _____.
7. How is rhythm achieved in a design?

Your Wardrobe

Objectives

After studying this section, you will be able to
- **choose** appropriate clothing for various activities and climates.
- **identify** styles, fashions, classics, and fads.
- **make** a wardrobe inventory.

Key Terms

wardrobe	fashion	fad
accessories	classic	wardrobe inventory
standards of dress		

Throughout history, the clothing people wear expresses the times in which they live. For instance, before the twentieth century, women rarely wore pants. It was considered in poor taste. It is hard to imagine that view today when women probably wear pants more often than skirts or dresses. When the views of a society change, so does the acceptable clothing.

The reasons people wear certain clothes does not change, however. Clothes must fit your activities and the weather. Your peers also affect what you wear.

Clothes to Match Your Lifestyle

Your **wardrobe** is all the clothes and accessories you have to wear. **Accessories** include belts, jewelry, scarves, gloves, hats, neckties, handbags, and shoes, **22-9**.

Consider your various activities. Attending school is probably your main activity. Unless you wear a uniform to school, most of your clothing and accessories must be appropriate for school. These clothes also work well for other activities, such as babysitting or shopping. If you play sports, such as tennis, field hockey, or volleyball, you need athletic clothes and shoes suitable for the sport.

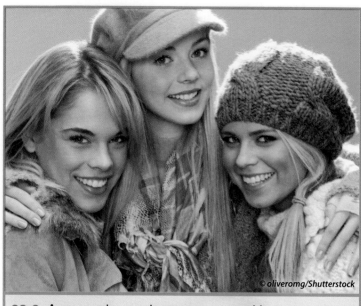
© oliveromg/Shutterstock

22-9 Accessories such as scarves and hats are very important to creating your desired look.

Clothing for Your Climate

The climate in which you live greatly influences the clothes you need, as do the seasons. For instance, you may not own a heavy coat if you live in Florida. In Wisconsin, a heavy coat is necessary in the winter. In some seasons or regions of the country, lightweight jackets and sweaters may keep you comfortable. Layering your clothing is sometimes a good option. The air trapped between the layers warms from a person's body heat. Adding or removing layers makes you comfortable in almost any temperature.

Standards of Dress

Standards of dress are the social influences determining appropriate dress. Standards of dress are written or unwritten. Most schools and workplaces have written dress codes. They vary from mandatory uniforms to only prohibiting T-shirts with objectionable designs. Standards of dress also vary by age groups. It is highly unusual to see a person in their sixties dressing like a teen.

Special Occasions

The right accessories can dress up a school outfit for some special events, **22-10**. Other events require dressier clothing. Men wear suits or tuxedos and women wear formal or cocktail dresses to weddings, formal parties, and elegant restaurants. Special-occasion clothing is often expensive. Consider exchanging formal dresses with friends to save money on clothing worn only once or twice.

Personal Style

Your *personal style* reflects your values and your sense of self. It is unique to you and includes not only how you act, but the clothing you wear. Your clothing makes a statement about you—even if you do not realize it. People you do not know make assumptions about you based on how you dress. Although it may not be fair, it is common. For instance, what is your first impression of a person in sloppy, ill-fitting clothing? Make sure your personal style reflects the best in you.

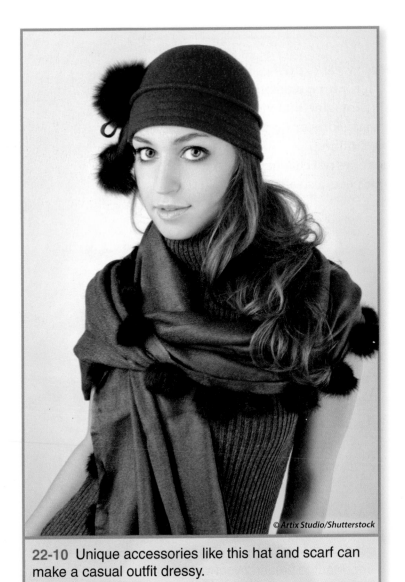

© Artix Studio/Shutterstock

22-10 Unique accessories like this hat and scarf can make a casual outfit dressy.

Style and Fashion

A garment's style is its design. A pullover sweater is different from a cardigan with an open front, **22-11**. Both are styles of sweaters. Styles of pants include jeans, cargo pants, and dress slacks. There are many styles of skirts. Common ones are A-line, pleated, pencil, and gathered.

A style popular at a certain time is called a **fashion**. Fashion trends change over time. Sometimes they even reappear. For instance, flared-leg jeans called bell-bottoms were a fashion trend in the 1970s. Thirty years later, they came back in fashion.

Classic

A **classic** style stays in fashion for a long time. The design only changes slightly from year to year. In any variation, the classic style is still recognized.

Tailored shirts, khaki pants, and blazers are classics. Classic clothing pieces are the basis of a good wardrobe. They are often well-made, more expensive garments. Because they are always in style, however, you wear them longer.

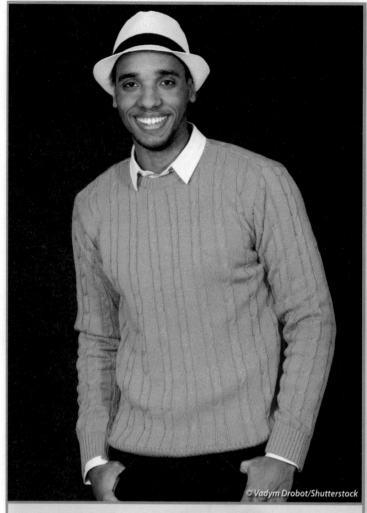

© Vadym Drobot/Shutterstock

22-11 This bright pink pullover style of sweater is also the outfit's emphasis.

Other classic clothing styles include jeans, business suits, tuxedos, and trench coats. Certain colors, fabrics, and patterns remain classics. Taupe and navy blue are classic colors that are always popular. Corduroy, denim, linen, and velvet seldom go out of fashion.

Fad

A **fad** is a clothing style only popular for a short time. Fads become popular fast and die out quickly. A fad's style is often unusual in design and/or color. Fad clothing or accessories are often less expensive and less durable. Wearing the latest fads can be fun and spice up a classic outfit. For instance, colorful ankle boots can make classic black pants more current. You do not wear fad items for very long, however, so limit your fad purchases.

Taking a Wardrobe Inventory

A *wardrobe plan* helps you organize your clothing and accessories. A good wardrobe plan starts with a **wardrobe inventory**, or an itemized list of all the clothes and accessories you own. Use the wardrobe inventory in **22-12** as a guide for taking your own inventory. Add or delete items as needed. After counting your clothes, group them into the following categories:

- Clothing you wear often
- Clothing you wear occasionally
- Clothing needing repairs or cleaning
- Clothing you no longer wear

Look at your entries under each garment type to determine what is missing. Do you have too many of one type of clothing and not enough of another? For instance, you may have too many casual sweatshirts but not enough nice sweaters for school. Do you have enough dressy clothes for the number of times you need them?

Wardrobe Inventory				
Clothes/Accessories	**Description (Colors/Fabrics)**	**Keep**	**Repair**	**Discard**
Jeans				
Pants				
Shirts/tops				
Sweaters				
Sweatshirts/sweatpants				
Suits				
Sport coats (guys)				
Dresses (girls)				
Skirts (girls)				
Jackets				
Coats				
Gloves				
Belts				
Shoes/boots				
Socks				
Underwear				
Jewelry				
Headwear				
Other:				

22-12 This sample wardrobe inventory can serve as the basis for completing your own inventory.

Decide if you need any new items. Also, consider what you want to do with the clothing you no longer wear. Options include giving them to a family member, friend, or a charity. You may also choose to recycle or redesign them for a different use.

Expanding Your Wardrobe

After taking a wardrobe inventory and evaluating it, you may wish to expand your wardrobe. Instead of buying new clothes, there are other ways to increase your wardrobe options. Mix and match current garments to make new outfits. Using accessories also changes the look of outfits.

Mixing and Matching

A wardrobe can seem larger by mixing and matching. Wear several garments in different combinations to create entirely new outfits.

Look at your current clothing items. Do you notice one basic color repeated in many of your clothes? If so, use this color as the basis for building your mix-and-match wardrobe, **22-13**. A few wise choices may create many new outfits.

Begin with clothes you already own before buying new ones. For instance, select a pair of pants and see how many of your shirts, sweaters, and jackets go with them. You may find some new, unexpected combinations.

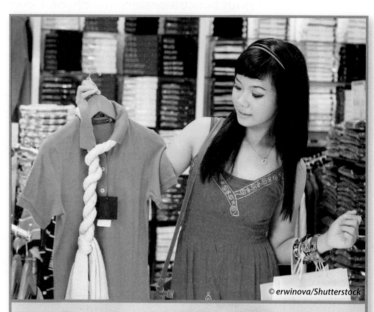
© erwinova/Shutterstock

22-13 Remember your mix-and-match theme when buying new clothes for your wardrobe.

Using Accessories

Accessories add variety to a wardrobe. Different accessories change the same outfit. Most plain or classic outfits can be dressed up or down. For instance, a girl might dress up an outfit with a fun scarf and higher heels. The same outfit can have a more casual look by switching to sweater and cowboy boots. A guy might add a tie to khakis and a tailored shirt for a dressier occasion. Accessories are an inexpensive way to keep up with the latest fashions. Some accessories are fads, though, so spend less money on those.

Reading Review

1. Give five examples of accessories.
2. A style that is popular at a certain time is a(n) _____.
3. How do layered outfits provide warmth?
4. List three things a wardrobe inventory helps you decide.
5. What is the advantage of having a mix-and-match wardrobe?

Shopping for Clothes

Objectives

After studying this section, you will be able to

- **analyze** the different places and ways to shop for clothing and accessories.
- **identify** different types of sales to save money on purchases.
- **explain** how the information on labels and hangtags help consumers make clothing decisions.
- **evaluate** price, quality, and fit before purchasing wardrobe additions.

Key Terms	
irregular	hangtags
labels	alterations

Clothing and accessories can be expensive. Good shopping skills are required to get the most for your money, **22-14**. Smart consumers buy only the clothes they need, will wear, and can afford. Shopping for clothes involves deciding where to shop, reading labels and hangtags, judging garment quality, and checking for proper fit.

Shopping Hints

- Make a shopping list before you leave home.
- Comparison shop before you buy.
- Resist impulse buying. Follow your wardrobe plan and stick to your shopping list.
- Resist buying expensive fad items.
- Shop at stores that accept returns. Know the return policies.
- Save all sales slips and hangtags.
- Watch for end-of-season sales to find bargains. Plan to buy then. Avoid buying sale items you do not need, however, just because they are on sale.
- Consider the upkeep for anything you plan to buy. Dry cleaning is expensive.
- Check for good quality fabrics and garment construction.
- Buy accessories that will go with many outfits.

22-14 Use these hints to develop your shopping skills and make the most of your clothing budget.

Make a list of the clothes and accessories you need to fill the gaps in your wardrobe inventory. Consider your budget and decide which wardrobe additions are most important. It is a good idea to spend most of your money on items you need and will wear often. For instance, if you need a winter coat, you may want to put that first on your list. You can add more casual clothes to your wardrobe later.

Where to Shop

Now that you know what to buy, the next step is deciding where to buy it. Stores range from one extreme to another in terms of clothing prices, quality, and return policies. It is a good idea to become familiar with the available options.

Department Stores

Department stores offer a variety of clothes in a wide range of styles, qualities, and prices. Services such as gift wrapping, mailing, delivery, and alterations are often available in department stores. Because of these extra services, the department stores prices are often higher than those in other types of stores. Some department stores carry less expensive brands, however, and reduce prices at certain times.

Specialty Stores

Shopping centers and malls are good places to find specialty stores. These stores are also called *boutiques* because they sell just one category of clothing, **22-15**. They may sell only sportswear, shoes, or children's clothing. Specialty stores often have unique items you cannot find in other stores. Because boutiques offer one type of clothing, the salespeople know the merchandise well. The quality of clothes varies by store, but prices are often in the middle to higher price range.

Discount Stores

Discount stores carry a wide range of clothing and household items. These stores have fewer customer services than department stores and specialty shops. They are located in large, spare buildings. The quality

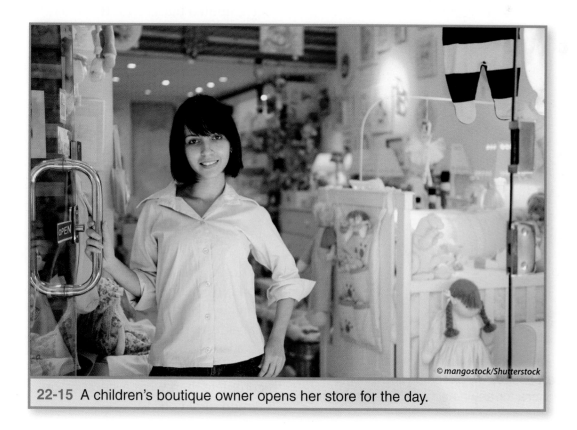

© mangostock/Shutterstock

22-15 A children's boutique owner opens her store for the day.

of clothing and accessories can range from high to low. Customers serve themselves and pay for their purchases at checkout counters when exiting. These differences allow discount stores to have lower prices.

Factory Outlet Stores

Factory outlet stores are discount stores owned by manufacturers. They sell goods directly from the factory to consumers so the prices are lower. These stores are often located together in an *outlet mall*. Factory outlets often sell clothes from past seasons at discounted prices. Some manufacturers may produce lines just for their outlet stores.

Many factory outlets offer first-quality items and irregulars. An **irregular** means there is some *defect* or flaw in the garment. The flaws are often minor. The garment's price tag indicates if it is an irregular. Before buying an irregular garment, look carefully for the defect. The flaw may be in a spot that would not show when wearing it. Some defects only require minor repair, such as a missing button or a ripped seam.

Thrift Stores and Yard Sales

Thrift stores sell some new, but mostly preowned, clothing and other household items for very low prices. Charities often own thrift stores as fundraisers, using them to sell donated merchandise.

A family or a group of neighbors can sell things they own, but no longer need or use. These sales take place in their yards or garages and usually last one or two days.

You can find good quality, useful clothing for greatly reduced prices at both of these places. Buying second-hand clothes is trendy and can be fun, especially on a limited budget, **22-16**. Items such as prom dresses and clothes for growing children could be good buys. Before buying clothes at a thrift shop or garage sale, look carefully at each item because returns are not accepted.

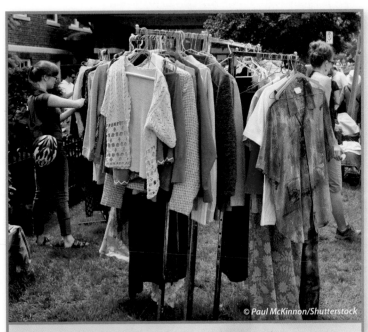

© Paul McKinnon/Shutterstock

22-16 It is rewarding to find high-quality preowned clothing and accessories for extremely low prices. Remember to check for any defects before purchasing.

Catalogs and Electronic Shopping

You can shop at home through catalogs, on websites, or home-shopping television shows. These options are convenient because you browse and purchase when you have the time. Items for sale have descriptions, pictures, fabric choices, sizes, colors, and prices. The information may be more complete than what a salesperson would give you.

The biggest benefit to shopping online is the ability to compare prices and shipping fees. Many websites offer free shipping. Prices are often lower than in department stores. Payment is nearly always by credit or debit card. When ordering over the Internet, only buy from secure websites, which begin with https://.

The drawback is you cannot try on a garment before buying. Some clothing fits differently and what you receive may not fit you right. Also, you may find slight color differences when the garment arrives. Exact colors are difficult to match on paper, TV, or a computer screen.

Sales

A *sale* is the selling of goods at reduced prices. Sales can be for a limited time or the merchandise can be permanently marked down for faster selling. Sales are good for both the stores and customers. Stores need to sell their current products and consumers want to save money on their purchases. Knowing when to shop is just as important as where to shop. Stores have different types of sales. *Clearance* and *end-of-season sales* make room for new merchandise, **22-17**. For instance, swimsuits are often priced lower in September than in May because the wearing time is shorter.

Inventory sales happen before a store spends the time and money to count current stock. They reduce the number of items a store has on hand, taking less time to count. You can save money at inventory sales if you do not care about having the newest styles.

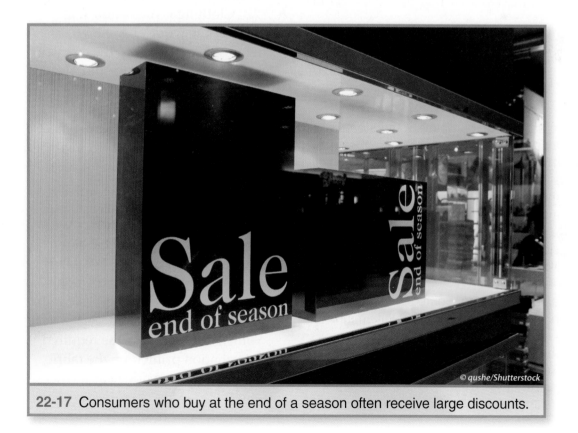

© qushe/Shutterstock

22-17 Consumers who buy at the end of a season often receive large discounts.

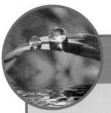

Go Green

Labels for Organic Textiles

Organic textiles are also called *eco-textiles* because they are produced with minimal effect on the natural environment. Little to no pesticides or other chemicals can be used in fiber or textile production. There are certain standards in North America, Europe, Japan, Australia, and India for labeling apparel made from organic textiles. Organic label standards apply to the country where the garments are sold, not where they are produced.

In general, apparel labels are required to list the fabric's organic fibers and the percentage of each. The fibers must be certified as organic by a recognized organization. In the United States, it is the National Organic Program (NOP). There are many in the European Union. In Japan, it is the Japanese Agricultural Standard. The Global Organic Textile Standard and the International Wool Textile Organization certify organic textiles across the world.

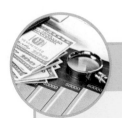

Financial Literacy Connections

Is It Really a Bargain?

When is a sale a true bargain? Some stores hold phony sales. This means, for instance, they may advertise a $100 item for 50% off the retail price, making it $50. This appears to be a good value. If you comparison shop, however, you find that the item's full retail price is in the $50 range everywhere else. Therefore, the store's sale is not a bargain. The store temporarily priced the item that usually sells for $50 at $100 to make a 50% discount look good. This is not only misleading for the consumers, but against the law. It is *false advertising*. Some stores continue the practice, however, even though lawsuits might happen. They are betting on the consumer *not* to comparison shop. Before you buy something on sale, make sure you know if the advertised discount is real.

Shopping during sales provides an opportunity for you to be a smart consumer and stretch your clothing budget. Before buying sales items, learn the store's return policy, because some sales are final.

Labels and Hangtags

Labels and hangtags help you make smart clothing decisions. They tell you what to expect from a garment and how to care for it properly.

Labels

Labels are cloth tags providing legally required information about the garments. By U.S. law, labels must state the fiber content, manufacturer, country of origin, and care instructions. They may also list the fabric construction, special finishes, performance standards, size, and brand name.

Clothing is made and sold all over the world. Labeling requirements apply to the country in which the apparel is sold, not made. For instance, a shirt is produced in China, but sold in Canada. The shirt label must meet Canada's label laws, not China's.

Labels are a permanent part of a garment and must be secure enough to withstand cleaning. Labels are not visible during wear. They are usually at the back of the neckline or along a side seam of shirts, tops, and dresses. Look for labels at the center back of the waistband of skirts and slacks. Some garments have the required information printed on the fabric, usually on the inside near the neck.

Hangtags

Hangtags are small, detachable signs providing size, price, style number, guarantees, and special features. They are on the outside of a garment. Hangtags are not a legal requirement, but often include some label information. Most manufacturers use hangtags as marketing pieces to explain an item's benefits to consumers. Always remove hangtags before wearing garments.

Compare Price, Quality, and Fit

Comparison shopping means comparing similar garments and prices online and in different stores before purchase. By taking the time to comparison shop, you can get the best clothing value for your money. The Internet is a good resource for comparison shopping. Then when you view newspaper ads or visit stores, you are ready to compare pricing. If the online price is less, you may decide to purchase the item through a website after trying it on in a store. Compare nationally advertised brands with lesser-known brands. Lesser-known brands often cost less. If the quality is the same, the lesser-known brand might be a better buy.

In clothing, *quality* refers to the construction of a garment and the way it performs during wearing. Terms describing levels of quality are *high*, *medium*, and *low* (or *poor*). A garment of poor quality will not perform as well as a high-quality one. Higher-quality garments have better construction, fit well, and last longer. Quality is often, but not always, related to price. A *bargain* is buying the highest quality item for the lowest price.

Decide which level of quality meets your needs. An expensive, but well-made, coat is a good buy if you plan to wear it for several seasons. On the other hand, you will most likely only wear a fad shirt for a short time. In that case, one of lower quality and price is probably your best buy.

Evaluating Fit

A garment may look great in an ad or store display. If it does not fit you well, however, it is not a good buy because you will not wear it. The only way to know how a garment fits you is to try it on. Try clothes on with the underclothes and shoes you plan to wear with them.

Look at all views in the dressing room mirror. Move around and sit down to check the feel and look. Can you reach and stretch without straining the fabric? Is the garment too tight or too loose in some areas? Do the armholes dig into your body?

Because sizes vary by manufacturer, you may need to try on several sizes to find the proper fit. Some quality guidelines for evaluating quality and fit are in **22-18**.

Guidelines for Evaluating Quality and Fit

Guidelines for buying shirts and tops

When trying on shirts and tops, check to see that

- there is ample room across the chest or bust, back, and shoulders.
- shoulder seams come to the end of the shoulder bone.
- sleeves are the correct length.
- the neckline is comfortable; not too tight or too loose. When the neckline is buttoned, you can slide the index finger easily between the collar and neck.
- armholes are large enough for arms to move freely.
- collars have even, sharp points.
- topstitching is smooth and straight.
- buttons are sewn on securely and placed directly under well-made buttonholes.
- cuffs are neat, even, and fit comfortably around wrists.
- pockets are sewn securely and are flat without wrinkles.

Guidelines for buying dresses and skirts

When trying on dresses or skirts, check to see that

- the fabric feels good on your body.
- you can bend over and sit comfortably in it.
- it hangs straight from the waistband without cupping under the hips.
- the garment's waist fits snugly at your natural waistline.
- the waistline does not roll up—it rolls when too tight in the hip area.
- if darts are present, they point toward the highest point of the bust.
- zippers work smoothly and have a lock tab.
- the seams and hems are straight and wide enough to alter, if necessary.

Guidelines for buying pants and jeans

When trying on pants and jeans, check to see that

- the seat area fits smoothly without bagging or binding.
- you can walk and sit comfortably in them.
- the crotch length is appropriate.
- the waistband has a double thickness of fabric.
- there is reinforced stitching at bottom of zipper and corner of pockets.
- any topstitching is straight.
- the zipper has a locking pull tab so it will not unzip by itself.
- seams are straight and without puckers.
- the length is attractive for your height and for current fashion.

22-18 Use these guidelines to find quality garments that fit you well.

Alterations

What if you find a garment you really like, but it does not fit well? You may be able to alter it for a better fit. Changes made in the size, length, or style of a garment are **alterations**. You may be able to make a garment longer, shorter, smaller, or larger. If you sew, lengthening or shortening a garment, shortening sleeves, or taking in seams are simple alterations. If you want to purchase a garment needing minor alterations, check the following:

* To increase the size of a garment, the seams must be wide enough to let them out.
* To make a garment longer, the hem width must be ample to let it down.

Some stores offer alterations as a paid customer service, **22-19**. Major alterations, such as changing a neckline or adjusting a garment for shoulder width, may not be worth the alteration cost.

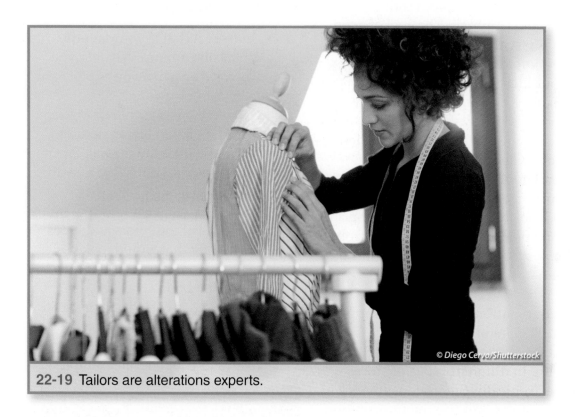

© Diego Cervo/Shutterstock

22-19 Tailors are alterations experts.

Reading Review

1. List one advantage and one disadvantage of shopping for clothes on the Internet.
2. Stores that sell just one type of clothes are _____.
3. True or false. You may not be able to return clothes you purchase on sale.
4. What information is required by law on a garment label?
5. Name three factors to evaluate when making a clothing purchase.

Chapter Summary

Section 22-1. The elements of design are color, line, texture, and form. Choose colors that enhance your natural skin tone and hair color. All of the design elements can be used in fashion design to create certain looks and illusions. Select garments with lines, textures, and forms that flatter your body type. The principles of design are balance, proportion, rhythm, and emphasis. The goal of good design is visual harmony.

Section 22-2. You need clothes to suit your lifestyle, activities, and climate or seasons. Knowing how to identify and choose styles, fashions, classics, and fads helps you achieve a well-rounded wardrobe. Complete a wardrobe inventory to analyze the clothes and accessories you have and what you need. Choosing garments that mix and match helps you expand your wardrobe. Different accessories dress an outfit up or down.

Section 22-3. You get the most from your clothing budget by shopping wisely. This involves knowing the advantages and disadvantages of shopping in different types of stores and electronically. Smart consumers watch for sales and use the information on garment labels and hangtags. Comparison shopping is necessary to know the general cost of items and help you find bargains. Learn to recognize quality and proper fit in the clothes you buy.

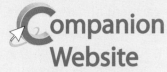

Companion Website
www.g-wlearning.com

Check your understanding of the main concepts for Chapter 22 at the website.

Critical Thinking

1. **Analyze.** What is your favorite article of clothing? What do you like to wear when you really want to be comfortable?

2. **Debate.** Why is such importance placed on name-brand clothing? What role does the media play in name-brand hype? What role do celebrities play?

3. **Produce.** Create a folder containing examples of the colors and types of clothing that would look best on you. Consider your skin tone, hair color, body type, and the illusions you wish to create. Write a short description about why each element or principle of design relates to your chosen examples.

Common Core

College and Career Readiness

4. **Reading.** Read the labels and hangtags, if you kept them, for the clothing in your closet. Make sure you

understand the care instructions so you do not ruin the garment by cleaning it improperly.

5. **Math.** Think of several articles of clothing for which you remember the prices you paid for them. Pick one that you wear often and one that you seldom wear. Estimate how often you wear each piece in a year. (*Hint*: if you wear a pair of pants twice each week, you wear them about 104 times [2 x 52 = 104].) Then divide the cost of the item by the number of times you think you wear it to find the *cost per wearing*. Using the same example, if you paid $55 for the pants, the cost per wearing in a year is $.53 ($55 ÷ 104 = $.53). Compare the cost per wearing of the garment worn more often to the one worn less often.

6. **Writing.** Use online or print resources to find pictures of six garments that could be mixed and matched. Mount the pictures on paper. Determine all the outfits you could make from combining them differently. List accessories you could use to give different looks to each outfit.

7. **Speaking and Writing.** Help your family members take an inventory of their wardrobes. If possible, ask them to give you any clothing they no longer wear. Donate all the clothing to a charitable organization, or hold a rummage sale and donate the proceeds to a local charity.

Technology

8. **Online research.** Practice comparison shopping online for a garment or accessory you want. Determine the website with the best pricing and lowest delivery fee. How does it compare to the price you would pay in a store?

Journal Writing

9. Write an entry in your journal about your favorite colors. Examine why you like them. How do they make you feel? Have your favorite colors changed over time? If so, why?

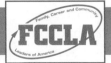 ## FCCLA

10. Use the *FCCLA Planning Process* to plan a fashion show that displays positive and negative examples of dress for different occasions, such as dressing for job interviews. Ask local retail organizations to donate clothing in exchange for free advertising. Charge a fee for the event and donate the funds to a local organization that provides clothes for homeless and/or unemployed people. Apply for national recognition through the *FCCLA National Community Service Program Award*. See your adviser for information as needed.

Chapter 23
Fibers, Fabrics, and Sewing Tools

Sections

College and Career Readiness

Reading Prep
Make a list of everything you already know about the topic of this chapter. As you read each section, check off the items on your list that are covered in the chapter.

Concept Organizer

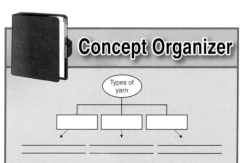

Use a diagram like the one shown to list the types of yarn and how they are made.

Companion Website
Print out the concept organizer for Chapter 23 at the website.

Companion Website
www.g-wlearning.com

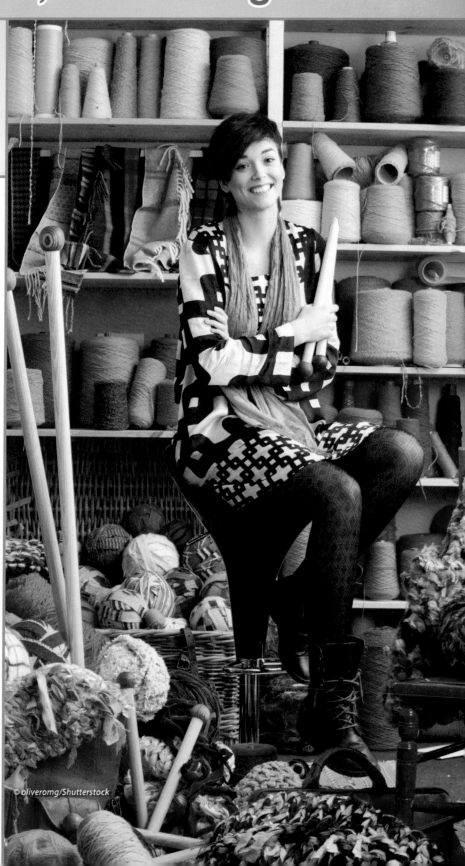

© oliveromg/Shutterstock

Fibers and Fabrics

Objectives

After studying this section, you will be able to
- **classify** fibers as natural or manufactured.
- **determine** how different fabrics are constructed.
- **explain** the functions of various fabric finishes.

Key Terms

fibers	protein fibers	combination
yarns	manufactured fibers	weaving
fabrics	spinneret	knitting
natural fibers	microfibers	finish
cellulose	blend	

Why does your wool sweater feel warmer than your cotton shirt? Why is denim stronger than satin? Why do some garments wrinkle and others do not? Answers to these questions can be found in this chapter. By learning about fibers and fabrics, you will be able to make wise clothing decisions.

Fibers

Fibers are hairlike strands that can be twisted together to form yarns. **Yarns** are continuous strands of fibers. **Fabrics** are the different materials made by weaving or knitting yarns or pressing fibers together.

Look closely at a piece of loosely knit fabric to see how fibers, yarns, and fabrics are related, **23-1**. First, pull a *thread* from the fabric. This is a yarn. Then untwist the yarn. These hairlike strands are the fibers. Fibers may be continuous strands called *filaments* or short lengths called *staple fibers*.

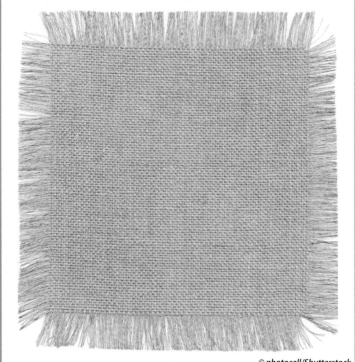

© photocell/Shutterstock

23-1 This piece of burlap clearly shows the yarns in the fabric's weave.

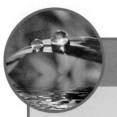

Go Green

Natural-Fiber Fabrics

Fabrics made from natural fibers and raw materials are considered much more environmentally friendly than those made from chemicals. One reason is that natural fibers are *biodegradable*, meaning they eventually decay into very small parts by natural processes. Biodegradable materials help keep the landfills small and contribute much less to pollution. Man-made manufactured fibers primarily use petroleum-based chemicals that behave more like plastic and are not biodegradable.

The characteristics of fibers determine the quality of the yarn and the fabrics. Fibers have certain properties that influence the strength, texture, absorbency, warmth, and shrinkage of fabrics. The properties of a fiber depend on its source. Fibers come from both natural and man-made chemical sources.

Natural Fibers

Natural fibers are those from plant or animal sources. The quality of natural fibers can vary depending on the type of plant or animal and the growing conditions. All natural fibers must go through cleaning and processing before they are made into yarns. Natural fibers have special properties that cannot be exactly duplicated by science, **23-2**.

Cellulosic fibers are those from plant sources because **cellulose** is the substance forming the main part of all plants' cell walls. Cellulose is used in making various products, including paper from wood. Cotton, flax, and ramie are the primary natural cellulosic fibers used to make clothing fabrics.

Fibers from animal sources are called **protein fibers**. Wool and silk are the primary protein fibers. Natural fibers are staple length, except for silk, which is a long filament fiber obtained from unraveling the cocoons of silkworms.

Other protein fibers are called *specialty hair fibers*. These include mohair and cashmere from the goat family; angora from the rabbit family; and camel, llama, alpaca, vicuna, and guanaco hair from the camel family. Because specialty hair fibers are hard to obtain, the fabrics they are made into are more expensive than wool.

Manufactured Fibers

Manufactured fibers are made in a laboratory through chemical processes. The two types of manufactured fibers are cellulosic and noncellulosic. Rayon, acetate, and lyocell are cellulosic manufactured fibers because they are made with cellulose from cotton linter or wood pulp.

Noncellulosic fibers are also called *synthetics* because they are man-made using chemical compounds. Nylon, polyester, and acrylic are examples of these. Different raw materials and chemicals produce manufactured fibers with distinct characteristics, **23-3**. The following process is basically the same for most manufactured fibers:

1. Solid raw materials are changed to a liquid form.
2. The liquid is forced through a **spinneret**, which is a small nozzle with many tiny holes.
3. The forced liquid hardens in a long filament form.

\multicolumn{4}{c}{**Natural Fibers**}			

Fiber	Source	Advantages	Disadvantages
\multicolumn{4}{c}{**Cellulosic Fibers**}			
Cotton	Boll of cotton plant	Inexpensive Comfortable—cool in warm weather Absorbent Withstands high temperature Dyes and prints well	Wrinkles easily unless a special finish is added Shrinks in hot water if not treated Mildews if put in damp storage area or put away damp
Linen	Flax plant	Strongest natural fiber Comfortable Smooth, lustrous Withstands high temperature Durable	Can be expensive Wrinkles easily unless treated Creases hard to remove Shines if ironed on right side Poor resistance to mildew and perspiration
Ramie	China grass plant	Strong and durable Naturally resists stains and bacteria Lustrous Dries quickly	Wrinkles easily Stiff and wirelike Coarse
\multicolumn{4}{c}{**Protein Fibers**}			
Wool	Sheep fleece	Warmest of all fibers Highly absorbent Wrinkle resistant Creases well Durable	Will shrink and mat when heat and moisture are applied Special care needed—most fabrics must be dry cleaned Attracts insects like moths
Silk	Cocoon of the silkworm	Luxurious look and feel Strong, but lightweight Very absorbent Resists wrinkling	Usually requires dry cleaning Yellows with age Spotted by water unless specially treated Expensive

23-2 This table summarizes advantages and disadvantages of the primary natural fibers.

Microfibers are extremely fine filaments that make extra smooth, soft, and silky fabrics. Because the filaments can be packed so close together, they form an effective wind barrier in clothing. Fabrics made from microfibers allow moisture vapor to escape, but keep the wearer dry and comfortable. Most of the manufactured fibers can be made into microfibers.

Yarns

A yarn is made by combining staple fibers or filaments into thicker strands. Yarns vary in size, stretch, and texture. There are three types of yarns—spun yarns, monofilament yarns, and multifilament yarns, **23-4**.

564 Unit 7 The Clothes You Wear

Manufactured Fibers

Cellulosic Fiber	Advantages	Disadvantages
Rayon (the first manufactured fiber)	Inexpensive Comfortable Dyes and drapes well	Poor strength Sensitive to heat May shrink or stretch; should be dry cleaned Wrinkles unless treated
Acetate	Inexpensive Luxurious feel and appearance Dyes and drapes well	Sensitive to heat Needs special cleaning care Poor strength
Lyocell	Soft and comfortable Strong and absorbent Biodegradable Dyes and drapes well	Can be machine washed and dried May mildew Wrinkles somewhat
Noncellulosic Fiber	**Advantages**	**Disadvantages**
Nylon	Strong and durable, yet lightweight Elastic, but keeps its shape Quick drying; does not need ironing Dyes easily	May pill Builds up static electricity Does not absorb moisture Sensitive to heat
Polyester	Resists wrinkling Strong and durable Resists moths, shrinking, and sunlight Dyes easily	Does not absorb moisture Does not breath, so uncomfortable May pill Builds up static electricity Holds oily stains
Olefin	Lightweight Resists wrinkling Resists soil, mildew, and insects Strong and durable	Difficult to dye Sensitive to heat Does not absorb moisture
Acrylic	Soft and warm Retains shape Resists wrinkles Resists sunlight and chemicals	May pill Builds up static electricity Does not absorb moisture
Modacrylic	Flame resistant Resists shrinking and chemicals Retains shape Quick drying Dyes and drapes well	Sensitive to heat Builds up static electricity Does not absorb moisture
Spandex	Elastic and durable Retains shape Resistant to sunlight, oil, insects, and perspiration Quick drying	Sensitive to heat Sensitive to chlorine

23-3 This table lists the advantages and disadvantages of the most common manufactured fibers.

Spun yarns are made by using short, natural fibers or manufactured fibers cut to staple lengths. Spun yarns have surfaces because some of the fiber ends stick out, creating a fuzzy look.

Filament yarns are made by twisting filaments together and winding them onto spools. *Monofilament yarns* are made from a single filament. Silk is the only natural filament fiber that can be made into monofilament yarn. *Multifilament yarns* are made from 5 to 100 filaments spun into yarns that tend to be stronger and more durable.

Fabrics

Fabrics are made with yarns from natural or manufactured fibers—and often from both types. Some yarns are made from a **blend** of two or more very different fibers. A **combination** contains two or more yarns that vary in fiber composition, content, and/or twist level.

Blends and combinations create fabrics with better performance features. For instance, cotton is cool and comfortable, but it wrinkles easily and shrinks. Polyester resists wrinkles, but is uncomfortable to wear in hot weather. A shirt that is a polyester/cotton blend combines the positive traits of both fibers, which creates a cool, comfortable shirt that does not wrinkle.

Wovens and Knits

Weaving and knitting are the most common fabric construction techniques. **Weaving** is the process of interlacing yarns at right angles to each other to produce a fabric. Weaving is done on machines

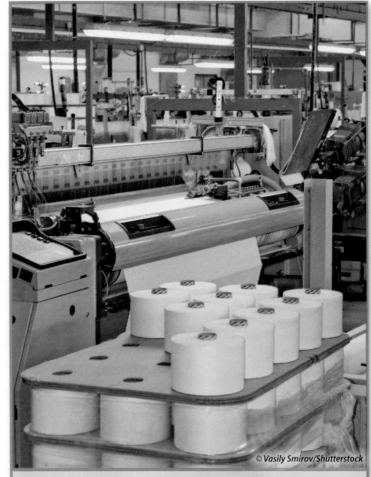
© Vasily Smirov/Shutterstock

23-4 Fibers are spun and twisted into yarns. The spools of yarn are then ready for dyeing or manufacturing fabrics.

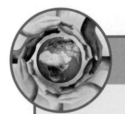

Global Connections

Egyptian Linen

Scientists believe that linen has been used since 5000 B.C. based on discoveries of linen fabrics and looms in ancient tombs. Ancient Egyptians used linen exclusively for their clothing, as well as for embalming their dead—known today as *mummies*. Cotton was unavailable and flax plants were abundant throughout the area.

From records left by ancient Egyptians, it is known that they made linen from the stalks of hardy flax plants growing along the Nile River. The stalks were soaked in water to release the fibers, which were beaten until soft enough to be twisted into yarn. The flax yarn was then woven into fabric on wooden looms. Egypt is still known for its fine linen fabrics today.

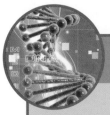

Science Connections

Interfacing Fabrics

Interfacing fabrics are materials inserted between layers of a garment to thicken or stiffen it. Practically all consist of manufactured fibers, but a few have natural fibers. Most are nonwoven fabrics having no grain, so pieces can be cut in any direction. Many are *fusible*, meaning they have a chemical resin on one side that melts and secures the interfacing to a fabric when pressed with a warm iron. Fusible interfacings are also used as stabilizers for embroidery.

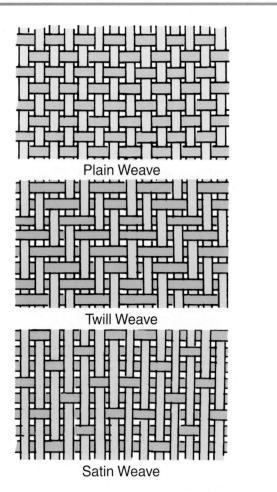

Plain Weave

Twill Weave

Satin Weave

© Goodheart-Willcox Publisher

23-5 Different patterns of interlacing yarns are used to create the three basic weaves.

called *looms*. Many different weaving effects can be created. The three basic weaves are the plain, twill, and satin weaves, **23-5**.

The *plain weave* uses an over one, under one pattern. Most plain weave fabrics are durable and strong. They are usually easy to sew.

The *twill weave* is made when yarns in one direction float (pass) over two or more yarns in the other direction. Each float begins one or more yarns over from the last one. This creates a diagonal line or wale in the fabric. Twill weave fabrics are durable and resist wrinkles.

The *satin weave* is created by floating a yarn from one direction over four or more yarns from the other direction and then under one yarn. Each float begins two yarns over from where the last float began. This creates a fabric with a very smooth, shiny surface. The satin weave is not very durable and it tends to snag.

Knitting is done by looping yarns together. These loops can be varied to create different patterns and textures. Knitted fabrics are versatile. They can be made from any fiber and any yarn. They are usually comfortable, easy-care fabrics. Knitting by hand using long knitting needles is a popular hobby.

Nonwoven fabrics are made by pressing fibers together with heat, pressure, or chemicals. Yarn is not used, and nonwovens have many uses, such as in upholstery and filtration. Some are disposable. Nonwoven fabrics used in clothing include felt, faux fur, and vinyl.

Finishes

A **finish** is a treatment that is given to fibers, yarns, or fabrics that can improve the look, feel, or performance of a fabric. Finishes can be added to yarns or fabric, depending on the final use of the garment. Some common finishes are described in **23-6**.

Fabric Finishes	
Finish	**Purpose**
Antistatic	Prevents static electricity so clothes will not cling during wear
Crease-resistant, durable press, permanent press	Help fabrics resist wrinkles
Flame resistant	Cuts off the oxygen supply or changes the chemical makeup of fibers as fabric burns
Mildew resistant	Prevents mildew
Mercerization	Improves the luster, strength, and absorbency of cotton and rayon fabrics
Moth-repellent	Repels moth larvae and some other insect pests
Preshrunk	Prevents shrinkage beyond three percent, unless otherwise stated
Sanforized®	Prevents shrinkage beyond one percent in either direction
Scotchgard®	Repels oil and water
Soil-release	Allows fabrics to be more easily *wetted* to help detergents release soil
Water-repellent	Helps fabrics resist water

23-6 Different finishes provide various functions on fabrics. Some finishes are created mechanically and others are made with chemicals.

Reading Review

1. How do the characteristics of fibers determine the quality of a fabric?
2. List the steps of producing manufactured fibers.
3. List the three types of yarns.
4. What is a finish?

Sewing Tools and Equipment

Objectives

After studying this section, you will be able to
- **identify** measuring, marking, cutting, and sewing tools.
- **explain** how and when to use the different measuring, marking, cutting, and sewing tools.
- **point out** the parts of a sewing machine.
- **discuss** the functions of different parts of a sewing machine.

Key Terms		
sewing gauge	thimbles	overlock stitches
shears	sergers	

Just as a builder uses certain tools to construct a house, you need certain tools to construct a sewing project. These include all the sewing tools and mechanical equipment you use to make a garment or project. Each piece helps you perform the various tasks involved. Measuring, marking, cutting, sewing, and pressing are all tasks that require a sewing tool or specific piece of equipment.

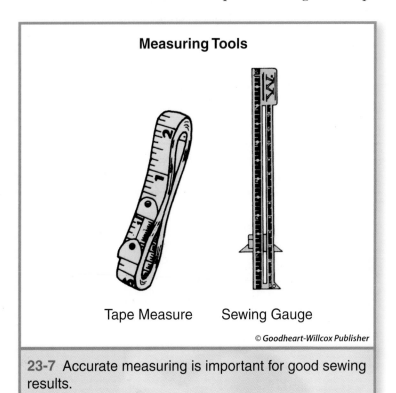

Measuring Tools

Tape Measure   Sewing Gauge

© Goodheart-Willcox Publisher

23-7 Accurate measuring is important for good sewing results.

Measuring Tools

For accurate sewing, measuring tools are a must. Some measuring tools include both standard and metric measurements. Helpful measuring tools include a tape measure and sewing gauge, **23-7**.

A *tape measure* is used to take body measurements. It is also used to measure fabric and pattern pieces. Tape measures are 60 inches long and made of plastic or strong fabric that does not stretch or tear.

A **sewing gauge** is a six-inch ruler with a sliding marker. It is used to measure short distances such as hems. A sewing gauge is a very useful measuring tool you may find you often need.

Marking Tools

Tracing wheels, dressmaker's carbon paper, tailor's chalk, and *tailor's pencils* are marking tools, **23-8.** They are used to transfer pattern markings to the fabric. These markings help you put the pattern pieces together correctly.

When using a marking tool, choose one with a similar color to your fabric yet still visible. This prevents the color from showing through on the right side. Make sure the marks you use can be washed out of the fabric. Use light pressure on tracing wheels to avoid damaging work surfaces and tearing your pattern.

Cutting Tools

Shears, scissors, pinking shears, and seam rippers are all cutting tools, **23-9.** Many people think shears and scissors are the same. They are not. **Shears** have extra-long blades and larger, bent handles for comfort and holding your fabric flat for more accurate cutting. Use shears to cut pattern pieces from fabric.

Scissors are usually short. The handles have small, matching holes. They are used to trim seams, clip around curves, and open buttonholes.

Pinking shears have a zigzag cutting edge. They are used to give seam edges a finished look. They can also be used to achieve a decorative look on nonwoven fabrics. Do not use pinking shears to cut garment pieces from fabrics. The uneven edge would be difficult to follow when sewing.

A *seam ripper* can be used to undo mistakes in sewing or to remove basting stitches. Since seam rippers are sharp, use them with care. They can injure you or cause damage to fabric.

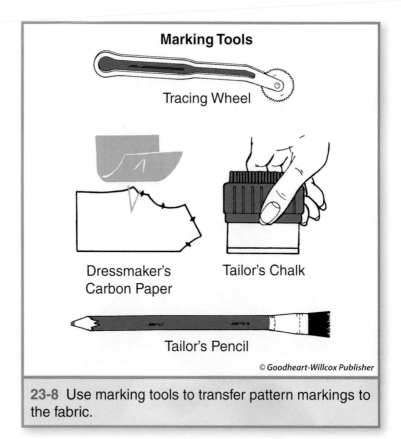

Marking Tools

Tracing Wheel

Dressmaker's Carbon Paper

Tailor's Chalk

Tailor's Pencil

© Goodheart-Willcox Publisher

23-8 Use marking tools to transfer pattern markings to the fabric.

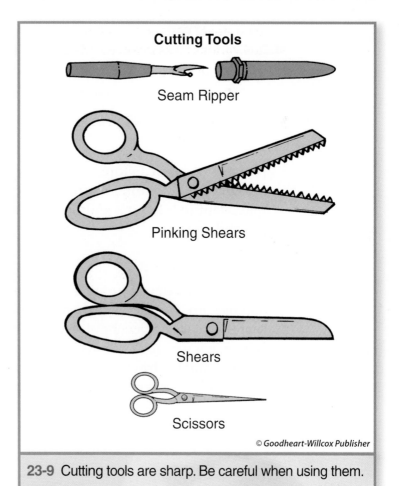

Cutting Tools

Seam Ripper

Pinking Shears

Shears

Scissors

© Goodheart-Willcox Publisher

23-9 Cutting tools are sharp. Be careful when using them.

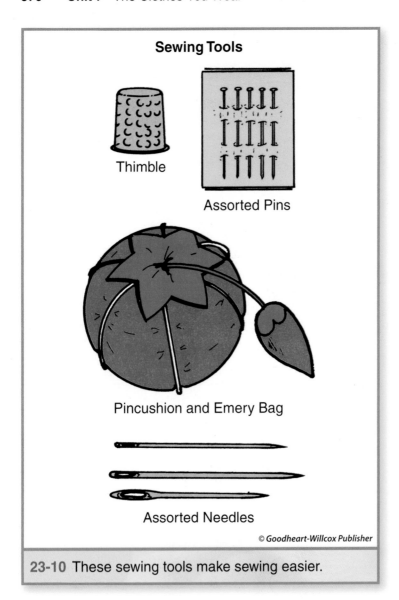

Sewing Tools

Thimble

Assorted Pins

Pincushion and Emery Bag

Assorted Needles

© Goodheart-Willcox Publisher

23-10 These sewing tools make sewing easier.

Sewing Tools

Sewing tools are the items you use as you stitch your project's fabric pieces together. These items include needles, pins, pincushions, and thimbles, **23-10**.

Needles

Needles are used for hand sewing. They come in many sizes and types. A package of assorted sizes would be a good choice to meet your hand-sewing needs. Fine needles are for delicate fabrics. Medium needles are for medium-weight fabrics. Coarser (large) needles are for heavier-weight fabrics.

Needles range in size from 1 to 12. The smaller numbers are coarser needles, and the larger numbers are finer needles. A size 1 needle is larger than a size 12 needle. For most hand-sewing tasks, a size 7 or 8 needle works well depending on the fabric.

Pins

Straight pins are used to hold patterns to fabric before and during cutting. They also hold pieces of fabric together before sewing. Pins come in boxes or in paper folders. You may want to buy pins with large plastic or glass heads. They are easy to see and use.

Pincushions

If you have ever dropped pins, you know how difficult they are to find and pick up. *Pincushions* are a handy place to store pins. They come in many shapes and sizes. Never put pins in your mouth. A wrist pincushion is a convenient way to keep pins handy.

The small, strawberry-shaped bag attached to some pincushions is an *emery bag*. An emery bag is used to remove rough spots or a dull point from a needle or pin. Do this by pushing the needle or pin into the bag several times.

Thimbles

Thimbles are used to help push the needle through thick or tightly woven fabrics when hand sewing. A thimble should be worn on your middle finger on your sewing hand. It should feel comfortable—not too snug and not too loose. The dents on thimbles hold the end of the needle as it is pushed through the fabric. Thimbles used for sewing are made of metal or plastic.

Sewing Equipment

The most important piece of sewing equipment is the sewing machine. Sewing machines vary. There are different models and brands, and some have special features. Pressing equipment is also needed when finishing a project.

Life Connections

Using Sewing Tools and Equipment for Crafts

Crafting activities involve making things in a skillful way by using your hands. Many people enjoy crafting, which is different from sewing clothing, but usually requires some of the same tools. Crafts can include small sewing projects, such as making place mats, table runners, toys, wearable art, blankets, pillows, totes, scarves, or holiday décor—to name just a few. They are sometimes referred to as *do-it-yourself* projects. Crafts are a fun and creative way to design and make useful items for yourself or to give as gifts.

Research Activity

The Internet has many websites with excellent craft ideas and instructions. Do some online research to find a project that interests you. Determine the materials, tools, and equipment you will need to complete it. If you complete the project, bring it in for display.

The Sewing Machine

It is important to learn how your sewing machine works. This also includes how to use it safely and maintain it properly. Start by reading the use and care manual for the sewing machines in your lab. This manual shows you the parts of the sewing machine, explains their functions, and describes how they work. It describes your machine's special features. The manual also provides information on how to prepare and maintain your machine for best sewing results.

All conventional sewing machines have the same basic parts. Some sewing machine basics include threading the machine, controlling the speed, and stopping at the desired point. Your instructor will help you learn how to thread your machine, wind bobbins, and create basic stitches.

Getting to Know the Sewing Machine

A sewing machine is a complex machine. Knowing the names of the parts and their functions are keys to understanding how a sewing machine works.

The parts of a sewing machine are shown in **23-11**. As you read the following descriptions, use the numbers in parentheses to locate each part in the diagram.

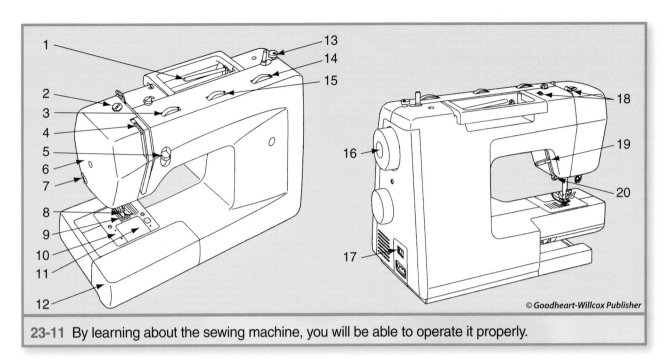

© Goodheart-Willcox Publisher

23-11 By learning about the sewing machine, you will be able to operate it properly.

The *head* is the top part of the machine. It holds most of the moving parts that help the machine operate.

The *spool pin* (1) holds the spool of thread.

The *presser foot pressure adjustment* (2) controls the amount of pressure the presser foot places against the feed system.

The *needle thread tension dial* (3) lets you set the tension for your particular project. Your fabric, stitch, and thread will determine the tension setting you need.

The *take-up lever* (4) controls the flow of needle thread. It must be at its highest position each time you start to sew. If it is not, the thread will be pulled away from the needle as the lever rises. Then you will have to thread the needle again.

The *reverse-stitch button* (5) lets you stitch backward.

The *face plate* (6) swings open for access to the movable parts and the light.

The *thread cutter* (7) is on the back of the presser bar for convenience.

The *presser foot* (8) holds fabric against the feed system teeth.

The *feed dog* (9) moves fabric under the presser foot.

The *needle plate* (10) has guidelines to help you sew straight, even seams. It also supports the fabric during sewing.

The *bobbin plate cover* (11) covers the bobbin and bobbin case.

The *removable extension table* (12) lets you change from flat bed to free arm. This feature is convenient for stitching tubular pieces such as cuffs and pant legs.

The *bobbin winder* (13) guides the thread when filling the bobbin with thread.

The *stitch length dial* (14) controls the length of the stitches.

The *stitch width dial* (15) controls the width of zigzag stitching. It also positions the needle for straight stitching.

The *handwheel* (16) controls the movement of the take-up lever and needle. It turns as the machine runs. You can move the needle up and down by turning the wheel with your hand.

The *power and light switch* (17) turns on the machine and sewing light at the same time.

The *thread guides* (18) lead the thread to the needle.

The *presser foot lifter* (19) allows you to raise and lower the presser foot.

The *needle clamp* (20) holds the needle in place.

Sewing machines use two threads: the needle thread and the bobbin thread. The needle thread runs from the spool pin. It goes around the tension discs and through the take-up lever, thread guides, and needle. The bobbin thread runs from the bobbin plate up through the throat plate. As you sew, these two threads interlock to hold fabric pieces together.

Before sewing your project, practice sewing on some fabric scraps to get the feel of sewing on material. Because most sewing is done with two layers of fabric, practice with two scraps.

Sergers

Sergers are high-speed sewing machines that stitch, trim, and finish seams in one step. Originally used by professionals, smaller sergers are now available for home use, too. Sergers are popular with home sewers because they save time. While sewing a seam, it also removes extra fabric and keeps the edges from unraveling by making **overlock stitches**.

A home serger uses from two to five threads and one or two needles. They differ from sewing machines, which use just one needle and one spool of thread. Sergers vary in their designs and operations, **23-12**.

Pressing Equipment

If you press as you sew, your garment will have a neat, professional look. The steam iron and ironing board are the basic items of pressing equipment. Most steam irons have a wide range of temperature settings. Make sure to use the correct temperature for the fabric you are pressing. Avoid ironing over pins. They can scratch the bottom of the iron. The ironing board should be sturdy and covered with a tight-fitting, padded cover.

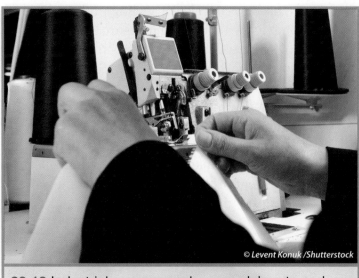

© Levent Konuk /Shutterstock

23-12 Industrial sergers can be very elaborate and utilize up to 100 thread spools.

Reading Review

1. Name four types of marking tools.
2. How are needles sized?
3. What is the purpose of the use and care manual that comes with a sewing machine?
4. Why should you avoid ironing over pins?

Chapter Summary

Section 23-1. The clothes you wear are made from a variety of fibers. Some fibers are natural fibers and come from plant, animal, and mineral sources. Other fibers are manufactured fibers and are made in a laboratory. Each fiber has certain characteristics that affect the appearance, feel, and care requirements of your garments. Fibers are formed into yarns. The yarns are then woven or knitted into fabrics. Different types of weaves and knits are used to create different kinds of fabrics. Fabrics may be treated with finishes to achieve certain characteristics.

Section 23-2. Many different tools are used to complete a sewing project. Some tools are used to measure. Other tools are needed to mark and cut fabric and put fabric pieces together. Still other tools are used to press sewing projects to give them a neat, finished look. You need to know what each tool does and how to use it correctly. This is especially true of the sewing machine. Using sewing equipment properly will make sewing easier and give you better results.

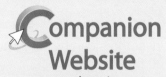

Companion Website
www.g-wlearning.com

Check your understanding of the main concepts for Chapter 23 at the website.

Critical Thinking

1. **Analyze.** Would you buy clothes made from animal skins and furs? Why or why not?
2. **Determine.** Make a list of your activities. Then decide what type of fiber/fabric would be the best choice for garments worn for those activities.
3. **Assess.** Imagine you are creating a mini sewing kit, and you can only choose four sewing tools. Which tools would you choose? Why?

Common Core

College and Career Readiness

4. **Compare.** Check the care labels in six of your garments. Make a list of all the fibers used for each garment. Compare your list with your classmates' lists. What seems to be the most popular fiber?
5. **Reading.** Study a use and care manual to find all the parts on a sewing machine in your classroom. Read about the purpose of each part.
6. **Speaking.** Imagine you work for the sewing machine manufacturer of the sewing machines in your lab. Demonstrate the use of the sewing machine to the class.

7. **Listening.** Interview a sewing machine sales associate about the features on various sewing machines.

Technology

8. **Electronic presentation.** Research computerized sewing machines. Prepare an electronic presentation about how they compare to standard sewing machines. Describe any advantages and disadvantages.

Journal Writing

9. Check the tags in several pieces of your favorite clothing to determine which fabrics you like most. What types of fabrics do you prefer? What types of fabrics do you least like? As a journal entry, compare the fabrics from your comfortable clothes with those you wear for special occasions.

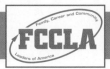

FCCLA

10. Research advancements in fiber or fabric technology, such as microfibers or nanofibers. Use the speaking and presentation guidelines in the *FCCLA Dynamic Leadership* program to develop an oral and visual presentation about your chosen fiber or fabric to share with the class. See your adviser for more information.

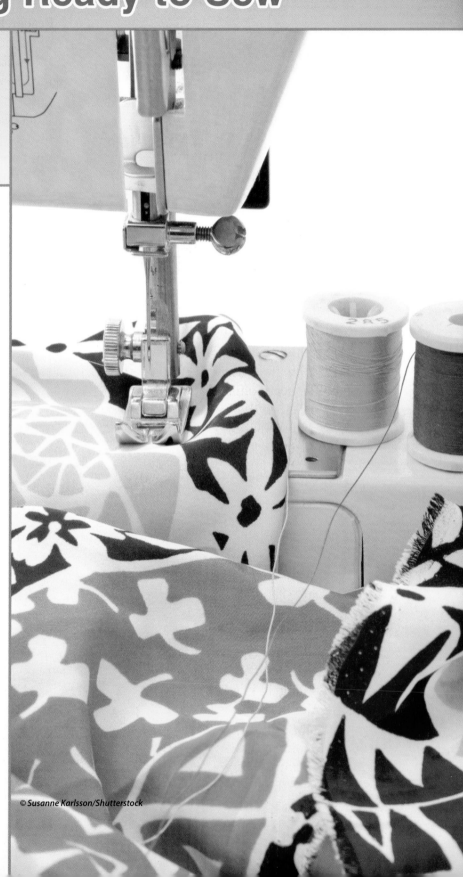

Chapter 24
Getting Ready to Sew

Sections

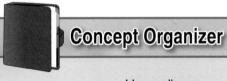

College and Career Readiness

● Reading Prep

Rewrite each chapter objective as a question. As you read, look for the answers to each question. Write the answers in your own words.

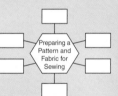

Concept Organizer

Preparing a Pattern and Fabric for Sewing

Use a diagram like the one shown to list the six steps for preparing a pattern and fabric for sewing.

Companion Website

Print out the concept organizer for Chapter 24 at the website.

Companion
Website
www.g-wlearning.com

© Susanne Karlsson/Shutterstock

Planning Your Project

Objectives

After studying this section, you will be able to
- **choose** a pattern and fabric to match your interests and skills.
- **organize** your sewing materials based on pattern envelope information.
- **understand** the directions on a pattern's guide sheet.
- **prepare** patterns and fabrics for sewing.

Key Terms

pattern	cutting lines	grain
multisized patterns	grain line	selvages
notions	adjustment lines	on-grain
fasteners	notches	off-grain
guide sheet	dots	

Sewing, like adding music to your personal media player or creating a drawing with CAD software, is a step-by-step process. Planning and preparing ensures your project is successful. First, you must decide what you are going to make. Next, gather the tools you need to complete your project. Selecting a special fabric helps make your project unique. Finally, you can put your sewing skills to practice.

Your First Sewing Project

Making your first sewing project can be a lot of fun. The item may likely be something you keep for a long time. You can plan to make something to wear, an accessory, or a decoration for your living space. Regardless of what you make, it is good to learn the basics of sewing as a life skill. You can apply the skills you learn to mending garments and creating new ones. Doing so can save money. If you are good at sewing, perhaps this skill can lead to a money-making business.

Global Connections

Different Cultures, Different Clothing

One of the best things about sewing your own clothes is that they can truly reflect you, often better than buying clothing off the rack. Patterns for any piece of clothing you imagine can be found on the Internet and sometimes in fabric store catalogs. If you are interested in making clothes that reflect a certain historical period or culture, there are many options for buying patterns online. Search for traditional or ethnic garments, such as Japanese kimonos, Austrian dirndls, Siberian parkas, the Moroccan burnoose, or even Navajo blouses and skirts. Depending on what you want, another good search term is *vintage patterns*. Happy pattern hunting and creating your personal look!

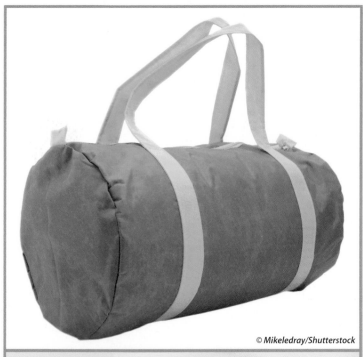

© Mikeledray/Shutterstock

24-1 Kit projects come ready to sew to make a professional-looking item like this gym bag.

Choosing a Project

Your first sewing project may be one your teacher chooses for everyone to learn the essential skills of sewing. You and your classmates will be able to work on the same steps or problems. Through your choice of fabric, notions, and design details, however, you can give your project a one-of-a-kind look.

In some sewing classes, a kit project may be the first item you sew. Using kits is a great way to practice following directions and using a sewing machine. They have everything you need to complete a project using step-by-step directions. You can choose kits that match your sewing skills, and you can learn new techniques as you progress.

Examples of kit projects include shorts and jams, stuffed animals, pillows, blankets, and sports bags, **24-1**.

A **pattern** is a basic model that helps you put together a garment or project. When selecting, look for one that is simple. *Jiffy, Simple to Sew, Very Easy, Step-by-Step,* or *For Beginners* are labels you may see on easy patterns. Often, these patterns have few pattern pieces, and fit loosely. They do not have collars, cuffs, pockets, or pleats. As you gain experience and confidence with sewing, your ability to sew more difficult projects will increase.

Taking Body Measurements

Your *body measurements* are the dimensions of your body. Taking accurate body measurements helps you choose the best garment pattern type and size for you. Taking your own body measurements accurately is extremely difficult, so ask a trusted adult to help you take your measurements. Have the person use a fabric tape measure or string tied snugly around the body area measured, **24-2**. Different measurements are taken for females and males depending on the garment.

- For females, use the bust measurement when choosing a pattern for a dress, blouse, or jacket for best fit. For skirts, slacks, and shorts, use hip measurements. Waistlines are easier to adjust.
- For males, select patterns for slacks or shorts using the waist measurement. To choose shirt patterns, males should use the neck and bent-arm measurements.

Figure Types and Pattern Sizes

People come in a variety of shapes and sizes, and so do patterns. The most important part of choosing a pattern is getting one that fits.

Pattern companies group patterns under *figure types* according to height and proportion. Look at your body profile in a full-length mirror. Then compare your figure with the pattern-catalog descriptions. Decide which figure types and measurements are most like yours and choose your type.

Once you know your figure type, you can easily figure out your pattern size. Just look at the measurement chart in the pattern catalog. Choose pattern sizes by using bust or chest, waist, and hip or seat measurements. There are different sizes in each figure type. Choose the size that matches or is closest to your measurements.

Almost all patterns are multisized. **Multisized patterns** have several sizes printed on the pattern tissue. You simply cut the size that best fits your body measurements. If necessary, you can choose different sizes for different body areas.

The Pattern Envelope

The pattern envelope is more than just a container for your pattern. It offers information you need to know about the pattern. The front of the envelope shows the pattern number, figure type, and size. It also shows a sketch or photograph of the garment or project you plan to make, **24-3**. Sometimes it shows more than one view. These views give you an idea of different designs, details, and fabrics to use.

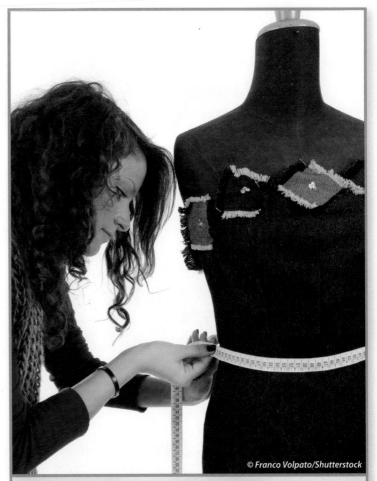

© Franco Volpato/Shutterstock

24-2 Dressmakers also use the same body measurement technique to ensure correct sizing.

Reading Connections

Exploring Patterns

Choosing just the right pattern can be the key to sewing success. Each major pattern company has its own catalogs. The catalogs are often similar in format and size, but the available patterns are different. Sometimes reading about the pattern differences and comparing them can help you choose the best ones for your sewing ability.

A measurement page in the back of a catalog shows all the charts for different pattern sizes. Helpful illustrations show how to take body measurements correctly to select the correct figure type and pattern size. The major pattern companies also sell patterns online. Visit their websites to read about the different types of patterns offered. Patterns are mailed to you after purchase.

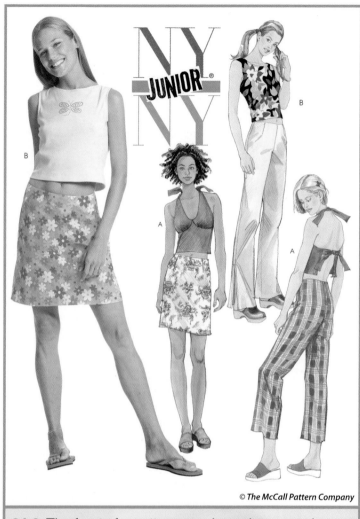

© The McCall Pattern Company

24-3 The front of a pattern envelope shows you how the finished garment or project should look.

For instance, a shirt pattern may show short sleeves, long sleeves, or no sleeves. The envelope contains pattern pieces for all these designs. You can make the one you prefer.

Choosing Fabric and Notions

A chart on the pattern-envelope back tells you how much fabric the pattern requires for making the garment. The chart lists various fabric widths so you can easily find the length you need. It also gives suitable fabric suggestions, and notes any fabrics and designs that are not suitable. See **24-4** to identify other types of information on the back of the pattern envelope.

In addition to fabric, the pattern envelope also indicates the notions needed to finish the project. Notions are the items that become a part of a garment or project. Thread, buttons, snaps, zippers, tapes, trims, and elastic are notions. Buy your project's notions at the same time you buy the fabric to match colors correctly. This way, everything you need is on hand.

Thread

Thread comes in a wide variety of colors and types. If you are using a solid-color fabric, try to select thread that is slightly darker. Thread usually looks lighter when it is stitched into fabric. If you are using a print or plaid fabric, select thread that matches the main color in the print.

The fiber content of thread is just as important as the fiber content in fabric. There are two basic types of thread available. These are polyester or polyester/cotton blend thread and *mercerized cotton* thread. Polyester or polyester/cotton thread is an all-purpose thread that works well with almost all fabrics. It is often used for knits and stretch fabrics because it is strong, stretchable, and prevents seams from breaking during wear.

Mercerized cotton thread is recommended for use on woven fabrics made of natural fibers. Although it sews well, it has limited stretching ability.

Fasteners

Fasteners include zippers, buttons, hooks and eyes, snaps, and hook and loop tape. The type of fastener and amount you need is listed on your

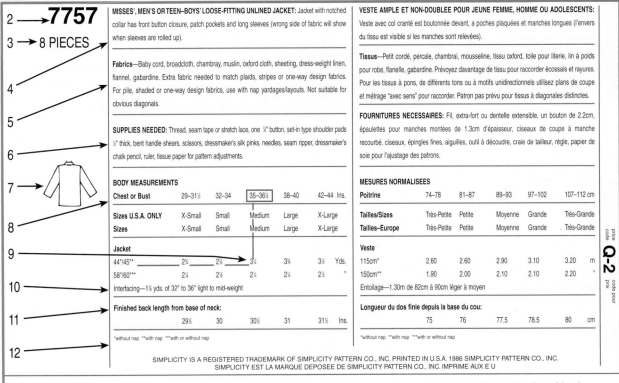

[2] **7757**

[3] 8 PIECES

[4] **MISSES', MEN'S OR TEEN–BOYS' LOOSE-FITTING UNLINED JACKET:** Jacket with notched collar has front button closure, patch pockets and long sleeves (wrong side of fabric will show when sleeves are rolled up).

[5] **Fabrics**—Baby cord, broadcloth, chambray, muslin, oxford cloth, sheeting, dress-weight linen, flannel, gabardine. Extra fabric needed to match plaids, stripes or one-way design fabrics. For pile, shaded or one-way design fabrics, use with nap yardages/layouts. Not suitable for obvious diagonals.

[6] **SUPPLIES NEEDED:** Thread, seam tape or stretch lace, one ⅞" button, set-in type shoulder pads ½" thick, bent handle shears, scissors, dressmaker's silk pinks, needles, seam ripper, dressmaker's chalk pencil, ruler, tissue paper for pattern adjustments.

[7] **BODY MEASUREMENTS**

Chest or Bust	29–31½	32–34	35–36½	38–40	42–44	Ins.
Sizes U.S.A. ONLY [8]	X-Small	Small	Medium	Large	X-Large	
Sizes	X-Small	Small	Medium	Large	X-Large	
Jacket						
44"/45"* [9]	2¾	2⅞	3¼	3⅜	3½	Yds.
58"/60"***	2⅛	2⅛	2¼	2¼	2½	"

[10] Interfacing—1⅜ yds. of 32" to 36" light to mid-weight

[11] **Finished back length from base of neck:**

	29½	30	30½	31	31½	Ins.

[12] *without nap **with nap ***with or without nap

VESTE AMPLE ET NON-DOUBLEE POUR JEUNE FEMME, HOMME OU ADOLESCENTS: Veste avec col cranté est boutonnée devant, a poches plaquées et manches longues (l'envers du tissu est visible si les manches sont relevées).

Tissus—Petit cordé, percale, chambrai, mousseline, tissu oxford, toile pour literie, lin à poids pour robe, flanelle, gabardine. Prévoyez davantage de tissu pour raccorder écossais et rayures. Pour les tissus à pons, de différents tons ou à motifs unidirectionnels utilisez plans de coupe et métrage "avec sens" pour raccorder. Patron pas prévu pour tissus à diagonales distinctes.

FOURNITURES NECESSAIRES: Fil, extra-fort ou dentelle extensible, un bouton de 2.2cm, épaulettes pour manches montées de 1.3cm d'épaisseur, ciseaux de coupe à manche recourbé, ciseaux, épingles fines, aiguilles, outil à découdre, craie de tailleur, règle, papier de soie pour l'ajustage des patrons.

MESURES NORMALISEES

Poitrine	74–78	81–87	89–93	97–102	107–112	cm
Tailles/Sizes	Très-Petite	Petite	Moyenne	Grande	Très-Grande	
Tailles–Europe	Très-Petite	Petite	Moyenne	Grande	Très-Grande	
Veste						
115cm*	2.60	2.60	2.90	3.10	3.20	m
150cm**	1.90	2.00	2.10	2.10	2.20	"

Entoilage—1.30m de 82cm à 90cm léger à moyen

Longueur du dos finie depuis la base du cou:

	75	76	77.5	78.5	80	cm

*without nap **with nap ***with or without nap

price code **Q-2** code pour prix

SIMPLICITY IS A REGISTERED TRADEMARK OF SIMPLICITY PATTERN CO., INC. PRINTED IN U.S.A. 1986 SIMPLICITY PATTERN CO., INC.
SIMPLICITY EST LA MARQUE DEPOSEE DE SIMPLICITY PATTERN CO., INC. IMPRIME AUX E U

1. Foreign language (French) translation.
2. Pattern number.
3. Number of pattern pieces in the envelope. Garments with few pattern pieces are usually easier to make than garments with many pieces.
4. The garment description explains details. You may not be able to see all of these in the photograph or sketch.
5. These fabrics have been selected by the designer as the best ones to use with this pattern. This section also warns you of any problems you may have with certain fabrics. Read it carefully before you select fabric. You may need extra fabric if you choose a large plaid or design that will have to be matched. The salesperson or your teacher can often help you make this decision.
6. These are notions and sewing tools needed to complete your garment. Buy them when you buy your fabric. You can easily match colors of thread, zippers, seam tape, and buttons at that time.
7. The back view shows you how the back will look.
8. Double-check the list of body measurements to be sure you buy the right size.
9. This tells you how much material to buy. Draw a line down from your pattern size. Draw a line across from the view you like and the width of your fabric. Where the lines cross is how much you need.
10. If linings or interfacings are needed, the yardage you need will be listed here.
11. Finished garment measurements.
12. Nap indication.

24-4 The back of a pattern envelope gives you important information. *© Simplicity Pattern Company*

pattern envelope. When you need to use zippers, choose the type and length specified on your pattern. The color of the zipper should match the fabric.

Buttons can be decorative or functional. A button's size is its diameter. Two common types of buttons are *sew-through* buttons and *shank* buttons. Sew-through buttons have holes in them for sewing through with thread. Shank buttons have a loop on the underside of the button through which the thread is sewn. This loop is called the *shank*.

Hooks and eyes and snaps come in various sizes. These sizes are indicated by smaller or larger numbers. Hooks and eyes and snaps usually come in black and silver. Black is recommended for dark-colored fabrics and silver for light-colored fabrics.

Go Green

Recycling Buttons and Fasteners

Before you throw away that ripped sweater or shirt, remove the buttons and other fasteners for future use. Recycling fasteners not only saves money, but helps reduce landfills. Most buttons and fasteners are made from plastic or metal, which are not biodegradable. Always keep the extra buttons that come with new garments, because even if you never need them for that garment, they may be useful for others. Designate a nice-sized container for all your extra buttons and other fasteners. This helps you easily find exactly what you need when making a new garment or repairing an existing one.

Hook and loop tape is a fastener made of two nylon strips that, when pressed together, stick to one another. One strip has tiny hooks. The other one has a looped pile. Hook and loop tape is often called by the band name Velcro®. It comes in precut shapes and is also available by the yard, **24-5**.

Elastic is used to provide fit to garments. Elastic can be used in a *casing* (an enclosure to hold elastic) or stitched directly to a garment. When buying elastic, read the label so you get the correct type listed on the pattern.

The Guide Sheet

The **guide sheet** is a detailed, step-by-step directions on how to cut and sew your garment. Guide sheets are always included inside the envelope with the pattern pieces. The guide sheet begins with suggested fabrics and cutting layouts, explanations of marking symbols, and a few basic sewing instructions.

Step-by-step instructions for putting all the pieces together follow on the back of the guide sheet. These instructions also include detailed sewing techniques.

Pattern Pieces

The pattern pieces consist of tissue paper. Study a pattern piece. You will notice terms and markings that may be unfamiliar. Descriptions for many of them are on the front of your guide sheet. These symbols show how to cut, mark, and sew pieces together correctly. Knowing what these symbols mean helps you avoid mistakes during assembly of your project.

Information printed on each pattern piece includes the pattern number, size, and view number. The name of the piece, an identification letter, and many symbols are also used. The bold, solid outlines around each piece are the **cutting lines**. Multisized patterns have several cutting lines. Choose the one for your size.

The heavy line with arrows on both ends identifies the **grain line**. This line helps you lay your pattern straight on the fabric. Instead of a grain line, some pieces may use the phrase *place on the fold*. Align these pieces with the fold of the fabric.

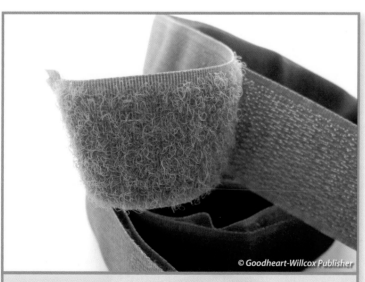

© Goodheart-Willcox Publisher

24-5 Hook and loop tape has tiny hooks that intermesh with pile loops making it an effective fastening option.

A number of other lines may appear on pattern pieces. **Adjustment lines** show you where to lengthen or shorten the pattern piece to change the fit of the garment. *Hemlines* show the location of the garment bottom after you finish it. Other lines indicate the placement of pockets or trims that go on the outside of the garment.

Notches are the diamond-shaped symbols along the cutting line. They indicate exactly where to join pieces together. **Dots** also aid in matching seams and other construction details. See Figure **24-6**.

Preparing the Pattern and Fabric

Before you begin sewing, you need to prepare your pattern and fabric. This may involve adjusting your pattern, preshrinking your fabric, and checking the grain. It also involves laying out the pattern pieces, pinning, cutting, and marking your fabric pieces.

The first step in preparing your pattern is to look at the sketch on the guide sheet. Determine which pieces you need for your project. Then refold the others and put them back in the envelope. Write your name on each pattern piece. If your pattern pieces are badly wrinkled, press them with a dry, warm iron.

Adjusting Pattern Length

Compare your measurements with the chart on the back of the pattern envelope. If they are not the same, you may need to adjust, or alter, your pattern. Altering a pattern is much easier than altering a finished garment. A finished garment might not have enough extra fabric in the seams to make the changes you need.

The most common pattern adjustment is for length. Always lengthen or shorten the front and back pieces the same amount. Some pattern-piece labels say *lengthen or shorten here.* You may find these words at the bottom cutting edge of a pattern piece. If you need to lengthen the piece, tape a piece of paper below the cutting line. Measure the desired amount from the original cutting line. Draw a new line that is parallel to the original. Fill in the seam lines and cutting lines. To shorten a pattern piece at the bottom edge, measure the desired amount up from the original line. Draw a new cutting line parallel to the original and cut off the excess length.

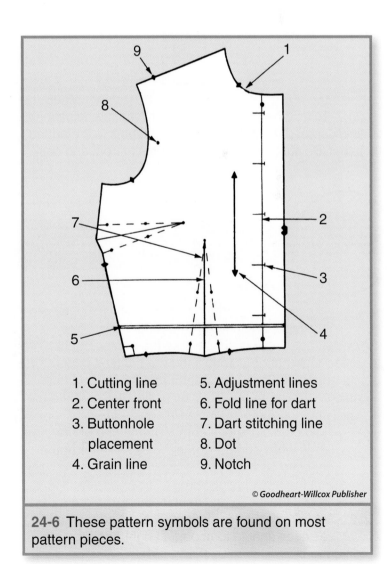

1. Cutting line
2. Center front
3. Buttonhole placement
4. Grain line
5. Adjustment lines
6. Fold line for dart
7. Dart stitching line
8. Dot
9. Notch

© Goodheart-Willcox Publisher

24-6 These pattern symbols are found on most pattern pieces.

Sometimes the middle of the pattern requires an adjustment. Look for two parallel lines that are close together. These are the adjustment lines. The phrase *lengthen or shorten here* will be next to them. If you want to lengthen a pattern piece, cut between the two lines and spread the pieces apart. Place a piece of paper under the pattern and tape it to one side, **24-7**. Measure and mark the additional length. Be sure the distance between the lines is the same from one side of the piece to the other. Then tape the other pattern piece to the paper. Be sure the cutting lines at the sides still form a straight line. If you want to shorten the pattern, make a fold between the adjustment lines. Then fold up half the amount you need to shorten.

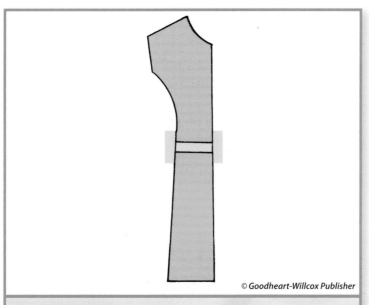

© Goodheart-Willcox Publisher

24-7 To lengthen a pattern, cut between the adjustment lines, spread the pattern open, and tape it to the added paper. Be sure to add equal amounts to front and back.

Preshrinking the Fabric

Some fabrics go through a preshrinking process during manufacturing to help keep them from shrinking during washing or cleaning. When you buy fabric, check the label on the end of the bolt. If the label does not indicate the fabric is preshrunk, it is a good idea to do it yourself.

Preshrinking fabric is easy. Just treat it the same way as a finished garment. If a garment requires machine washing and drying, then machine wash and dry the fabric. Press the fabric if needed. Some fabrics require dry cleaning; check the care label on the fabric bolt before purchase.

Checking the Fabric Grain

The direction yarns run in a fabric is called the **grain**. In woven fabrics, there are two sets of yarns that run over and under each other. When your pattern refers to the straight grain or *grain line*, it means the *lengthwise grain*, **24-8**. To find the lengthwise grain, simply look for the selvages of the fabric. The **selvages** are the smooth, closely woven edges that do not ravel. The lengthwise grain runs in the same direction as the selvages (vertically). The yarns that run across the fabric from one selvage to the other (horizontally) are called the *crosswise grain* of the fabric.

Math Connections

Finding Right Angles When Checking Grain

It is important to know that a right angle is a *90° angle*, meaning it is shaped like the printed capital letter "L." What do you do if the right angles on the cut edges and selvages do not match? You may be able to straighten the fabric by pulling it. Complete the following activity to straighten fabric grain:

- Hold both sides of a corner at one end of the fabric while someone else holds a corner at the opposite end.
- Pull the fabric diagonally.
- Refold the fabric and double-check the grain again to see if it is straight. The cut edges and selvages should form perfect right angles.

Fabric is **on-grain** when the crosswise and lengthwise yarns are at right angles to each other. **Off-grain** fabrics look crooked and are hard to handle because the fabric yarns do not cross at right angles. Garments made with off-grain fabrics may twist, pull to one side, and hang unevenly. The fabric grain must be straight to make a garment look right.

The first step in checking the grain is to straighten the cut edges. Near the edge of the fabric, find a crosswise yarn and pull it. Push the fabric along the pulled yarn. This will leave a straight, open line you can use as a cutting line. What do you do if the yarn breaks in the middle of the fabric? Cut as far as you can see the open line. Then pick up the yarn and pull it again. Do this until you have cut all the way across the fabric, **24-9**.

The next step is to lay the fabric on a flat surface. Bring the two selvages together to make a lengthwise fold. If the grain line is straight, the cut edges on each end will match and so will the selvages. The cut edges and the selvages will form a right angle.

Laying Out the Pattern

Refer to the guide sheet that came with your pattern. It suggests many cutting layouts. *Cutting layouts* show you how to lay your pattern pieces on the fabric. Find the one that matches your project or view, fabric width, and pattern size. It is a good idea to draw a circle around it so you can easily refer to it.

Place the fabric on a smooth, flat surface such as a table. Fold the fabric according to the instructions on your guide sheet. The fabric is usually doubled before cutting. This is because most pieces need to be cut twice. Check each piece to be sure. The label on some pieces may say *cut one* or *cut four*.

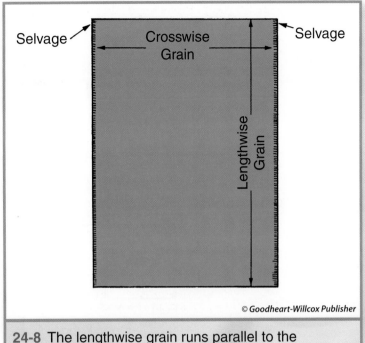

© Goodheart-Willcox Publisher

24-8 The lengthwise grain runs parallel to the selvages. The crosswise grain runs between selvages.

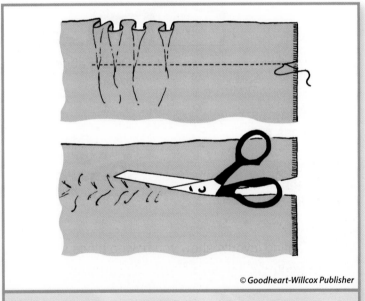

© Goodheart-Willcox Publisher

24-9 To find the straight crosswise grain of woven fabric, you can pull a filling yarn, leaving an open, straight line for cutting the fabric.

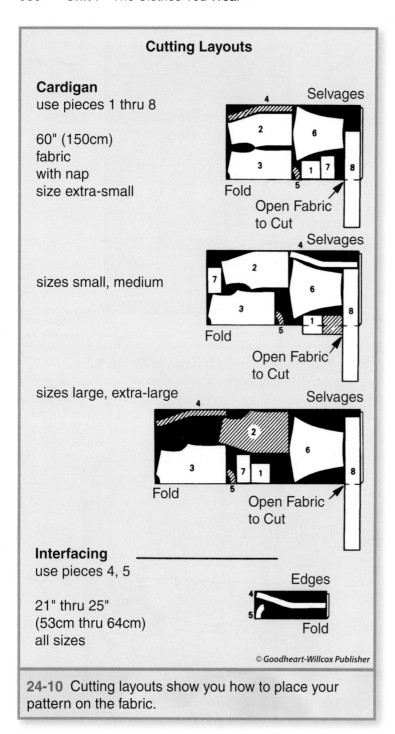

Cutting Layouts

Cardigan
use pieces 1 thru 8

60" (150cm)
fabric
with nap
size extra-small

sizes small, medium

sizes large, extra-large

Interfacing
use pieces 4, 5

21" thru 25"
(53cm thru 64cm)
all sizes

© Goodheart-Willcox Publisher

24-10 Cutting layouts show you how to place your pattern on the fabric.

Most pattern pieces are placed on the fabric with the printed side up. These pieces appear white on the cutting layouts. Place shaded pieces printed side down. Be sure to lay and pin all the pattern pieces on the fabric before you cut to make sure you have enough fabric. See **24-10**.

Pinning

Locate the grain line on each pattern piece. The grain line is a straight line with an arrow at each end. Place this line on the lengthwise grain of the fabric. Insert a pin at each end of the arrow. Then measure from the point of each arrow to the lengthwise edge of the fabric. The two distances should be equal. If they are not, make an adjustment. Then measure again. Repeat this process until the grain line is straight. See **24-11**.

If the pattern piece requires placement on a fold, this is noted along the edge of the pattern piece. Place that edge on the folded edge of the fabric. Pin along the folded edge first, placing the pins at right angles to the fold.

Once the pattern pieces are on-grain, pin the other areas of the pattern pieces. Insert the pins about six inches apart. Insert them closer together on edges with curves. Always insert pins at right angles to the cutting lines. Pin diagonally in the corners. Never pin across cutting lines.

Cutting

Use bent-handled shears to cut out fabric pieces. The design of these shears allows the blade and the fabric to lie flat on the table as you cut. This helps you cut exactly along the cutting lines, **24-12**.

As you cut, make long, smooth strokes with the shears. Take care not to cut inside the cutting line. Cut slowly enough to be aware of notches. As you approach a notch on your cutting line, cut the notch outward. Be sure to leave the pattern pieces pinned to the fabric after cutting to easily transfer the pattern markings.

Marking

After cutting out your project, transfer the necessary pattern markings to the fabric. These markings serve as a guide in putting your garment together. Markings to transfer include center front, center back, darts, dots, buttons, buttonholes, pockets, and the tops of sleeves.

You can transfer markings to fabrics in several ways. One of the most common methods is using a *tracing wheel* with *dressmaker's carbon paper*. Use care with this method of marking. Before you begin, test the carbon on a fabric scrap. Make sure the markings are visible on the wrong side of the fabric, but do not show on the right side. Use only light colors of carbon paper on light fabrics. Dark carbon paper shows through on the right side of light-color fabrics.

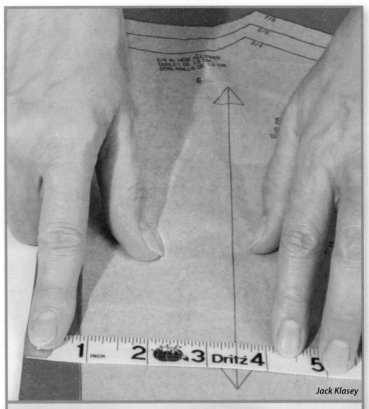

Jack Klasey

24-11 Measure from each end of the arrow to make sure the pattern is placed on the fabric grain.

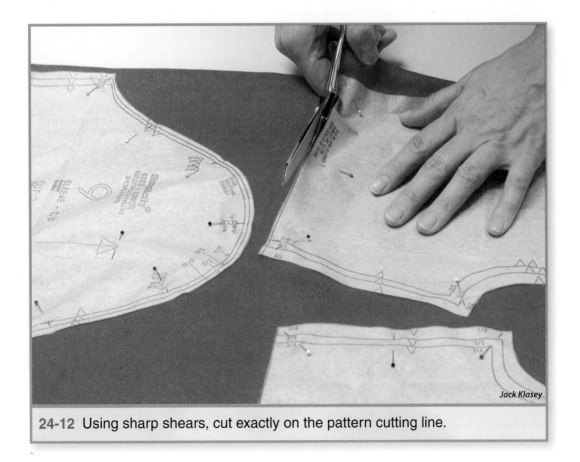

Jack Klasey

24-12 Using sharp shears, cut exactly on the pattern cutting line.

Place the colored, waxy side of the carbon paper next to the wrong side of the fabric. Then roll the tracing wheel along the markings you need to transfer. Use a ruler to help mark straight lines. Apply just enough pressure to make the markings show on the fabric. Too much pressure may result in marks showing on the right side. Tailor's chalk, soap slivers, chalk pencils, water-soluble marking pens, and pencils could also be used to mark fabric, **24-13**.

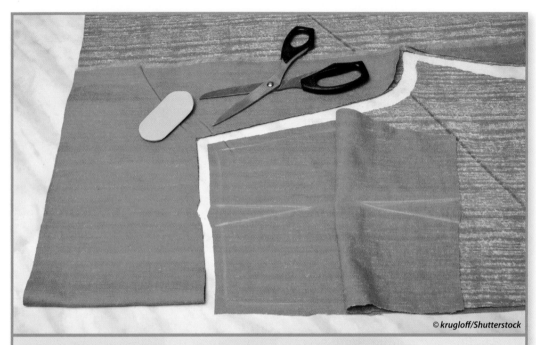

© krugloff/Shutterstock

24-13 Tailor's chalk was used to mark the new stitching and dart lines on the wrong side of this fabric.

Reading Review

1. A(n) _____ is a basic model that helps you put together a garment or project.
2. What is the most important part of choosing a pattern?
3. List four examples of notions.
4. What is the purpose of the grain line?
5. Which pattern markings are necessary to transfer to the fabric?

Section 24-2

Sewing Skills

Objectives

After studying this section, you will be able to
- **perform** basic construction steps using a sewing machine.
- **identify** basic seam finishes.
- **demonstrate** how to make facings, casings, and attach fasteners.
- **demonstrate** how to mark, finish, and hand stitch a hem.
- **demonstrate** how to make simple clothing alterations.

Key Terms

backstitching	seam	notching
staystitching	seam allowance	facings
basting	trimming	understitching
easing	grading	casing
gathering	clipping	hem
darts		

Reading and talking about sewing is not quite as exciting as actually sewing. Using your skills to transform a pattern, fabric, and notions into a garment is a great experience. You get a feeling of pride when you say "I made it myself!" Like playing a musical instrument or swimming, sewing is a learned skill. By learning basic sewing techniques and following the directions on the guide sheet, you can achieve sewing success.

Machine Sewing

You are now ready to begin the construction of your project. This means sewing the pieces together. The most common way to do this is with a sewing machine, **24-14**.

Before sewing, check the spool and bobbin threads on the machine. They should be pulled about five inches behind the presser foot. This will keep the thread from tangling at the beginning of the seam. Make sure the take-up lever of the machine is at its highest point. If it is not, the thread could pull out of the needle as you begin to sew.

Place the fabric under the presser foot, keeping most of the fabric to the left of the needle. This is so you can see the seam guides on the throat plate. Suppose you are sewing a ⅝-inch seam. The fabric edges should lie exactly on the ⅝-inch seam guide line on the machine.

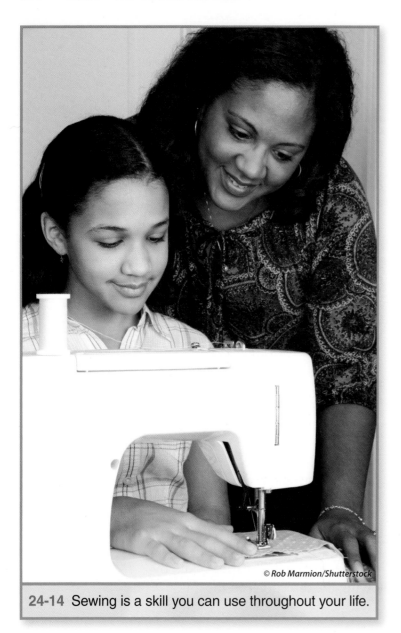

24-14 Sewing is a skill you can use throughout your life.

© Rob Marmion/Shutterstock

Hold the fabric with your left hand. With your right hand, turn the hand wheel and lower the needle into the fabric. Then lower the presser foot.

Begin to stitch. Maintain a slow, constant speed. Guide the fabric by keeping both hands lightly on the fabric. Watch the seam guide as you sew to produce an even seam. Remember to follow sewing safety rules.

Backstitching

Backstitching secures the threads at the start and end of each seam. To backstitch, take four or five stitches forward with the machine. Then sew in reverse, exactly over the first stitches. Finally, sew forward again to secure the thread.

As you sew, remove each pin as the presser foot comes to it. If you sew over the pins, the needle could bend or break if it hits a pin. This can cause an injury.

To turn a corner while stitching, stitch to within ⅝ inch of the corner and stop. Make sure the needle remains down in the fabric. Lift the presser foot. Turn the fabric. Lower the presser foot. Continue to sew.

Once the seam is made, move the take-up lever to its highest point by turning the hand wheel. (*Note:* With some newer machines, the take-up lever stops at the highest point when you stop the machine.) Next, raise the presser foot and pull the fabric to the back of the machine. Cut the threads, leaving four to five inches extending from the machine.

Staystitching

Staystitching is a line of regular machine stitches on a single thickness of fabric. It is done to prevent garment pieces from stretching out of shape. Staystitching is sewn ½ inch from the cut edge of the fabric. Use it on curved and bias edges such as necklines and armholes. When staystitching, use the same thread you use to make the garment.

Loosely woven or less sturdy fabrics require staystitching. Staystitching is not always necessary on other fabrics because the yarns are *locked* into position with finishes.

Basting

Basting refers to long, loose stitches. The major purpose of basting is to check the fit of a garment. Basting stitches are useful for easing and gathering, too. You can make basting stitches by hand or machine. To hand baste, sew along the seam line, making your stitches about ¼-inch long.

To machine baste, set the stitch length control to the longest stitch length on your machine. Sew along the regular seam line. Do not backstitch or knot the thread ends.

Easing and Gathering

Use **easing** and **gathering** stitches to make extra fabric fit into a smaller space. Gathers are fuller than easing. Easing produces a smoother line than gathering. For instance, gathers are used to make a full skirt, and easing is used to make set-in sleeves.

To ease or gather, sew two parallel rows of basting stitches. With the right side of the fabric facing up in the area to ease or gather, sew one row of basting stitches on the seam line. Sew another row ¼ inch from the first row inside the seam allowance. Do not backstitch. Leave long threads at both ends.

Next, turn the fabric to the wrong side so the bobbin threads are facing up. Place a pin at one end of the stitches as shown in **24-15**. Wrap the threads at that end around the pin in a figure eight motion to secure them. Gently pull the two bobbin threads from the other end. Pull extra fullness across the rows of stitching. When you have enough gathers, place a pin at the other end and wrap the threads around it. Arrange the gathers evenly across the rows of stitching. With right sides together, pin the fabric edges every 2 to 3 inches, matching notches, markings, and seams.

Darts

Darts give shape and fullness to a garment so it fits the curves of the body. Darts point to the fullest part of body curves. On slacks and skirts, for example, darts begin at the waistline and taper to the hipline. This allows extra fullness around the hips. The darts used in jackets, blouses, and shirts taper to the fullest part of the bust or chest.

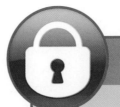

Safety Connections

Sewing Lab Safety

- When machine sewing, keep your fingers away from the presser foot and needle while holding the fabric securely. If your machine has a finger guard attachment, use it for safety. Do not lean your face too close to the machine while stitching.
- Place pins and needles in a pincushion; do not leave them on a table or put them in your mouth.
- Keep scissors closed when not in use, and hand to others with the handles facing them.
- Unplug all electrical equipment when not in use. Make sure cords are wrapped around equipment and not hanging loose.
- Always rest an iron on its heel.
- Keep your sewing area and floor clean and swept free of scraps and threads.

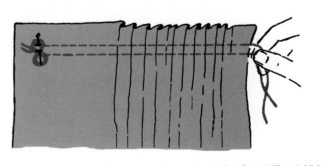

© Goodheart-Willcox Publisher

24-15 Secure threads by wrapping them around a pin. Then pull the other ends to ease or gather.

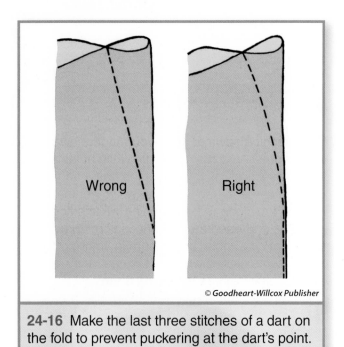

24-16 Make the last three stitches of a dart on the fold to prevent puckering at the dart's point.

Darts are made before seams in a garment. This is because they cross over seam lines. To make a dart, begin at the widest end of the dart and sew to the point. Make the last three stitches of the dart on the fold to prevent the fabric from puckering at the dart point, **24-16**. After stitching, tie the threads ends securely at the dart point. Do not backstitch to avoid puckers at the dart point.

To press darts, press along the stitching line from the widest end to the point. Press vertical darts toward the center front or center back. Press horizontal darts downward. Darts that are wide or made of bulky fabric can be cut open to within 1 inch of the point. They can then be trimmed to ⅝ inch and pressed open.

Making a Seam

A **seam** is a row of stitches that holds two pieces of fabric together. The fabric between the stitching and the fabric edge is the **seam allowance**. The width of a standard seam allowance is ⅝ inch, **24-17**.

The *plain* seam is the most common seam in garment construction. With right sides of the fabric facing together, match the cut edges and notches and pin. Sew along the seam line, carefully removing the pins before you make the stitches.

Finishing Seams

To keep fabrics from raveling, you can apply a seam finish. Your choice of seam finishes depends on the weight, texture, and thickness of the fabric. See **24-18** for several types of seam finishes.

A *pinked seam finish* looks nice, but it does not prevent raveling. Use this type of seam finish only on fabrics that do not ravel. To produce a pinked seam finish, sew the seam. Next, press it flat and use pinking shears to trim the seam allowance edges. Then press the seam open.

A *turned and stitched seam finish* prevents raveling and gives a neat appearance. Use this finish on the edges of facings for sheer and lightweight fabrics. Because it is bulky, avoid using this finish on medium and heavyweight fabrics. To produce this seam finish, press the seam open. Turn the edges under ¼ inch. Stitch close to the fold.

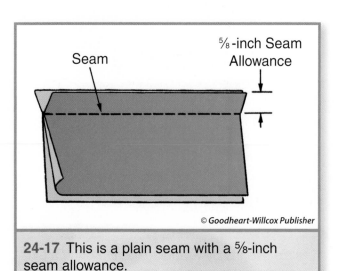

24-17 This is a plain seam with a ⅝-inch seam allowance.

Most sewing machines have a zigzag setting. A *zigzag seam finish* is quick and easy, and it prevents raveling. It puckers less than a line of straight stitches because it has more *give* or flexibility. It works best on medium and heavyweight fabrics. To produce a zigzag finish, press the seam open and zigzag stitch close to the edge of the seam allowance through a single layer of fabric.

Trimming, Grading, Clipping, and Notching Seams

Trimming, grading, clipping, and notching are techniques to reduce fabric bulk in seams, allowing them to lie flat. **Trimming** is done on lightweight fabrics. To trim a seam, cut away part of the seam allowance.

Trim the corners to make the points lay flat, **24-19**. To trim a corner with a right angle, cut diagonally across the seam allowances. Cut close to the stitching. If the corner has a sharper point, cut diagonally across the seam allowance as before. Then make another cut on each side of the corner to remove extra fabric.

Grading is useful on heavier fabrics or seams with three or more layers. To grade a seam, press the seam allowances to one side. Trim each layer to a different width, **24-20**. For a smooth, flat seam, trim the layer closest to the garment less than the other layers.

Use **clipping** on seams that form an inward curve to help them lie flat. Armhole, neckline, and waistline seams form inward curves. Clip such seams by cutting straight into the seam allowance without cutting through the seam line. Clip about every ½ inch along the curve, **24-21**.

Like inward curves, inside corners also require clipping. Clip diagonally into the corner without cutting through the stitching. This will allow a sharp, flat corner when you turn the garment right side out.

Rounded collars and pockets have seams that form outward curves. To make these seams lie flat, you need to notch the seam allowance. **Notching** means cutting V-shaped sections from the seam allowance, **24-22**.

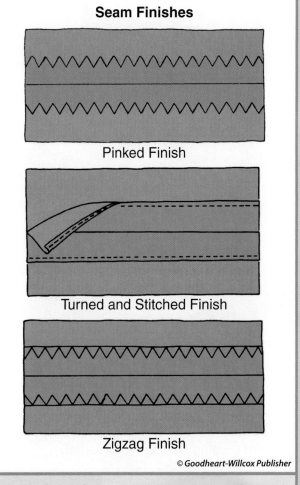

Seam Finishes

Pinked Finish

Turned and Stitched Finish

Zigzag Finish

© Goodheart-Willcox Publisher

24-18 Seam finishes help prevent raveling and provide a neat look to the inside of a garment.

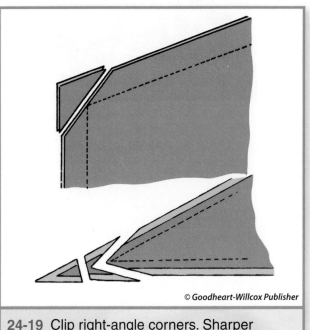

© Goodheart-Willcox Publisher

24-19 Clip right-angle corners. Sharper corners need to be graded and clipped.

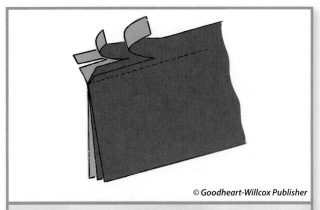

24-20 Grade a seam by cutting each seam allowance to a different width.

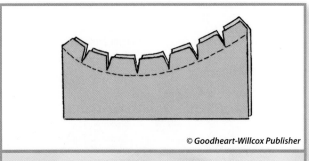

24-21 Both inside curves and inside corners require clipping so seams will lie flat.

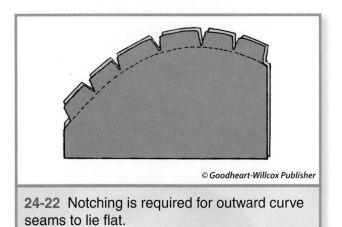

24-22 Notching is required for outward curve seams to lie flat.

Facings and Interfacing

Some garment parts are not visible. Instead, they form part of the garment inside to add structure and support. Facings and interfacings are examples of *hidden* garment pieces.

Facings

Facings are found at garment openings, such as armholes and necklines, 24-23. They are usually not visible on the outside of the garment. The main purpose of a facing is to cover the raw edges. Facings also add firmness to the open areas and keep them from stretching out of shape.

The two main types of facings are extended facings and fitted facings. An *extended facing* is cut as part of the garment pattern piece. The facing section is then folded to the inside.

A *fitted facing*, also called a *shaped facing*, is cut as a separate pattern piece. A fitted facing has the same shape as the raw edge. It is stitched to the edge and turned to the inside of the garment. After the facing is stitched to the garment, grade and clip the seam allowance for a smooth flat finish. Grade the seam layers first, and then clip the curved areas of the seam.

Press a facing seam toward the facing and understitch it. **Understitching** is a line of stitching along the edge of a facing to keep it from rolling to the outside. As you understitch, sew on the right side of the facing. Be sure to keep the seam allowances turned toward the facing.

Interfacing

Interfacing material adds support, shape, and stability to areas such as collars, waistbands, and cuffs. It also adds strength to areas of stress such as around buttonholes. Interfacings are placed between the garment fabric and the facings.

Interfacings are either sewn in or (if using a fusible interfacing) ironed on to the wrong side of garment pieces. Trim ½ inch of the interfacing seam allowances off before fusing it to the garment fabric. This keeps the stiffened fabric from making the seam areas of the garment bulky.

Casings

A **casing** is an enclosure for elastic or a drawstring that gathers the garment snugly to the body. A casing is a useful waistline treatment for garments that pull on, **24-24**. You may also use casings on sleeve and leg edges.

A casing may be formed in one of two ways. A *self-casing* forms when you fold the edge of the garment to the inside and stitch it. An *applied casing* requires use of a separate piece of fabric or bias tape to form the casing. An opening is left to insert the elastic or drawstring in both types of casings.

You need to determine the length of elastic or drawstring to use in the casing. Hold the elastic around the body where the casing is located. Do not pull it too tight. Add one inch to this amount to overlap the ends. A drawstring needs to be long enough so it will not slip through when it is untied.

To insert elastic, attach a safety pin to one end. Push the pin through the casing and overlap the elastic ends. Secure the elastic ends by stitching across them several times. Distribute garment fullness evenly. Stitch the opening closed where the elastic was inserted.

Fasteners

Fasteners are useful for closing openings on garments. They include zippers, buttons, hooks and eyes, snaps, and hook and loop tape. Zippers are sewn into garments with a sewing machine. The easiest types of fasteners to attach are buttons, hooks, and snaps, which are hand sewn. View the steps for sewing on buttons in **24-25**. The steps for sewing on hooks and eyes and snaps are in **24-26**. Hook and loop tape is either sewn on or has adhesive backing.

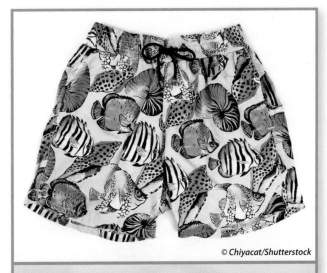

© Goodheart-Willcox Publisher

24-23 Use facings to cover the raw edges of garments. This facing is ready to be trimmed, clipped, and turned to the inside.

© Chiyacat/Shutterstock

24-24 These drawstring shorts with a casing are easy to make.

Hems

Hemming is one of the final steps in sewing a garment. A **hem** produces a finished edge on a garment. The hemline should always be smooth, even, and nearly invisible.

Sewing on Buttons

(A) **Button placement:** Close garment opening. To mark placement of the button, place a pin through buttonhole. Slip the buttonhole over the pin to open.

(B) **Sew-through button:** Place a pin or toothpick on top of the button. Bring the needle and thread through the fabric and button, over the toothpick and back through the fabric. Repeat five or six times.

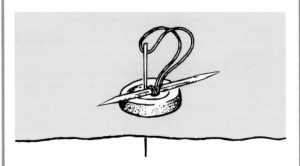

Remove the toothpick and pull the button up. Bring threaded needle between garment and button. Wind thread around stitches several times to make a shank. (Shanks raise buttons from the garment to allow room for the button hole to fit smoothly beneath it.) Pass the thread to the garment underside and fasten securely.

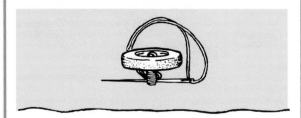

(C) **Shank button:** Shank buttons need an additional thread shank, but it can be smaller than the shank for sew-through ones. Sew the button on loosely. Then wind the thread under the button to form the thread shank.

24-25 Follow these steps for attaching buttons.

Sewing on Hooks and Eyes

Use the bar eye for edges that lap.

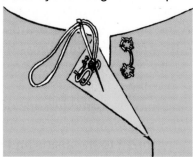

Use the round eye for edges that meet.

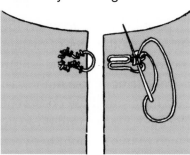

Insert the needle through the fabric and one ring of the hook. Bring the thread under the point of the needle. Loop the thread in the same direction for each stitch and pull it tight. Repeat this for the other rings of the hook and eye. Also, take two or three stitches in the bill of the hook to hold it in place.

Sewing on Snaps

Use snaps for closings where there is very little strain.

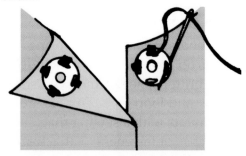

Using a needle and thread, stitch over the edge of the snap and into the fabric several times. Stitches should be close together. Insert the needle under the snap and into the next hole. When the stitching is complete, secure the thread on the wrong side under the snap.

24-26 Follow these steps for attaching hooks and eyes and snaps.

Marking a Hem

After completing all other sewing steps, you are ready to mark the hem. Try on the garment with the shoes you plan to wear with it. Standing in front of a full-length mirror, test several different lengths. Choose the length that is best for you and mark it with a pin. The best way to mark a hem evenly is to have someone help you. As you stand straight and still, the other person can move around you. Use a yardstick for this task. Place pins parallel to the floor about 3 inches apart.

Next, fold the fabric up at the marked line and pin it. Move the pins so they are at right angles to the cut edge of the hem. Match the seam lines in the hem to the seam lines in the garment. After pinning the hem, hand baste close to the folded edge to temporarily hold the hem secure.

Your pattern will suggest a hem width. Use this as a guide. See **24-27** for the steps in pinning and measuring the hem width. Use a ruler or sewing gauge to measure the desired distance up from the hemline. Mark the line with tailor's chalk. Cut along the marked line. Be careful to cut only the extra hem allowance, not the garment.

Finishing Hems

A hem finish is much like a seam finish. See **24-28** for types of hem finishes. For fabrics that do not ravel, machine stitch ¼ inch from the cut edge. Then pink the edge. Finish fabrics that ravel in other ways. Zigzag or overcast hem finishes produce very flat hems.

For some hems, it is possible to use a turned and stitched hem. Turn the cut edges under ¼ inch and stitch close to the fold. This method is bulky. For this reason, use it only on straight hems of medium- or lightweight fabrics.

For straight hems of medium- or heavyweight fabrics, seam binding is a good choice. With the right side of the fabric facing up, lap the tape over the hem edge ¼ inch. Stitch close to the tape edge and through the hem allowance.

Securing Hems

Securing a hem means to sew it into place. This is usually sewn by hand using a fine needle with a single thread. Hold the garment so the hem allowance is on top and facing you. If you are right-handed, stitch from right to left. If you are left-handed, stitch from left to right. For a neat look, evenly space the hand stitches. To prevent puckering, do not pull the stitches too tight.

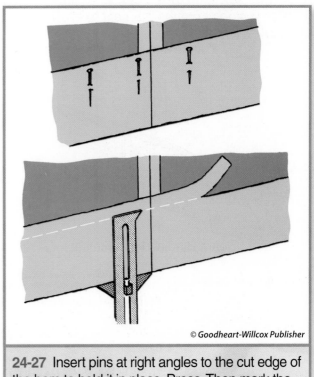

© Goodheart-Willcox Publisher

24-27 Insert pins at right angles to the cut edge of the hem to hold it in place. Press. Then mark the desired width of the hem and cut off extra fabric.

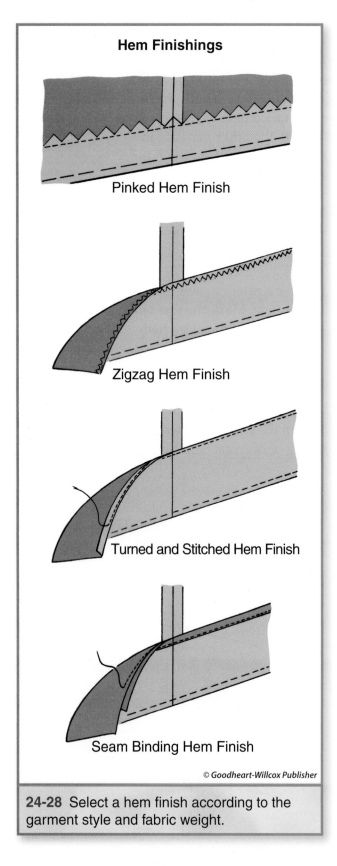

Hem Finishings

Pinked Hem Finish

Zigzag Hem Finish

Turned and Stitched Hem Finish

Seam Binding Hem Finish

© Goodheart-Willcox Publisher

24-28 Select a hem finish according to the garment style and fabric weight.

The *hemming stitch* is a strong stitch that is useful for hems with almost any type of finish. To make this stitch, secure the thread in the hem edge with a knot or small backstitch. Pick up a yarn from the garment. Then bring the needle straight up through the hem allowance. Move about ¼ inch to the left and pick up another yarn from the garment fabric. Repeat making stitches across the hem edge.

The *slip stitch* barely shows on either side of the garment. The thread is hidden under a fold along the hem allowance edge. Since a fold is needed, the slip stitch is used for hems with either a turned and stitched finish or a seam binding hem finish.

To make the slip stitch, secure the thread in the hem edge. Pick up a yarn from the garment. Bring the needle straight up and into the fold of the hem allowance, then across about ¼ inch inside the fold. Next, bring the needle straight down, and pick up another yarn from the garment. Repeat around the hem.

The *blind stitch* shows even less than the slip stitch. This is because the thread lies between the hem allowance and the garment. This is an advantage because it prevents the thread from wearing and snagging. The stitches are loose to allow the two layers of fabric to move slightly without pulling.

To make the blind stitch, secure the thread in the hem edge. Fold the hem edge up, away from the garment. Pick up a yarn from the garment. Move the needle diagonally up and to the left about ¼ inch. Pick up a yarn from the hem allowance. Move the needle diagonally down and to the left, and pick up a yarn from the garment. Make the stitches loose. Repeat this process around the hem.

Another method of securing a hem is *topstitching* or making a line of stitching on the outside of a garment close to a seam. Straight, zigzag, and decorative stitches can be used for different looks.

A fusible web material can also be useful in securing hems. The heat from an iron melts the web and bonds the hem to the garment. This method is quick and easy, but take extra care when using it. Be sure to read the manufacturer's directions. Since this type of hem is permanent, make sure the garment is the right length. Do not let a hot iron touch the fusible web material. If it melts onto the iron, it is difficult to remove.

Altering Your Clothes

Suppose you made or purchased a garment that no longer fits well. Perhaps you have lost weight or grown several inches. By altering your clothes, you can achieve a good fit. Alterations can decrease or increase the length or width of a garment. A simple alteration often makes a garment fit better so you wear it more often.

Altering Hems

One of the easiest alterations is adjusting the hem length of a garment. To lengthen a garment, check the hem allowance to see if there is enough fabric for the extra length. If you want to make a garment shorter, you may need to trim away some of the hem depth.

To alter the hem of a garment, carefully remove the hem stitches. Press out the crease. Then try on the garment. Ask someone to pin the hem in place. Hem again as described.

Altering Seams

Changing the width of a garment can be an easy or complex job. Perhaps all you need to do is move a button or hook. Other times you may need to let out or take in the seams of a garment. Letting out makes a garment larger, while taking in makes a garment smaller. Depending on the garment's construction, you may need to adjust both sides or the front and back of a garment.

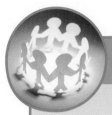

Life Connections

Better Fitting Clothes

When altering a garment's width for a better fit, pin the new seams in place first. Be sure to evenly distribute the decrease or increase among all seams. Try on the garment after pinning the seams to check the fit before sewing them.

When letting out a garment, sew the new seam in the seam allowance of the old seam. Always check the width of a seam allowance to be sure it is wide enough to sew a new seam. When taking a garment in, sew the new seam inside the garment's original seam. After sewing the new seams, remove the old stitches, press the seams open, and give the garment a final press.

Math Activity

Choose a garment to alter for yourself or another person to ensure a better fit. Determine the amount every seam needs to be either let out or taken in. Practice measuring and marking all the new seams using the proper measurement tools.

Reading Review

1. What is the purpose of backstitching?
2. Why are darts made before seams in a garment?
3. What is the width of a standard seam allowance?
4. List four techniques to reduce fabric bulk in seams, allowing them to lie flat.
5. When securing a hem, how do you prevent puckering?

Chapter Summary

Section 24-1. Choosing a sewing project that matches your skill level will help assure your success. If you choose to make a garment, you need to use care in selecting a pattern. Choose a size that fits your body measurements. Make use of information found in pattern catalogs and on pattern envelopes. Once you select your pattern, prepare it and your fabric before you can begin to sew. Use information on your guide sheet and pattern pieces to help you pin, cut, and mark your project pieces.

Section 24-2. Using basic construction steps and a sewing machine, you can transform your pattern, fabric, and notions into a garment. Making seams and finishing them, as well as making facings, casings, and attaching fasteners are all part of constructing a garment. Once the garment is constructed, the hem must be marked, finished, and hand stitched. Sometimes garments require changes to achieve a good fit. This is when alterations become necessary.

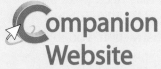

Companion Website
www.g-wlearning.com

Check your understanding of the main concepts for Chapter 24 at the website.

Critical Thinking

1. **Determine.** What ways could you provide winter coats for people who cannot afford them? What service-learning project could you and your classmates do to meet this need? What sewing skills might you use for this project?

2. **Identify.** If you were a clothing designer and were offered the position of developing an entire wardrobe for one character from a television show, what character would you choose and why?

3. **Analyze.** Check out a garment you are wearing. Analyze the sewing techniques that went into constructing the garment. Which of the techniques do you know how to do? Which would you like to learn how to do?

Common Core

College and Career Readiness

4. **Writing.** Gather patterns and pictures of items and garments that would be easy sewing projects for beginners. Make a display for a bulletin board or showcase. Write reasons these projects would be good for beginners to attempt.

5. **Speaking.** Imagine you work at a sewing center. Your customers are eager to learn new skills. Demonstrate the following sewing preparation tasks:
   A. adjusting pattern length
   B. checking fabric grain
   C. laying out and pinning a pattern
   D. transferring pattern markings

6. **Reading.** Research the history of the sewing machine. Find out about the part it played in the Industrial Revolution.

7. **Speaking.** Imagine you are a family and consumer sciences teacher. Your students are learning basic sewing skills. Demonstrate the following sewing skills to the class:
   A. hand basting
   B. sewing seams with the sewing machine
   C. seam finishes
   D. hem stitches
   E. sewing on buttons and other fasteners

Technology

8. **Use new technologies.** Have your class design patterns for a quilt using CAD or other computer technology. Each student should design and sew a square to add to the quilt. Consider embellishing some of the squares using a computerized sewing machine with embroidery features. Then display the quilt at a school or civic function. If possible, hold a silent auction to sell the quilt to the highest bidder. Donate the proceeds to a charitable organization that provides clothing to children in need.

Journal Writing

9. Create a notebook displaying samples of the various sewing techniques you have mastered. Include samples of basic seams, seam finishes, hemming stitches, and fastener applications. Under each one, write about how each technique was done.

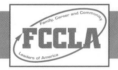 ## FCCLA

10. Apply fashion construction skills to create a *Fashion Construction STAR Event*. Create a display board that illustrates the construction process, the final product complete with accessories, a fabric profile, a cost analysis, and a time log of events. Use the *FCCLA Planning Process* to plan and execute your project. See your adviser for information as needed.

Chapter 25
Caring for Clothes

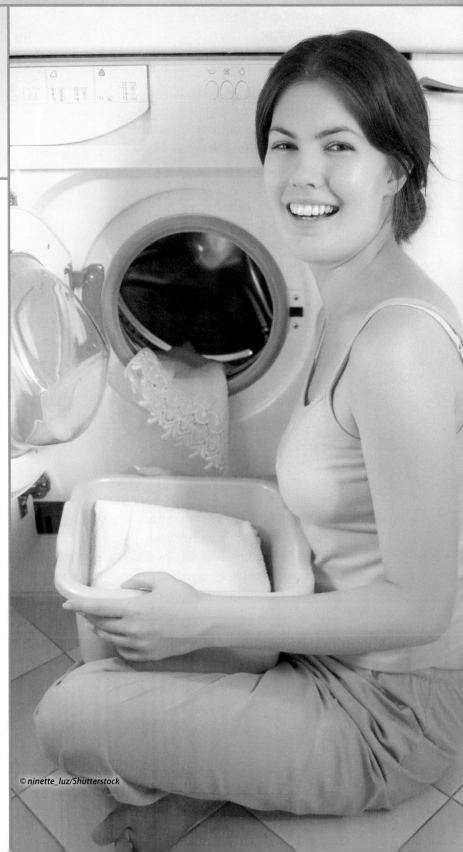

Reading Prep

College and Career Readiness

Arrange a study session to read the chapter with a classmate. After you read each section independently, stop and tell each other what you think the main points are in the section. Continue with each section until you finish the chapter.

Concept Organizer

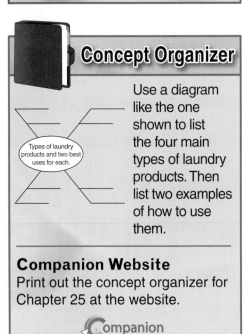

Types of laundry products and two best uses for each.

Use a diagram like the one shown to list the four main types of laundry products. Then list two examples of how to use them.

Companion Website

Print out the concept organizer for Chapter 25 at the website.

Companion Website
www.g-wlearning.com

© ninette_luz/Shutterstock

602

Routine Clothing Care

Objectives

After studying this section, you will be able to
- **develop** a daily clothing care routine.
- **determine** how to clean clothes properly based on care label information.
- **operate** washing machines, dryers, pressing, and ironing equipment properly.
- **demonstrate** how to sort, launder, and dry clothes.
- **summarize** how to properly store clothing.

Key Terms

care labels	permanent press	dry cleaning
stain	tumble drying	pressing
tannin	line-drying	ironing
sorting	flat-drying	moths

Keeping your clothes in good condition involves creating a clothing care routine and sticking to it. The few extra minutes it takes for routine care now can save time later. It can also help you to avoid problems. You will avoid worrying about not having anything to wear because your clothes are dirty, wrinkled, or need repair, **25-1**.

Daily Clothing Care

As you dress and undress, be careful to avoid damaging your clothes. For instance, remove your shoes when stepping into your pants. Rips, tears, missing buttons, and broken zippers can occur from carelessness.

After wearing clothes, inspect them for dirt, stains, rips, or missing buttons. Take care of these promptly. If clothes are clean and in good repair, hang them on hangers. Fasten buttons and close zippers so the garments will keep their shapes and stay on the hangers. Use a lint brush to remove any lint or pet hair.

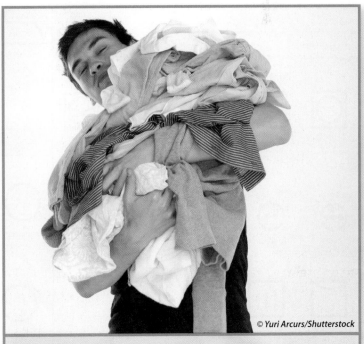

© Yuri Arcurs/Shutterstock

25-1 Because clothes can be expensive, it is smart to take care of them so you can wear them for a long time.

Neatly fold clean knitted garments, such as sweaters and knit shirts, and place them on a shelf or in a drawer. If you hang knits on a hanger, they may stretch out of shape.

Laundry Basics

Laundering your clothes is a basic part of caring for them. Removing stains and sorting your clothes before washing helps assure thorough cleaning.

Reading Care Labels

The first step in laundering your clothes is to read the garment's care label. **Care labels** describe how to clean garments without damaging the textiles. These labels are a legal requirement on all clothing. They may use certain symbols instead of words, **25-2**.

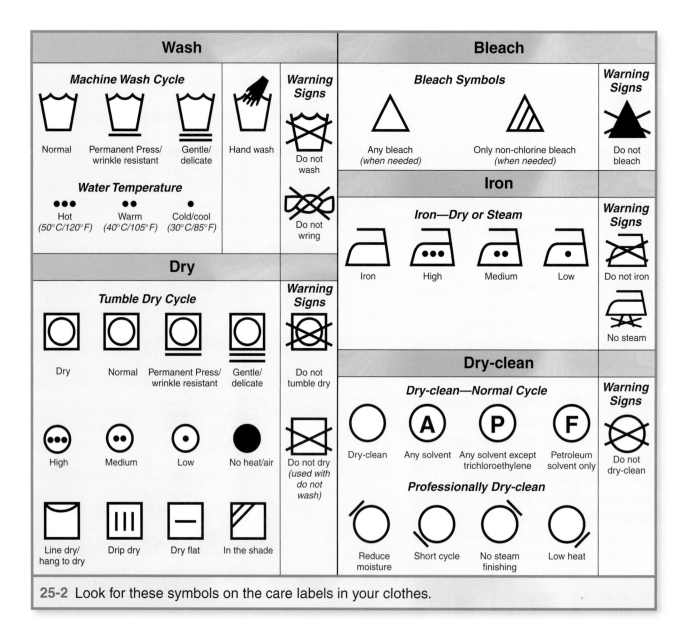

25-2 Look for these symbols on the care labels in your clothes.

Care labels include the following information:

- method of cleaning (hand or machine wash; dry cleaning)
- water temperature (cold, warm, or hot)
- method of drying (machine, hang, or lay flat)
- drying temperature (low, medium, or high)
- type of bleach that can be used safely
- ironing or pressing temperature (cool, warm, or do not iron)

What is *not* on a care label is also important. You can often use a product or procedure by following normal practices—as long as the label does not specifically warn against it. For instance, if dry cleaning is *not* indicated on a label, you should be able to safely dry-clean the garment. You will see the words *dry-clean only* when an item cannot be laundered safely.

Care labels reduce the guesswork in doing laundry and ensure your clothes remain wearable. Figure **25-3** explains the meaning of different care label instructions. By leaving the labels in place, you can refer to them each time a garment needs cleaning. The center-back neckline, a seam, or the front facing of a garment are typical locations for care labels. Tagless garments have the required information permanently stamped on the inside of the item.

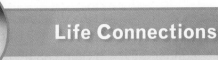

Life Connections

Basic Stain Removal Tips

Treat stains as soon as you notice them and before laundering. It is easier to remove a fresh stain than an old one. Stubborn stains may require several rounds of treatment. Follow the garment's care instructions carefully. Heat will set some stains permanently, yet is needed to remove others.

Protein-based stains often have some dried areas that need to be brushed or scraped off first. Use only cool water for washing and rinsing. Heat sets proteins into the fabric and can make them permanent.

Oil-based stains need to be pretreated or presoaked in detergent and washed in the hottest water temperature safe for the fabric. Double check that the stain is removed. If not, continue treating before placing in the dryer.

Dye-based stains are the most difficult to remove even when caught early. Unlike protein-based stains, dye-based stains respond better to hot water. Depending on the stain, and if treated quickly enough, you might remove it by running it under hot water. If the stain has set, rub the area with detergent or oxygen bleach and soak for 20 minutes. Repeat as necessary. Sometimes lemon juice works as an eco-friendly presoak, too.

Fresh *tannin-based* stains are usually easy to remove. Run the stain under cold water and then launder with the hottest temperature of water safe for the fabric. Set-in tannin-based stains, however, need pretreatment. Never use soap (only use detergent) on tannin-based stains because soap sets those stains permanently.

Science Activity

Test stain removal techniques by creating four different types of stains on spare material scraps. Compare how effective the different techniques are for each stain type.

Stain Removal

A **stain** is a spot or discoloration on a garment that is hard to remove. Each type of stain needs a particular removal process. The best way to remove a stain

When Label Reads		It Means
Machine Washable	Machine wash	Wash, bleach, dry, and press by any customary method including commercial laundering and dry cleaning.
	Home launder only	Same as above, but do not use commercial laundering.
	No chlorine bleach	Do not use chlorine bleach. Oxygen bleach may be used.
	No bleach	Do not use any type of bleach.
	Cold wash Cold rinse	Use cold water or cold washing machine setting.
	Warm wash Warm rinse	Use warm water or warm washing machine setting.
	Hot wash	Use hot water or hot washing machine setting.
	No spin	Remove wash load before final machine spin cycle.
	Delicate cycle Gentle cycle	Use appropriate machine setting; otherwise wash by hand.
	Durable press cycle Permanent press cycle	Use appropriate machine setting; otherwise use warm wash, cold rinse, and short spin cycle.
	Wash separately	Wash alone or with like colors.
Nonmachine Washing	Hand wash	Launder only by hand in lukewarm (hand comfortable) water. May be bleached, may be dry-cleaned.
	Hand wash only	Same as above, but do not dry-clean.
	Hand wash separately	Hand wash alone or with like colors.
	No bleach	Do not use bleach.
	Damp wipe	Clean surface with damp cloth or sponge.
Home Drying	Tumble dry	Dry in tumble dryer at specified setting—high, medium, low, or no heat.
	Tumble dry, remove promptly	Same as above, but in absence of cool down cycle, remove at once when tumbling stops.
	Drip dry	Hang wet and allow to dry with hand shaping only.
	Line dry	Hang damp and allow to dry.
	No wring No twist	Hang dry, drip dry, or dry flat only. Handle to prevent wrinkles and distortion.
	Dry flat	Lay garment on flat surface.
	Block to dry	Maintain original size and shape while drying.
Ironing or Pressing	Cool iron	Set iron at lowest setting.
	Warm iron	Set iron at medium setting.
	Hot iron	Set iron at hot setting.
	Do not iron	Do not iron or press with heat.
	Steam iron	Iron or press with steam.
	Iron damp	Dampen garment before ironing.
Misc.	Dry-clean only	Garment should be dry-cleaned only, including self-service.
	Professional dry-clean only	Do not use self-service dry cleaning.
	No dry-clean	Use recommended care instructions. No dry cleaning materials to be used.

25-3 This table will help you understand the instructions on garment care labels.

is to know the material that caused the stain so the proper technique is used. The main stain categories are

- *protein-based*, which includes blood, dairy products, body soils, baby formula, mud, eggs, and baby food.
- *oil-based*, which includes butter, makeup, oil, mayonnaise, deodorant, gasoline, and collar and cuff stains from natural body oils.
- *dye-based*, which includes some inks, fruit, grass, flavored drink mixes, and mustard.
- *tannin-based*, which includes tea, coffee, soft drinks, berries, fruit juices, and alcoholic beverages. **Tannin** is a reddish, plant-based acid occurring naturally in various foods and drinks.

Simple laundering may remove some stains from washable garments, especially fresh ones. It is best, however, to pretreat stains and then launder as usual. *Prewash*, or pretreatment, products work using enzymes or oxygen formulas activated by water to loosen the stain's hold on fibers. Never press with an iron over a stain. Heat often makes stains impossible to remove.

Stains on non-washable garments should be dry-cleaned as soon as possible. Tell the dry cleaner the cause of the stain, if you know it. Dry cleaners use solvents to remove oil-based stains, such as grease or makeup. Chemical solvents are often referred to as *cleaning fluids*. Some are flammable and can be poisonous. Dry cleaners must use chemical stain-removal solvents in well-ventilated places.

Laundry Products

Check out the many types of laundry products now available for purchase, **25-4**. Your product choices depend on the types of fabrics and

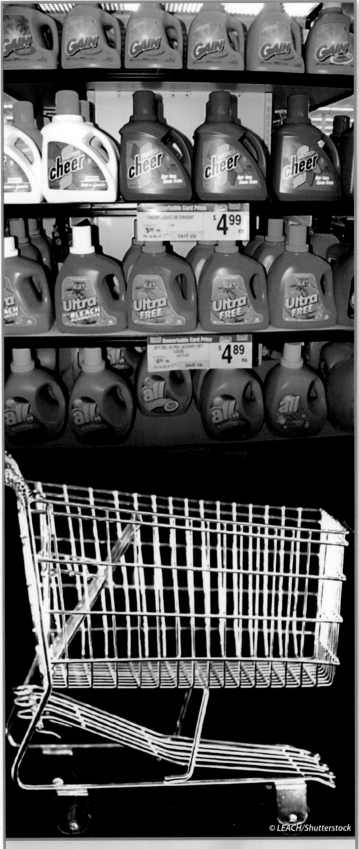

© LEACH/Shutterstock

25-4 There are many laundry products on the market. Knowing which ones to buy and how to use them is important.

the amount of soil in your laundry loads. Each laundry product is designed for a certain function and may not work well for all fabrics. For this reason, be sure to read the product labels carefully to obtain good results.

Prewash Products

Prewash products can help remove some stains and heavy soil, especially in fabrics made from manufactured fibers. Prewash products come in liquid, spray, and stick forms. Apply to the stained area for pretreatment and allow the product to remain on the stain for several minutes before washing. Follow the product's instructions, as they can differ.

Detergents

Detergents remove soil from fabrics using chemical cleaning agents. They are available in powdered and liquid forms. Some are all-purpose detergents and others are light duty. They work well in hard or soft water. Some detergents are high-sudsing and others are low-sudsing. Use either type with a top-loading washer. Measure detergent correctly and add to a top-loading machine while it fills with water and before adding the laundry.

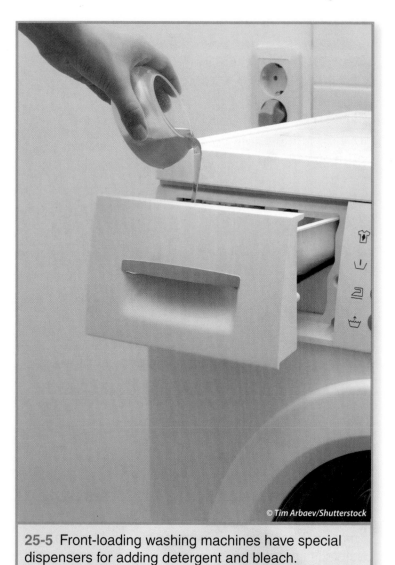

© Tim Arbaev/Shutterstock

25-5 Front-loading washing machines have special dispensers for adding detergent and bleach.

Front-loading, high efficiency (HE) washing machines require special low-sudsing detergents labeled *HE*. Because detergents differ in concentration and are added differently, it is important to follow your washing machine's directions carefully, **25-5**.

Bleaches

Liquid and dry bleaches remove stains and whiten and brighten fabrics. There are two kinds of bleach—chlorine and oxygen. *Chlorine bleach* disinfects and deodorizes fabrics, but is not safe for all fabrics. Chlorine bleach can also remove dyes that will change the color of your garment, so it is best for white and light-colored cotton fabrics. Read a garment's care label to find out if chlorine bleach can be used. *Oxygen bleach* is safe for most colored fabrics.

For best results, follow the directions on the bleach container. Never pour bleach directly onto garments. Instead, add the bleach to the water according to your washing machine's directions and before adding the clothes.

Fabric Softeners

Fabric softeners can be used to make laundry soft, clean-smelling, and reduce wrinkling and static cling. Depending on the brand, fabric softener can be added at the beginning of the laundry cycle at the same time as the detergent or during the rinse cycle. Fabric softener also comes in heat-activated sheets for the dryer.

Doing Your Laundry

Before washing your clothes, sort the items by how they are to be washed. Sorting is grouping clothes by fabric weight, color, degree of soil, fabric construction, and size of item. See Figure **25-6** for a guide for sorting clothes. Sorting clothes properly prevents laundry problems, such as darker fabrics bleeding dye into light-colored fabrics.

As you sort clothes, inspect each garment carefully. Remove all items from the pockets, especially pens, gum, coins, and tissues. Close buttons, zippers, hooks and eyes, and snaps to prevent them from damaging other items. Do not launder ripped or torn garments because the agitation will worsen the rip or tear and make it harder to mend.

Using the Washing Machine

Depending on the machine type and brand, several selections are required for each load of laundry. The most common selections for top-loading washers are wash cycle, wash and rinse water temperatures, and water level. If you are washing just a few items, use a low water level. This saves energy and water.

Many front-loading, high efficiency washers automatically adjust the water level by the size or weight of the load. The water temperatures in these models are also adjusted automatically based on the selected cycle.

Guide for Sorting Clothes		
Sort by fabric weight and garment construction		
Sturdy cloths	Knits	Delicate items, sheers, loosely woven fabrics
Sort by color		
Whites, solid pastels, light prints	Medium and bright colors	Dark or bright colors that might run
Sort by degree of soil		
Heavily soiled	Normal soil	Less soil
Sort by fabric construction and size of item		
Lint-producing fabrics, such as towels	Lint takers, such as corduroy and synthetic fabrics	Mix large and small items
25-6 Keep this guide in mind as you sort clothes.		

Go Green

High Efficiency (*HE*) Washing Machines

While top-loading washing machines are more common and less expensive, front-loading washers are significantly more energy efficient. The initial purchase price is higher, but the cost savings throughout the life of the appliance saves money over time. Benefits of frontloading machines include

- spins clothes faster to extract more water, saving energy and lowering electric bills because drying takes much less time.
- uses less water, which lowers utility bills.
- uses less special *HE* detergent due to less water, so detergent lasts longer.
- tumbles clothes in an up-and-down motion similar to hand washing, which causes less wear and tear on clothing.
- can be stacked with a dryer on top to conserve space.

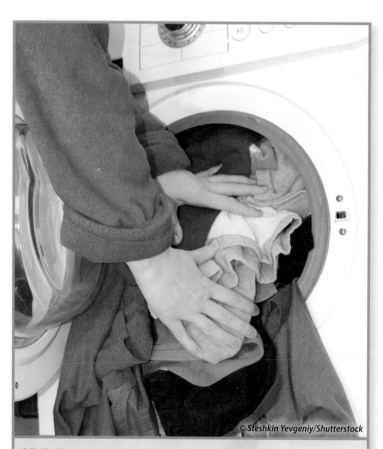

©Steshkin Yevgeniy/Shutterstock

25-7 If you cannot easily close the door of your washing machine, it is overloaded and the laundry will not clean properly.

Always read the care labels on items to learn the recommended wash and rinse water temperatures. For instance, **permanent press** shirts, or those requiring no ironing, do best in a washer's *permanent press cycle* with a cold water rinse. This helps avoid wrinkles.

When washing lingerie, silks, woolens, embroidered or embellished fabrics, lace, and baby items, select a *delicate cycle* with a warm or cold water rinse. This gentle cycle uses a low agitation and delicate spin cycle, allowing you to get the appropriate wash for those items.

Select a *permanent press cycle* if you want a basic wash with delicate spin cycle. This cycle works well for fabrics such as polyester, flannel, and knitted fabrics. These fabrics need a strong agitation to thoroughly clean the fabric. Then, end with a slower spin to prevent the fabric from stretching out of shape.

Use a *normal cycle* for cottons, T-shirts, denims, towels, and other sturdy fabrics. Also, use this cycle for heavily soiled garments that require a more vigorous cleaning. The stronger agitation, along with a faster spin, cleans fabrics thoroughly without leaving residue. White towels need a normal cycle with hot water.

Take care not to overload a washer, **25-7**. For good cleaning results, clothes need room to move freely in the water and laundry product.

Hand Washing

Many loosely woven, knitted, and wool garments have care labels that recommend hand washing. Garments with delicate trims or colors that run when washed also often require hand washing. Use a detergent product recommended for clothing washed by hand. Cold or lukewarm water are the safest water temperatures for hand washing clothing.

Add detergent in the amount the product label suggests. Dissolve the detergent by swishing it in the water with your hand before adding the garment. Force the water through the garment by gently squeezing it several times with your hands. This dissolves soil and releases it from the garment into the water.

Rinse the garment several times to remove all the detergent and the water is clear. Then roll it in a large towel and press with your fingers to remove most of the water. Finally, continue drying according to the care label instructions.

Drying Clothes

You can tumble dry most washable clothing in an automatic dryer. Some clothes need to dry on a flat surface, however, and others must be hung to dry. Always refer to the garment care labels for drying instructions.

Tumble Drying

Tumble drying clothes in an automatic dryer is the quickest way to dry them. Be careful not to overload the dryer with clothes. Overloading causes wrinkling and overworks the dryer's motor, **25-8**.

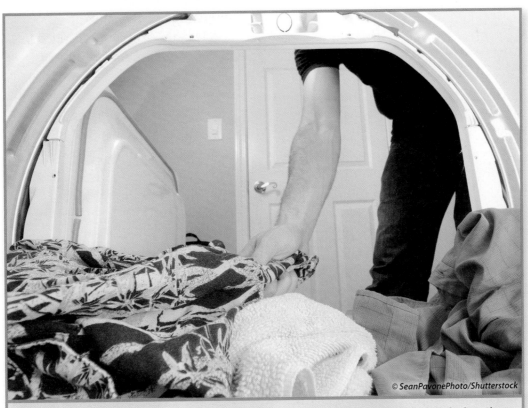

© SeanPavonePhoto/Shutterstock

25-8 Overloading a dryer reduces energy efficiency by increasing the drying time.

Be sure to set the correct drying time and temperature based on care label directions. For instance, sturdy, cotton garments can withstand higher temperatures than manufactured-fiber fabrics. High temperatures can shrink some clothes, however. Fabrics with wrinkle-resistant finishes need lower temperatures because heat dissolves the chemicals used.

An average load of clothes needs about 25–30 minutes of drying time. Items such as towels and sweatshirts may require more time. Delicate, lightweight garments require a lower temperature and about 10–15 minutes of drying time.

As soon as the dryer stops, remove the clothes to minimize wrinkling. Hang garments, such as shirts, blouses, dresses, and pants on hangers. Fold flat items, such as socks, underwear, and towels. Damp clothes can cause mildew and odors. Be sure clothes are completely dry before you put them away.

Line-drying

Line-drying is required for some garments made with fabrics that will shrink from a dryer's heat. Many care labels will say "Hang to dry." Hang these items on plastic hangers, smoothing out the wrinkles and straightening the seams. You can line-dry clothes outdoors or inside over a towel rack or other drying device, **25-9**.

Some garments may require *drip-drying*. Lift these garments from the rinse water and place them on plastic hangers. Do not squeeze, wring, or twist them.

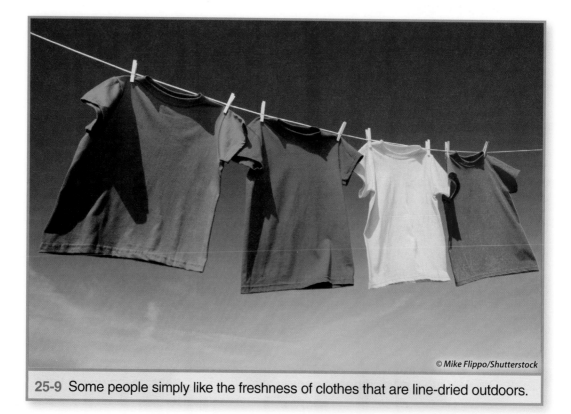

© Mike Flippo/Shutterstock

25-9 Some people simply like the freshness of clothes that are line-dried outdoors.

Flat-drying

Some care labels suggest garments should be dried on a flat surface. Garments that may shrink or stretch out of shape, such as sweaters, often require flat-drying. **Flat-drying** requires first removing much of the rinse water by wrapping the garment in a towel. Roll the garment in the towel and press it with your hands. Unroll and shape the garment on a clean, flat, absorbent surface away from direct heat. This drying method helps garments retain their shapes.

Dry Cleaning

Dry cleaning is a process of cleaning clothes using chemical solvents instead of water. Check the care labels on garments to see if they require dry cleaning instead of laundering. Garments such as suits, coats, and some dresses often need dry-cleaning.

Professional dry cleaners try to remove stains before cleaning garments. If possible, name the stain, and be sure to point out any stains that are light in color. Overlooking these stains may cause them to turn dark during the dry-cleaning process.

Professional dry cleaners are skillful in cleaning special materials such as fur, leather, suede, and their imitations. Some offer other services, such as alterations. If requested, they may remove some buttons and trim before cleaning to prevent chemical solvent damage. Buttons are sewn in place after cleaning the garment. Dry cleaners also press most garments after cleaning, using special pressing equipment.

Home dry-cleaning kits are also available for use in a dryer. These kits contain stain removal solution for pretreatment, heat-activated dry-cleaning sheets, and heat-resistant plastic bags. Place the clothing item and cleaning sheet in the sealable bag. Set the dryer to the instructed heat setting and time according to the directions.

Pressing and Ironing

You may ask "What is the difference between pressing and ironing? Aren't they the same task?" The answer is *no*.

Pressing is the process of removing wrinkles from clothing using a lifting motion and steam. Pressing seams as you sew helps give a professional finish to the seam. Seams are often pressed open. Pressing on the wrong side of fabrics prevents shine on the outside of the garment.

Go Green

Safer Dry-Cleaning Options

Some dry cleaners use a toxic chemical called *perchloroethylene*, or *perc*, to clean clothing. Perc is a hazardous air pollutant under the federal pollution standards. If it seeps into drinking water supplies, it is extremely difficult to remove.

While dry cleaners are subject to emission laws, the most environmentally friendly option is to locate a *green* dry-cleaning business. Green dry-cleaning businesses replace perc with liquid carbon dioxide (CO_2 is a natural substance used in sodas) or a silicone-based solvent used in modified dry-cleaning machines. A third, less reliable method is wet cleaning (using soap and water) in computer-controlled washing machines.

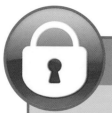

Safety Connections

Iron Safety

Although everyone knows that touching a hot iron causes a bad burn, there are some other important safety precautions to remember.

- Insert the iron's plug firmly into the outlet and unplug it by grasping the plug. Never yank the cord because this will eventually weaken it and potentially cause a fire.
- Always disconnect an iron from an electrical outlet when filling with water, emptying the water, and when not in use.
- Do not allow the cord to touch the hot iron surface.
- Do not operate an iron with a damaged cord, if it has been dropped, or if it appears damaged in any way.
- Let the iron cool completely and loop cord loosely around it before storing.

Ironing is also a process of removing wrinkles with heat, but requires a *gliding* motion instead of a lifting motion. As you iron, start with the smaller sections such as collars, sleeves, and cuffs. Then move to larger sections of the garment, such as the back and front shoulder areas. This prevents wrinkling of sections already ironed. Always iron with the grain of the fabric to help prevent stretching the garment.

Most irons have temperature control settings according to fabric types. Use these settings to prevent scorching fabrics or melting some synthetic fabrics. If you think the heat may damage a garment, press an unnoticeable seam as a test. Press or iron all delicate or low-temperature garments first. This saves time spent waiting for a hot iron to cool.

Clothing Storage

The most important thing to remember when storing any clothing is to store only *clean* clothes. Always launder or dry-clean garments before storage. Sometimes you cannot see soil spots in a garment. Suppose you store a garment with a soft drink spill that does not show. It may turn yellow or brown during storage and be impossible to remove later.

Everyday Storage

Keeping your clothes wrinkle free and easily available are the two primary reasons for learning proper storage techniques. Place like items, such as pants, shirts, or dresses together in one place. For instance, if you keep all your T-shirts folded neatly in the same drawer, you can find the one you want quickly.

Use drawers for storing smaller items and knits so they do not stretch and lose their shape. Make sure the garments hanging in your closet are not crushed together. Give your clothing enough closet space to prevent wrinkling. This also makes it easier to locate items for wearing.

Traditional wire hangers may work for some pieces of hanging clothing, but will give pants unsightly creases. They can also cause bumps in shoulders. Flimsy clothing can slip off wire hangers. Special hangers are available to help different garments keep their shapes. They are easy to find and often inexpensive.

Seasonal Storage

In many regions of the country, seasonal clothing is necessary. Coats and sweaters are needed in winter, but are put in storage in the summer. During the summer, warm-weather clothing such as shorts and swimsuits are brought out of storage. Proper storage keeps your clothing in good condition from season to season.

Wool garments require special care to look nice for years to come. **Moths** are insects that feed on woolen garments. They lay eggs on clothing. When the eggs hatch, the larvae eat the wool. Dry cleaning destroys any moth eggs or larvae. Moth repellents are also available. Use them according to the manufacturer's directions. Many moth repellents have an odor, so it is important to air out clothes before wearing them. You can also use natural moth repellent substances, such as lavender, cedar, or cinnamon sticks.

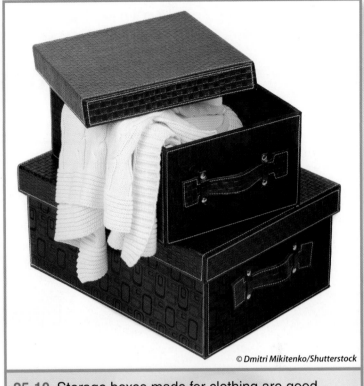

© Dmitri Mikitenko/Shutterstock

25-10 Storage boxes made for clothing are good choices for seasonal storage.

Select a storage area that is dry and away from direct sunlight. Attics are usually better than basements. Dampness in a basement can cause mildew and musty odors that are difficult to remove. Cedar chests, closets, storage bags, and boxes are good containers for storing out-of-season clothes, **25-10**. Seal bags and boxes tightly with tape to keep dust and insects out.

Reading Review

1. What does keeping your clothes in good condition involve?
2. What information is included on care labels?
3. When doing laundry, how are clothes grouped when sorting?
4. Differentiate between pressing and ironing.
5. What is the most important thing to remember when storing any clothing?

Repairing, Redesigning, and Recycling Clothes

Objectives

After studying this section, you will be able to
- **demonstrate** how to perform simple clothing repairs.
- **demonstrate** how to extend the life of an old garment by redesigning it.
- **identify** options for recycling clothes.

Key Terms	
appliqué	redesign
snag	resale shops

From time to time, garments may need some type of repair. Repairs can be easy and use many of the sewing skills you already have. Maybe you have simply outgrown a garment or it seems out of style. There are many options for old clothing other than discarding them.

Repairing Your Clothes

Suppose your jeans have a rip or tear. Maybe you need to replace a button on a shirt. Perhaps your favorite sweater was caught in a zipper. Instead of setting these garments aside and forgetting about them, repair them. This allows them to remain a part of your wardrobe, and saves your clothing budget money.

Ripped Seams and Tears

You can repair rips and tears by machine or by hand. Try to match the color of the thread to the fabric in the garment. If this is not possible, choose a darker shade of thread rather than a lighter one.

To mend a ripped seam, turn the garment inside out. Pin the seam together and sew with short stitches. Extend your line of stitching a little past the rip in both directions. If you are hand sewing, do not pull the stitches too tight. Tight stitches may break again under stress. Repair rips in areas that receive a lot of stress with a double row of machine stitches. These areas include crotch seams on pants and armhole seams on shirts. If the seam edges are frayed, trim the loose threads and add a row of stitching close to the edge.

Patching Tears

To mend a tear, clip loose threads from the frayed area to ready it for patching. To patch a tear, apply the patch to the outside of the garment using machine or hand stitches, **25-11**. The patch can match the garment fabric or it can be a different fabric completely. Think of jackets and blazers with patches sewn on the elbows.

Another method is to apply a piece of an *iron-on patch* in a similar color to the underside of the tear (on the inside of the garment). The tear is mended by ironing the patch, which allows the heat to melt the resin and fuse the tear. Carefully follow the directions on the package of the iron-on patching material.

Consider using an **appliqué**, or decorative cutout made from material or embroidery, to patch a small hole. Appliqués can also be ironed on or sewn on, depending on the type you purchase.

Fixing Fasteners

A loose or missing button or a broken zipper can cause embarrassment. Tape and safety pins will do in an emergency, but they are only a temporary solution. Replace or repair fasteners as soon as possible.

If a zipper breaks, carefully remove it. Press the zipper area flat. Choose a new zipper that is the same size and color as the old one. Pin the new zipper in place. Machine stitch the zipper along the original stitching lines, removing the pins as you sew.

When you first notice a loose button, resew it immediately. If you do not have time, remove it and put it in a safe place until you can resew it. If a button is lost, it is often difficult to find an identical replacement. If that is the case, all the buttons on the garment may need replacement so they match, **25-12**.

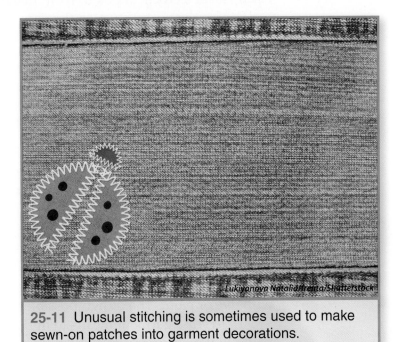

© Lukiyanova Natalia/frenta/Shutterstock

25-11 Unusual stitching is sometimes used to make sewn-on patches into garment decorations.

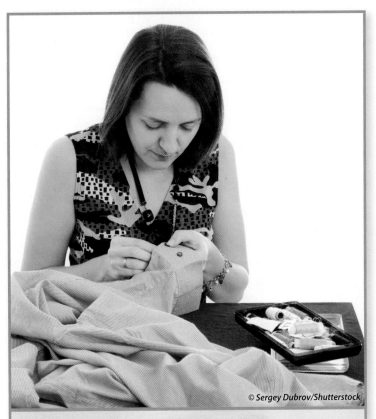

© Sergey Dubrov/Shutterstock

25-12 Save the extra buttons that come with garments so if you lose any, you only have to replace one.

Snags

Snags are usually a quick and easy repair. A **snag** is a loop of yarn pulled out of fabric. If a snag occurs, never cut the loop of thread. Instead, use a *snag repair tool* or a crochet hook to fix it. Insert the hook from the inside of the garment to the outside. Grasp the snag with the hook and pull it back through to the inside of the garment. Then gently stretch the fabric to smooth the area where the snag occurred.

Redesigning and Recycling

To **redesign** means to change the appearance or function of a garment. Redesigning includes restyling, adding decorative features, painting, or changing the color of a garment. For instance, you can restyle an old pair of pants by cutting off the lower part of the legs to make a pair of *cut-offs* or shorts. You can also use the remaining leg fabric to turn the shorts into a skirt.

Adding decorative trims, appliqués, embroidery, or buttons can give old clothes a new look. Dyeing, stamping, or painting also changes the look of a garment. A plain white T-shirt can become any color you want by adding color with dye or paint. The design possibilities are almost endless.

To *recycle* a garment means to find a new purpose for it. For instance, you might give outgrown clothing to a younger relative or a charitable organization. You might donate clothing, shoes, and accessories to a *thrift shop* for resale. Charities often operate thrift shops as fundraising ventures.

Global Connections

Recycle Clothing to Third World Countries

The term *Third World* was coined in the 1950s to describe developing nations with little industry. Many of these countries are in Africa, Asia, and Latin America. Consider recycling your unwanted clothing by donating them to charitable organizations that send them to Third World countries.

Some organizations simply give clothing to certain countries. Others sell your donated clothes inexpensively to clothing dealers in various Third World countries. The dealers then sell the clothes for a small profit and turn unwanted items into rags for other uses. Recycled items provide affordable clothing to needy people and help the environment by lessening the production of new clothes.

Use the Internet to investigate organizations in your area that send donated clothing to Third World countries. Before donating your clothes, wash and repair them to ensure they are in good shape with no tears, major stains, or missing zippers.

Another option is to sell your garments through a consignment shop. A consignment shop sells wearable preowned clothing for the original owners, receiving a percentage of the selling price. This is a good way to recycle your clothing and make some money at the same time.

Some specialty **resale shops** purchase expensive items for low prices, such as bridal gowns and other formal wear, and resell them for a profit. The prices are still less than those in department stores, making formal wear affordable for more people. It also benefits the sellers because they make money on expensive items sitting in their closets that were only worn once.

A wide variety of creative sewing projects result from recycling old garments into completely different items. Consider using the fabric from old garments to make clothes for children or their dolls. You can also create patchwork pillows or quilts, computer covers, or small tote bags from old pieces of fabric. Use your imagination to come up with new and different uses for old clothes, **25-13**. Recycling clothing is a good way to conserve resources and save money.

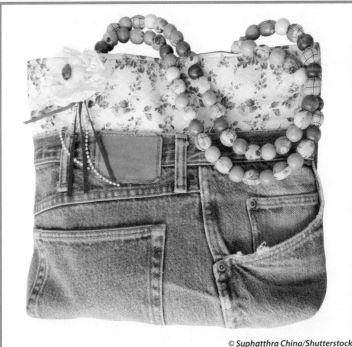

© Suphatthra China/Shutterstock

25-13 This unique purse was made using two fabrics from old clothing and adding beads for the handles.

Reading Review

1. If a garment has a rip or tear, why is it important to repair it and not set it aside and forget about it?
2. When repairing ripped seams or tears, which seams should have a double row of machine stitches?
3. When you first notice a loose button, why should you resew it immediately or remove it and put it in a safe place until you can resew it?
4. How do you repair a snag in a garment?
5. What can you do with clothes you no longer wear?

Chapter Summary

Section 25-1. You can get more wear out of your clothes if you care for them properly. Basic clothing care starts with keeping your clothes clean. Care labels in garments will tell you what laundry products to use and what procedures to follow. Sort clothes according to their laundering requirements. Garments will either need to be machine-washed, hand washed, or dry-cleaned. Garments cleaned at home may be tumble-dried, line-dried, or flat-dried. Once garments are clean, press or iron them and store them carefully to keep them looking neat.

Section 25-2. Making simple repairs and when they are needed will allow you to wear your clothes longer. Repairing seams or tears, sewing on buttons, and fixing snags are easy repair jobs that should be done as soon as possible. Taking a few minutes to do these clothing care tasks will extend your wardrobe and the life of your clothes. If you can no longer wear certain items, you can recycle or redesign them to extend their usefulness.

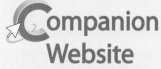

Companion Website
www.g-wlearning.com

Check your understanding of the main concepts for Chapter 25 at the website.

Critical Thinking

1. **Draw conclusions.** Think about what steps you can take to be more responsible about your clothing. How can taking these steps help you to get the most out of the clothing you have?
2. **Analyze.** Consider your clothes-buying habits. When you buy clothes, do you consider the type of care they require? If a garment requires hand washing or dry cleaning, will you still buy it? Explain your answer.
3. **Evaluate.** Look through your clothing. Check each garment to determine what care and repairs each garment requires. Evaluate the care and repair each garment needs and how and when you will accomplish these tasks.

Common Core

College and Career Readiness

4. **Writing.** Prepare a stain removal guide to use in your laundry room. Next to each type of stain, write instructions for how to remove it.
5. **Math.** Prepare a table listing various laundry products. Calculate the cost per load of using each product.

6. **Reading.** Read the use and care manuals for a washer and dryer either in the classroom or at home. What helpful information did you learn from reading these manuals?

7. **Speaking.** Demonstrate for the class how to repair a seam or tear and how to sew on a button. Answer any questions class members may have.

Technology

8. **Investigate new technologies.** Learn about new technologies in laundering by searching laundry products and equipment on the Internet. You may also want to read current consumer journals and reviews. Prepare a report about your findings and the websites and journals you explored.

Journal Writing

9. Write about your daily clothing care routine. What techniques extend the life of your clothes? What could you do to adjust your routine to better maintain your clothes? What recycling and redesigning options could you use for clothes you no longer wear?

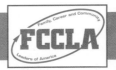

FCCLA

10. Design a new garment that uses scraps from recycled fabrics or garments for a *Recycle and Redesign STAR Event*. Create a display that includes a storyboard showing reconstruction of the new product, a time log of events, and a cost analysis. See your adviser for information as needed.

11. In teams, create an *FCCLA STAR Event Entrepreneurship* project. Develop a plan for a small business that provides alterations, embroidery, or other related services to faculty, parents, and students for a small fee. Use the FCCLA Planning Process to create a business plan, organizational chart, and budget. Identify any codes and regulations your business must follow. Use profits for scholarships for students who are pursuing a career in fashion and textiles. See your adviser for information as needed.

Unit 8
Housing and Transportation

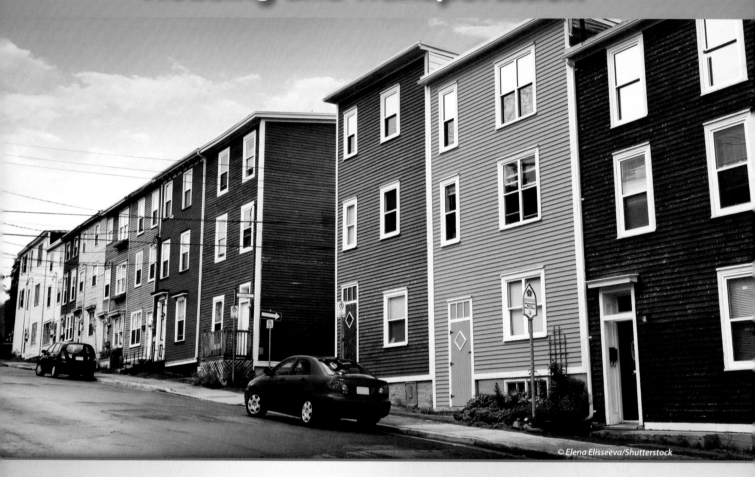

© Elena Elisseeva/Shutterstock

Chapter 26 Your Personal Living Space
Chapter 27 Transportation Options

Unit Essential Question

What are your values related to the personal space you call home?

Exploring Career Pathways

Housing and Interiors Careers

What catches your eye about the dwellings and buildings around you? Is it the design details, or other aspects that make one property more inviting to sell or buy than others? The following includes just a few housing and interiors careers you may find rewarding.

Real Estate Broker or Sales Agent

Real estate brokers or agents require knowledge of zoning laws and real estate financing, the ability to do a market analysis, and strong negotiation skills. Brokers are licensed to manage their own businesses. Agents work for brokers who pay them a commission for each property they sell. Some specialize in residential or commercial real estate. A high school diploma, 30 to 90 hours of classroom instruction in real estate, and passing a written exam are necessary for licensing. Additional training and experience are needed to obtain a broker's license.

Interior Design Assistant

Interior design assistants have a 2- or 3-year certificate or associate's degree to obtain an entry-level position in interior design. They may work in furniture stores or at an interior design firm. Most work with interior designers and do administrative tasks such as reviewing catalogs and ordering samples. Ability to use computer-aided design software and create hand-drawn designs is necessary. Good verbal and listening skills are essential for knowing client and designer needs and wants. After several years of quality experience and excellent performance, interior design assistants may move into designer positions.

Interior Designer

Creativity, superior knowledge of design, ability to read blueprints, and strong understanding of building codes are just a few of the duties of an interior designer. They also create design plans, estimate costs, and specify finishes, materials, and furnishings. Designers develop project deadlines and work with other contractors to carry out design plans for their clients. Use of design software is essential. Interior designers may choose to specialize. A bachelor's degree and formal apprenticeship are required for licensing. Eligibility to take the *National Council for Interior Design Qualification (NCIDQ)* exam requires a total of 6 years of formal education and interior design experience.

Is this career path for you? Use the following activities to determine your interest in or ability for a housing and interiors career.

- Investigate the design process for interior design. Then create a simple design plan for a room in your home or someone else's home, choosing samples for all materials, finishes, furnishings, and accessories. Share your designs with the class.
- Talk with your school guidance counselor about taking the O*NET *Ability Profiler* assessment to see if you have the ability for an interior design career.

Chapter 26
Your Personal Living Space

Sections

Reading Prep

College and Career Readiness

Before you read this chapter, find an area that is quiet and without distractions. Be sure you have adequate lighting to avoid eyestrain, as well as a comfortable chair.

Concept Organizer

Types of accidents in the home	
CAUSE	**EFFECTS**
1.	
2.	
3.	
4.	

Use a diagram like the one shown to identify one cause and effect for the four most common accidents occurring in the home.

Companion Website

Print out the concept organizer for Chapter 26 at the website.

Companion Website
www.g-wlearning.com

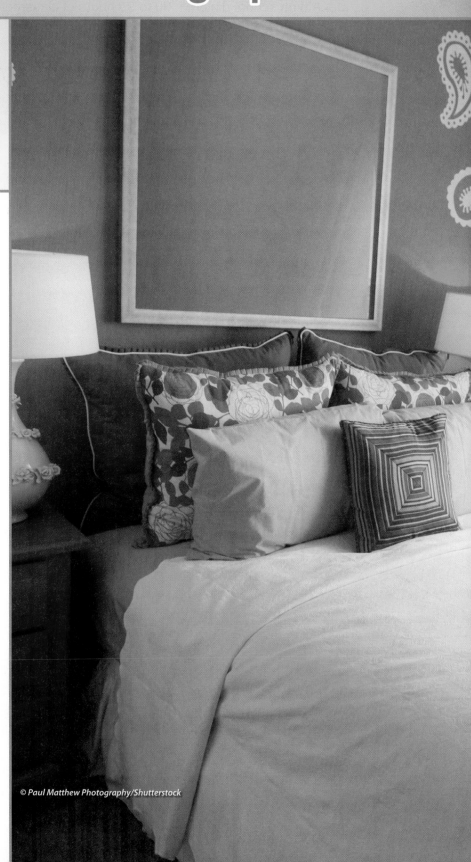

© Paul Matthew Photography/Shutterstock

Homes Fulfill Needs

Objectives

- **explain** how homes fulfill physical, emotional, and social needs.
- **determine** how housing needs change throughout the lifespan.
- **give examples** of the different types of housing.
- **evaluate** housing choices and their associated costs.

Key Terms		
social needs	single-family house	lease
amenities	town houses	mortgage
rural	residential properties	trustees
multiple-family housing	landlords	

What comes to mind when you think of home? You might think of a small house, condo, or tall apartment complex. You might think of having meals with your family in a happy, cozy kitchen. You might recall playing games with your brother or sister in the backyard. You might think of a big overstuffed chair in a quiet corner that is your favorite place to relax. These are the experiences and memories that make a place a home.

Housing Fulfills People's Needs

People define *home* many different ways. Some might say a home is where food, clothing, and shelter are provided to keep a family safe, healthy, and happy, **26-1**. Others might say it is a place to relax, entertain, and do what they please. In short, the home is a place that fulfills people's physical, emotional, and social needs.

Physical Needs

One of the most basic physical needs is shelter. Everyone needs a place for protection from severe weather, such as storms and extreme heat or cold. A home provides protection and safety for a family. Both inside and outside the home, spaces should be arranged and cared for with protection and safety in mind. Everything you need for your personal care and health are often located and stored somewhere in your home.

Emotional Needs

Emotional needs are associated with feelings. They include the need to belong and feel accepted, the need for comfort, and the need for self-confidence.

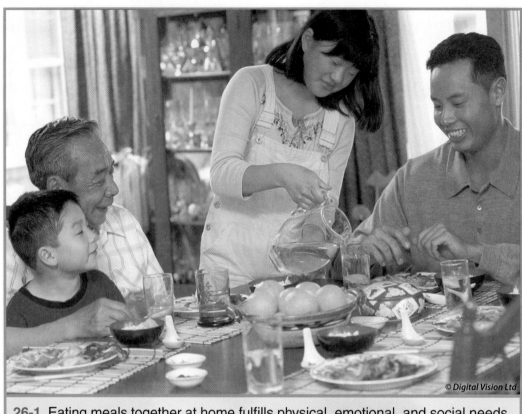

26-1 Eating meals together at home fulfills physical, emotional, and social needs.

Your home can be comfortable without great expense. When family members have a spirit of caring and cooperation, everyone feels more comfortable. Your family and home help you meet your need for self-confidence. Expressing your own personality and special talents at home can help you gain self-confidence in other areas of your life, too.

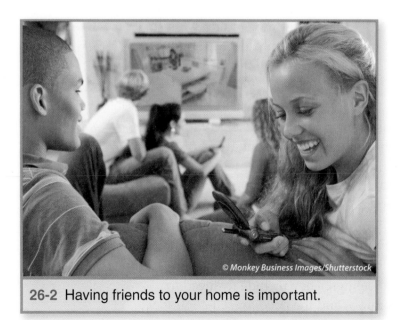

26-2 Having friends to your home is important.

Social Needs

Social needs are those related to interacting with people. Living spaces in a home should meet people's needs to interact with others. *Shared spaces* are those used by all the family members and for entertaining guests. Kitchens, dining, living, and family rooms are all shared spaces, 26-2. The need for family members' privacy should also be respected. This means choosing times and places for private activities that do not cause problems for the rest of the family. By using good communication skills, family members are more likely to reach compromises when sharing spaces together.

Housing Needs Change

Depending on a family's size, the members' ages, and their priorities, families' housing needs will change at different times during their lives. For instance, a young family with three children under the age of six will need a very different type of home than a retired couple in their 70s. There are many considerations when choosing housing to best meet needs.

- **Family size and ages.** This is one of the more important considerations because it determines the amount and types of space a family needs. Families with more children need more space and **amenities**, which are things that make life easier and more pleasant. Children grow older, and family sizes can increase or decrease. These circumstances also affect housing decisions. Some families may grow out of their homes with the addition of new family members. When children move out, however, families may choose to decrease their home size. Single people often want different housing and amenities depending on their ages. The environment a 26-year-old may want probably differs from what a 62-year-old wants.

- **Housing budget.** Most experts suggest between one-quarter and one-third of your monthly income should be budgeted for housing expenses. For renters, that includes your rent and renter's insurance. For homeowners, that includes your mortgage payment, property taxes, home repairs, and insurance. Your income directly affects the type of home you can afford.

- **Location.** Many people choose their housing based on convenience of location. Some may want to be closer to their jobs or live in a certain school district. Length of commute time is a big consideration because it can decrease both time and money spent on transportation.

Life Connections

Universal Design

When looking for a home, consider the ages and needs of the family members. Also, think about how long you plan to remain in the home. *Universal design* is an approach to design that provides equal access to everyone using the product. In the case of home design, it applies to creating living spaces that meet all family members' needs throughout the lifespan.

From the arrangement of the rooms to the heights of counters and types of flooring, many details go into the creation of accessible spaces. For instance, wide hallways, larger and more easily accessible bathrooms, and full-length mirrors appeal to families with young children, as well as older adults. Spiral staircases may seem appealing at one stage in your life, but may be dangerous for children and older adults.

Aging in place is the term for the ability to remain in one home throughout a person's life. With more and more baby boomers becoming older adults, universal design in homes becomes even more important. When choosing or remodeling a home, keep the universal design concepts in mind.

Writing Activity

Conduct online research about universal design and write a one-page paper about how architects and interior designers plan to create homes using the concepts. Explain which universal design concepts are the most important considerations in home design and why.

Families with children may value the reputations of some schools over others, so they would move into that district's neighborhood or town, **26-3**.

- **Lifestyle.** Do you want to live in a big city for the fun and excitement or a smaller town where it is easy to know all your neighbors? Do you want an office in your home or access to a big swimming pool? Perhaps you might choose to live in a **rural**, or country, area for activities like horseback riding or golf. These types of preferences indicate your lifestyle, which also has bearing on where you choose to live.

- **Environmental priorities.** You may choose a type of home that is environmentally friendly, which could mean a number of things. It may have energy-saving appliances and features. It may have solar heating, or it may be so close to your work and other activities that you do not have to use your car.

- **Any special needs.** Some families have members with limited *physical mobility*, or the ability to move freely. For instance, a person using a wheelchair will need wider hallways and doors or possible ramps if there are stairs. There are many forms of special needs, including *visual impairments*, or the inability to see clearly, and reduced hearing capacity. Any special need will affect the type of home a family chooses.

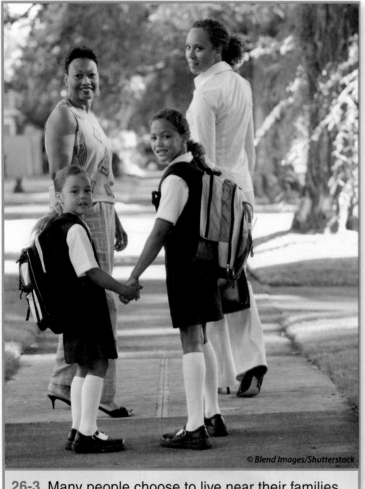

© Blend Images/Shutterstock

26-3 Many people choose to live near their families for support.

Housing Types

Think about your current home. Is it in a building with other similar housing units? If so, you live in a type of **multiple-family housing**. If you live in a freestanding house, you are in a **single-family house**. These are the two primary types of housing.

Multiple-Family Housing

Multiple-family housing can range from a *duplex*, which is two living units attached by a common wall, to a large building with many living units. Your neighbors are very close to you and there are often shared amenities. Sometimes the shared amenities are simply common indoor or outdoor areas. Two or more large multiple-family buildings may be called *complexes*. Some multiple-family buildings and complexes offer health club-like facilities, such as swimming pools, saunas, sports courts, or party rooms as amenities.

The cost of living in buildings or complexes with many amenities is often higher than those with fewer amenities.

Another benefit of multiple-family housing is that people other than the residents handle the maintenance and upkeep. While this provides more free time and less work for the residents, the maintenance cost is part of the rent or additional owners' fees.

Apartments are one-level units in buildings that are rented. Those that are available for purchase are *condominiums* or *condos*. **Town houses** are two- or three-level-homes in a row attached by common walls. They are also called *row houses*, **26-4**.

Single-Family Houses

While multiple-family housing units have common walls, single-family houses do not. Unattached homes give the residents more privacy and yard space, but they are usually more expensive due to the construction, building materials, and land costs. In addition, the owners are responsible for all maintenance and upkeep, which may be extensive for older homes. Single-family dwellings include the following:

- *Custom-built homes* are designed entirely to the specifications of the owners. They tend to be the most expensive types of homes.
- *Tract homes*, also called *mass-produced homes*, are built using a standardized set of floor plans for each home in a subdivision. Builders only allow owners to make slight modifications to the floor plans. To make the homes more affordable, builders often use lower-priced materials, appliances, and fixtures.
- *Manufactured homes* are the least expensive freestanding dwellings because the home pieces are built in factories and then transported to the site for assembly. The land is rented, not owned. Manufactured homes are also called *mobile homes* because they can be moved.

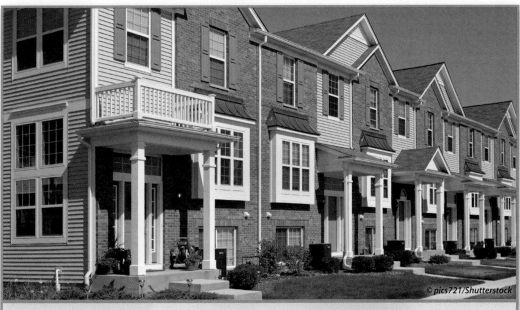

© pics721/Shutterstock

26-4 Town houses and duplexes have private entries on the ground level.

Housing Options

All housing types are residential properties that someone owns. Most people live in the homes they own, but some owners may rent to others for specific periods of time.

Renting a Home

The owners, or landlords, of rental homes or apartments can be individuals, companies, or corporations, **26-5**. The owners usually consider them *investment properties*, meaning they will make money on the rent paid to them over time. There are many benefits to renting, including the amenities, less responsibility, no added maintenance costs, and the ability to move more easily.

Renters must sign a legal document called a lease agreeing to pay the rent on time and keep the property in good shape. Owners often request a security deposit to cover any renter damage to the home. The security deposit is returned when the lease ends—less any expenses to fix damages. Owners usually ask for payment of the first and last month's rent up front to ensure the renters do not leave before the lease ends. Renters cannot paint or otherwise alter their home without the owner's permission.

Disadvantages of renting are that you do not own the property and must find a new place when your lease expires. Some people like the flexibility of moving without the hassle of selling a home. Renters also give up the possibility of making money when their home sells, however, depending on how long they have owned it.

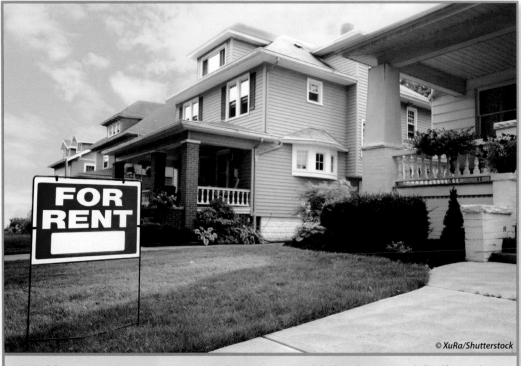

© XuRa/Shutterstock

26-5 Many rentals are less expensive on a monthly basis, especially if you have roommates to share the costs.

Buying a Home

Buying a home provides owners with the security of always knowing where they will live. They only have to move when it suits them. Owners can alter, remodel, and decorate their house, town house, or condominium exactly as they want. There is more freedom in home ownership, but it is also more costly. Property taxes, homeowner's insurance, and repairs are necessary expenses. Owners also assume the risk that their home will be worth more than it cost them when they sell it.

Buying a home is the biggest expense most people will ever have. Therefore, buying a home with cash is rare. The type of long-term loan taken out for home purchase is a **mortgage**. Mortgage loans generally have from 15- to 30-year terms, although other options are available. Lenders require a 5–10 percent down payment. Many owners, however, will make larger down payments to lower the amount financed and their monthly payments.

Cooperative, Condominium, and House Ownership

Many owners opt for purchasing a condominium or a cooperative unit because they do not want to spend time on yard work or home repairs, **26-6**. Cooperatives (co-ops) are similar to condos, but differ in the structure of ownership. Co-ops are real estate corporations formed by the building's unit owners who own the building jointly. The owners' shares in the corporation depend on how much space they occupy. The co-op owners elect a board of **trustees** to manage the building's maintenance funds and

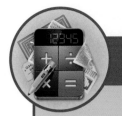

Math Connections

Tax-Deductible Interest

A mortgage's interest rate depends on the type and length of loan chosen, the current economy, and the borrowers' credit histories. Another benefit of home ownership is that mortgage interest paid is tax deductible yearly when submitting an itemized tax return. This tax savings can make owning a home more attractive than renting to some, despite the higher costs of owning.

For instance, approximately how much interest would the Riveras be able to deduct from their yearly taxes if they have a $150,000 mortgage at 4.00% interest for 30 years?

(*Answer:* multiply $150,000 by .04 to get an approximate amount of mortgage interest on the loan, which is $6,000.)

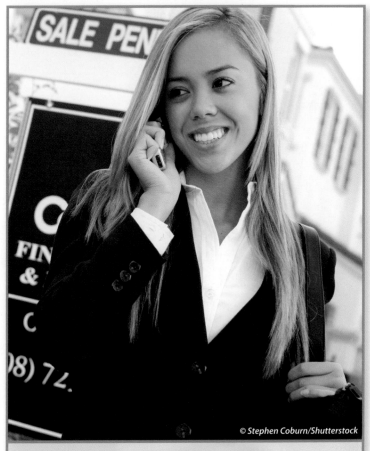

© Stephen Coburn/Shutterstock

26-6 Most people use a real estate agent to help them buy and sell their homes.

other property issues. The co-op board must approve a potential new buyer to join in ownership. The co-op does not own any land, just the building.

In contrast, each condominium owner holds a deed to his or her unit and obtains an individual mortgage. This approach means that individual owners are responsible for mortgage payments and property taxes associated with their units. Generally, a building or complex's unit owners gather to form a condo association. The condo association elects trustees who are responsible for the management and oversight of the buildings. The owners agree to pay monthly maintenance fees in addition to their mortgages. Unlike co-ops, anyone can buy a unit in a complex or building without approval of other owners. Condo owners own their units, plus a portion of the land.

Owning a single-family home is similar to owning a condo. All maintenance, repairs, and other fees are the owner's responsibility, however. The house and land are legally documented on the owner's deed of trust. Residential properties that include more land are worth more than similar properties with less land, **26-7**.

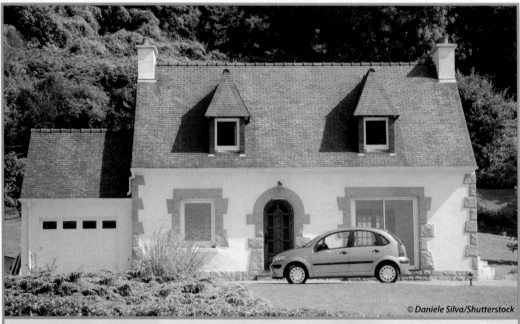

© Daniele Silva/Shutterstock

26-7 Another option for home buyers is to purchase undeveloped land and build their own custom houses.

Reading Review

1. What are social needs?
2. List considerations that need to be made when choosing housing to best meet needs.
3. Distinguish between multiple-family housing and single-family housing.
4. What is a lease?
5. What is a mortgage?

Designing Your Space

Objectives

After studying this section, you will be able to
- **apply** the elements and principles of design to your personal space.
- **give examples** of appropriate home décor products, furniture, and accessories.
- **organize** personal space for improved storage options.
- **create** scale floor plans for different rooms.
- **use** a floor plan to determine efficient room arrangement and traffic patterns.

Key Terms

décor	antique	pegboard
fixtures	drapery	scale floor plan
functional	duvet	traffic patterns

Your personal space belongs more to you than it does to anyone else in your home. One space is most likely your bedroom. Even if you share a bedroom, part of the room is yours. It may be where you relax, visit with friends, or study. It might be your favorite place to go for privacy. Wherever your favorite spaces are, they should be comfortable and useful to you, **26-8**. Important design considerations are your budget, color preferences, furniture, storage, and accessories.

Making the Most of Your Personal Space

Most likely, there are limits to how you could improve your personal space. Within those limits, you can organize your space so you can use it in many ways. You might have permission to paint your space

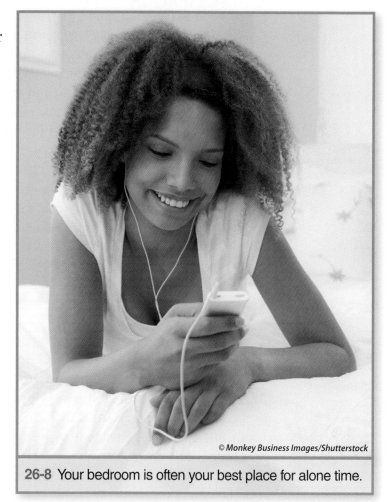

© Monkey Business Images/Shutterstock

26-8 Your bedroom is often your best place for alone time.

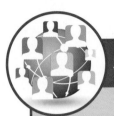

and change the look of it entirely. Once you have determined the goals for your space and talked with your parents about any necessary limits, you can make a plan for your room. As you think about changes, keep the elements and principles of design in mind.

Using the Elements and Principles of Design

The design elements of *color, line, texture, form,* and *space* are integral to achieving your design goal. For instance, use cooler, pale colors to make your room feel relaxing. Vertical lines give the illusion of more space by making your ceiling appear higher. Shiny textures brighten a room by reflecting light. Simple, rectangular forms in a room with little clutter make it feel organized and orderly. Larger pieces of furniture help fill large spaces. Many other effects are possible depending on how you use the elements of design.

The principles of *balance, proportion, rhythm,* and *emphasis* are important considerations when using the various design elements. For instance, a large item, such as a bed or dresser can be balanced with a few smaller items, such as a group of plants. Proportion means choosing items that do not look oversized or tiny in your room. For instance, a canopy bed looks best in a room with a high ceiling. Repeating a color in your room's accessories is a good use of the principle of rhythm. You may choose to make the room's emphasis a unique piece of artwork or painted furniture. These are just a few of the many ways to utilize the principles of design.

Using the elements and principles of design properly can give your room *harmony*, or an overall pleasing, comfortable arrangement. A finished room should easily lead your eyes from one item to the next and look as if everything belongs together.

Home Décor

You can express your personality through your choices of room **décor**, which is the style and layout of interior furnishings. By following some basic guidelines, you can make any room more attractive and functional. Backgrounds, furniture, fixtures, window coverings, and accessories are all home décor choices. **Fixtures** include those permanent pieces installed in a room, such as ceiling and wall lighting, door and window handles, faucets, and other built-ins.

Backgrounds

Backgrounds set the stage for the furnishings, accessories, and other design choices in a room. Walls, floor, and ceiling make up your room's background. No matter where you look in your room, you will see at least part of a background.

Painting is one of the least expensive, easiest ways to change your walls and ceiling. Wallpaper can be fairly inexpensive and it comes in a wide variety of styles and colors. Fabric can cover walls and soften sounds by absorbing them. Remember that darker colors make rooms seem smaller and light colors are expanding. Use two opposite colors from your palette for more contrast. You might even use one color or a design from a specific artist on just one wall for emphasis. Hardware and home improvement stores provide information on how to apply paint, wallpaper, and other materials to walls.

Furniture and Fixtures

Does your room's furniture fit your needs and match your style? Furniture is both decorative and **functional**, meaning having a practical use. While your bed is primarily the place you sleep, it can be the easiest way to redecorate by just changing its coverings and pillows. You might be able to paint some of your existing furniture for a new look.

Perhaps a few new pieces of furniture are all you need. If you decide to buy furniture, there are many inexpensive options, **26-9**. You can find both old and new furniture listed on the Internet and in newspapers. For instance, director's chairs are not very expensive and are available in a variety of colors.

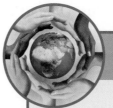

Global Connections

Ethnic Backgrounds

Backgrounds are great places to try different *color palettes* (groups of colors used together) and designs reflecting an ethnicity attractive to you. Many home design books, magazines, and websites have ideas to help you choose colors and prints. For instance, deep reds, golden yellows, purples, and fiesta prints are identified with Latin America. Scandinavian colors include neutral grays and tans, light blues, stark white, and large contemporary prints. Design motifs associated with Africa are bright oranges, greens, blues, and wildlife prints.

Floors are harder to change than walls and can be more expensive. If you have a wood or tile floor, small area rugs with ethnic designs are inexpensive and easy to find. If you can change wall-to-wall carpeting, look for strong and durable replacement carpet. Neutral tans or grays go well with nearly every color and do not show dirt easily. Neutrals allow you to change the look of your room later without replacing your carpet.

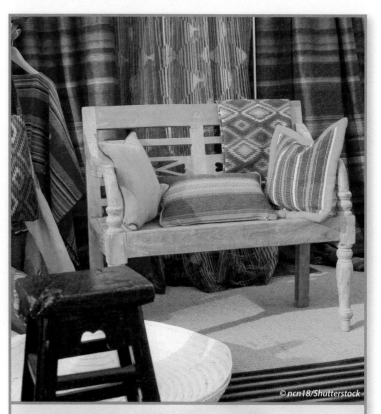

© ncn18/Shutterstock

26-9 You can find some great bargains at garage sales, flea markets, and used furniture stores.

Select furniture and fixtures that fit your personality and decorating scheme. Contemporary furniture and fixtures usually have simple shapes and can be more colorful. More traditional or antique styles have features belonging to an earlier period, style, or fashion. There are no defined rules for furniture or fixture styles. You may want furniture or fixtures in the same style or a mixture of several styles.

Before buying a piece of furniture or particular fixture, check the quality carefully. Be sure it is sturdy enough for its use. Look for minor flaws, such as scratches or dents. Make sure they are either hidden or not obvious. You may be able to get furniture or fixtures with minor flaws at lower prices.

Window Coverings

Window coverings shade light and provide privacy, but they also decorate your room. You can use shades, blinds, shutters, or curtains to cover windows. People often use shades or blinds to keep the sun out, **26-10**. You can use almost any kind of fabric to make shades. The different types of fabric shades include variations on the classic Roman shade and the balloon shade. *Venetian blinds* are strips of wood, plastic, or metal you can turn to let light in or keep it out.

Drapery is the term used for full-length, formal window treatments that are lined. Drapery refers to the beautiful way they *drape* from the curtain rod to the floor. *Curtains* are less formal, unlined, and can be either short or long. You can buy curtains or make them to coordinate with your bedspread or other fabrics. For instance, you can use sheets as curtains. Just place the curtain rod through the hem on the sheet. You may need to cut and hem the sheet to your window's length.

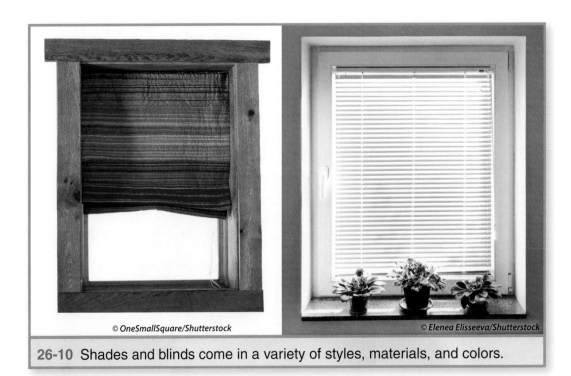

© OneSmallSquare/Shutterstock   © Elenea Elisseeva/Shutterstock

26-10 Shades and blinds come in a variety of styles, materials, and colors.

Accessories

Accessories are the accents that make a room more attractive, comfortable, and convenient. Your choice of accessories will not be exactly like anyone else's. Some accessories are functional, such as window coverings, pillows, wastebaskets, and lamps. Other accessories, such as wall hangings or plants are simply decorative.

Making accessories or purchasing older ones at garage sales and flea markets can be much less expensive than buying new ones. With a little work, you can redesign some to fit the style of your room. For instance, you could paint an old picture frame with bright enamel color. Turning inexpensive table linens into festive pillow covers can save you a lot of money and become a centerpiece of your bed.

How to Use Accessories

Accessories should harmonize with the furniture and backgrounds in your room. The elements and principles of design also apply when choosing and arranging accessories. You are limited only by your imagination in the kind of accessories you can create or buy.

Your bed's covering is one of the most noticeable accessories and might easily become the focal point of your room, **26-11**. There are bed covers to fit every design style and budget—from bedspreads and quilts to blankets and comforters. You might choose a **duvet**, which is a washable, removable bed cover that encloses a comforter. A duvet cover can be changed when you want to give your room a new look. Pillows are great accents on your bed, on chairs, or as seating spaces.

Pictures and wall hangings can also express your personality, and the possibilities are endless. You can purchase or create any type of posters, paintings, drawings, and photographs. You can make hanging *collages* in which you arrange various objects on a flat surface. Objects you might use in the collage include paint, cardboard, sand, keys, feathers, or almost any small object.

Plants can add color and life to any room. You can buy small plants at a greenhouse or store for very low prices and repot them in decorative containers. Plants do need care, however. If you want to grow plants, be sure to learn and follow the care directions for each plant.

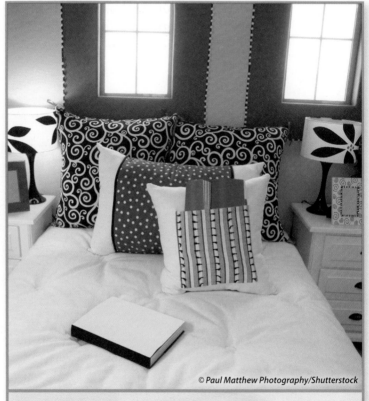

© Paul Matthew Photography/Shutterstock

26-11 Pillows are versatile accessories that can be made or bought in any shape, size, and fabric.

Improving Storage Space

You might feel there is not enough space for all your belongings. If you organize your space properly, however, you can find much more room for storage. When items are stored correctly, they are also easier to remove and replace. When organizing space for improved storage, think about how often you use the items. Store items used daily, such as school supplies and personal care items, where you can reach them easily and quickly. Under-bed storage containers are handy for seasonal items, such as snow boots and swimsuits, or other items used infrequently.

Closets

Closets often have unused or *dead space*. A few simple changes can increase the amount of usable space. For instance, mount two rods, one above the other, to double the amount of your hanging space for clothes. Securely attach hooks on closet walls to hang hats, belts, or other accessories. Hang a shoe bag on the wall or closet door for more shoe storage.

There are many closet organizing systems on the market today, **26-12**. Some are fairly inexpensive. The systems consist of various types of storage units and racks you can combine in different ways. The combinations depend on what you are storing and where. Another option is using boxes or shelves to create your own customized closet organization.

Walls and Furniture

If you still need more storage in your room, look to your walls. You can hang single or multiple shelves or pegboard on empty wall spaces. **Pegboard** is a particle-wood board with small holes in it. You can attach

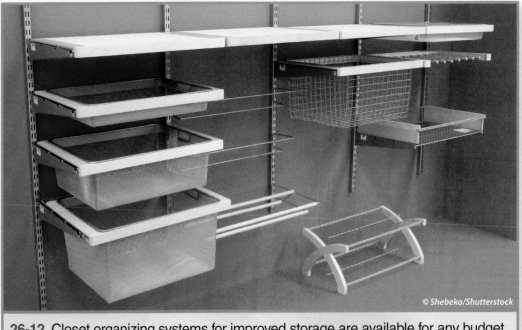

© Shebeko/Shutterstock

26-12 Closet organizing systems for improved storage are available for any budget.

and remove hooks easily from pegboard. Sports equipment, souvenirs, jewelry, and other items can be easily stored on the hooks.

You could add furniture created specifically for storage to your room. Cabinets with drawers and shelves are available in many sizes, styles, and price ranges. You can stack cubes or crates to create your own storage units that could easily be changed as your needs change. Baskets, cubes, and crates are also available in many sizes, materials, and colors, **26-13**.

Rearrange or reorganize your existing furniture drawers for better use of space. Make drawer compartments with smaller plastic or cardboard boxes. Using compartments to hold similar items, such as socks or T-shirts, allows for better storage and improved identification and retrieval.

Functional Rooms

You should be able to move through a room without feeling cramped or running into anything. Functional rooms make activities as easy as possible through logical placement of furniture and accessories. For instance, doing homework in your room is easier if your computer is close to paper, pencils, and books. Making a floor plan can help you to have a more functional room.

Making a Scale Floor Plan

A **scale floor plan** is a flat drawing of a room's floor corresponding to the actual room's size and shape. For instance, one-half inch on the floor plan might

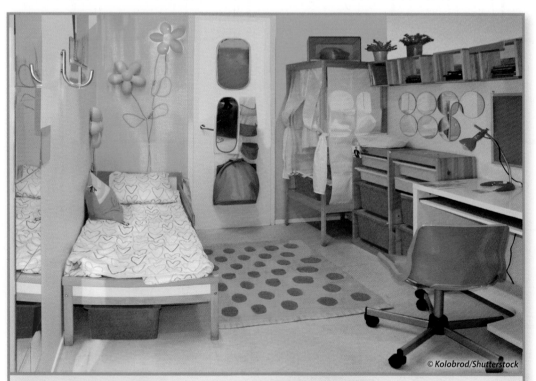

© Kolobrod/Shutterstock

26-13 This room was specifically designed for efficient storage. How many different forms of storage can you identify in the picture?

represent one foot in the room. Use graph paper for drawing a scale floor plan. Assign each square on the graph paper a measurement of your room's floor. For instance, you might decide that one square equals six inches. Therefore, if the room you are drawing is 10 feet by 12 feet, the scale is 20 squares by 24 squares.

To make an accurate floor plan, measure the dimensions of your floor first. Draw the outline of the floor to scale on paper. Then mark the location of doors, windows, closets, air vents, and electrical outlets.

Once your floor plan is complete, try different furniture arrangements on it, **26-14**. You can use pieces of paper to represent your furniture. Measure the outside of each furniture piece. Then draw it to scale as you did with the room dimensions. Cut out the furniture pieces and move them around to find the best arrangements. This activity is called *space planning*, and is used by professional interior designers and decorators.

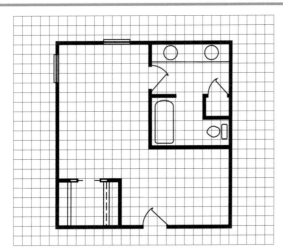

Step 1. Draw the dimensions of the bedroom on graph paper. Show windows and doors in their correct positions.

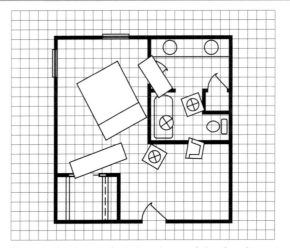

Step 2. Make scaled drawings of the furniture to be placed in the room and cut them out.

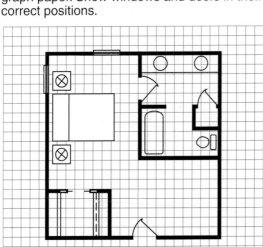

Step 3. Place the bed first.

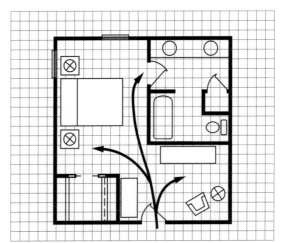

Step 4. Placed the remaining furniture, keeping circulation paths clear.

26-14 You can save much effort by trying out different furniture arrangements on a scale floor plan.

Arranging Furniture

There are many factors to think about when arranging furniture. You need to consider the types of activities you will do in the room, the amount of space you need for each piece of furniture, and optimal traffic patterns. **Traffic patterns** are the paths you take to get to different parts of your room. Good traffic patterns do not have anything blocking the way. For instance, you should not have to walk around a chair to get from your bed to your door. You should not have to squeeze past a bookcase to get from your closet to your bed. Arranging for good traffic patterns makes a room comfortable and safe.

Grouping furniture for certain activities helps organize your space. You can use some areas for more than one activity. A study area could include a desk, chair, and bookcase, **26-15**. You might also use this area for working on a hobby. You can keep a computer in this area, too. A nightstand or table and lamp by your bed will allow you to read in bed.

You need to allow space around some pieces of furniture, such as your bed. You will not have enough room to make your bed if one side is against the wall. You need to have room in front of dresser drawers and closet doors to open them. You also need room to pull a chair out from a desk. Having a dressing area is convenient. Place your chest of drawers and any other furniture that holds clothes near your closet.

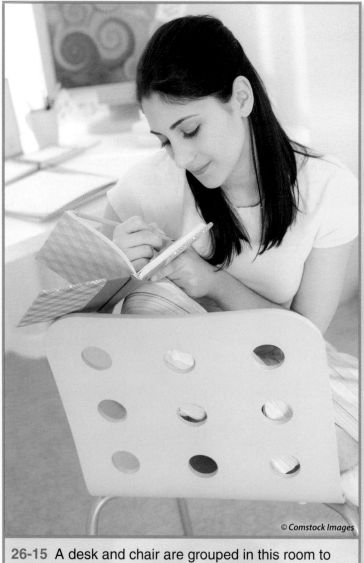
© Comstock Images

26-15 A desk and chair are grouped in this room to form a study area.

Reading Review

1. What design elements are integral to achieving your design goal?
2. What are the principles of design?
3. List five home décor choices.
4. What is space planning?
5. Describe optimal traffic patterns.

Keeping Your Home Clean and Safe

Objectives

After studying this section, you will be able to

- **describe** home maintenance.
- **plan** a cleaning schedule for your family or yourself.
- **help choose, organize, and use** appropriate cleaning supplies for your home.
- **explain** ways to make your home safe and prevent accidents.

Key Terms

routine jobs	loose dirt	disinfectant cleaner
cleaning schedule	adhesive dirt	electrical hazard
cleaning agents		

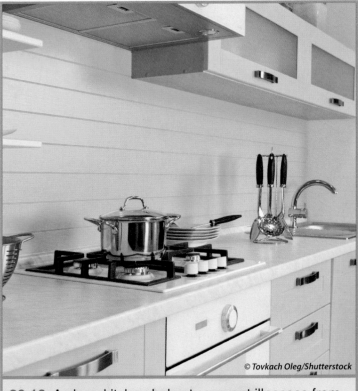

26-16 A clean kitchen helps to prevent illnesses from unsanitary food conditions.

Keeping your home neat and clean can help you feel comfortable in your home. It can also keep you safe from germs, pests, and falls. Most people do not want to spend all their time cleaning, so families need to work together to care for their homes. You can help by doing your share to keep your home clean and safe.

What Clean Means

First, your family needs to agree on cleaning standards. What is clean and neat to one person may not be to another person. Some people need to have everything in place and spotless most of the time, **26-16**. Clutter and dust may not bother others as much. There are minimum standards people should meet to keep their home safe and sanitary, however. A sanitary home is clean enough to prevent diseases or other health problems. Beyond that, standards can vary quite a bit.

Setting family cleaning standards helps avoid frustration and arguments about cleaning. It also creates a feeling of cooperation among family members. Your family's standards of clean should be agreeable to the whole family, especially in shared parts of the home. Members may need to raise or lower their standards a little, however. For instance, your mother might prefer no eating in the living room because food can spill on the carpet. You might want to take snacks in any time. You could compromise by agreeing to always use plates, napkins, and trays when eating in the living room.

When to Clean

Routine jobs are done daily as a part of your regular activities. Washing dishes and making your bed are examples of routine jobs, **26-17**. Routine cleaning helps prevent clutter and dirt from accumulating. It makes bigger cleaning jobs go more quickly and easily.

Weekly jobs might include dusting and vacuuming. Thorough kitchen and bathroom cleanings are often weekly jobs as well. Plan to set aside a few hours for weekly jobs.

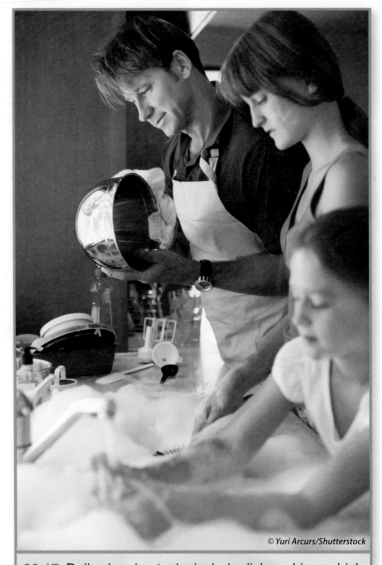

© Yuri Arcurs/Shutterstock

26-17 Daily cleaning tasks include dishwashing, which goes quicker when more than one person does it.

Occasional jobs might be done every few months or once or twice a year. These jobs might include washing windows, walls, and woodwork or cleaning out closets. Although you do not do these tasks often, they can take much time and work to complete. Some families may set aside a day for doing occasional cleaning jobs.

A Cleaning Schedule

A **cleaning schedule** is a plan for organizing the work of cleaning a home. After the routine (or daily), weekly, and occasional tasks are defined, specific schedules can be determined. Family members often feel better about household cleaning when they share the work. Therefore, including all members in the planning is important. A written schedule can provide a good checklist for completed work.

Assigning Jobs

In many families, each person takes care of his or her personal space. Family members often divide cleaning jobs for shared spaces, however. Shared spaces include the kitchen, dining room, living room, family room, bathroom, and yard.

When assigning jobs, consider the jobs that family members enjoy doing. For instance, one person might not mind washing the dishes or vacuuming. The same person may dislike mopping floors or lawn mowing. Also, consider members' abilities when assigning jobs, **26-18**. In most cases, though, practice is all a person might need to improve ability.

There are certain cleaning jobs that no one likes, and some jobs can take longer. Rotating these jobs ensures fairness. For instance, a different family member cleans the bathroom each week. Families may choose to rotate all jobs or only the most unpopular ones. When creating a cleaning schedule, consider the schedules of each member. If you have softball practice after dinner three nights a week, doing dinner cleanup on those nights would be difficult. You might need to do more jobs on the weekend instead. Every family is different.

Sometimes, keeping a positive attitude is more important than getting the work done in the quickest, best way. For instance, perhaps your three-year-old brother wants to help you mop the floor. You may need to let him hold the handle and move slowly. Even if the job takes longer, you are helping your brother feel good about himself and about cleaning.

Cleaning Supplies

Having the right supplies on hand makes cleaning much easier. Once you have the right supplies, keep them organized. This also saves time and effort as you work, **26-19**.

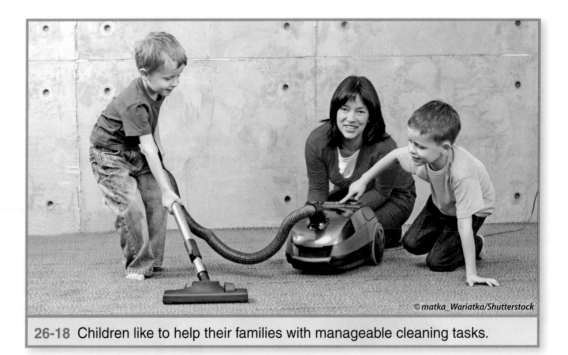

© matka_Wariatka/Shutterstock

26-18 Children like to help their families with manageable cleaning tasks.

Cleaning Agents

Cleaning agents are the substances or chemicals used to clean household surfaces. A large number of cleaning agents are on the market today. You may find it hard to decide which products you need and which work best. Cleaning is possible with a minimum of cleaning agents. Water with a mild detergent is a good, inexpensive cleaning product. It dissolves many kinds of dirt. You might prefer agents designed for special uses.

The best way to use products safely is to follow the manufacturer's directions. These directions are on product labels and should not be removed. They provide information about how to best use the product. They may also warn of possible hazards from using the product incorrectly.

Cleaning Equipment

Having the right cleaning equipment makes cleaning jobs easier. You can use most equipment for more than one job. Therefore, you really only need a few basic items.

The following items could be part of your cleaning supplies:
- broom and dustpan
- vacuum cleaner
- dust mop
- wet mop and bucket
- clean cloths
- sponges
- rubber gloves

After use, you should clean, discard, repair, and properly store equipment as necessary. This prevents using dirty or broken equipment for your next cleaning job. If you clean with a used cloth, for instance, you may end up mixing cleaning agents that have soaked into the cloth. You may also spread grime from a dirty used cloth onto the surface you are trying to clean.

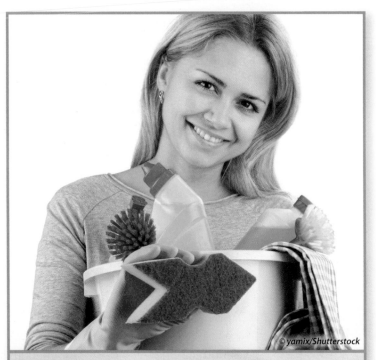

© yamix/Shutterstock

26-19 The container should be large enough to hold all your cleaning supplies.

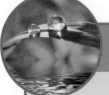

Go Green

Cleaning Green

Concern for the environment has prompted the creation of many new nontoxic, biodegradable cleaning agents. These products are available in most stores, although they tend to cost slightly more than traditional chemical-based cleaners. Most are made from renewable natural resources (not petroleum). You can also choose to make your own environmentally friendly cleaning solutions. Both vinegar and baking soda are nontoxic, inexpensive materials you can use to clean almost anything. Mix 3 Tbsp of either one in 1 qt. of warm water for an all-purpose, gentle cleaner.

Baking soda absorbs odors naturally. Instead of air freshening products that use chemicals to mask odors, put open boxes of baking soda in odor-producing spaces to eliminate them. Some good places to use baking soda include refrigerators, garbage areas, animals' spaces, or laundry rooms. Another tip for keeping a garbage disposal smelling fresh is to occasionally run several pieces of a freshly cut lemon through it with plenty of water.

Having one neat storage area helps keep supplies organized. A cleaning caddy or kit is also helpful. You can carry the caddy with you as you clean. You can use almost any sturdy container as a caddy.

Doing the Cleaning

Once organized, you are ready to get to work. Each cleaning task is a little bit different because there are different kinds of dirt and surfaces to clean. The two main types of dirt are loose dirt and adhesive dirt. Figure **26-20** shows some tips for cleaning different surfaces.

Cleaning Household Surfaces		
Surfaces	**Supplies**	**Methods**
Floors		
Carpeting	Vacuum cleaner Vacuum cleaning attachments Carpet cleaner	Vacuum carpeting using long, slow strokes. Move furniture when necessary. Use attachments to clean baseboards and corners. If carpeting is soiled, a stain-removing carpet cleaner may be necessary.
Throw rug	Washing machine Mild detergent Broom	Throw rugs may be cleaned in washing machine (check care label first), swept clean, or shaken outside to remove loose dirt.
Vinyl	Broom Dry mop Vacuum Mild detergent and water Sponge Water-based wax Acrylic floor coating	Sweep, dry mop, or vacuum vinyl to remove loose dirt. Mild detergent solution and sponge may be used to wash vinyl. Wax or acrylic coating may be applied as directed after cleaning to restore finish.
Tile	**Glazed:** Wet mop Mild detergent and water	Moisten mop with mild detergent solution. Use long, smooth strokes to clean floor. Rinse and let dry.
	Unglazed: Wet mop Special product for unglazed tile surfaces	Follow directions on cleaning product.
Wood	Broom Dustpan Damp or dust mop Water	To remove an excess of loose dirt, sweep wood floor with broom using small, low strokes. Pick up accumulation of dirt with dustpan. For mild cleaning, mop wood floor with slightly moistened mop to remove dirt and dust. Use long, smooth strokes and frequently rinse mop while cleaning. *(Continued)*

26-20 Different cleaning methods and agents should be used for different types of surfaces.

Cleaning Household Surfaces *(Continued)*		
Surfaces	**Supplies**	**Methods**
Finished Counter Tops Granite, formica, tile, etc.	Sponge Mild detergent Water	Moisten sponge with mild detergent solution. Wipe away loose dirt; scrub away adhesive dirt. Rinse if necessary.
Glass Windows and mirrors	Window or glass cleaning product Clean, lintless cloth Paper towels	Using a clean, lintless cloth or paper towel, follow directions on cleaner. Wipe window or mirror in one direction to prevent streaking.
Bath Fixtures Porcelain	Clean cloth Dry or spray all-purpose cleaner Toilet brush Toilet bowl cleaner	Follow directions on cleaning product. Dampen cloth and surface before using dry cleaner. For toilet bowl, use brush to scrub stains and area under the rim.
Fiberglass	Clean, soft cloth Nonabrasive cleaner	Follow directions on cleaning product. Fiberglass fixtures scratch easily, so do not use abrasive cleaning pads or products.
Nonwood Furniture Upholstered furniture	Vacuum cleaner Vacuum cleaner attachments	Use appropriate attachments to dust and clean fabric on furniture.
Vinyl furniture	Clean cloth Polish cleaning product	Using clean cloth, follow directions on cleaner. Wipe in one direction to prevent streaking.
Woodwork Wood cabinets	Clean cloth Mild detergent Water Wood cleaning product Polish Wax	Moisten clean cloth with mild detergent solution. Wipe cabinet to remove surface dirt and dust. A wood cleaning product may also be used according to label directions. If cabinets have been polished or waxed before, polish or wax again as directed.
Wood furniture	Clean cloth Wood cleaning product Polish Wax	With clean cloth, use wood cleaning product as directed. If furniture has been polished or waxed before, polish or wax again as directed.
Painted wood surfaces	Moistened cloth Sponge Mild detergent Water Clean cloth Wood cleaning product	Moisten cloth or sponge with mild detergent solution. Wipe a small area to prevent softening or damaging the paint. Using a clean cloth and a wood cleaning product designed for painted surfaces is also effective.

Loose Dirt

Dust and crumbs are examples of **loose dirt**. Loose dirt is dry and not bound to a surface. Some loose dirt is carried in the air and settles on surfaces. People and pets leave other loose dirt. The equipment used to remove loose dirt includes brooms, vacuum cleaners, dust mops, and cloths. Some cleaning agents help pick up loose dirt. These include furniture polish, mild spray cleaners, and mild detergent solutions.

Many people like to clean a room from top to bottom to keep dirt from falling on a clean floor. If you are cleaning a lot of loose dirt, try to pick up as much as possible using a dry method. You might use a dry floor mop or a broom to sweep most of the dirt into a dustpan. After removing as much as possible, use a slightly damp cloth to pick up the rest.

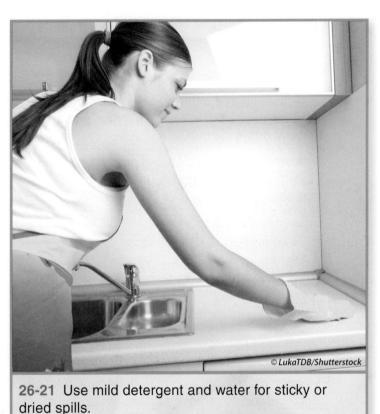

© LukaTDB/Shutterstock

26-21 Use mild detergent and water for sticky or dried spills.

Adhesive Dirt

Adhesive dirt sticks to surfaces. In most cases, it is harder to remove than loose dirt. Dried food and drinks are the most common sources of adhesive dirt. The best way to clean this kind of dirt is to wipe it up while still wet, **26-21**. You may also need a scrubbing pad or brush and some "elbow grease."

Oily dirt is a type of adhesive dirt that is especially hard to remove. Foods, cosmetics, and oil-based chemicals often leave this type of dirt. Some oily dirt results from spills and frying food, which causes oil to settle on surfaces throughout the kitchen. Mild detergent and water is not always strong enough to break up oil or grease. Depending on the surface, there are effective cleaning products for dissolving oily dirt.

Bathrooms

Because so much water is used in the bathroom, mold and mildew tend to grow on bathroom surfaces. To prevent this, family members should rinse the tub and sink when through using them. It also means hanging up wet towels and washcloths and cleaning shower curtains.

About once a week, though, bathrooms need a thorough cleaning, **26-22**. Many bathroom fixtures are made of smooth materials, such as porcelain, chrome, or brass. Using abrasive cleaners on these surfaces can scratch or dull them. Instead, use a disinfectant cleaner labeled safe for bathroom surfaces. A **disinfectant cleaner** kill germs and cleans surfaces. Disinfectant cleaners are used to clean toilet bowls, too. A long-handled toilet bowl brush also makes this job easier.

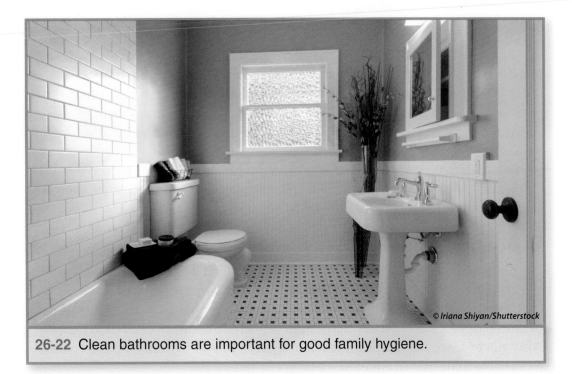

26-22 Clean bathrooms are important for good family hygiene.

© Iriana Shiyan/Shutterstock

Kitchen and Dining Areas

Adhesive dirt is also a cleaning challenge in the kitchen and dining areas. Clean up spills and messes when they happen; but a thorough weekly cleaning is also recommended. A good grease-dissolving cleaner is needed to remove oily dirt. Surfaces where food is prepared need special attention. A disinfectant cleaner ensures harmful germs do not transfer to foods.

Overflowing garbage cans are unsanitary because germs and odors develop and spread quickly. Unwashed dishes and food left on counters and floors can attract pests, such as ants, cockroaches, flies, or mice. Keeping your kitchen and dining areas clean on a daily basis prevents pests. Major pest problems may need professional pest removal.

Safety in the Home

Your home needs to be safe for everyone in the family. Keeping your home clean is one way to help prevent accidents. Simple planning can help reduce the dangers of falls, fires, electrical hazards, and poisonings in your home. Making sure you are safe when adults are not present is also important. Learn safety procedures for emergencies such as tornadoes, hurricanes, storms, and earthquakes. Find out where the safest places in your home are during emergencies.

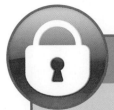

Safety Connections

Managing Clutter

Objects left in hallways and on stairs contribute to floor *clutter*, which can cause falls. The best way to avoid clutter is to put items away properly as soon as you are done with them. For instance, put up a coat rack to hang coats and other clothing items. Keep a laundry basket or hamper for dirty clothes. Designate storage units for loose items along walls in shared spaces. Easy-to-use storage encourages people to put items away rather than leave them on the floor.

Preventing Falls

Falls are the most common and easily preventable home accidents. Kitchens and bathrooms are the most likely places for falls due to water or other liquids spilling on floors. Bathtubs are slippery when wet, so place nonskid mats or decals in them. Nonskid rug pads are good for under small throw and area rugs. Use a sturdy step stool or small ladder when reaching for items in the kitchen. Never climb on counters or cabinets.

Make sure cords and wires are not located where people could trip on them. Use nightlights to effectively light hallways and bathrooms at night. Make sure outdoor walkways are clear. Keep them free of snow and ice in the winter.

Preventing Fires

You can take many steps to help prevent fires in your home. Some fires start in the kitchen from flaming cooking grease. Burning candles, incense, or tobacco products can spread fire to anything flammable, such as furniture, bedding, or carpeting. Never leave matches where children can reach them. Also, never leave burning candles unattended. Keep oily rags or other flammable materials in covered metal containers.

Carefully monitor any space heaters and turn them off promptly after use. Make sure your home has working smoke detectors and a fire extinguisher, **26-23**.

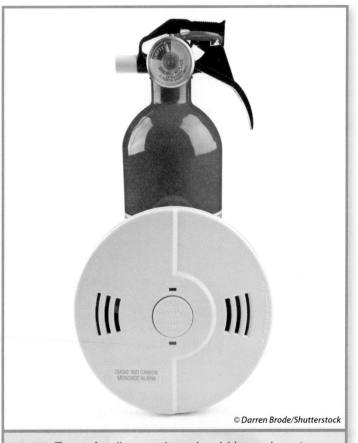

© Darren Brode/Shutterstock

26-23 Every family member should know how to use a fire extinguisher and understand smoke detectors.

Emergency Escape Plan

Talk with your family to determine at least two ways to escape from your home in an emergency. Always plan two exits in case one is blocked by fire or debris. Designate one meeting place after evacuating the house. If everyone meets in the same place, you can account for all family members.

Preventing Electrical Hazards

An **electrical hazard** is a danger from any form of electricity, such as electrical appliances and cords. Cracked or frayed wires and cords can cause fires. Replace any damaged cords and never run electrical cords under rugs or carpets. Plugging too many appliance cords into one electrical outlet will overload it, and break the circuit.

Shock is another very serious consequence of using electricity improperly. Never touch a frayed or exposed cord or wire. Place outlet plug covers on any open plugs to prevent electrocution, especially to keep curious children from inserting their fingers. Keep electrical appliances away from water and do not use them with wet hands. Be sure to unplug any electrical appliance when not in use.

Preventing Poisonings

It is important to know that some cleaning agents are harmful if swallowed, even in small amounts. Check the labels to see how safe your cleaners are. Be sure to wipe any strong cleaners completely off surfaces, especially those in the kitchen. Keep all medicines and products with chemicals away from children. Install *childproof locks and latches*, which are products for doors or cabinets allowing only adults to open them. These locks and latches prevent children from reaching potentially harmful products.

If an accidental poisoning does occur, follow the product's directions for how to treat an accidental poisoning and contact poison control. Call your doctor or 911 for immediate medical attention. Make sure you know exactly which product caused the poisoning because different products require different treatments.

Home Alone Safety Tips

- If a stranger calls or comes to the door, never let the person know you are home alone. Instead, tell the person your parents are busy and cannot come to the phone or door.
- Keep emergency numbers next to a telephone or posted in the kitchen.
- When you leave the house, check that all doors and windows are closed and locked.
- If you come home and find an open door or broken window, do not go inside. Go to a neighbor's home and call your parents. If you cannot reach them, call the police. The police will check the house for you.

Safety Connections

Use the Correct Lightbulb Wattage

Most light bases in your home require you to use 60-watt lightbulbs. The *wattage limit* is shown next to the socket for safety reasons. A 100-watt bulb fits in most sockets like a 60-watt bulb, but is just brighter. So, what is the issue if both bulbs fit the same? A 100-watt light bulb uses more power and gets much hotter than a 60-watt bulb. The socket contacts are *not* designed for this extra power load. As a result, the base will get hotter. An overheated lighting base can potentially cause a fire. For your safety, always check the recommended wattage and use the correct lightbulb in all light fixtures.

Reading Review

1. What is a sanitary home?
2. Give examples of routine, weekly, and occasional cleaning jobs in your home.
3. What is a cleaning schedule?
4. True or false. Falls are the most common and easily preventable home accidents.
5. List five safety rules that should be followed in a home.

Chapter Summary

Section 26-1. A home is a place that fills people's needs. Homes fulfill physical, emotional, and social needs. Housing needs change throughout the lifespan. There are various types of housing. Each type of housing option has advantages and disadvantages and associated costs.

Section 26-2. Your bedroom is your personal space in your home. You can decorate your room to reflect your personality using the elements and principles of design. When changing the look of your room, you should first consider the backgrounds, furniture, fixtures, window coverings, and accessories. These items should meet your needs and create a pleasing appearance in your room. Making a floor plan can help you arrange items in your room. You need to consider your activities, storage, and traffic patterns when deciding how to arrange a room.

Section 26-3. A neat, clean home is comfortable. Each family has its own cleaning standards. A cleaning schedule helps to organize the cleaning of a home. Choosing, organizing, and using appropriate cleaning supplies can help keep your home clean. Following safety procedures can make your home safe and prevent accidents.

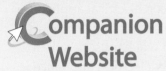

Companion Website

www.g-wlearning.com

Check your understanding of the main concepts for Chapter 26 at the website.

Critical Thinking

1. **Evaluate.** If you were old enough to move into your own apartment, what would you want it be like in terms of cleanliness, design, and security?
2. **Assess.** How could you improve your cleaning skills?
3. **Analyze.** Visit a supermarket or grocery store and analyze various cleaning products. List five products you have never seen. Record the names and uses and report them to the class.

Common Core

College and Career Readiness

4. **Writing.** As a class, brainstorm a list of tips that teens could use to make cleaning their bedrooms easier. Use the list to develop a brochure. Make copies of the brochure and pass them out to students in your school.

5. **Math.** Create a scale floor plan of your room. Make scale outlines of your furniture. Arrange the furniture pieces on your floor plan, taking your activities and traffic patterns into consideration.

6. **Listening.** Interview two friends outside of your class who share their rooms. Ask them to describe techniques they have found helpful in getting along with their roommates. Use these interviews to write a two-page report on the topic of privacy.

7. **Speaking.** Choose a cleaning product and create a television commercial for the product. Demonstrate the use of the product to the class.

Technology

8. **Design project.** Imagine you are a professional decorator or interior designer. Using space planning software, create a floor plan of your room. Make a printout of the floor plan. Use shapes to represent the furniture in your room. Arrange the furniture, keeping in mind activities, space needs, and traffic patterns. Highlight the traffic patterns in the room.

Journal Writing

9. Write about your own cleaning standards. Describe what clean means to you. Explain how your cleaning standards are similar or differ from family members or friends. Describe how you keep your room clean now. How well do you think you would keep your home clean 10 years from now?

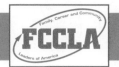 ## FCCLA

10. Design the interior of a space in which you live for an *Interior Design STAR Event*. Create a display board that includes a floor plan, an elevation, furniture plan, fabric samples, and a cost analysis. Present your project in class. See your adviser for information as needed.

Chapter 27
Transportation Options

Sections

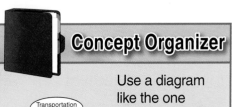

College and Career Readiness

Reading Prep
Before you read this chapter, review the vocabulary terms in each section. Make a list of terms you do not recognize and look them up in the glossary or dictionary. Boosting your vocabulary is a good way to broaden your understanding of new material.

Concept Organizer

Transportation Types

Use a diagram like the one shown to list the two primary forms of transportation and at least four examples of each type.

Companion Website
Print out the concept organizer for Chapter 27 at the website.

Companion
Website
www.g-wlearning.com

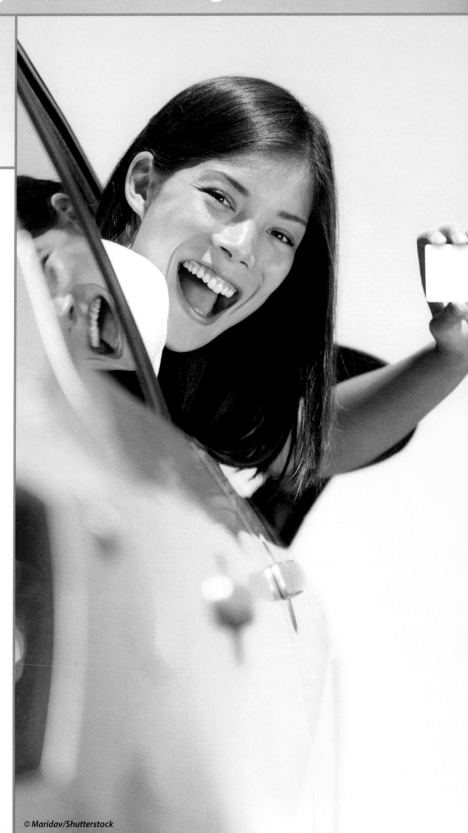

Section 27-1

History of Transportation

Objectives

After studying this section, you will be able to
- **summarize** the history of transportation.
- **discuss** the growth and importance of the U.S. aviation industry.
- **identify** current transportation choices.
- **compare and contrast** personal and public transportation options.
- **evaluate** transportation needs.

Key Terms

transcontinental railroad	assembly line	public transportation
internal combustion engine	buoyant	personal transportation
	aeronautics	
	NASA	motor scooters

Getting from one place to another has always been a necessity throughout history. Until the invention of the wheel in 3500 B.C., walking or riding on animals and in boats were the only transportation choices. The wheel added new transportation options, such as carts, chariots, wagons, and carriages. Transportation did not change much again until the inventions of the steam engine and the bicycle in the mid-19th century. After that, new technology changed transportation choices very quickly. No one in 1799 could have believed men would land safely on the moon only 170 years later.

Transportation choices now are many. They partly depend on where you live. Areas with greater populations often have several forms of mass transit. Trains, buses, streetcars, subways, ferries, or taxis may be available to you. In areas with lower concentrated populations, the choices are fewer or you may have to rely on family-owned vehicles.

Transportation in America

People first came to America by ships and canoes and settled along seas, lakes, and rivers. Cities grew by waterways because that was the most efficient form of mass transit at the time. People could transport raw materials and finished goods for sale by boats along canals and rivers. Less efficiently, they could move goods by using horse-drawn wagons on dirt roads, **27-1**.

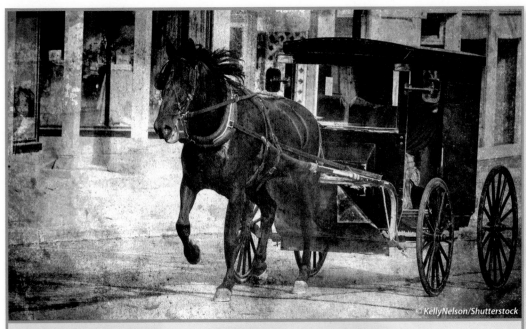

© KellyNelson/Shutterstock

27-1 Horses and horse-drawn carriages were the primary means of transportation for individuals.

The Industrial Revolution, the invention of commercial steam and locomotive engines, and the railroads changed America forever. In the early 1800s, American engineer, Robert Fulton built the first successful steamboat. By the mid-1800s, people were transporting freight across the Atlantic Ocean. Commercial railroads appeared in the 1830s. The first American **transcontinental railroad**, which spanned from one end of the country to the other, was completed in 1869. This made travel time from coast to coast much shorter.

The First Automobiles

The next big leap in transportation happened with the invention of the internal combustion engine in the 1860s. An **internal combustion engine** is one that creates mechanical power by the burning of a fuel (usually a fossil fuel) when exposed to air in an internal chamber. In Detroit, Michigan, in the 1890s, Henry Ford built the first American automobiles to use internal combustion engines, **27-2**.

© James Steidl/Shutterstock

27-2 The first public use of the term *automobile* was in 1897. Until then, cars were often called *horseless carriages*.

Henry Ford is also credited with inventing the assembly line for efficient automobile manufacturing. An **assembly line** is a line of machines, equipment, and workers in a factory that builds a product by passing work from one station to the next until the product is finished. The workers or machines at each station perform the same functions repeatedly.

Ford's assembly lines greatly decreased the cost and time it took to produce his cars, making them affordable for most people. The assembly line concept was so profitable that it spread to nearly every form of manufacturing, and is still in use today.

Air Travel

Ever since humans observed birds flying, they dreamed of traveling through the air. Until the first hot air balloon carrying passengers in a basket took flight in 1783 France, air travel was simply impossible. Filling the balloons with heated air (and later helium) made them **buoyant**, meaning they had the ability to float. About 100 years later, this concept helped develop *airships* that use an engine to propel a very large, football-shaped balloon. These massive vehicles carried many passengers and were sometimes called *dirigibles* or *Zeppelins*. Today they are known as *blimps* and do not carry passengers. You may see them occasionally with advertising messages in the sky.

The Wright Brothers

Orville and Wilbur Wright were pioneers in **aeronautics**, the art or science of flight. From 1899–1905 in North Carolina, they experimented with making a piloted, heavier-than-air machine fly. The Wrights observed the principles of *aerodynamics*, or the way air moves around objects, by determining the wing structures and movements of birds in flight. Next, they applied those principles to a series of wooden gliders that flew when lifted by the wind. In 1905, the Wright brothers carried aerodynamics further to design and fly the first motor-powered airplane. They formed The Wright Company and became the first to manufacture airplanes.

U.S. Aviation

Initially, people would fly planes mostly in traveling exhibitions meant to entertain the public. There were few trained pilots. Then World War I (1914–1919) demanded increased airplane production, which would lead to a new way to fight wars. During the 1920s, U.S. commercial airlines were formed and larger airplanes became very important both for human and freight transportation.

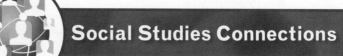

Social Studies Connections

The Hindenburg Disaster

Airships were awkward, easily affected by the weather, and quite dangerous. There were many accidents and deaths, but one of the worst happened in the United States in 1937. A German Zeppelin, the *Hindenburg*, had crossed the Atlantic Ocean and was attempting to land in New Jersey during bad weather. It caught fire, crashed, and killed 36 of the 97 passengers and crew while hundreds of spectators watched. That disaster ended airships as means of air travel.

Global Connections

The International Space Station

Although the U.S.S.R. launched the first rocket into space, the U.S. space program landed six separate manned missions on the moon by 1972. The space race ended amicably and construction on the International Space Station began in 1998. Now, 16 countries utilize and maintain the International Space Station. While trained *astronauts* are the only people allowed to man the space station, experts foresee the day when space travel will be safe enough and affordable for many.

When the world went to war again in World War II (1939–1945), much of the fighting took place in the air. The countries raced to increase their airplanes' technology and gain advantage in the war, **27-3**. The result was the creation of a more powerful and faster turbojet propulsion engine that is still in use today.

World War II made aviation the top U.S. industry for many years, producing over 300,000 military aircraft for America and its war allies. The sheer number of superior aircrafts contributed greatly to winning the war. Despite the huge aviation effort in both world wars, however, the United States Air Force did not officially form until 1947.

In 1958, President Dwight D. Eisenhower established the National Aeronautics and Space Administration (NASA) and the space race began. It was President John F. Kennedy, however, that coined the term *space race*. He was describing the competition between the United States and the United Soviet Socialist Republic (U.S.S.R., but now Russia and its surrounding countries) to explore space.

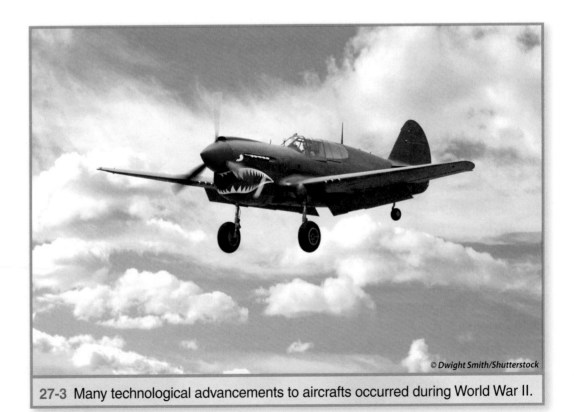

© Dwight Smith/Shutterstock

27-3 Many technological advancements to aircrafts occurred during World War II.

Today's Transportation

Due to the many advances in transportation in the last 100 years, people have never had more choices for getting around. The two primary categories are public and personal transportation. **Public transportation** such as buses, trains, subways, trolleys, ferries, and taxis use regular routes at fixed times to transport many people. **Personal transportation** options include vehicles you can operate either alone or with several people, such as a car, motorcycle, bicycle, or scooter.

Public Transportation

Public transportation, also called *mass transit*, is generally less expensive than car ownership. People who use public transportation may be able to save even more money by purchasing fare in bulk amounts, such as a monthly pass or set number of tokens. Larger cities tend to offer more mass transit choices. For instance, every type of public transportation is available in New York City. Not every large city, however, has a subway system or ferries, **27-4**. Many trains only run from suburban areas into the cities and back again.

City-operated public transportation such as buses, trains, and subways have set schedules for pickup and drop off times and places. Schedules should be available at a city's website on the Internet.

Advantages and Disadvantages

Depending on the city, or sometimes even the neighborhoods within it, mass transit options can be safe and reliable. Using them can have many advantages over driving. You can avoid driving in crowded rush-hour traffic, and you can even read or listen to music during the ride. You will also not have to worry about finding a safe place to park your car for the day. Parking fees in larger cities tend to be high, so public transportation saves money on fuel, parking, and highway tolls. It also cuts down on environmental pollution.

Mass transit can also have disadvantages. You must follow their schedules, and that may be inconvenient. You will have to walk or drive to the mass transit station or stop. You may have to pay for parking at the station. Depending on the time of day, mass transit may be crowded and uncomfortable. In some areas, it might also be unsafe.

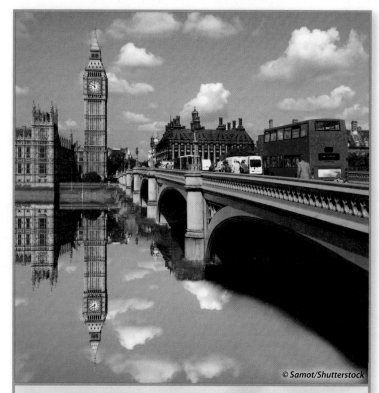
© Samot/Shutterstock

27-4 When visiting an unfamiliar city, it is a good idea to research the best forms of public transportation available to help you get around efficiently.

Taxis may be a perfect solution in large cities or for short-term specific trips. Remember that taxis also have disadvantages. They can be expensive, depending on the length of the ride, and availability is uncertain. If possible, it is better to call ahead for a taxi to meet you when and where you need it. Some hotels have shuttles to airports or train stations, which are very good options if they fit your needs.

Personal Transportation

Owning a car means having the freedom to go where you want whenever you want. A car or other personal vehicle may be necessary for people whose other transportation options are limited. While some people may enjoy owning their own car, others may not want the responsibility or added costs. Cars are expensive to buy and maintain. Fuel and insurance are necessary expenses. Parking is another expense many people do not consider when weighing the options of purchasing a car with other forms of transportation. If you live in an area with high traffic, you can spend quite a bit of time getting back and forth to school or work.

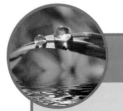

Go Green

Car Pools

A *car pool* is two or more people who commute together in one of the members' vehicles. Each member contributes to the fuel and additional costs such as parking. By sharing the driving and commuting costs, carpoolers save money and the wear and tear on their own cars. Car pools are good for the environment. Fewer cars on the road mean less pollution emissions. It also means using less fossil fuels, which saves the planet's nonrenewable resources.

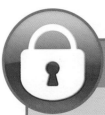

Safety Connections

Motorcycle Safety

Motorcycles can be dangerous because there is no bodily protection from a fall or accident. There are very specific laws about helmets, eye protection, headlights, earphones, and passengers by age for on-road versus off-road riding. These laws vary greatly by state, so research your state's requirements before purchasing or riding one. It is advised to wear a protective helmet and eyewear for safety—whether required by law in your state or not.

Two-Wheel Vehicles

Bicycles, scooters, or motorcycles save energy and have little to no polluting emissions. They are considered environmentally friendly transportation choices. Compared to other options, bicycles are inexpensive and there are many choices. Bicycling is also a physical activity that improves a person's health. Paying attention to designated bike paths, especially on streets, is central to the biking experience.

Motor scooters can be an inexpensive choice for transportation, but they are low-powered vehicles and work better for local trips. Laws for scooters vary by city and state. Investigate your state's laws to see age restrictions, helmet laws, and what types of permits, licenses, and insurance are required.

Motorcycles come in many different models and sizes. If you need a vehicle for short commutes, a basic motorcycle may be sufficient. More expensive features may be unnecessary for your purposes.

Insurance is also more expensive for motorcycles due to the increased safety risk. Unlike scooters, motorcycles are generally considered motor vehicles because they have the same speed capabilities as cars.

Evaluating Your Transportation Needs

Every person has different transportation needs at different times in their lives. Answering the following questions may help you choose the best options for you at any given time:

- How far and how often do you need to travel?
- What is your budget for transportation?
- What options are available to you? Can you use public transportation? Do you or your family own a vehicle you could use? Is there someone with whom you could carpool?
- What are the short- and long-term costs, such as car repairs, fuel increases, and mass transit fare increases? Compare the costs for each of your options for one year and three years.
- What form of transportation is most convenient to you? Is one closer to your home, school, or work? Is weather an issue?
- Which of your options is safest? Are there any that are unsafe?
- Do you value your time? comfort? the environment? Your values impact your decisions about transportation.

Reading Review

1. Why did people who first came to America settle along seas, lakes, and rivers?
2. Orville and Wilbur Wright were pioneers in _____, the art or science of flight.
3. List two primary categories of transportation.
4. List two advantages and two disadvantages of public transportation.
5. Why are bicycles, scooters, or motorcycles considered to be environmentally friendly?

Buying Your First Car

Objectives

After studying this section, you will be able to

- **explain** the process of financing a car.
- **list** the expenses of owning a car.
- **determine** your budget, needs, and wants for a car.
- **identify** different types of car sellers.
- **summarize** how to test-drive a car.
- **outline** car maintenance and servicing criteria.

Key Terms	
credit report	certified pre-owned cars
cosigner	options
leasing	
vehicle identification number (VIN)	

If you decide to buy a car, you should first learn as much as you can about the process. Think about what you need in a first vehicle and how much you can afford to spend. Establish a budget based on your income and estimated expenses. Unless you have saved enough money to buy your car with cash, financing will be necessary. Teens or college students with no established credit history may find some challenges to financing their first car.

Financing a Car

Learning how financing works can help you make the best decisions. It is important to know how much your car will really cost after you pay off a loan. Usually, you cannot get a car loan unless you are at least 18 years old, earn income from a full-time job, and have a good credit history. Having a good credit report is an important factor to all lenders. A **credit report** is a detailed report of an individual's credit history prepared by a credit bureau and used by lenders to determine a loan applicant's ability to repay the loan, **27-5**.

Obtaining Financing

Banks, credit unions, car dealerships, and finance companies all offer car loans. Gather as much information as possible so you can compare the interest rates and other terms before making a decision.

Car loans are *installment loans*, which people repay by making the same monthly payment until the loan balance is zero. The loan's repayment period and monthly payment depend on the amount borrowed and the rate of interest charged by the lender. The more money you borrow, the more interest you will pay over time. It is wise to put as much cash toward the down payment as possible. If you choose to make larger monthly payments, it will take less time to pay off the loan and you will pay less interest.

If you do not qualify for a loan by yourself, an adult family member with a good credit report may need to be your cosigner. A **cosigner** is a person named as a partner on the loan who is legally bound to repay it if the other signer does not make payments. Because a cosigner is legally responsible for the loan, his or her name should also be listed on the vehicle's title as a co-owner. Cosigning a loan for a younger person is often risky, so there are many people who refuse to cosign loans.

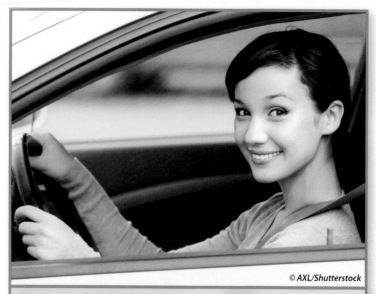
© AXL/Shutterstock

27-5 It is important to know that lenders typically give better (lower) interest rates to borrowers with the best credit reports.

Leasing

Leasing is another word for renting. Many people choose to lease their cars instead of buying. Leasing is generally less expensive than buying a car. The lessee makes a down payment and installment payments over time. Monthly lease payments are usually much lower than loan payments. At the end of the lease period, however, the lessee does not own the car and must return it.

When you sign a lease, make sure you know and understand all the terms of the contract. Check the requirements for returning the car, such as the condition of the vehicle. Also, check for issues that will incur penalties, such as mileage limits or early termination of the lease.

Vehicle Needs and Wants

After you establish a budget and before you begin shopping for a vehicle, think specifically about what you need and want in a car.

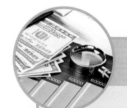

Financial Literacy Connections

Estimating Total Car Costs

The cash purchase price or down payment and financing charges of a car are only the beginning of car ownership expenses. Consider the following additional expenses for owning a car:

- taxes and fees
- insurance premiums
- licensing and registration (paid every year)
- fuel and other operating costs
- maintenance costs (oil changes, new tires and tire rotation, battery replacement, etc.)
- car repair costs
- parking

Answer the following questions to help steer you toward the type of car best suited to your needs:

- How far will you need to travel, and how often?
- What kind of roads will you be traveling?
- How large does the vehicle need to be?
- What features do you need? want?
- What is the vehicle's safety record?
- What is the vehicle's fuel efficiency or miles per gallon (mpg)?
- What type of warranty would you prefer?
- What make, model, and color would you like at this time?

Life Connections

Car Buying Research

Before you buy your first car, it is a good idea to conduct research to narrow down your options. Following are several helpful car buying resources:

- *Kelley Blue Book* and *Edmunds* both list the estimated resale values and purchase prices of new and pre-owned cars.
- *The National Automotive Dealers Association (NADA) Official Used Car Guide* has general information on cars by the make, model, and year.
- *The National Highway Traffic Safety Administration (NHTSA)* provides recall and crash test information on various car models.

At times, you may find online research challenging because there are so many sources available. Learning how to use search terms effectively can help you find the information you need with just a few simple keystrokes.

When conducting a search on the Internet, think about the terms you should use. Search terms should be specific and relate exactly to the material you need. Use quotation marks to limit your search results to only pages containing that exact wording. For instance, use the search term *"Kelley Blue Book used car values"* to learn more about pricing of used cars.

Writing Activity

Use the Internet to conduct your own car buying research. Before you begin, write a specific search term that will help you focus on the information you want to find. Check at least three websites to evaluate the effectiveness of your search. Write a brief paragraph depicting the results and information available on each site. Share with the class any helpful research tips you learned from completing this exercise.

Shopping for a Car

Because there are so many options for buying a car, you may need the advice of an experienced adult. Are you looking for a new or pre-owned (used) car? Do you think a traditional dealership offers more choices, but may also have salespeople who pressure you to buy immediately? Would you prefer to use a competitive auto superstore? Do you want to buy a car directly from a current owner? Would you ever consider using the Internet as a car-buying tool? Any of these options may help you find the best car for the least amount of money.

Traditional Dealerships

Traditional dealerships sell new and pre-owned cars. Dealerships can also provide financing for the purchase. They usually have service departments available to make repairs and perform routine maintenance.

To protect consumers, the Federal Trade Commission (FTC) requires all cars sold by dealers have *Buyers Guide* window stickers with specific information about the vehicle. The stickers provide details about the car and helpful information for the consumer.

Pre-owned Cars

Depending on the year, make, model, and mileage, a pre-owned car is usually less expensive than a new car. If a pre-owned car needs many repairs, it can eventually become more expensive than buying a new car, **27-6**. The used car Buyers Guide is a standard federal form that specifies any warranty coverage and lists "some major defects that may occur in pre-owned motor vehicles." It also recommends that an independent automotive technician inspect a pre-owned car.

There are various ways to check on the status of a car. Every car has a **vehicle identification number (VIN)**, which is a unique number the automobile industry assigns to each vehicle. Manufacturers place the VIN on the dashboard and on a sticker on the driver's side doorjamb.

You can use the VIN to find history reports on a particular pre-owned car. The records will include important information such as accidents involving the car, theft, and odometer records. If you buy a pre-owned car, get a *Vehicle History Report* on the VIN and have a reputable mechanic inspect the car for potential problems. Carefully inspect any available service records.

Certified pre-owned cars are late-model used vehicles (usually less than five years old) that the manufacturers put through a demanding inspection and repair process. They are often for sale at higher prices because dealers add an extended warranty and other extras. Certified pre-owned cars are popular choices because they cost less than the new models and give the buyers peace of mind.

Auto Superstores

Auto superstores offer new and pre-owned cars for fixed prices. You can use the superstore's computer system to search for attributes you want in your car. These may include price, model, and certain options. Superstores often offer financing and servicing.

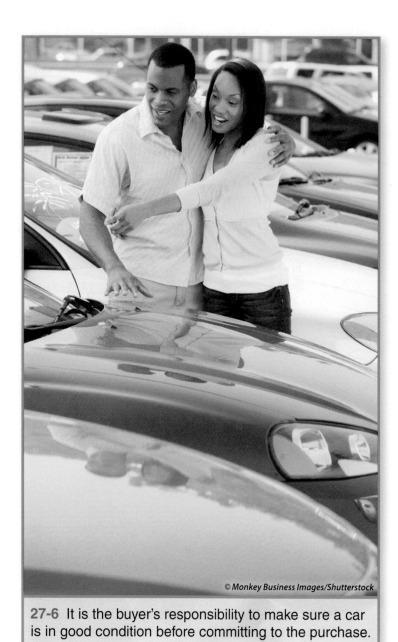

© Monkey Business Images/Shutterstock

27-6 It is the buyer's responsibility to make sure a car is in good condition before committing to the purchase.

Private Sellers

Many people buy pre-owned cars from private sellers because the prices are better. Pre-owned cars are more expensive at dealerships because of the dealer's overhead and sales commissions. Unfortunately, buying a car from its owner means there is no warranty unless the original warranty is still in effect. If you plan to buy a car from a private seller, arrange to have it checked by a reliable service technician, **27-7**.

The Internet

The Internet is the most efficient way to find nearby dealers or private sellers who are selling the car you want. The Internet can save you time by immediately showing the most current information on available cars. You can also search online for information about different features on vehicles and compare prices.

Making a Final Choice

The basic features on a new car are referred to as *standard equipment*. **Options** are additional features that may be added for appearance, safety, performance, or convenience. Standard equipment is included in the base price of the car. All options add to the total price of the car. New cars and certified pre-owned cars have warranties. Some parts have full coverage while others have limited coverage. It is likely that the owner will have to meet requirements outlined in the warranty. This usually involves following scheduled maintenance recommendations.

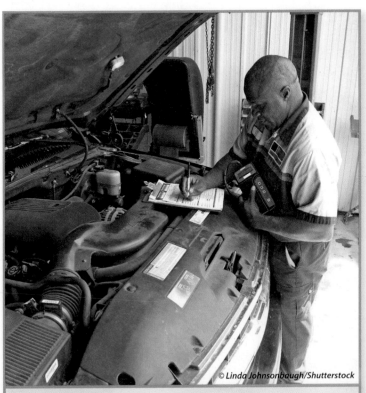

© Linda Johnsonbaugh/Shutterstock

27-7 When buying a car *as is*, be sure to find out about any problems before you commit to the purchase.

Test-Driving

When you have decided on the details, it is time to *test-drive* the car to evaluate its performance. First, are you comfortable in the driver's seat? Are all controls within reach, and do you have good visibility? When driving the car, how does it handle? Test the car on the open road and in neighborhood driving. Test all the equipment so you understand how everything works. If you are buying a pre-owned car, you will want to have the engine and all fluid levels checked. Check the amount of wear on the tires. Listen for noises and smoothness of the drive. These can help indicate if there are problems.

Maintaining Your Car

Regular maintenance will ensure your car's safety and performance. A well-maintained car should need fewer repairs and ultimately save you money. The owner's manual for the car indicates typical schedules based on mileage for oil changes, tire rotation, and other routine servicing. Some newer cars even have regular maintenance indication lights on the dashboard that tell you which service you need.

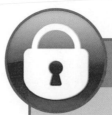

Safety Connections

Keep Vehicles Safe

In most cars, warning lights notify you of potential problems with your vehicle, such as the *check engine* light. Other signs of problems are unusual sounds, leaks, and odors. If you notice a problem with the way the car is driving, have it checked. Watch the dashboard gauges to make sure they are within normal parameters. Getting a problem checked as soon as it appears can improve vehicle safety and possibly save lives.

Servicing

When choosing a repair center for car servicing, you will want to find one that is convenient for you. The location should be close to your home or job and equipped to service your car's make and model. Learn if you need to make appointments or if they will take the car at any time. The hours of operation should also work with your schedule. Sometimes you may have to leave your car for several hours, or possibly overnight, while repair work is done.

Servicing your car can be very costly. You will want to make sure you trust the service technicians to make only necessary repairs. Reputable mechanics can be found in dealerships, independent auto service centers, some gas stations, and chain auto service centers. Before choosing a service center, you may want to ask friends and family members if they have experience with that center. You can also find out if they have a Better Business Bureau (BBB) rating by checking the BBB website.

You may wish to choose a repair center that meets the standards of the American Automobile Association (AAA) and has been endorsed by this organization. You can also check to see that the mechanics are *ASE certified*. This means they are trained and passed the National Institute for Automotive Service Excellence testing.

Reading Review

1. A(n) _____ is a person named as a partner on a loan who is legally bound to repay it if the other signer does not make payments.
2. List three requirements for getting a car loan.
3. Why do some people choose to lease cars instead of buying?
4. What is a VIN?
5. What is the difference between standard equipment and options?

Chapter Summary

Section 27-1. From the invention of the wheel to the invention of the automobile and air travel, transportation has been evolving. People have many transportation choices. Public and private transportation offer advantages and disadvantages. By evaluating your transportation needs, you can choose the best option for your needs. Your choice may depend on factors such as cost, convenience, time, safety, and environmental concerns.

Section 27-2. If you buy or lease a car, the process of financing a car takes some consideration. When shopping for a car, consider your needs and wants. Cars are available new or pre-owned from a variety of sellers. Once you have selected a car, take it on a test drive to evaluate it. Regular car maintenance and servicing will ensure safety and performance.

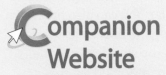

Companion Website

www.g-wlearning.com

Check your understanding of the main concepts for Chapter 27 at the website.

Critical Thinking

1. **Summarize.** Prepare a timeline of the various modes of transportation used throughout history.

2. **Assess.** Compare local public transportation options available to you. How do these compare to private modes of transportation?

3. **Apply.** Imagine you are buying a car. What are some do's and don'ts to consider when buying a car?

Common Core

College and Career Readiness

4. **Reading.** Read a book about a person who played a major role in the development of transportation. Prepare a book report and share it with the class.

5. **Speaking.** Role-play a situation involving a teen buying his or her first car from a sales associate who wants to make a sale. What questions should the teen ask? How should the teen respond to various sales tactics?

6. **Writing.** Prepare an evaluation sheet a person could use when test-driving a vehicle. Compare your evaluation sheet with those of classmates and create a master evaluation sheet.

7. **Listening.** Visit an automotive repair shop. Ask the technician for some maintenance tips that will help ensure the safety and performance of a car.

Technology

8. **Internet research.** Search the Internet for a car that interests you. Create a table indicating the types of information you find on each website. Then search online for a car loan calculator. Enter in the cost of the car and other information requested to determine monthly payments for a loan. Share your findings with the class.

Journal Writing

9. Write about your *dream car*. Describe how it looks and what features you want. Also, describe the responsibilities involved in owning the car.

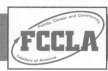 ## FCCLA

10. As a team, choose one of the following units from the "FCCLA Families Acting for Community Traffic Safety (FACTS)": *Think SMART*, *Buckle Up*, *Arrive Alive*, *Speak Up*, or *Bridge the Gap*. Complete activities provided with each FACTS unit. Then you and your team members should create an innovative project related to your unit topic. Share your project with the class. Consider submitting your project for national recognition. See your adviser for information as needed.

Glossary

A

abdominal thrust. A procedure that can dislodge a piece of food or other item that is stuck in a choking victim's throat. Also called the *Heimlich Maneuver*. (15-3)

abilities. Skills developed through training or practice. (9-1)

abstinence. Choosing not to have sex. (3-3)

accessories. Accents to clothing, including belts, jewelry, scarves, gloves, hats, neckties, handbags, and shoes. (22-2)

acne. A skin disorder that results in the appearance of blemishes on the face, neck, scalp, upper chest, or back. (15-1)

acquaintances. People you have met, but do not know well. (3-1)

acquired traits. Traits that develop as a part of the environment. (1-1)

active listening. A communication technique in which the listener shows a clear understanding of what a person is saying. (4-1)

adhesive dirt. Dirt that sticks to surfaces. (26-3)

adjustment lines. Lines that show where to lengthen or shorten the pattern piece to change the fit of the garment. (24-1)

adolescence. The stage between childhood and adulthood. (1-2)

adoptive family. Family that forms when an adult brings a child from another family into his or her own family through legal means. (2-1)

advertisement. A paid public announcement about goods, services, or ideas for sale. (7-1)

aerodynamics. The way air moves around objects. (27-1)

aeronautics. The art or science of flight. (27-1)

affirm. To positively validate an action or thing. (14-1)

agenda. Outline of items to consider or do in a meeting. (11-2)

aggressive communication. Expressing yourself in a forceful way that may step on the rights of others. (4-2)

AIDS (acquired immune deficiency syndrome). A disease caused by HIV (human immunodeficiency virus) that weakens the immune system and leads to death. (3-3)

alcoholism. Disease a person has when he or she is addicted to alcohol. (15-2)

al dente. To cook pasta until it has a slight resistance in the center when chewed. (20-2)

alterations. Changes made in the size, length, or style of a garment. (22-3)

alternatives. Options. (5-4)

ambition. A desire or drive to achieve and succeed. (8-1)

amenities. Things that make life easier and more pleasant. (26-1)

analogous color scheme. Colors that are next to each other on the color wheel. (22-1)

annual percentage rate (APR). The yearly credit cost the lender charges. (6-3)

anorexia nervosa. An eating disorder that causes people to starve themselves. (16-3)

antiperspirant. A product that reduces the flow of perspiration and controls body odor. (15-1)

antique. Styles with features belonging to an earlier period, style, or fashion. (26-2)

apartment. One-level units in buildings that are rented. (26-1)

appliance. Piece of equipment run by gas or electricity that is used to store, process, or cook food. (19-2)

appliqué. A decorative cutout made from material or embroidery. (25-2)

aptitudes. Natural talents with which you were born. (9-1)

ascorbic acid. The acidic juice in citrus fruits that prevent cut slices from browning. (20-1)

assembly line. A line of machines, equipment, and workers in a factory that builds a product by passing work from one station to the next until the product is finished. (27-1)

assertive communication. Expressing thoughts, feelings, and beliefs in open, honest, and respectful ways. (4-2)

ATM card. Card that enables customers to use an ATM to make deposits, withdraw money, or transfer money from one account to another. (6-2)

attitudes. Feelings and opinions about someone or something. (1-1)

authority figures. People who help guide the behaviors of others in the community by creating and enforcing rules designed to help and protect you and all other citizens in the community. (1-3)

automated teller machine (ATM). A computer terminal that allows customers to complete transactions with their financial institutions. (6-2)

B

babbling. Repeating a string of one-syllable sounds such as *da-da-da* or *be-be-be*. (12-1)

backstitching. Stitching used to secure the threads at the start and end of each seam. (24-2)

bacteria. One-celled organisms that live in soil, water, and the bodies of plants and animals. (19-1)

bait and switch. When advertisers promote a product at a low price to get your attention, but then try to persuade you to buy a more expensive item. (7-1)

bakeware. Items used to cook food in an oven. (19-2)

balance. One of the principles of design that shows equal visual weight on both sides. (22-1)

bank statement. A record of all the financial transactions you make during the month. (6-2)

basal metabolism. The energy used to support the basic functions that keep you alive. (16-3)

basting. Long, loose stitches. (24-2)

batter. Mixture of ingredients that is liquid enough to be poured into a pan. (20-2)

binge-eating disorder. Type of eating disorder that involves repeatedly eating great amounts of food and feeling powerless to stop. (16-3)

birth order. The order of birth that indicates whether you are the first, middle, or youngest child in your family. (1-1)

blend. Yarn made of two or more very different fibers. (23-1)

blog. An online journal or diary. (6-4)

body composition. The proportion of body fat to lean mass in your body. (16-3)

body language. Form of nonverbal communication that involves the sending of messages through body movements. (4-1)

budget. A written plan for spending your money wisely. (6-2)

buffet service. Serving dishes set on a separate table allowing people to help themselves. (21-1)

bulimia nervosa. Type of eating disorder that involves uncontrollable urges to eat large amounts of food followed by behavior to avoid weight gain, including forced vomiting. (16-3)

bullying. When a person hurts or threatens another person. (3-2)

buoyant. Ability to float. (27-1)

burping. Gently patting or rubbing a baby's back to help expel excess air from feeding. (12-2)

buyers. People in fashion merchandising who select which clothes and accessories will be sold in a store. (9-2)

C

CAD programs. Computer aided design used in jobs with artistic elements. (11-1)

cafeteria style. Food service where people choose their foods along a counter and carry it to a table for eating. (21-2)

calamine lotion. A zinc oxide mixture with a small amount of ferric (iron) oxide used to help reduce itching. (15-3)

calories. Units of energy of body fuel provided by carbohydrates, fats, and proteins in food. (16-3)

carbohydrates. The body's main source of energy. (16-1)

carbon dioxide. Gas bubbles. (20-2)

career. The sequence of jobs you have over a period of years. (8-1)

career and technical student organizations (CTSOs). Groups that help students develop leadership skills and prepare them to work in certain jobs. (11-2)

career clusters. Sixteen groupings of careers based on common knowledge and skills. (9-1)

care labels. Small labels on clothing describing how to clean the garment without damaging the textiles. (25-1)

carryout. Food that is prepared at a restaurant, but is brought home to eat. (21-2)

casing. An enclosure for elastic or a drawstring that gathers the garment snugly to the body. (24-2)

cellulose. The substance forming the main part of all plants' cell walls. (23-1)

certificate of deposit (CD). A savings tool that requires you to deposit a certain amount of money for a specified period of time. (6-2)

certification. A special standing within a profession as a result of meeting certain educational and work requirements. (9-1)

certified pre-owned cars. Late-model used vehicles (usually less than five years old) that the manufacturers put through a demanding inspection and repair process. (27-2)

character. A description of a person's good qualities, which often include moral strength, honesty, and fairness. (5-2)

child abuse. Harm to a child that is done on purpose, which may be physical, emotional, or sexual. (14-2)

childless family. A married couple without children. (2-1)

child neglect. Failure to meet a child's needs. (14-2)

childproofing. Making the home safe for children by keeping potential dangers away from them. (12-3)

children in self-care. Children who stay home by themselves while parents work. (8-2)

chronic. Sicknesses that continue for a long time and may be life threatening. (2-3)

citizen. A member of the community. (1-3)

citizenship. Your status as a citizen with rights and responsibilities. (1-3)

classic. Style that stays in fashion for a long time. (22-2)

cleaning agents. Substances or chemicals used to clean household surfaces. (26-3)

cleaning schedule. A plan for organizing the work of cleaning a home. (26-3)

climate change. Any significant change in measures—such as temperatures, precipitation, and wind—of the Earth's climate lasting for an extended period of time. (7-2)

clipping. Technique used on seams that form an inward curve to reduce fabric bulk and help the garment lie flat. (24-2)

clique. A group that excludes other people. (3-2)

cognitive disabilities. Intellectual disabilities. (12-3)

combination. Two or more yarns that vary in fiber composition, content, and/or twist level. (23-1)

committee. A group of people working together for a special purpose. (11-2)

communication. The process of sending and receiving information. (4-1)

community resource. Resources that are found locally, such as schools, libraries, stores, theaters, parks, zoos, and museums. (5-3)

comparison shopping. Looking at competing brands and models of a product in several stores to compare quality, features, and prices before buying. (7-1)

complementary color scheme. Two colors that are directly across from each other on the color wheel. (22-1)

complex. Two or more large multiple-family buildings. (26-1)

composting. The natural breakdown of organic, or *biodegradable*, material. (7-2)

compromise. A way of resolving a conflict that is fair to all where both sides give up some of what they want in order to settle the conflict. (4-2)

condominiums. Apartments available for purchase. (26-1)

conflicts. Disagreements or problems in a relationship. (4-2)

conformity. Looking and behaving like the other members of a group. (3-2)

consequences. Results of your decisions. (5-4)

conserve. To use carefully in order to prevent loss or waste of resources. (7-2)

constructive criticism. Information given that helps describe where or how a person could improve or learn new tasks. (4-2)

consumer. A person who buys or uses goods and services. (7-1)

consumer advocates. People or organizations that support the rights of the consumer to obtain safe goods and services at fair prices. (9-2)

consumerism. The promotion of the consumer's interests. (9-2)

contaminants. Harmful substances. (19-1)

convection oven. A conventional oven with the addition of a fan that circulates the hot air. (19-2)

cookware. Pots and pans used on top of the range. (19-2)

cool colors. Blue, green, purple, and their different variations. (22-1)

cooperate. To work well with others. (11-2)

cooperation. When everyone works together and does their share to reach goals. (2-2)

cooperative extension agents. People who provide practical and research-based information to agricultural producers, business owners, youth, consumers, and others in rural areas and communities of all sizes. (9-2)

cooperative play. Form of play in which preschoolers join together to play a group activity. (13-2)

cosigner. A person named as a partner on a loan who is legally bound to repay it if the other signer does not make payments. (27-2)

cover. The table space in front of a person's seat. Also called a *place setting*. (21-1)

credit. Buying or borrowing now and paying later. (6-3)

credit report. A detailed report of an individual's credit history prepared by a credit bureau and used by lenders to determine a loan applicant's ability to repay the loan. (27-2)

creole foods. Cooking style found mainly in New Orleans that has roots in French, Spanish, African, and Native American cultures. (17-1)

crisis. A difficult situation that becomes very serious. (2-3)

critic. A person who criticizes people, items, or events. (4-2)

critical thinking. Looking at all sides of an issue to analyze the situation and solve problems. (11-1)

criticize. To make judgmental remarks without having sufficient knowledge. (4-2)

cross-contamination. Bacteria transferred to food by people, insects, rodents, pets, unclean utensils, or other unsanitary objects. (19-1)

crosswise grain. The yarns that run across the fabric from one selvage to the other (horizontally). (24-1)

cruciferous vegetables. Strong-flavored vegetables that include Brussels sprouts, cauliflower, turnips, onions, broccoli, and cabbage. (18-3)

culture. Beliefs and customs of a particular racial, religious, or social group. (2-1)

curdle. A lump of milk protein. (20-3)

cutting lines. The bold, solid outlines on each pattern piece. (24-1)

cyberbullying. Cruel and hurtful messages you receive or witness online. (6-4)

D

Daily Values. References used on food labels to show consumers how food products fit into an overall diet. (18-2)

dandruff. Flakes of dead skin cells on the scalp. (15-1)

darts. A stitched fold that gives shape and fullness to a garment so it fits the curves of the body. (24-2)

dating. Participating in an activity with a friend of the opposite sex. (3-3)

debit card. Card that enables you to perform transactions at ATMs or make purchases at stores. The amount is immediately deducted from your checking account. (6-2)

decision. A choice. (5-4)

decision-making process. A step-by-step approach to help you make a decision, reach a goal, or solve a problem. Steps include stating the decision to be made, listing all possible alternatives, evaluating alternatives, choosing the best alternative, acting on a decision, and evaluating the decision. (5-4)

décor. The style and layout of interior furnishings. (26-2)

deductions. Amounts of money that an employer subtracts from your paycheck before you receive it. (6-2)

deficiency. A shortage. (16-1)

deodorant. A product that controls body odor by interfering with the growth of bacteria, but does not stop the flow of perspiration. (15-1)

dependable. Being trusted to do or provide what is needed. (11-3)

depressant. A drug that slows down activity in the brain and spinal cord. (15-2)

dermatologist. A skin specialist. (15-1)

destructive criticism. Criticism that uses negative comments to poke fun at a person and is not helpful. (4-2)

developmentally appropriate activities. Activities that take into account the level of physical, social, emotional, and intellectual development of children at certain ages. (13-2)

developmental tasks. Certain skills and behavior patterns that should be achieved within each stage of life. (1-2)

diabetes. A disease that limits or prevents the body's ability to properly use energy from food. (16-4)

diet. All the foods you regularly eat and drink. (16-1)

Dietary Guidelines for Americans. A publication by the United States Departments of Agriculture and Health and Human Services that serves as a basis for many nutrition programs and sources of information in the United States. (16-2)

Dietary Reference Intakes (DRIs). A set of dietary standards for the United States that recommend how much of each nutrient is needed in the diet. (16-1)

dietetics. Field of study that applies the principles of food, nutrition, business, social, and basic sciences in different settings to promote nutritional health. (9-2)

dieting. Restricting your food intake. (16-3)

dinnerware. Plates, cups, saucers, and bowls. (21-1)

disability. A functional limitation that interferes with a person's ability. (12-3)

disinfectant cleaner. Product that kills germs and cleans surfaces. (26-3)

domestic violence. Physical or emotional abuse of a family member. (2-3)

dots. Symbols used in a pattern piece to aid in matching seams and other construction details. (24-1)

double boiler. A small pan that fits inside a larger pan used for cooking delicate foods. (19-2)

dough. A stiff, thick mixture that cannot be poured. (20-2)

drapery. Term used for full-length, formal window treatments that are lined. (26-2)

drug abuse. Using a drug for a purpose other than one for which it was intended. (15-2)

dry cleaning. Process of cleaning clothes using chemical solvents instead of water. (25-1)

dual-career family. Families where both parents work. (8-2)

duplex. Two living units attached by a common wall. (26-1)

duvet. A washable, removable bed cover that encloses a comforter. (26-2)

dysfunctional family. Family where a member does not do his or her part to fulfill responsibilities to the family unit. (2-1)

E

early brain development. The most critical period of human development that occurs from conception until around the third birthday. (12-1)

easing. A smooth stitch used to make fabric fit into a smaller space. (24-2)

eating disorder. An illness that results in abnormal eating patterns which can be life threatening. (16-3)

eating pattern. All the foods you regularly eat and drink. (17-2)

E-commerce. Shopping online. (7-1)

ecosystem. All of the living and nonliving things existing in a particular environment. (7-2)

egg poacher. Kitchen tool used to prevent poached eggs from separating. (20-4)

egg separator. A kitchen tool that allows the white part of an egg to slide away as the yolk remains in the cup. (20-4)

electrical hazard. A danger from any form of electricity, such as electrical appliances and cords. (26-3)

elements of design. Color, line, texture, and form. (22-1)

emotional changes. Changes that affect how you feel about situations and how you express those feelings. (1-2)

emotional development. The way in which a person develops and expresses emotions. (12-1)

emotions. Feelings about people and events in your life. (1-2)

empathy. Ability to understand another person's emotions and see from his or her point of view. (3-2)

emphasis. One of the principles of design that shows the center of interest in a design. (22-1)

employability skills. Basic skills you need to get, keep, and succeed on a job. Sometimes called *transferable skills*. (11-1)

empty nest. When the last child in the household leaves home. (2-3)

endorse. To sign your name on the back of a check. (6-2) To publicly express support or approval. (7-1)

energy balance. When calories taken in (from food) equal calories used (for physical activity, digestion, and basic functions). (16-3)

entrepreneurs. People who start and manage businesses of their own. (9-2)

environment. Everything and everyone around you, including family, home, friends, school, classmates, teachers, coaches, and community. (1-1)

ethics. The strong beliefs about what is morally right and wrong that guide your behavior. (5-2)

etiquette. Polite and proper behavior in social settings. (6-4)

evaluate. To judge the value of something. (5-4)

evaporated milk. Form of canned milk made from whole milk, from which 60 percent of the water has been removed. (18-5)

exchange. To substitute one item for another. (7-1)

expenses. The ways you spend your money. (6-2)

extended family. Relatives other than parents (or stepparents) and children living together in one home. May include grandparents, aunts, uncles, or cousins. (2-1)

F

fabrics. Different materials made by weaving or knitting yarns or pressing fibers together. (23-1)

facings. Pieces of fabric used to cover raw edges in garment openings, such as armholes and necklines. (24-2)

fad. Clothing style only popular for a short time. (22-2)

fad diets. Unsafe diet plans that promise quick weight loss in a very short period of time. (16-3)

family. Group of two or more people related to each other, including by blood (birth), marriage, and adoption. (2-1)

family-friendly policies. Company rules that affect the family positively. (8-2)

family life cycle. Changes that occur within families in six basic stages: beginning stage, childbearing stage, parenting stage, launching stage, mid-years stage, and aging stage. (2-3)

family service. Passing serving dishes around the table for diners to fill their own plates. (21-1)

fashion. A style popular at a certain time. (22-2)

fasteners. Zippers, buttons, hooks and eyes, snaps, and hook and loop tape. (24-1)

fasting. A form of fad dieting that requires going without food for a certain amount of time. (16-3)

fats. Concentrated sources of energy found in both animal and plant foods. (16-1)

FCCLA planning process. A set of five steps used to help make decisions, reach goals, and solve problems. The steps include identifying concerns, setting your goal, forming a plan, acting on the plan, and then following up. (5-4)

feedback. Letting the speaker know you receive the message correctly. (4-1)

fetal alcohol syndrome (FAS). A condition that causes permanent physical and cognitive disabilities in children. This syndrome occurs when alcohol is consumed during pregnancy. (14-2)

fibers. Hairlike strands that can be twisted together to form yarns. (23-1)

filaments. Continuous strands of fibers. (23-1)

finance charge. The dollar amount you pay for credit. (6-3)

finish. A treatment that is given to fibers, yarns, or fabrics that can improve the look, feel, or performance of a fabric. (23-1)

fixed expenses. The regular expenses you cannot avoid. (6-2)

fixtures. Permanent pieces installed in a room. (26-2)

flat-drying. Drying garments on a flat surface. (25-1)

flatware. Forks, knives, and spoons. (21-1)

flexible expenses. Costs that can vary from time to time, and do not occur regularly. (6-2)

flextime. Freedom to work hours that are convenient to an employee's personal situation. (8-2)

follow-up letter. A professional letter written to your interviewers thanking them for the interview opportunity and expressing continued interest in the job. (10-2)

food additive. Any substance added to a food to improve the final product. (18-2)

food allergy. When a food protein you have eaten triggers a response by your body's immune system. (16-4)

foodborne illness. Sickness caused from eating contaminated food. (19-1)

food intolerance. A reaction to food that is unpleasant, but not the result of an immune response. (16-4)

food science. The study of the production, processing, storage, preservation, and safety of food. (9-2)

form. One of the elements of design that refers to the shape of an object. (22-1)

formula. A special milk mixture designed to meet the nutritional needs of infants. (12-2)

fortify. When certain vitamins or other nutrients are added into food. (16-1)

fossil fuels. Resources formed by the decomposition of animals many millions of years ago and contain large amounts of carbon. They include coal, petroleum (oil), and natural gas. (7-2)

foster family. Family that temporarily takes care of children because their parents are unable to do so. (2-1)

freezer burn. A white or gray-colored spot where food has dried out because of exposure to air in the freezer. (18-6)

fringe benefits. Benefits offered to full-time employees, including paid vacation and holiday time, sick leave, health and life insurance plans, and retirement benefits. (8-2)

functional. Something that has a practical use. (26-2)

functional family. Family where each member contributes to the family unit by fulfilling his or her roles and responsibilities. (2-1)

G

gang. A group of people that join together for a variety of reasons and may be violent. (3-2)

garnishes. Foods that decorate a dish or plate. (17-2)

gathering. A heavier stitch used to make fabric fit into a smaller space. (24-2)

gelatinization. The process of starches absorbing very hot liquid, making the product soft and thick. (20-2)

generic products. Products that have no brand names and usually cost less than both national and store brands. (18-1)

genes. Sections of the DNA molecule found in a person's cells that determine the characteristics that will appear as a person grows and develops. (1-1)

geography. The location and climate of a land. (17-1)

gifted children. Children who show outward signs of high achievement or potential for high achievement in skill or intelligence. (12-3)

glassware. All types of drinking glasses. (21-1)

gluten. A protein found in many grains that provides structure for baked goods. (18-4)

goals. What you endeavor to do or achieve. (5-2)

grading. Technique used on heavier fabrics or seams with three or more layers to reduce fabric bulk and help the garment lie flat. (24-2)

grain. The direction yarns run in a fabric. (24-1)

grain line. Heavy line with arrows on both ends on the pattern piece. (24-1)

grief. Emotions felt such as sadness, loss, anger, and guilt when someone you know or love dies. (2-3)

grooming. Taking the best care of yourself and trying to always look your best. (15-1)

gross income. The income you earn before deductions. (6-2)

growth spurts. Rapid periods of growth. (1-2)

guidance. Words and actions parents or guardians use to affect their children's behavior. (14-2)

guide sheet. Detailed step-by-step directions on how to cut and sew your garment. (24-1)

H

hangtags. Small, detachable signs providing size, price, style number, guarantees, and special features. (22-3)

hard-cooked eggs. Eggs cooked in the shell until both the white and yolk are firm. (20-4)

harmony. The goal of good design, which is the result of using the principles of design properly. (22-1)

hem. A finished edge on a garment. (24-2)

heredity. The passing of traits from one generation of family to the next. (1-1)

HIV (human immunodeficiency virus). A virus that is spread through sexual contact or blood. (3-3)

hormones. Chemicals produced in the body that influence the way you grow and develop. (1-2)

house rules. Specific rules that apply to the family's household and the members who live there. (13-1)

hue. The name of a color. (22-1)

human resources. Resources that come from within yourself or from relationships with other people. Also called *personal resources.* (5-3)

hybrids. Automobiles that have a gasoline engine and an electric motor. (6-4)

I

identity theft. The illegal use of someone's personal information to obtain money or credit. (6-4)

illusions. Images that appear different from what they are. (22-1)

immunizations. Treatments that help people's bodies develop antibodies to resist certain diseases, such as polio, tetanus, measles, mumps, and rubella. (15-3)

implement. To carry out a plan. (5-4)

impulse buying. An unplanned or spur-of-the-moment purchase, which often leads people to buy items they do not really need. (7-1)

income. The money you earn. (6-2)

independence. A state of being in which people are responsible for their own actions and provide for their own needs and wants. (1-3)

individual retirement account (IRA). An investment option providing tax benefits to those workers saving money for retirement. (6-2)

infant. Term used to describe a baby that is between birth to twelve months old. (12-1)

infatuation. An intense feeling of attraction that begins and ends quickly. Sometimes called a *crush*. (3-3)

ingredients. Food items needed to make a certain food product. (17-3)

inherited traits. Traits you receive from your parents and ancestors. (1-1)

in season. Foods that during their time of harvest are most plentiful and at a peak flavor. (18-1)

installment credit. A cash loan you repay with interest in regular payments. (6-3)

intellectual changes. Changes that take place as you learn more about the world around you. (1-2)

intellectual development. Development of the mind, including the ability to think, reason, use language, and form ideas. (12-1)

interest. An amount of money paid to you for the use of your money. (6-2)

interests. Things you enjoy learning about or doing. (9-1)

internal combustion engine. Machine creating power by the burning of a fuel (usually a fossil fuel) when exposed to air in an internal chamber. (27-1)

internships. Supervised, practical job experiences at the postsecondary level. (9-1)

interview. A meeting between an employer and a job applicant. (10-2)

ironing. Process of removing wrinkles with heat using a gliding motion. (25-1)

irregular. A garment that has a defect or flaw. (22-3)

J

job shadowing. Spending time at work with someone whose career interests you. (9-1)

job sharing. When two people do the same job, but work at different times of the day or week. (8-2)

job trends. General patterns of whether hiring is increasing or decreasing in certain job sectors. (9-1)

joint account. A bank account with more than one person that allows each person in the account access to the money. (6-2)

K

kitchen utensil. A handheld, hand-powered tool used to prepare food. (19-2)

knead. To work dough with your hands. (20-2)

knitting. Looping yarns together. (23-1)

L

labels. Cloth tags providing legally required information about the garments. (22-3)

landfills. Places where trash is compacted and buried underground. (7-2)

landlords. Owners of building property. (26-1)

leader. Person who guides a group toward a common goal. (11-2)

lease. A legal document that renters must sign agreeing to pay the rent on time and to keep the property in good shape. (26-1)

leasing. Renting. (27-2)

leavening agent. Product that produces carbon dioxide through a chemical reaction with other ingredients, causing the bread or cake to rise. (20-2)

legumes. The edible seeds of plants. (18-3)

lengthwise grain. The straight grain or *grain line* in a fabric. (24-1)

letter of application. A letter that accompanies your résumé expressing interest in a position and providing more information about your qualifications. (10-1)

letter of recommendation. A document written by one of your references you can show to any prospective employer testifying to your abilities. (10-1)

line. One of the elements of design that gives direction to a design. (22-1)

line-drying. Hanging the garment to dry either outdoors, over a towel rack, or with a special type of drying device. (25-1)

linens. The table's place mats, napkins, and tablecloths. (21-1)

long-term goals. Major accomplishments you are trying to achieve that may take many months, a year, or several years. (5-2)

looms. Machines used for weaving fabrics. (23-1)

loose dirt. Dry dirt not bound to a surface. (26-3)

love. A strong feeling of affection between two people. (3-3)

loyalty. A quality that shows strong support for a friend. (3-1)

M

maître d'. (Pronounced may tra de'). A host or hostess that seats guests at a restaurant. (21-2)

major. The academic subject chosen in college as a field of specialization. (9-1)

malnutrition. When a person's diet lacks needed nutrients over a period of time. This can be caused by not eating the right amount or selection of foods. (16-1)

management. Using your resources to reach a goal. (5-4)

management process. A method used to achieve a goal using available resources. Steps include setting a goal, making a plan, implementing the plan, and evaluating it. (5-4)

manners. Rules for proper conduct. (4-1)

manufactured fibers. Fibers made in a laboratory through chemical processes. (23-1)

marbling. The fat that is mixed in with the muscle part of the meat. (18-6)

mass transit. System that is used for moving large numbers of people on buses, trains, or subways. (7-2)

mediator. A person not involved in the conflict, but who leads the parties through the steps of conflict resolution. (4-2)

mentor. A trusted person that guides someone's career. (9-1)

microfibers. Extremely fine filaments that make extra smooth, soft, and silky fabrics. (23-1)

microwaves. High-frequency waves used to cook food. (19-2)

minerals. Type of nutrient needed for a healthy body. (16-1)

mixed messages. When people's actions send one message and their words say something else. (4-2)

money market account. A type of savings account that offers a higher rate of interest, but the rate changes daily. (6-2)

monochromatic color scheme. Variations of a single hue on the color wheel. (22-1)

monofilament yarns. Yarns made from a single filament. (23-1)

mortgage. Long-term loan taken out for home purchase. (26-1)

moths. Insects that feed on woolen garments. (25-1)

motivation. Feeling the need or desire to do something. (11-2)

motor scooters. Low-powered two-wheeled vehicles similar to a motorcycle. (27-1)

multifilament yarns. Yarns made from 5 to 100 filaments spun into yarns that tend to be stronger and more durable. (23-1)

multiple-family housing. Building containing similar types of housing that is home to more than one family. (26-1)

multisized patterns. Sewing patterns with several sizes printed on the pattern tissue. (24-1)

multitasking. Accomplishing more than one task at a time. (19-3)

MyPlate. A food guidance system created by the United States Department of Agriculture (USDA) to help people apply the messages from the *Dietary Guidelines* to their daily life. (16-2)

N

NASA. National Aeronautics and Space Administration. (27-1)

natural fibers. Fibers created from plant or animal sources. (23-1)

natural leaders. People who can get group members to easily follow their lead and do what they ask. (11-2)

natural resources. Materials found in nature and shared by everyone. (7-2)

needs. Basic items you must have to live. (5-1)

net income. The amount of money you earn after deductions. (6-2)

netiquette. Proper behavior when using the Internet. (6-4)

networking. Making contacts with people who may be able to help you find a job. (10-1)

neutrals. White, gray, ivory, and black, which are not true colors. (22-1)

newborn. The first month after birth of an infant's life. (12-1)

nicotine. A colorless and odorless drug found in tobacco. (15-2)

nonassertive communication. A manner of speaking that is unclear or easily misunderstood. Also called *passive communication*. (4-2)

nonhuman resources. Resources that include money, community resources, and possessions. (5-3)

noninstallment credit. Amount you repay in one payment. (6-3)

nonrenewable resources. Natural resources that have formed very slowly and are limited in supply, such as minerals and fossil fuels. (7-2)

nonverbal communication. Type of communication that includes any means of sending a message that does not use words, such as facial expressions, gestures, and posture. (4-1)

notches. Diamond-shaped symbols along the cutting line in a pattern piece indicating exactly where to join pieces together. (24-1)

notching. Cutting V-shaped sections from the seam allowance to reduce fabric bulk and help the garment lie flat. (24-2)

notions. Items that become a part of a garment or project, such as thread, buttons, snaps, zippers, tapes, trims, and elastic. (24-1)

nuclear family. A married couple and their biological children. (2-1)

nutrient dense. Foods and beverages that provide vitamins, minerals, and other substances that may have positive health effects with relatively few calories. (16-2)

nutrients. The substances in food that are used by your body to grow and function properly. (16-1)

nutrition. The study of how your body processes and uses the foods you eat and drink. (16-1)

O

obsolete. A device that is no longer useful. (6-4)

occupation. Job. (8-1)

off-grain. Fabric that does not have the crosswise and lengthwise yarns crossing at right angles. The fabric will look crooked and is hard to handle. (24-1)

on-grain. Fabric that has the crosswise and lengthwise yarns at right angles to each other. (24-1)

open dating. A method used to help store employees and consumers know when a food product is fresh. (18-2)

optimists. People who have positive attitudes. (1-1)

options. Additional features that may be added to a vehicle for appearance, safety, performance, or convenience. (27-2)

organic foods. Foods raised without the use of pesticides, fertilizers, and drugs that are commonly used for crops and livestock. (18-2)

overlock stitches. Type of stitch used on the serger for seams. (23-2)

over-the-counter medications. Drugs sold legally without a prescription. (14-2)

P

parallel play. Toddlers that play near each other, but not with each other. (13-2)

part-time job. A job that is fewer than 40 hours per week. (10-2)

pasta. Products made by rolling out and shaping flour dough. (18-4)

pasteurization. A process in which products are heated to destroy much of the harmful bacteria they contain. (18-5)

pattern. A basic model that helps you put together a garment or project. (24-1)

peer pressure. The influence that your peers have on you. (3-2)

peers. People who are about the same age as you. (3-2)

pegboard. A particle-wood board with small holes in it. (26-2)

permanent press. Garments requiring no ironing. (25-1)

personal identification number (PIN). A security number that allows you to use your debit card for purchases and withdrawals at ATMs. (6-2)

personality. Combination of traits that makes you the person you are, including habits and feelings. (1-1)

personal space. The area around you. (4-1)

personal transportation. Privately owned modes of transportation, such as a car, motorcycle, bicycle, or scooter. (27-1)

pessimists. People who have negative attitudes. (1-1)

photosynthesis. How plants turn carbon dioxide into oxygen. (7-2)

physical changes. Changes that occur as your body grows and matures. (1-2)

physical dependence. When a person is addicted to a drug and his or her body begins to require the drug to function. (15-2)

physical development. Growth or change in body size and ability. (12-1)

physical needs. Your most basic needs, including food, water, clothing, shelter, and sleep. (5-1)

plaque. An invisible film of bacteria that forms on your teeth. (15-1)

plate service. Filling plates in the kitchen and then serving them to each seated guest. (21-1)

poison. Any substance that harms the human body. (15-3)

portfolio. An organized collection of your work showcasing your talents and skills. (10-1)

positive discipline. Intentional methods parents or guardians use to teach their children acceptable behavior. (14-2)

postsecondary. Additional schooling beyond high school. (9-1)

potluck. A meal where families eat together and each family brings one or two dishes for everyone to enjoy. (17-1)

preheat. To turn on the oven before beginning to cook. This allows the oven to heat to the correct temperature before you place food in it. (17-3)

prejudices. Opinions people form without complete knowledge. (4-2)

preschooler. Children ages three, four, and five. (12-1)

pressing. The process of removing wrinkles from clothing using a lifting motion and steam. (25-1)

prewash. Pretreatment of clothing stains before laundering. (25-1)

principles of design. Guides for using the elements of design including balance, proportion, rhythm, and emphasis. (22-1)

priority. What is most important to you. (5-2)

privileges. Rights to certain benefits. (13-1)

procrastination. Putting off difficult or unpleasant tasks until later. (6-1)

produce. Fresh fruits and vegetables. (18-1)

professional organizations. Recognized associations that unite and inform people who work in the same occupation or industry. (10-1)

proportion. One of the principles of design that shows how the sizes of parts relate to each other and to the whole. Also called *scale*. (22-1)

protein. A nutrient needed for growth, maintenance, and repair of tissues. (16-1)

protein fibers. Fibers created from animal sources. (23-1)

psychological dependence. When a person craves a drug for the feeling it provides or because it provides an escape from reality. (15-2)

psychological needs. Needs related to your mind and feelings, including the needs to feel safe, secure, loved, and accepted. (5-1)

puberty. The time when the body begins to mature sexually. (1-2)

public transportation. Transportation using regular routes at fixed times to transport many people. Also called *mass transit*. (27-1)

punctual. On time. (11-3)

R

racism. An extreme type of prejudice with the belief that one culture or race is superior to another. (4-2)

recipe. A set of instructions used to prepare a food product. (17-3)

recipe conversion. Changing a recipe's yield up or down. (17-3)

recycled. Materials that are reprocessed resources and are reused in a different form. (7-2)

redesign. To change the appearance or function of a garment. (25-2)

redress. To correct something that is wrong. (7-1)

references. People who know you and your work habits well, but are not relatives. (10-1)

reflexes. Reactions that happen automatically. (12-1)

refund. Repayment of a product's purchase price. (7-1)

Regrets only. A phrase written on an invitation that means the host only wants to hear from those who cannot attend. (21-1)

rehydrated. Dried foods that have been restored to their natural state by adding water before cooking. (20-1)

relationship. A special bond or link between people. (2-2)

renewable resources. Natural resources that simply exist or rebuild themselves fairly quickly after use, such as sunlight and fast-growing plants. (7-2)

resale shops. Stores that purchase expensive items for low prices and resells them for a profit. (25-2)

residential properties. All types of housing. (26-1)

resource. Anything that can help you reach a goal. (5-3)

responsibilities. Duties or jobs you must carry through. (1-3)

résumé. A short history of your education, qualifications, and work experience. (10-1)

revolving credit. A specified amount of money that is repeatedly available as long as you make regular payments each month. (6-3)

rhythm. One of the principles of design that creates a feeling of movement. (22-1)

R.I.C.E. A simple treatment that involves *rest, ice, compression,* and *elevation* used to relieve swelling, bruising, joint or muscle pain, or difficulty moving the injured area of a sprain or strain. (15-3)

role. A pattern of expected behavior. (1-2)

routine jobs. Tasks done daily as a part of your regular activity. (26-3)

RSVP. A French abbreviation, *répondez, s'il vous plaît,* that means *please respond.* (21-1)

rural. Country. (26-1)

S

sacrifice. To give up time or a belonging to benefit someone or something else. (14-1)

sanitation. The process of making conditions clean and healthy. (19-1)

scalding. Heating to just below the boiling point. (20-3)

scale floor plan. A flat drawing of a room's floor corresponding to the actual room's size and shape. (26-2)

schedule. A written plan for reaching your goals within a certain time. (6-1)

scientific principles. Practices used to examine a problem, research possible solutions, and analyze potential outcomes. (11-1)

seam. A row of stitches that holds two pieces of fabric together. (24-2)

seam allowance. The fabric between the stitching and the fabric edge. (24-2)

secondhand smoke. When you are near people who are smoking and breathe in smoke. (15-2)

self-actualization. To fully realize your own potential. (5-1)

self-concept. The mental image you have of yourself. (1-1)

self-confidence. Assurance you have in yourself and your abilities. (1-1)

self-dressing features. Clothing characteristics that make dressing easier for children. (12-2)

self-esteem. How you feel about yourself; how you view your worth as a person. (1-1)

selvages. (24-1) Smooth, closely woven edges that do not ravel on a fabric. (24-1)

separation anxiety. Anxiety that infants feel when they are separated from their caregivers. (12-1)

sergers. High-speed sewing machines that stitch, trim, and finish seams in one step. (23-2)

sewing gauge. A six-inch ruler with a sliding marker. (23-2)

sexually transmitted infections (STIs). Illnesses that spread through sexual contact. Also known as *sexually transmitted diseases (STDs)*. (3-3)

Shaken Baby Syndrome (SBS). A form of physical abuse characterized by severe trauma to the brain. This can occur if a parent violently shakes a baby out of frustration for inconsolable crying. (14-2)

shared space. Areas in the home used by all the family members and for entertaining guests. (26-1)

shears. Sewing tool that has extra-long blades and larger, bent handles for comfort and holding a fabric flat for more accurate cutting. (23-2)

shellfish. Any fish that live inside shells. (20-4)

shelters. Places that provide food, clothing, and housing to families who do not have anywhere else to go. (2-3)

short-term goals. Goals you hope to achieve in the near future. (5-2)

sibling. Brother or sister. (1-3)

sibling rivalry. Competition between brothers and sisters. (2-2)

single-family house. A freestanding house that is home to only one family. (26-1)

single-parent family. One parent and one or more children. (2-1)

skillets. Kitchen utensils used for panfrying, panbroiling, and braising foods. Also called *frying pans*. (19-2)

snag. A loop of yarn pulled out of fabric. (25-2)

social changes. Changes that occur as you meet more people and learn how to get along with them. (1-2)

social development. Learning to communicate and get along with others. (12-1)

socialization. Teaching children about the culture of the society in which they live. (2-1)

social needs. Human need to interact with people. (26-1)

soft-cooked eggs. Eggs cooked in the shell until they have a firm white, but a runny yolk. (20-4)

sorting. Grouping clothes by fabric weight, color, degree of soil, fabric construction, and size of item. (25-1)

soul food. Cooking style based on the food customs of African Americans in the South. (17-1)

spinneret. A small nozzle with many tiny holes used in the production of fibers. (23-1)

sprains. Injuries that result from tearing ligaments and tendons, usually at a joint such as a knee, elbow, or ankle. (15-3)

spun yarns. Yarns made by using short, natural fibers or manufactured fibers cut to staple lengths. (23-1)

stabilizers. Additives that maintain an ice cream's smooth, creamy texture. (18-5)

stain. A spot or discoloration on a garment that is hard to remove. (25-1)

standards. The way you measure what you have done. (5-2)

standards of dress. The social influences determining appropriate dress. (22-2)

staple fibers. Short lengths of fibers. (23-1)

starch. The complex carbohydrate portion of grain plants, such as wheat, corn, barley, oats, or rice. (20-2)

staystitching. A line of regular machine stitches on a single thickness of fabric used to prevent garment pieces from stretching out of shape. (24-2)

stepfamily. A family that forms when a single parent marries. Also called *blended family*. (2-1)

stepparent. Person who marries a child's mother or father. (2-1)

stereotype. A fixed belief that all members of a group are the same. (4-2)

sterility. The inability to conceive a child. (3-3)

stir-frying. Frying quickly over high heat in a lightly oiled pan while stirring continuously. (20-1)

strains. Injuries that result from overstretching muscles. (15-3)

stress. The mental or physical tension you feel when faced with a challenge. (15-1)

substance abuse. The misuse of drugs, alcohol, or some other chemical to a potentially harmful level. (2-3)

sudden infant death syndrome (SIDS). When an apparently healthy infant dies suddenly without warning or cause. (14-2)

superheating. Heating liquid beyond its boiling point with no bubbles being produced. (19-2)

superior. An employee's boss. (11-1)

support groups. Group of people who meet regularly to discuss common challenges and to help one another cope. (2-3)

support system. People who provide aid and assistance for individuals. This includes emotional and instrumental support. (8-2)

sweetened condensed milk. Type of milk made from whole milk and sugar that has about 60 percent of its water removed. (18-5)

T

tactful. Being careful not to offend or upset other people. (11-3)

tannin. A reddish, plant-based acid occurring naturally in various foods and drinks. (25-1)

tartar. When plaque remains on the teeth and becomes a hard, crusty substance. (15-1)

tasks. All the smaller duties you perform throughout the day. (8-1)

T-commerce. Shopping through television. (7-1)

teamwork. The effort of a group of people acting together to do something or to reach a goal. (11-2)

technology. The use of scientific knowledge to improve the quality of life. (6-4)

telecommuting. A work program in which an employee works at home by connecting electronically to a central office. (8-2)

telephone hotlines. An immediate source of support for people coping with a crisis. (2-3)

temperature danger zone. Temperatures between 40°F and 140°F, where bacteria multiply rapidly and the risk for foodborne illness increases. (19-1)

tenderize. To make tough meats softer by pounding, marinating, or adding powdered tenderizers to the meat. (20-4)

texture. One of the elements of design that describes how a fabric feels and looks. (22-1)

thimbles. Sewing tool used to help push the needle through thick or tightly woven fabrics when hand sewing. (23-2)

tip. Extra money paid for the service you receive that shows your gratitude. (21-2)

toddler. Children between the ages of one and three years. (12-1)

toilet learning. The process by which children develop bladder and bowel control and successfully learn how and when to use the toilet. (12-2)

town houses. Two-or three-level-homes in a row attached by common walls. Also called *row houses*. (26-1)

trade-off. An exchange of one thing in return for another. (5-4)

traditions. Customs that are passed from generation to generation. (17-1)

traffic patterns. The paths you take to get to different parts of your room. (26-2)

traits. Qualities that make you different from everyone else. (1-1)

transcontinental railroad. Railway spanning from one country to another. (27-1)

translucent. Something that is clear enough to allow light to pass through, but is not transparent. (20-1)

trimming. Technique used on lightweight fabrics to reduce fabric bulk in seams. (24-2)

trustees. A group of members that manage a building's maintenance funds and other property issues. (26-1)

trustworthy. Quality describing someone's honesty. (11-3)

tumble drying. Technique used to dry clothes in automatic dryers. (25-1)

U

ultra high temperature (UHT) milk. Milk sterilized by heating it to a very high temperature for a few seconds. (18-5)

unconditional love. Love given freely without conditions or limits. (14-1)

understitching. Line of stitching along the edge of a facing to keep it from rolling to the outside. (24-2)

unit price. The cost for each measure of a product. (18-1)

universal product code (UPC). The group of bars and numbers that appears on product packaging. (18-2)

U.S. savings bonds. A type of savings in which you loan the government money for at least a year. When the loan is due, the government will repay you the full amount of the bond, plus interest. (6-2)

V

value. The lightness or darkness of a color. (22-1)

values. The beliefs, feelings, and experiences you consider important. (5-2)

vegetable brush. Tool with stiff bristles on the end used to remove some dirt from vegetables. (20-1)

vegetarianism. An eating pattern that excludes some or all animal products. (16-4)

vehicle identification number (VIN). A unique number the automobile industry assigns to each vehicle. (27-2)

verbal communication. Type of communication that involves the use of words to send information. (4-1)

vitamins. Substances needed by the body for growth and maintenance. (16-1)

W

wants. Items you would like to have, but do not need. (5-1)

wardrobe. All the clothes and accessories you have to wear. (22-2)

wardrobe inventory. An itemized list of all the clothes and accessories you own. (22-2)

warm colors. Red, yellow, orange, and their different variations. (22-1)

warranty. A written statement provided by a manufacturer that guarantees a product is in good condition. (7-1)

weaving. The process of interlacing yarns at right angles to each other to produce a fabric. (23-1)

webcams. Small video cameras used to show live images of the callers. (6-4)

wellness. Total health related to your physical, mental, and social well-being. (15-1)

work. Paid jobs. (8-1)

work-based learning. Programs that provide opportunities for students to learn about jobs through direct work experience as part of their school courses. (9-1)

work ethic. A person's belief about work based on his or her values. (11-3)

work plan. A list of preparation tasks, who is assigned each task, the time each task should be performed, and the equipment or supplies needed. (19-3)

work triangle. The area in the kitchen between the refrigerator, sink, and range. (19-3)

Y

yarns. Continuous strands of fibers. (23-1)

yeast. A single-celled organism in the fungi family that causes bread to rise. (20-2)

yield. The number of servings the recipe produces. (17-3)

Index